CURRENT CLINICAL ONCOLOGY

Maurie Markman, MD, SERIES EDITOR

Squamous Cell Head and Neck Cancer

SQUAMOUS CELL HEAD AND NECK CANCER

*Recent Clinical Progress
and Prospects for the Future*

Edited by

DAVID J. ADELSTEIN, MD

*Department of Hematology and Medical Oncology,
Cleveland Clinic Foundation, Cleveland, OH*

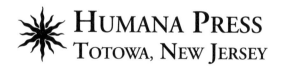

HUMANA PRESS
TOTOWA, NEW JERSEY

© 2005 Humana Press Inc.
999 Riverview Drive, Suite 208
Totowa, New Jersey 07512

humanapress.com

For additional copies, pricing for bulk purchases, and/or information about other Humana titles, contact Humana at the above address or at any of the following numbers: Tel.: 973-256-1699; Fax: 973-256-8341; E-mail: orders@humanapr.com; or visit our Website: www.humanapress.com

Due diligence has been taken by the publishers, editors, and authors of this book to assure the accuracy of the information published and to describe generally accepted practices. The contributors herein have carefully checked to ensure that the drug selections and dosages set forth in this text are accurate and in accord with the standards accepted at the time of publication. Notwithstanding, as new research, changes in government regulations, and knowledge from clinical experience relating to drug therapy and drug reactions constantly occurs, the reader is advised to check the product information provided by the manufacturer of each drug for any change in dosages or for additional warnings and contraindications. This is of utmost importance when the recommended drug herein is a new or infrequently used drug. It is the responsibility of the treating physician to determine dosages and treatment strategies for individual patients. Further it is the responsibility of the health care provider to ascertain the Food and Drug Administration status of each drug or device used in their clinical practice. The publisher, editors, and authors are not responsible for errors or omissions or for any consequences from the application of the information presented in this book and make no warranty, express or implied, with respect to the contents in this publication.

This publication is printed on acid-free paper. ∞
ANSI Z39.48-1984 (American National Standards Institute)
Permanence of Paper for Printed Library Materials.

Production Editor: Nicole E. Furia
Cover design by Patricia F. Cleary
Cover Illustration: Figure 1 from Chapter 14, "Postoperative Treatment of Locally Advanced Head and Neck Cancers," by Jacques Bernier and Søren M. Bentzen; Figure 1 from Chapter 8, "Intensity-Modulated Radiation Therapy in the Management of Head and Neck Cancer," by Theodore S. Hong, Wolfgang A. Tomé, and Paul M. Harari;and Figure 1 from Chapter 2, "Laryngeal Preservation Surgery," by Joseph Scharpf and Robert R. Lorenz.

eISBN 1-59259-938-9

Printed in the United States of America. 10 9 8 7 6 5 4 3 2 1

Library of Congress Cataloging-in-Publication Data

Squamous cell head and neck cancer : recent clinical progress and prospects
for the future / edited by David J. Adelstein.
      p. cm. — (Current clinical oncology)
  Includes bibliographical references and index.
  ISBN 1-58829-473-0 (alk. paper)
  1. Head—Cancer—Treatment. 2. Neck—Cancer—Treatment. 3. Squamous cell
carcinoma—Treatment. I. Adelstein, David J. II. Series.
  RC280.H4S68 2005
  616.99'49106—dc22
                                    2004024564

Preface

Although squamous cell head and neck cancer is a relatively uncommon malignancy in North America, it has been the focus of intensive clinical investigation, from all oncological disciplines, over the past 20 years. Surgical interest is high because of the unique and complex anatomic relationships in the head and neck region and their profound functional and cosmetic implications. Radiation and medical oncology interest has been driven by the remarkable sensitivity of this neoplasm to both of these interventions. As a result there has been considerable recent progress in our understanding of this disease and in the success of our treatments. Indeed, head and neck cancer serves as a good oncologic model for the benefits of multidisciplinary investigation and management.

Squamous Cell Head and Neck Cancer: Recent Clinical Progress and Prospects for the Future reviews recent progress made in the surgical, radiotherapeutic, and chemotherapeutic management of squamous cell head and neck cancer, with particular emphasis on the coordination of these treatment modalities. Several surgical issues are addressed including laser-based surgery, larynx preservation approaches, salvage surgery, and neck management after non-operative treatment. Definitive radiation for larynx cancer, brachytherapy, altered fractionation radiation, intensity-modulated radiation therapy, and the importance of tumor hypoxia are among current radiation therapy concerns and will be discussed. Chapters have also been included reviewing the role of chemotherapy in sequential, concurrent, and adjuvant multimodality treatment schedules.

A number of treatment approaches with significant promise for the future will also be presented. Interventions including gene therapy, targeted therapies, chemoprevention, and toxicity modification are discussed. The epidemiology of this disease, particularly in the non-smoker nondrinker is addressed as well as the quality of life and symptom management issues so important to this patient population.

Although this book's scope has been restricted to the relatively homogenous squamous cell head and neck cancers, Chapter 15 is devoted to the management of nasopharyngeal cancer in view of the worldwide epidemiologic importance of this disease and the recent success achieved with multimodality treatment approaches.

The organization of *Squamous Cell Head and Neck Cancer: Recent Clinical Progress and Prospects for the Future* reflects the advances that have been made on multiple fronts in the treatment of these conditions. It is meant to serve as both a review of recent success and a blueprint for future investigation of this disease.

David J. Adelstein, MD

Contents

Contributors

DAVID J. ADELSTEIN, MD • *Department of Hematology and Medical Oncology, Cleveland Clinic Foundation, Cleveland, OH*

ANESA AHAMAD, MD, FRCR • *Radiation Oncology, University of Texas MD Anderson Cancer Center, Houston, TX*

LEE M. AKST, MD • *Head and Neck Institute, Cleveland Clinic Foundation, Cleveland, OH*

K. KIAN ANG, MD, PhD • *Radiation Oncology, University of Texas MD Anderson Cancer Center, Houston, TX*

SØREN M. BENTZEN, PhD, DSc • *Department of Human Oncology, University of Wisconsin Medical School, Madison, WI*

JACQUES BERNIER, MD, PD • *Department of Radiotherapy, Oncology Institute of Southern Switzerland, Bellinzona, Switzerland*

DAVID M. BRIZEL, MD • *Department of Radiation Oncology, Duke University Medical Center, Durham, NC*

J. MARTIN BROWN, PhD • *Department of Radiation Oncology, Stanford University, Stanford, CA*

EZRA E. W. COHEN, MD • *Department of Medicine, Section of Hematology/Oncology, University of Chicago, Chicago, IL*

MELLAR P. DAVIS, MD, FACP • *Department of Hematology and Medical Oncology, Cleveland Clinic Foundation, Cleveland, OH*

GYPSYAMBER D'SOUZA MS, MPH • *Department of Epidemiology, Johns Hopkins Bloomberg School of Public Health, Baltimore, MD*

RAMON M. ESCLAMADO, MD • *Head and Neck Institute, Cleveland Clinic Foundation, Cleveland, OH*

KAM-WENG FONG, FRCR • *Department of Therapeutic Radiology, National Cancer Centre, Singapore*

AMATO J. GIACCIA, PhD • *Department of Radiation Oncology, Stanford University, Stanford, CA*

MAURA L. GILLISON, MD, PhD • *Sydney Kimmel Comprehensive Cancer Center, Johns Hopkins University, Baltimore, MD*

ROBERT I. HADDAD, MD • *Head and Neck Oncology Program, Dana-Farber Cancer Institute, Boston, MA*

EHAB HANNA, MD, FACS • *Department of Head and Neck Surgery, University of Texas MD Anderson Cancer Center, Houston, TX*

PAUL M. HARARI, MD • *Department of Human Oncology, University of Wisconsin Medical School, Madison, WI*

LOUIS B. HARRISON, MD • *Department of Radiation Oncology, Beth Israel Medical Center, New York, NY*

THEODORE S. HONG, MD • *Department of Human Oncology, University of Wisconsin Medical School, Madison, WI*

KENNETH S. HU, MD • *Department of Radiation Oncology, Beth Israel Medical Center, New York, NY*

ANDREW ISKANDER, MD • *Department of Otolaryngology—Head and Neck Surgery, Wayne State University, Detroit, MI*

FADLO R. KHURI, MD • *Winship Cancer Institute, Emory University, Atlanta, GA*

PIERRE LAVERTU, MD • *Department of Otolaryngology Head and Neck Surgery, University Hospitals of Cleveland, Cleveland, OH*

QUYNH-THU LE, MD • *Department of Radiation Oncology, Stanford University, Stanford, CA*

WALTER T. LEE, MD • *Head and Neck Institute, Cleveland Clinic Foundation, Cleveland, OH*

SWAN-SWAN LEONG, MRCP • *Department of Medical Oncology, National Cancer Centre, Singapore*

ROBERT R. LORENZ, MD • *Head and Neck Institute, Cleveland Clinic Foundation, Cleveland, OH*

WILLIAM M. MENDENHALL, MD • *Department of Radiation Oncology, University of Florida Health Science Center, Gainesville, FL*

CHARLES M. NORRIS, MD • *Head and Neck Oncology Program, Dana-Farber Cancer Institute, Boston, MA*

MARSHALL R. POSNER, MD • *Head and Neck Oncology Program, Dana-Farber Cancer Institute, Boston, MA*

DANNY RISCHIN, MD • *Division of Hematology and Medical Oncology, Peter MacCallum Cancer Institute, Melbourne, Australia*

DAVID I. ROSENTHAL, MD • *Radiation Oncology, University of Texas MD Anderson Cancer Center, Houston, TX*

NABIL F. SABA, MD • *Winship Cancer Institute, Emory University, Atlanta, GA*

JOSEPH SCHARPF, MD • *Head and Neck Institute, Cleveland Clinic Foundation, Cleveland, OH*

TANGUY Y. SEIWERT, MD • *Department of Medicine, Section of Hematology/Oncology, University of Chicago, Chicago, IL*

RAVI A. SHANKAR, MD • *Department of Radiation Oncology, Beth Israel Medical Center, New York, NY*

ALLEN C. SHERMAN, PhD • *Division of Behavioral Medicine, Department of Otolaryngology, University of Arkansas for Medical Sciences, Little Rock, AR*

STEPHANIE SIMONTON, PhD • *Division of Behavioral Medicine, Department of Otolaryngology, University of Arkansas for Medical Sciences, Little Rock, AR*

MARSHALL STROME, MD • *Head and Neck Institute, Cleveland Clinic Foundation, Cleveland, OH*

ENG-HUAT TAN, MRCP • *Department of Medical Oncology, National Cancer Centre, Singapore*

TERENCE TAN, FRCR • *Department of Therapeutic Radiology, National Cancer Centre, Singapore*

ROY B. TISHLER, MD • *Head and Neck Oncology Program, Dana-Farber Cancer Institute, Boston, MA*

WOLFGANG A. TOMÉ, PhD • *Department of Human Oncology, University of Wisconsin Medical School, Madison, WI*

TUNG T. TRANG, MD • *Department of Otolaryngology Head and Neck Surgery, University Hospitals of Cleveland, Cleveland, OH*

JOSEPH WEE, FRCR • *Department of Therapeutic Radiology, National Cancer Centre, Singapore*

LORI WIRTH, MD • *Head and Neck Oncology Program, Dana-Farber Cancer Institute, Boston, MA*

GEORGE H. YOO, MD • *Department of Otolaryngology–Head and Neck Surgery, Wayne State University, Detroit, MI*

1

Head and Neck Squamous Cell Cancers in the Nonsmoker-Nondrinker

Gypsyamber D'Souza, MS, MPH
and Maura L. Gillison, MD, PhD

1. INTRODUCTION

The vast majority of patients with head and neck squamous cell carcinoma (HNSCC) report a history of tobacco and alcohol use. The risk of oral cancer increases as a function of both intensity and duration of each exposure, indicating that alcohol and tobacco act synergistically to promote cancer development *(1–3)*.

In the absence of tobacco exposure, alcohol remains an important cause of HNSCC. Several case-control studies have evaluated the risk for HNSCC associated with alcohol use among nonsmokers (NS); only high levels of alcohol use (more than 5 drinks per day) were associated with increased risk of oral cancer (OR = 3.7–8.0) *(1–6)*. NS who drink less than 21 drinks per week do not have increased HNSCC risk compared with NS nondrinkers (ND) (OR = 0.7–1.5) *(1–6)*. Acetaldehyde, a metabolite of alcohol, may be responsible for the tumor-promoting effect of ethanol via free radical production and DNA damage *(7)*. Metabolism of ethanol to acetaldehyde is performed by alcohol dehydrogenases (ADHs) and oral microflora. ADH alleles that increase ethanol metabolism to acetaldehyde increase the risk of HNSCC *(8–11)*. In contrast to NS, studies consistently reported that smokers who have 1–14 drinks per week have increased HNSCC risk (OR = 1.6–3.7) compared with nondrinking smokers *(2,3,6,12–14)*. The effect of alcohol may be more pronounced in smokers because of an interaction between tobacco and alcohol. Smokers have higher salivary acetaldehyde concentrations than NS after exposure to the same amount of alcohol *(15)*, suggesting that the synergy between alcohol and tobacco may in part be attributed to increased exposure to carcinogenic salivary acetaldehyde. Therefore, although moderate alcohol use does not appear to be an important cause of HNSCC in NS, it may interact with tobacco to increase HNSCC risk in smokers.

1.1. Current Problems in the Definition of the "Nonsmoker–Nondrinker"

Despite the preponderance of HNSCC cases in individuals who smoke and or drink, cases do occur in individuals without either of these major risk factors. Estimates of the proportions of head and neck cancers that arise in the "nonsmoker and nondrinker" (NSND) depend on how this category is defined. Ideally, the definition would be based on a biologically or epidemiologically defined cutoff of exposure known not to be associated with elevated risk

From: *Current Clinical Oncology: Squamous Cell Head and Neck Cancer*
Edited by: D. J. Adelstein © Humana Press Inc., Totowa, NJ

for HNSCC. Currently, however, there is no consensus on the minimal duration or intensity of tobacco exposure associated with a significant increase in risk for head and neck cancer. Further complicating this issue is the considerable variability in measures of tobacco exposure (e.g., pack-years, cigarettes per day, years smoked, grams of tar per day, and so on) used in epidemiologic studies, as well as the variety of tobacco products available *(6)*, and the fact that associations may differ by anatomic site *(16,17)*. Significantly elevated risk for oral *(1,6,14,18–21)*, pharyngeal *(1,6,14,18–20)*, laryngeal *(18,22)*, and esophageal *(18,23)* cancers has been reported among individuals who smoke 1–15 cigarettes per day compared with never smokers. However, it is unclear whether exposures as low as 1, 5, or 10 cigarettes per day elevate risk. Those studies that estimate risk based on pack-years of exposure similarly group together individuals with less than 20 pack-years of exposure. A limited number of studies have explored risk associated with other sources of tobacco, including bidi, pan, and cigars, and have demonstrated elevated odds of oral cancer with exposures of less than 20 bidi per day, less than 5 pan per day *(13,20,24)*, and less than 4 cigars per day compared with never smokers *(14)*.

There are several common working definitions of the nonsmoker, including individuals who have a cumulative lifetime exposure of less than 100 cigarettes, or individuals who have smoked daily for less than a year, and the never smoker (an individual who has never used any form of tobacco). A strict definition of NSND as those who have never used alcohol or tobacco may underestimate the proportion of cases that could be attributed to non-traditional risk factors. Further complicating data interpretation are issues of data quality, including retrospective determination of tobacco and alcohol use by means of medical record review *(25–34)*, a method with limited accuracy that can differentially misclassify exposure and attenuate real differences between the NSND and the smoker-drinker. Even studies that use patient interviews *(35–40)*, can still have problems of differential recall bias among cases and controls that may accentuate differences.

To illustrate the effect of the definition of NSND on estimates of the proportion of HNSCC among NSND, results from several case series are presented in Table 1. In a case-series defining NSND stringently as no history of ever using tobacco or alcohol and excluding individuals with a history of immunosuppressive disease or medication, only 40 (2.4%) of 1648 HNSCC cases were NSND *(39)* (Table 1). This study probably underestimates the true proportion of individuals without alcohol- and tobacco-related risk by misclassifying individuals with very low tobacco and alcohol use as "users"; inferences are further limited by extraction of exposure data from medical records. The exclusion of individuals with immunosuppression may underestimate the proportion of cases among NSND because risk of infectious causes of HNSCC is greater among immunosuppressed individuals (e.g., HIV-infected individuals) *(41)*. In a case series of 48 oral cavity cases, the nonsmoker was defined as individuals with less than 1 pack-year of exposure and the nondrinker as an individual who took less than 0.1 shots per day. Use of these definitions, by comparison with the previous study, resulted in higher proportions of non-smoking patients (19%) and nonsmoking-nondrinking patients (8.3%) *(40)*. In a third case series of 129 patients with HNSCC, the researchers collected data from hospital charts and also interviewed patients and physicians as necessary to collect more complete exposure information. They defined NSND more loosely as those who never used, rarely used, or had stopped using tobacco and alcohol more than 20 yr ago and they found that a higher proportion (18.6%) were NSND *(36)*.

Table 1
Definitions of Nonsmokers (NS)-Nondrinkers (ND) in HNSCC Research and the Percent of Cases That
Were Considered NSND With Each of These Definitions

Author	Study design	Definition of NS, ND	% NSND
Limited tobacco-alcohol use definitions			
Koch et al., 1999 (47)	Case-series 305 HNSCC	MR: never used tobacco on regular basis; no or light alcohol use	14 HNSCC
Brennan et al., 1995 (36)	Case-series 129 HNSCC	MR&INT: never or rarely used or had stopped using alcohol and tobacco 20+ yr ago	19 HNSCC
Muscat et al., 1996[a] (37)	Case-control 1009 oral cavity or pharynx SCC matched with hospital controls with nontobacco conditions	INT: Never smoked cigarettes regularly; never drank or drank less than 1 alcoholic drink per week	Percent NS 10 Male cases 22 Male controls 24 Female cases 55 Female controls
Lazarus et al., 1996 (40)	Prospective case-series of 2 8 oral cavity SCC	MR or INT: less than 1 pack-year; less than 0.1 shots per day	14 HNSCC
Lazarus et al., 1995 (28)	Case-series 14 oral cavity SCC	MR: less than 1 cigarette per day; less than 0.1 shots per day	57 Oral cavity SCC
Schantz et al., 1988[a] (29)	Case-control 83 untreated HNSCC <40 yr old matched to 83 HNSCC >40 yr	MR: no history of cigarette use in medical chart	Percent NS 10 HNSCC > 40 yr 30 HNSCC < 40 yr
Rodriguez et al., 2004[a] (35)	Two case-control studies of 137 oral and pharyngeal cancers 46 yr old and 298 hospital controls	INT: report never having smoked in epidemiologic interview administered by interviewer	Percent NS 10 Oral and pharyngeal
Sorensen et al., 1997 (26)	Case-series 11 tongue invasive SCC <40 yr old	MR: no measurable exposure to tobacco or alcohol	55 Tongue
De Boer et al., 1997 (30)	Case-series 303 women >39 yr with oral cavity or oropharyngeal SCC	MR: never used tobacco or stopped 10+ yr ago; never or occasional alcohol use	50 Oral cavity 28 Oropharyngeal
Freije et al., 1996 (31)	Case-series 23 NS larynx SCC with evidence of GERD	MR: no history of smoking or quit 10+ yr ago; minimal alcohol use	Among NS: % ND 39 Larynx
Singh et al., 2002 (202)	Case-series 71 untreated HNSCC	MR: less than 2 pack-years smoking; less than 2 alcohol equivalents per day and no binge drinking	21 HNSCC
No tobacco-alcohol use definitions			
Constantinides et al., 1992 (32)	Case-series 10 NSND HNSCC >60 yr old	MR: no history of cigarette smoking or alcohol use	Limited to NSND
Wiseman et al., 2003 (39)	Case-series 1648 invasive HNSCC	MR and INT: documented definitive history of no cigarette use in registry and no alcohol use reported in survey	2.4 HNSCC

(continued)

Table 1 (continued)

Author	Study design	Definition of NS, ND	% NSND
Agudelo et al., 1997 (33)	Case-series 933 larynx SCC	MR: no history of alcohol or tobacco use	3.3 Larynx
Hodge et al., 1985[a] (25)	Case-series 945 HNSCC	MR: never used tobacco in any form	Percent NS 3.5 HNSCC
Fouret et al., 1997 (34)	Case-series 187 HNSSC	MR: no history of alcohol or tobacco use	5 HNSCC

Abbreviations: MR, exposure information collected from the medical record; INT, exposure information collected from interview or survey; HNSCC, head and neck squamous cell carcinoma; GERD, gastroesophageal reflux disease.
[a]Smoking status but not drinking status was reported. No measure of NSND reported.

1.2. Proportion of HNSCC That Are Nonsmokers-Nondrinkers

Population-based case-control studies provide the best estimates of the proportion of HNSCC cases that occurs among individuals without alcohol and tobacco exposure. However, it is difficult to estimate, even from these studies, the proportion of cases that occurs in the NSND, because the proportion of the cases that are both NS and ND is not usually reported. From these studies, it is estimated that approx 10 to 17% of oral cancer cases are never smokers, and approx 16% are nondrinkers. The best data come from population-based case-control studies, but these studies often do not report NSND results (42,43). The best NSND data came from two hospital case-control studies in which exposure data were collected by patient interview. In the first study, 1009 oral cavity and pharyngeal cancer cases were matched to 923 hospital controls on gender, age, race, and date of admission. Ten percent of male cases and 22% of female cases had never smoked cigarettes regularly, according to an interview-administered survey. A ND was defined as an individual who reported drinking 0–1 drinks per week and included 8.5% of male cases and 36.4% of female cases (37). The proportion of NSND was not reported. The second study included 137 oral cavity and pharyngeal cancers cases less than 46 yr old and 298 hospital controls matched for sex and age. Ten percent of cases reported during an interview-administered epidemiologic survey that they were never smokers, and 9.5% of cases reported being ND (35). Again, the proportion of the cases that were both NSND was not reported. Results from single-institution case series report an overall proportion of NSND of 2.4 to 19% among HNSCC cases (Table 1).

1.3. Prospective Measures of HNSCC Risk in Nonsmokers-Nondrinkers

Prospective data on HNSCC in NSND is limited, and only one estimate of HNSCC incidence in NSND is available. A cohort study of 34,439 British male doctors followed prospectively for 40 yr explored the mortality from upper respiratory cancers (mouth, pharynx excluding nasopharynx, and larynx) in smokers and nonsmokers (44). Annual upper respiratory mortality was 12 times lower in never smokers (1/100,000) than in those who currently smoked 1–14 cigarettes per day (12/100,000). Mortality rate increased with increasing level of tobacco use (18/100,000 and 48/100,000 in those who currently smoked 15–24 and ≥25 cigarettes per day, respectively). The lower HNSCC mortality rate in NS may represent a lower incidence of HNSCC in NS but could also be explained by improved survival in NS HNSCC cases.

1.4. Need to Study Risk Factors for HNSCC in Nonsmokers-Nondrinkers

Tobacco and alcohol account for most HNSCC cases, but there must be other factors leading to tumorogenesis in NSND. Important reasons for the study of risk factors for head and neck cancer among NS include the following:

- Studies that rely on adjustment for alcohol and tobacco use may report associations owing to residual confounding by these factors because of remaining issues with accurate assessment of exposure.
- The incidence of HNSCC in NSND will not decrease with behavioral modifications to reduce tobacco and alcohol consumption.
- Understanding nontraditional causes of HNSCC may also provide clues to the etiology of other cancer risks in the general population.

2. RISK FACTORS FOR HNSCC IN THE NONSMOKER-NONDRINKER

Nontraditional risk factors associated with HNSCC can best be evaluated in studies of never smokers-never drinkers. Two studies restricted to NSND have evaluated HNSCC cases, and although patient demographics were reported, other risk factors were not. The first was a case series of 10 NSND HNSCC patients older than 59 yr *(32)*, and the second included 40 NSND with a diagnosis of invasive HNSCC *(39)*. Patients were primarily female (78–90%), and the mean age was 60 yr (range 27–90 yr). Tumors occurred in the oral cavity (60–75%), oropharynx (20–30%), and larynx (5–10%) *(32,39)*. These studies suggest that NSND HNSCC cases occur predominately in the oral cavity and oropharynx and that women constitute a large proportion of NSND. However, the data are limited, and further research is needed to describe the demographics of the NSND case better.

2.1. Human Papillomavirus

Oral human papillomavirus (HPV) genomic DNA is more common in NSND HNSCC cases (17–50%) than smoker/drinker cases (8–23%) *(34,45–48)* (Table 2). This fact is unlikely to suggest that NSND are more likely to be infected with HPV or to develop HNSCC if infected, rather, the larger proportion of HPV-HNSCC among NSND cases probably occurs because HPV is a major cause of HNSCC among individuals without traditional risk factors and these individuals thus constitute a larger proportion of NSND cases.

Oral HPV infection is associated with increased HNSCC risk in NSND. Three case-control studies have demonstrated increased odds of HNSCC in NS among individuals seropositive for HPV16 L1 capsid antibodies compared with nonsmoking individuals who are HPV seronegative (OR = 1.6–5.5) *(38,43,49)*. This suggests that NS infected with oral HPV have increased risk of HNSCC. Increased risk of HNSCC was also recently demonstrated among NSND with an oral high-risk HPV infection compared with individuals without such an infection (OR = 2.3, 95% CI = 0.8–6.7) *(50)*. Oral HPV infection is therefore an important cause of HNSCC among NSND.

HPV-positive NS HNSCC cases are less likely to have mutations in *p53* or loss of heterozygosity (LOH) than NS HPV-negative cases *(34,47)*. This is likely because tobacco causes *p53* mutations in smokers, whereas NS HNSCC cases may have wild-type *p53* but impaired *p53* function owing to HPV infection.

2.2. Environmental Tobacco Smoke (Second-Hand Smoke)

One of the more established risk factors for HNSCC among NSND remains tobacco, in the form of environmental tobacco smoke (ETS). ETS consists of exhalations of smokers as well

Table 2
Human Papillomavirus (HPV) Prevalence in Nonsmokers-Nondrinkers (NSND) With Head and
Neck Squamous Cell Carcinoma (HNSCC) Compared With Smokers/Drinkers With HNSCC

	HPV prevalence in HNSCC cases		
Author	Nonsmoker-Nondrinker[b]	Smoker/Drinker[b]	P value[c]
Fouret, 1997	100 (4/4) oropharynx	8.5 (15/177) HNSCC	0.0001
Koch, 1999	59 (13/22) oropharynx	28 (15/54) oropharynx	0.01
Smith, 1998[a]	39 (7/18) oral, pharyngeal	15 (7/46) oral, pharyngeal	0.036
Smith, 2004	20[d] (7/35) oral, oropharynx	25[d] (16/67) oral, oropharynx	0.57
Snidjers, 1996	40 (2/5)[e] HNSCC	17 (4/24) HNSCC	0.25
Herrero, 2003[a]	9 (18/194) oral cavity	9 (95/1097) oral cavity	1.0
	33 (6/18) oropharynx	12 (26/220) oropharynx	0.01
Gillison, 2000[a]	88 (7/8) oropharynx	53 (27/51) oropharynx	0.062
	8 (2/24) other HNSCC	16 (26/168) other HNSCC	0.30
Dahlstrom, 2003[a]	69 (24/35) oropharynx	40 (17/35) oropharynx	0.015
	8 (2/25) other HNSCC	24 (6/25) other HNSCC	0.12
Scholes, 1997[a]	50 (4/8)[f] HNSCC	44 (4/9) HNSCC	0.81
Ringstrom, 2002[a]	25 (3/12) HNSCC	19 (9/48) HNSCC	0.64

[a]These studies only reported HPV prevalence in NS and did not report results for NSND.
[b]Results stratified by tumor site when available. Data are percent, with number/total in parentheses.
[c]Test for homogeneity of binomial proportions.
[d]Prevalence of high-risk oral HPV infection.
[e]Includes former smokers who are nondrinkers. Of six never smokers unstratified by alcohol use, only one (17%) was HPV positive.
[f]Includes former smokers (unknown alcohol use). Of three never smokers unstratified by alcohol use, only one (33%) was HPV positive.

as direct emissions from cigarettes, cigars, and pipes. ETS was classified as a human carcinogen by the Environmental Protection Agency in 1993. Three case-control studies have demonstrated increased odds of HNSCC in NS exposed to ETS. In a study of 173 HNSCC patients, never-smoking patients were more likely to have a history of ETS exposure than controls (OR = 2.2, 95% CI = 0.6–8.4). Furthermore, a dose-response relationship was observed. NS exposed to ETS both at work and at home had increased odds of cancer (OR = 4.3, 95% CI = 0.8–24) ($p = 0.008$) compared with NS exposed to ETS either at work or home (OR = 1.8, 95% CI = 0.5–7.3) and NS with no ETS exposure (51). Similar findings were reported in another study (52). A population-based case-control study in patients with nasopharyngeal carcinoma also reported increased odds of NPC among nonsmokers with a history of ETS during childhood (OR = 2.0, 95% CI = 1.2–3.4) as well as during adulthood (OR = 1.9, 95% CI = 1.1–3.2) (53). Because ETS exposure was not stratified by intensity of exposure, these studies probably underestimate the true magnitude of the association by including some individuals with low levels of exposure. It can be concluded from these data that ETS, either at work or at home, is associated with increased risk of HNSCC in NS.

2.3. Dietary Antioxidants

Whereas the data for a role for dietary micronutrients in reducing risk of HNSCC in smokers and drinkers are inconsistent, the data for a role for dietary nutrients in decreasing risk of HNSCC in NSND is compelling. NSND with high vegetable (OR = 0.4–0.7) and fruit (OR = 0.2–1.2) intake have decreased odds of oral and oropharyngeal cancer (54–57). Studies of NS laryngeal and nasopharyngeal cancer cases suggest a protective effect of carotenoids (OR = 0.14–0.17), particularly β-carotene *(58–60)*. Carotenes may be one of the antioxidants responsible for the observed association between high vegetable and fruit intake and decreased oral cancer risk in NSND. This research supports the hypothesis of an independent protective effect of fruit and vegetables on HNSCC risk.

2.4. Genetic Factors

Data on genetic alterations in HNSCC support the hypothesis that HNSCC in NSND may represent a distinct molecular disease compared with that of the smoker/drinker. Most of the molecular markers (*p53*, chromosomal LOH, and microsatellite alterations) we associate with HNSCC cases were defined in patients with tobacco exposure and occur less frequently in the NSND *(36,47)*. Common (tobacco-associated) *p53* mutations are found in 0–25% of NSND HNSCC *(26–28,36,40,47)* compared with 40 to 76% of smoker/drinkers *(26–28,36,40,47)* and an intermediate 33 to 43% in smoker/ND *(36,40)*. Some evidence suggests that *p53* mutations caused by spontaneous deamination of cytosine phosphate guanine dinucleotides sites are more common in NSND than in the smoker/drinker *(27,36)*. Among HNSCC cases with *p53* mutations, Brennan et al. *(36)* found a fourfold increased odds of cytosine phosphate guanine dinucleotide mutations in NSND than in smokers/drinkers. These studies suggest that *p53* mutations are less frequent in the NSND than the smoker/drinker and occur at different sites.

Most studies of LOH have analyzed HNSCC in smokers and drinkers, thus characterizing mutations caused by alcohol and tobacco. Case series suggest that NSND with HNSCC have a 60 to 80% reduction in odds of LOH compared with HNSCC tumors in smokers *(27,47)*. However, the reduced odds of LOH mutations reported may reflect lower odds of LOH at tobacco-associated sites. LOH at established sites in smoker/drinkers does not occur frequently in NSND and does not appear to play an important role in the genetic progression of HNSCC in NSND. Distinct LOH sites in NSND may exist but have not been identified.

Individuals with increased mutagen sensitivity, as measured by number of in vitro bleomycin-induced chromosomal breaks in blood lymphocytes *(61)*, are at increased risk of developing HNSCC. In a multicenter case-control study of 104 NS and 271 ND, increased odds of HNSCC were demonstrated among mutagen-sensitive NS (OR = 2.6, 95% CI = 0.9–7.6) and ND (OR = 3.5, 95% CI = 2.0–5.8) compared with those without mutagen sensitivity *(63)*. Other case-control studies demonstrate similar increases in odds of HNSCC in NSND with increased mutagen sensitivity *(62–64)*. Many mechanisms could account for differences in chromosomal sensitivity, such as increased susceptibility to DNA damage and defective DNA repair capability, but the specific molecular defects (with the exception of Fanconi's anemia; *see* **Subheading 3.4.3.**) remain to be identified. Mutagen sensitivity, if found to be hereditary, could be one explanation for the observed association between family history of HNSCC and increased HNSCC risk (*see* **Subheading 3.4.1.**). These data suggest that in the absence of tobacco and alcohol use, genetic susceptibility to other as yet unspecified mutagens is an independent risk factor for HNSCC.

3. STUDIES OF HNSCC RISK FACTORS THAT CONTROL FOR SMOKING AND ALCOHOL USE

The studies presented here include data from individuals with varying degrees of alcohol and tobacco use that were controlled for in the analyses. Residual confounding and interactions with tobacco and alcohol use may hamper evaluation of the independent effect of these factors on HNSCC risk. Differential recall bias among cases and controls may also influence tobacco and alcohol information collected and many accentuate differences between smoker/drinkers and NSND.

3.1. Characteristics of the Nonsmoker-Nondrinker

3.1.1. GENDER

Although there is a male predominance overall among patients with HNSCC (~75%), there appears to be a more equitable gender distribution among NSND HNSCC cases *(37,39,47)*. A population-based study of oral cavity and oropharyngeal cancer demonstrated a similar proportion of NS among male (15%) and female (18%) cases *(43)*. When both alcohol and tobacco use are considered, women constitute a higher proportion of NSND patients. Case series of HNSCC (oral cavity, oropharynx, larynx, and hypopharynx) demonstrate a higher proportion of women among NSND cases (41–90%) on average *(25,32,37,39,47)* compared with smokers with HNSCC (23–30%) *(37,47)*. This is probably because women traditionally have been less likely to smoke and drink than men, and thus women constitute a larger proportion of the NSND population than the smoking/drinking population. However, gender may also confound the definition of the NS: studies have reported that women have a significantly elevated risk of oral cavity and oropharyngeal cancer at lower cumulative exposure compared with men *(4,37)*.

3.1.2. AGE

The age distribution of NSND HNSCC cases has not been well characterized. The occurrence of HNSCC cancers in young NSND might suggest a genetic predisposition to cancer. Few studies have compared the age at HNSCC diagnosis in NSND and smoker/drinkers. A case series of 305 individuals with HNSCC of all sites found similar mean age at diagnosis of NS and smokers, although the NS category had more individuals at extremes of age (all six individuals <30 yr old and five individuals >85 yr old were NSND) *(47)*. However, another case series of 314 women over 40 yr of age with oral cavity or oropharyngeal cancers found that NSND were on average 15 yr older when the cancer was diagnosed than smoker/drinkers and yet were more likely to present with early-stage disease *(30)*. The older age of NSND at diagnosis in this study is not owing to a delay in diagnosis, as these NSND women also presented with early-stage disease. There is insufficient evidence to know whether NSND HNSCC patients are more likely to present at a different age than patients with traditional risk factors.

Most HNSCC cases occur in older individuals; 4 to 6% of cases occur in those less than 40 yr of age *(65)*. In recent years some attention has been focused on HNSCC in younger individuals in an attempt to explore genetic factors that may lead to increased risk of cancer *(65)*. Many of the studies on young HNSCC patients failed to report information on NSND cases or report information on smoking status and alcohol use separately without consideration of NSND as a single category *(37,66–69)*. Whereas some studies report low levels of smoking and drinking in young HNSCC patients *(26,28,68,69)*, other studies of young HNSCC patients report high levels of alcohol and tobacco abuse *(35,70,71)*. In a case series of 39 HNSCC (oral cavity, larynx, and pharynx) patients under 40 yr of age, all were smokers and drinkers with an average of 40 pack-years at diagnosis, and 64% were classified by the authors as alcoholics *(70)*. In a case-control study of 137 oral and pharyngeal patients younger than 46 yr, 63% smoked more than 15 cigarettes per day, 62% drank more than 6 drinks per day, and 47% abused both tobacco and alcohol at these levels *(35)*. Despite their younger ages, some of these patients may have been abusing alcohol and tobacco for 20 yr or more. The incidence of HNSCC in patients younger than 40 yr may still be owing to tobacco and alcohol exposure, and studies evaluating other causes of cancer in this population may be confounded by smoking and alcohol.

3.1.3. SURVIVAL

NSND patients have similar survival to that of smoking/drinking cases. In a case series of 40 NSND, the overall 5-yr survival of NSND HNSCC was estimated to be approx 70% *(39)*. Three case-series of HNSCC (oral cavity, oropharynx, hypopharynx, larynx) patients did not find a statistically significant difference in survival between NS and smoking cases *(29,47,69)*.

Although NS HNSCC patients do not appear to have improved overall survival, they do have lower rates of secondary primary tumors (SPTs). SPTs in the aerodigestive tract were observed less frequently in NS HNSCC (oral cavity, pharynx, larynx) cases (0–4%) than in smoking HNSCC (4–14%) cases *(29,69,72)* (length of follow-up not reported). The SPT tumor *rate* in NS was reported in only one study and was 16 per 154 person-years (1.0/10 yr) in NS compared with 74 per 433 person-years (1.7/10 yr) in current smokers ($p = 0.05$) *(72)*. If observed, improved survival among NS HNSCC cases could be attributed to the lower rate of secondary tumors and lack of other smoking-induced comorbidities. HPV-infected HNSCC patients have improved survival compared with HPV-negative cases *(73)*, so HPV status could also confound the analysis of survival and smoking status.

3.2. Environmental Causes of HNSCC

3.2.1. HUMAN PAPILLOMAVIRUS

HPV is an etiologic cause for a distinct subset of HNSCC, including approximately half of the squamous cell carcinomas that arise from the lingual and palatine tonsils. In numerous case series, HPV genomic DNA has been consistently detected in approx 20% of all HNSCCs *(34,43,48,45,74–79)* and approx 50% of oropharyngeal or tonsillar squamous cell carcinomas *(43,45,74,76–78,80–85)*. HPV16 is present in an overwhelming majority (~90–95%) of HPV-positive HNSCC cases (HPV-HNSCC) *(49)*. Studies demonstrate better survival in HPV-positive (OR = 0.59–0.83) than HPV-negative HNSCC cases *(45,47,83,86,87)*. HPV-associated cancers are distinguished by their predominance in the oropharynx, more frequent basaloid morphology, less frequent *p53* mutation, better survival *(45,86)*, and less frequent LOH *(88)*.

Extensive biological evidence supports a causal role of HPV in HNSCC carcinogenesis. Viral genomic DNA is specifically localized in tumor cell nuclei *(45,79)*, present in high-copy number *(89–92)*, frequently integrated *(45,79,81,89,93–96)*, and transcriptionally active *(78,81,82,93,95,97,98)*. Elevated levels of antibodies to HPV16 proteins E6 and E7 in individuals with HPV-HNSCC but not in HPV-negative HNSCC or controls provide evidence of viral oncoprotein expression specifically in HPV-HNSCC *(49,99)*. The presence of HPV16 L1 antibodies in precancer diagnosis sera strongly suggests that viral exposure precedes development of disease and is associated with an approx 14-fold increased risk of incident oropharyngeal cancer *(100)*.

HPV infection is associated with increased cancer risk in NSND as well as in smoker/drinkers. An independent increase in odds of HNSCC in those with HPV16 L1 capsid antibody is observed among smokers (OR = 2.0–9.2) and NS (OR = 1.6–5.5) *(38,43,49)*. These results suggest that oral HPV infection is associated with increased odds of cancer in both NS and smokers. Individuals who use tobacco have a higher risk of HNSCC owing to interaction between HPV infection and tobacco. Case-control studies of oral cavity and oropharyngeal cases that evaluated this interaction found that the presence of HPV16 L1 viral capsid antibody and tobacco use increased risk beyond that expected with either exposure alone, with two studies showing evidence for additive interaction *(49,50)* and one study supporting multiplicative interaction *(43)*. HPV infection is independently associated with increased HNSCC risk in NS and interacts with tobacco in smokers to increase HNSCC risk further.

3.2.2. EPSTEIN-BARR VIRUS

Epstein-Barr virus (EBV) is a herpesvirus, endemic worldwide, to which more than 90% of adults are exposed and carry as a life-long persistent latent infection of B lymphocytes. EBV infection is associated with several malignancies (Burkitt's lymphoma, Hodgkin's disease, non-Hodgkin's lymphoma, gastric cancer) and is accepted as an etiologic cause of nasopharyngeal carcinoma (NPC). EBV is clearly not a sufficient cause of NPC, and when oncogenesis occurs it is several decades after primary EBV infection. In nonindustrialized countries and low socioeconomic communities, primary infection usually occurs early in childhood and is asymptomatic. By comparison, in industrialized or wealthy countries, infection is often delayed until adolescence, at which time it often causes clinical symptoms of infectious mononucleosis. NPC incidence is high in parts of Asia, especially in southern China, where diet is believed to play a role in the higher incidence *(101)*. In areas with low NPC incidence such as Europe and North America, a smaller proportion of cases are EBV associated, and tobacco and alcohol abuse and thought to be more prominent causes *(102)*.

Extensive evidence suggests that EBV is an etiologic cause of NPC. EBV DNA has been localized to tumor cells in patients with NPC *(103)* and is clonal *(104)*. EBV-encoded latent genes are also expressed in the tumor cells and appear to contribute to the malignancy *(105)*. EBV is most consistently associated with the undifferentiated form of nasopharyngeal carcinoma (UNPC) but has also been associated with squamous cell NPC. There is little evidence that EBV plays an etiologic role for HNSCC outside the nasopharynx.

Smoking and alcohol have been associated with increased risk of NPC. Case-control studies show that the odds of NPC are reduced 30 to 50% in NS compared with smokers *(53,106–108)*. Individuals with more than 30 pack-years have 1.6–4.0-fold higher odds of NPC than NS *(53,106,107,109)*. Epidemiologic data on the interaction of tobacco and EBV infection in NPC risk is not available. Two case-control studies show no increase in the odds of NPC in those who drink alcohol compared with ND *(53,108)*, although at high levels of alcohol use (>20 drinks/wk), an association has been suggested by two other studies (OR = 2–7) *(106,109)*. Tobacco use and potentially high levels of alcohol use increase NPC risk.

3.2.3. WORKPLACE EXPOSURES

Many occupational exposures including asbestos, cement dust, wood dust, solvents, and varnish, have been suggested as causes of HNSCC. However, evidence is limited for most of these exposures.

Although there are several studies suggesting a positive association between asbestos (a known carcinogen) and laryngeal cancer, confounding by alcohol, tobacco, and additional job-related exposures, as well as contradictory negative studies, suggests there is insufficient evidence to conclude that asbestos is a cause of laryngeal cancer. A meta-analysis of 69 asbestos-exposed occupational cohorts reported an elevated laryngeal cancer standardized mortality ratio (SMR) among asbestos-exposed individuals. (SMR is a ratio of the observed number of deaths among exposed individuals over the expected number of deaths among unexposed individuals and is interpreted similarly to a RR.) The meta-SMR for laryngeal cancer was 133 (95% CI 114–155), suggesting that asbestos-exposed individuals have a 33% increase in risk of laryngeal cancer death compared with unexposed individuals *(110)*. Although the data are compelling, this increase in deaths from laryngeal cancer may be explained by residual confounding by smoking, age, and socioeconomic status, all of which may impact on laryngeal cancer risk. As detailed by Brown and Gee *(111)*, almost half of the existing cohort studies of asbestos exposure report an SMR of 1 or less, whereas studies with SMR more than 1 suffer from various flaws, including the use of comparison groups without comparable smoking and alcohol exposure history. Case-control studies also report marginally significant or nonsignificant associations of asbestos exposure with laryngeal cancer *(112–116)*. Asbestos exposure may be associated with an increase in laryngeal cancer risk; however, this association may also be explained by residual confounding by factors that are more strongly related to laryngeal cancer, such as smoking.

Three case-control studies have reported an association between cement dust exposure (OR = 2.4–4.4) *(117–119)* and laryngeal cancer. One of these studies included 257 laryngeal cancer cases and 769 population-based controls *(117)*. Exposure information was collected with an interview-administered survey that included a checklist of various suspected carcinogens, and specific questions about occupation and job related exposures. An increase was found in the odds of laryngeal cancer independent of tobacco exposure (OR = 2.4, 95% CI = 1.1–5.2) *(117)*. These studies suggest there may be a relationship, but confirmatory research is needed.

In 1994, the International Agency for Research on Cancer classified wood dust as a human carcinogen, based on strong associations between wood dust and sinonasal cancer (especially nasal adenocarcinomas) *(120)*. As reviewed by Blot et al., cohort studies of woodworkers and furniture workers in Europe (RR = 5–8) but not in North America (RR ~ 1) show increase nasal cancer in those with occupational wood dust exposure compared with the general population *(121–123)*. As in cohort studies, European case-control studies report strong associations (OR > 5) with nasal cancer, whereas North American studies report weaker (OR = 0.6–4.4) nonsignificant associations *(121,124)*. A pooled analysis of 12 case-control studies demonstrated that the increased risk associated with woodworking was limited to adenocarcinomas (pooled OR = 13.5, 95% CI = 9–20) with no increased risk of squamous cell nasal cancer (pooled OR = 0.8, 95% CI = 0.6–1.1) *(125)*. The risk of nasal adenocarcinoma varied from OR = 1.0 among unexposed men, OR = 1.2 (95% CI = 0.9–1.6) in men with moderate exposure, and OR = 45 (95% CI = 28–73) in men with high (>5 mg/m^3/d) wood dust exposure *(125)*, suggesting elevated risk only at high levels of exposure. Most of these studies did not control for tobacco and alcohol use, and in some the occupation was collected from medical records or death certificates instead of surveys, potentially biasing the exposure assessment. The increased risk for nasal adenocarcinomas among woodworkers in European but not North American studies may be owing to variability in wood type, exposure dose, workplace ventilation, and tobacco use between the populations studied *(121)*. A few studies have evaluated associations between wood dust and other cancers. A pooled analysis of five cohort studies found increased risk of nasopharyngeal cancer (SMR = 2.4, 95% CI = 1.1–4.5) in woodworkers. Increased odds of laryngeal cancer in those exposed to wood dust were reported in one study *(126)* but not in two others *(113,127)*.

Other occupational exposures that have been suggested as causes of laryngeal cancer include solvents, paint, laquers, and varnish, but there is insufficient evidence to support any of these associations at this time. Studies on these exposures present conflicting results and suffer from potential confounding. Some studies have suggested an association between laryngeal cancer and high levels of solvents *(113,128)*; however, other studies report no association *(115,116)*. Increased odds of laryngeal and oral cavity SCC were reported among those exposed to paint, laquer, and varnish in two studies *(129,130)* but not in other studies *(127,131)*. Although numerous occupational exposures have been proposed as potential causes of laryngeal cancer, the available evidence does not support associations with solvents, paint, laquer, and varnish. Occupational exposures that may be associated with increased cancer risk include cement dust and asbestos with laryngeal cancer and high levels of wood dust exposure with nasal adenocarcinomas.

3.2.4. SUN EXPOSURE

An association between lip cancer and sunlight exposure has been reported in several case-control studies based on increased risk among outdoor workers, those with high cumulative leisure exposure, and those with a fair complexion or sun-sensitive genetic diseases *(132–135)*. Smoking and alcohol were not well controlled for in some of these studies and confound the relationship. A population-based case-control study of 74 women with lip cancer and 105 controls found that among those with high lifetime solar radiation exposure, those with infrequent lip protection use had twice the risk of lip cancer than those who used lip protection regularly *(132)*. This supports the hypothesis of a causal association between sun exposure and lip cancer, but further research is needed.

3.3. Nonenvironmental Causes of HNSCC

3.3.1. DIETARY FACTORS

High consumption of fruits and vegetables or their antioxidant micronutrients has been associated with reduced risk of several cancers in case-control studies. These studies consistently found that high fruit and vegetable intake (defined as approx >10 fruit and vegetables per week) were associated with decreased odds of oral and oropharyngeal cancer (OR = 0.3–0.6) *(54,55,57,136–139)*. Decreased odds of oral and oropharyngeal cancer observed among NSND with high vegetable (OR = 0.4–0.7) and fruit (OR = 0.2–1.2) intake appear to be more pronounced than among smokers/drinkers *(54–57)*. This research supports the hypothesis of an independent protective effect of fruit and vegetables on HNSCC risk.

Several studies have evaluated which micronutrients may be responsible for the observed decreases in HNSCC risk. A nested case-control study of 28 individuals who developed oral and pharyngeal cancer and 112 matched controls reported lower serum levels of all carotenoids in cases than controls. Those in the highest tertile of carotenoid levels had one-third the risk of cancer than those in the lowest tertile of carotenoid level *(140)*. This and other studies suggest that the observed protective effect of high fruit and vegetable intake may be from carotenoids, particularly β-carotene *(58–60,140)*. This protective association was more pronounced among NS *(58–60)*. A prospective study of plasma nutrient levels in 25 healthy subjects, followed monthly for 11 months, studied intraindividual variation in mutagen sensitivity and diet. These researchers found that higher plasma carotene levels were correlated with lower monthly mean chromosomal breaks *(141)*.

The potential effect of nutrition appears to be real in NSND, but evaluation of the independent effect of nutrition on HNSCC risk has been hampered by interactions with tobacco and alcohol use. Interactions among smoking, alcohol, and dietary factors clearly exist *(140,142–144)*. A population-based cohort study demonstrated 16–40% lower dietary and serum carotenoids in smokers than never smokers *(142)*. An inverse association between alcohol use and dietary nutrient intake was found independently of smoking status, with 7–20% lower dietary and serum carotenoids in those with high alcohol use *(142)*. It has been suggested that the decreased antioxidant levels in smokers may be owing to depletion of antioxidant micronutrients from tobacco-generated oxidative stress *(145)*; however, this cannot be sufficiently evaluated with existing data: observed differences may also be explained by socioeconomic and demographic differences between smokers and nonsmokers that influence diet. The potential effect of β-carotene was evaluated in a large randomized control trial supplementing the diet of smokers with β-carotene and surprisingly resulted in increased lung cancer risk compared to placebo (this effect was not seen among nonsmokers) *(146)*. While the results may not apply to the head and neck, the study suggests that β-carotene may not be the antioxidant responsible for the decreased cancer risks observed in those with high fruit and vegetable intake. Antioxidants appear to have an independent protective effect for HNSCC, but it is unclear which antioxidants are important and the effect, if any, may be more prominent among NSND.

3.3.1.1. Iron Deficiency. Plummer-Vinson syndrome is a precancerous condition caused by chronic iron deficiency in women who have years of menstruation-related anemia. Iron and riboflavin deficiency can lead to epithelial hyperplasia, so it has been proposed that Plummer-Vinson syndrome could be a cause of HNSCC. Anecdotal data have suggested that the observed preponderance of lateral tongue cancers in nonsmoking women may in part be attributed to iron deficiency, but this remains a hypothesis with limited supporting data. Limited data are available on chronic iron deficiency in NSND, and the association of Plummer-Vinson with HNSCC is largely untested.

3.3.2. MOUTHWASH USE

Mouthwash use has been suggested as a possible cause of some oral and pharyngeal cancers. Listerine, for example, contains 27% alcohol, a higher alcohol content than wine or beer *(147)*. Most studies do not report an association between mouthwash use and oral and pharyngeal cancers *(148–152)*. However, possible effects may have been attenuated by grouping of both high and low alcohol content mouthwashes. A population-based case-control study reported increased risk (OR = 1.9, 95% CI = 1.1–3.3) in those who used high alcohol content (≥25%) mouthwashes after adjusting for alcohol and tobacco use *(153)*. Two case-control studies have indicated that the risk associated with mouthwash may be more pronounced in NS (OR = 1.9, 95% CI = 0.8–4.7) *(154)* and NSND (OR = 2.8, 95% CI = 0.8–9.9) *(155)*. It is certainly plausible that high-alcohol mouthwashes are associated with oral and pharyngeal cancers, given the known effects of alcohol. However, existing data are insufficient to support a causal association of mouthwash with oral and pharyngeal cancers.

3.3.3. ORAL HYGIENE

Numerous case-control studies suggest that poor oral hygiene and poor dental status are related to HNSCC risk. Measures of oral hygiene vary, and reported associations include significantly increased odds of oral cancer in individuals with poor dentition (few teeth) (OR = 2.4–7.6) *(8,156–158)*, broken teeth (OR = 1.3, 95% CI = 0.9–1.8) *(159)*, infrequent toothbrushing (OR = 2.3–6.9) *(8,157,159–161)*, and infrequent dental visits (OR = 2.1–12.6) *(156,160)*. The associations between poor oral hygiene and increased HNSCC risk are adjusted for tobacco and alcohol use, although residual confounding may remain. The association has not been evaluated among NSND. Wearing dentures has consistently been shown not to be associated with increased risk of oral cancer (OR = 0.3–1.3) *(8,148,153,157,159,162)* in case-control studies. These data support the hypothesis that poor oral hygiene, but not denture wearing, is associated with increased HNSCC risk; further research is needed.

3.3.4. GASTROESOPHAGEAL REFLUX DISEASE

Gastroesophageal reflux disease (GERD) is defined as the movement of gastric acids into the esophagus. Often called heartburn, it is a common complaint among US adults. GERD has been proposed as a possible cause of some laryngeal SCC. It has been suggested that the gastric acid carried by frequent reflux from GERD could damage laryngeal mucosa and thus cause laryngeal cancer, but there are no data to support this proposed mechanism.

Smoking and drinking are major causes of laryngeal cancer, so the effect, if any, of GERD is best evaluated among NSND. Several small case series have reported high rates of GERD in NSND laryngeal cancer cases *(31,163,164)*. One case series reported development of laryngeal carcinoma in 19 NSND individuals after a "long GERD clinical history" *(163)*. The common presence of GERD in NSND laryngeal cancer cases may support future studies of the topic, but the coexistence of these diseases does not provide evidence for an association. A case series of 31 laryngeal cancer patients found abnormal pH levels in 71% of cases, although only 34% had symptomatic GERD *(165)*, suggesting the possibility that gastric acid may play a role in some individuals who have "silent" GERD. This hypothesis was supported by a study of 72 laryngeal cancer patients without GERD symptoms, which demonstrated silent GERD based on pH monitoring in 37% of the cases *(166)*. The potential effect of abnormal pH levels on laryngeal cancer risk needs to be explored further.

The best evaluation of the role of GERD in laryngeal cancer was a large case-control study of 17,520 laryngeal cases and 70,080 controls from the computerized records of the Department of Veterans Affairs. GERD was independently associated (OR = 2.4, 95% CI = 2.1–2.7) with laryngeal cancer after controlling for age, gender, ethnicity, smoking, and alcohol use. GERD was also associated with increased odds of pharyngeal cancer (OR = 2.0, 95% CI = 1.9–3.0) *(167)*. This is compelling data that remains to be confirmed.

3.3.5. IMMUNE DEFICIENCY

Two case series have described HNSCC cases in HIV-seropositive patients and suggested that clinical outcomes may be poorer and cases may occur at a younger age in HIV-positive patients *(168,169)*. These studies had small sample sizes, did not control for HPV infection, and were confounded by smoking and alcohol use, so limited conclusions about differential risk for HIV positive individuals can be made.

Oral HPV infection is three times more prevalent among HIV-infected individuals and is further associated with CD4 count below 200 (OR = 2.6, 95% CI = 1.0–6.2) *(41)*. Thus, an increase in HNSCC risk in HIV-seropositive individuals could be owing to increased oral HPV infection or increased HPV persistence in HIV-infected individuals. This hypothesis is supported by an AIDS registry study of 309,365 individuals with HIV that reported larger than expected rates of tonsillar cancer (RR = 2.6, 95% CI = 1.8–3.8) among HIV-positive men *(170)*. The malignant potential of oral HPV infection may be higher in immunosuppressed individuals, who may represent a particularly vulnerable group in which an epidemic of HPV-associated HNSCC might appear, associated with increased longevity from highly active antiviral therapy.

A few reports have described cases of HNSCC in patients with other causes of immunosuppression. One case report described an 18-yr old NSND patient who had a history of renal transplant and later developed HPV-positive HNSCC *(171)*. Oropharyngeal cancers were reported in patients with immunosuppression owing to bone marrow and solid organ transplantation (172,173). Other possible contributing factors may include graft-vs-host-disease and preparative regimens for bone marrow transplant. At this time it is unclear whether individuals who are immunosuppressed (from HIV or transplants) are at higher risk of HNSCC, independent of HPV infection-related HNSCC.

3.3.6. ORAL LICHEN PLANUS

Oral lichen planus (OLP) is a chronic inflammatory disease of unknown etiology, in which T lymphocytes accumulate beneath oral mucosal epithelium, leading to increased differentiation of the stratified squamous epithelium. Evidence suggests that OLP can develop into squamous cell carcinoma and thus can be considered to have malignant potential (174–176). The malignant potential of OLP is supported by data demonstrating that the carcinoma develops within the site of the existing OLP and occurs after OLP diagnosis (176). It is not know what causes OLP or why some OLP cases become malignant.

The frequency with which OLP develops into SCC has been evaluated in several studies. Few of the OLP patients who progress to SCC are smokers (~10%) (177), suggesting a malignant potential of OLP independent of tobacco use. A summary of several OLP case-series found that 2.5% of OLP patients developed SCC (177), with a mean time to transformation of 5 yr (175). A retrospective case series reported that eight patients with OLP progressed to SCC within 10 yr, with a mean transformation time of 4.5 yr. (The total number of OLP patients during this period was not reported [176].) However, a literature review of 26 studies evaluating the malignant potential of OLP found that only 34% of reported transformations had sufficient clinical and histopathologic documentation of the OLP diagnosis to be rigorously considered malignant transformations of OLP (175). OLP can develop into OSCC, but reports have overestimated the true frequency with which this occurs.

OLP cases that progress to cancer have some genetic distinctions. Individuals with OLP and dysplastic epithelium have a higher frequency of genetic mutations such as LOH than OLP cases without dysplasia. As dysplasia increases and SCC develops, LOH frequency increases (46% in moderate dysplasia, 81% in severe dysplasia, and 91% in SCC) (178,179). This suggests that nondysplastic OLP may have a different molecular profile and malignant potential than dysplastic OLP.

3.4. Genetic Causes of HNSCC

3.4.1. FAMILY HISTORY

Family history of HNSCC has been explored to evaluate whether there may be inherited genetic causes of HNSCC. Six recent case-control studies evaluated whether there are increased odds of HNSCC in individuals with a first-degree relative with HNSCC. Five of the studies reported significant (180–182) or marginally significant (183,184) increased odds of HNSCC in patients with a first-degree relative who had HNSCC, and one reported nonsignificant results (185) (Table 3). Higher odds of HNSCC were also reported in those with siblings who had HNSCC (OR = 2.7–3.8) (181–183). Results were adjusted for alcohol and tobacco use in the cases. Only one of these studies (182) controlled for tobacco and alcohol use in both the cases and their relatives, so residual confounding by environmental tobacco smoke may be a problem. Case-control studies adjusting for alcohol and tobacco use suggest that individuals with a first-degree relative with HNSCC have increased odds of HNSCC, but studies in NSND are needed to determine whether there is truly an independent association.

Table 3
Increased Odds of Having HNSCC if Patient Has a First-Degree Relative or a Sibling
Who Had HNSCC

Author	Study type	Collected smoking/ alcohol	No. (cases/ control)	OR first-degree relative	OR in siblings
Foulkes, 1995	Case-control	Yes/Yes	754/1507	3.7 (2.0–6.8)	8.6 (2.7–27)
Brown, 2001	Case-control	Yes/Yes	342/521	2.6 (1.4–4.8)	2.7 (1.1–6.7)
Copper, 1995	Case-control	Yes/No	617/618	3.4 (0.8–13.7)	2.8 (0.2–34)
Foulkes, 1996	Case-control	Yes/Yes	1429/934	3.8 (1.1–13)	
Mork, 1999[a]	Case-control	No/No	127/629	2.0 (0.9–4.4)	
Goldstein, 1994	Case-control	Yes/Yes	1066/1183	1.2 (0.7–2.3)	
Li, 2002	Cohort	No/No	2302	1.4 (1.0–2.0)	
Hemminki, 2004	Cohort	No/No		1.6 (1.0–23)	

[a]This study included population based controls. Only HNSCC cases < 45 yr of age were included.

Associations between family cancer history and HNSCC risk were also evaluated in two cohort studies. These registry-based cohort studies reported marginally significant increased odds of upper aerodigestive tract (UADT) cancers in those with first-degree relatives with UADT cancers (RR = 1.4–1.6) (186,187). One of these study reported the effect of family history among NSND (defined as <10 cigarettes per day, <8 drinks per week). They found a nonsignificant increase in the odds of oral cavity and pharyngeal cancer among NSND with a family history of UADT compared with NSND cases without a family history (OR = 1.8, 95% CI = 0.6–5.6). Conclusions cannot be formed from a single study, and it is possible that a nonsignificant result was observed owing to the small numbers of NSND. There were significant increases in cancer risk in NS drinkers (OR = 11.5, 95% CI = 3.2–41), ND smokers (OR = 12.3, 95% CI = 3–51), and smokers/drinkers (OR = 61, 95% CI = 21–174) with a family history of UADT cancer compared with NSND without a family history. Comparison of those with similar alcohol and tobacco use but without a family history of UADT cancer also showed increased cancer risk in NS drinkers (OR = 5.5, CI not reported), ND smokers (OR = 2.9, CI not reported), and smokers/drinkers (OR = 5.0, CI not reported) (181). These data provide some evidence for an effect of familial (genetic) factors on HNSCC risk, independent of alcohol and tobacco use. However, the studies suffer from potential recall bias, confounding by alcohol and tobacco, and overall marginally significant results. It is not clear whether NSND with a family history of HNSCC have increased risk of HNSCC.

It has also been suggested that HNSCC patients with a family history of HNSCC are at increased risk of SPTs. One study that evaluated this association compared 97 HNSCC patients who developed SPT and 100 HNSCC patients without SPT 6 yr after treatment. They demonstrated increased odds of developing SPT in HNSCC patients with a first-degree relative with respiratory or upper digestive tract (RUDT) cancer (OR = 3.8, 95% CI = 2.0–7.6) (188). All the subjects in this study reported some history of smoking, but no information on amount of tobacco use or any information on alcohol use was collected, so confounding is possible. A second study of 1429 "exposed" relatives of HNSCC cases and 934 "unexposed" relatives of the HNSCC cases' spouses reported increased odds of HNSCC (RR = 3.8, 95% CI = 1.0–12) and of SPT (RR = 7.9, 95% CI = 1.5–42) in those with a family history of HNSCC after adjusting for alcohol and tobacco use (182). HNSCC cases with a family history of HNSCC appear to be at an increased risk for multiple primary tumors.

3.4.2. METABOLISM

3.4.2.1. Alcohol Dehydrogenase . Although the risk of HNSCC increases with increasing alcohol use among nonsmokers *(5)*, ethanol itself is neither mutagenic nor carcinogenic. Acetaldehyde (a metabolite of alcohol) may be responsible for the tumor-promoting effect of ethanol via free radical production and DNA damage *(10)*. The metabolism of ethanol to acetaldehyde is performed by ADH and cytochrome P-450E1 (CYP-E1), both of which are present in upper aerodigestive tract mucosa *(189)*. ADH alleles that increase ethanol metabolism to acetaldehyde *(11)* may increase the risk of HNSCC *(12–14)*.

The potential effect of ADH allele on HNSCC risk was explored in three case-control studies. The ADH_3*2 allele has been shown to reduce the rate of ethanol oxidation by 2.5-fold compared with the ADH_3*1 allele *(190)*. Thus, it has been hypothesized that the ADH_3*1 (rapid) allele may be associated with increased risk for alcohol-related cancers because the rapid oxidation of ethanol would result in higher tissue levels of the potential carcinogen acetaldehyde. A study of 182 HNSCC cases and 202 hospital controls found there was no increased cancer risk in ND (OR = 1.1, 95% CI = 0.3–4.6) or drinkers (OR = 2.0, 95% CI = 0.5–8.1) with the ADH_3*1/1 (rapid) or *1/2 genotype compared to ND with the ADH_3*2/2 (slow allele) genotype after controlling for age, sex, and tobacco use *(191)*. Two studies of oral cavity and oropharyngeal cancers reported nonsignificantly lower odds of oral cavity SCC in ND (OR = 0.4, 95% CI = 0.1–1.8) *(192)* and (OR = 0.6, 95% CI = 0.3–1.6) *(12)* with the ADH_3*2/2 (slow) allele after controlling for gender and tobacco use. These studies do not support a strong protective role for the ADH_3*2/2 (slow) allele in ND.

3.4.2.2. Glutathione-*S*-Transferase. Glutathione-*S*-transferases (GST) are enzymes that detoxify carcinogens and protect cells against DNA damage and adduct formation. There are several different families of GST isozymes, including GSTM1 and GSTT1, which have null alleles that commonly occur in the population and have no enzyme activity. These null genotypes lead to decreased detoxification of carcinogens, for example from tobacco, and have been hypothesized to increase the risk of tobacco-related cancers. As summarized by Geisler and Olshan, studies evaluating GSTT1 allele type and HNSCC risk have reported inconsistent findings. Eight studies reported no effect (OR = 0.5–1.2), whereas six other studies suggested increased odds (OR = 1.4–2.6) of HNSCC in those with the GSTT1 null allele *(193)*. Inconsistent results have also been reported for the GSTM1 null allele, with 13 studies reporting nonsignificant associations (OR = 0.9–1.3) between the presence of GSTM1 allele and HNSCC risk. Eight other studies reported marginally significant or significantly increased odds of HNSCC (OR = 1.3–3.9) *(193)*. The evidence regarding GSTM1 and GSTT1 allele type and HNSCC risk is inconclusive.

Two studies evaluated the effect of GST allele among NS. A matched case-control study of 162 HNSCC patients and 315 healthy controls reported that NS with the GSTM1 (OR = 1.35, $p = 0.17$) or GSTT1 (OR = 3.2, $p = 0.002$) null genotype had higher odds of HNSCC. Increased odds of HNSCC were also reported among ND with the GSTM1 (OR = 1.6, $p = 0.03$) or GSTT1 (OR = 1.8, $p = 0.12$) null genotype *(194)*. Adjusted OR were not reported for NS or ND, although an independent increase for GSTM1 (OR = 1.5, 95% CI = 1.0–2.2) and GSTT1 (OR = 2.3, 95% CI 1.4–3.6) null alleles, adjusted for age, sex, and tobacco and alcohol us, was reported in the study population overall. This study suggests that the GST null genotypes may be associated with increased HNSCC risk in NSND. However, another case-control study of 182 HNSCC cases and 202 hospital controls found increased odds of HNSCC in smokers (OR = 4.7, 95% CI = 1.8–21) but not among NS (OR = 1.3, 95% CI = 0.3–46) with null GSTM1 *(195)*. The evidence for a role of GSTM1 and GSTT1 null alleles in HNSCC risk among NSND is inconclusive.

3.4.3. Fanconi's Anemia

Fanconi's anemia (FA) is an autosomal recessive disorder caused by mutations in DNA repair genes that lead to bone marrow failure and increased risk for multiple malignancies, including HNSCC. Inactivation of any of the seven FA genes is associated with cellular hypersensitivity to oxidative stress and DNA crosslinking agents, chromosomal instability, increased DNA double-strand breaks, loss of telemere integrity, and cell cycle prolongation. A registry-based cohort of 754 individuals with FA reported that most (85%) FA patients with HNSCC have no history of alcohol or tobacco use (196). FA is a genetic disorder associated with increased HNSCC risk.

Individuals with FA have an approx 500-fold increased risk of HNSCC compared with the general population (196–199). In a recent study, HPV16 DNA was detected by real-time polymerase chain reaction in specimens from 15 of 18 FA patients with HNSCC (200). FA-associated HPV-HNSCC was distinguished from HPV-HNSCC in non-FA patients by lower patient age (median 31 yr), location in the anterior tongue and oral cavity, and a poorer prognosis. Similarities included development in NS and wild-type p53 (200,201). These data suggest that the increased cancer rate in individuals with FA is owing to an inherited susceptibility to HPV-induced carcinogenesis. Individuals with other bone marrow failure syndromes (e.g., congenital dyskeratosis) may also have elevated risk for HNSCC (Blanche Alter, personal communication).

4. SUMMARY

Further research is required on the exact amount of tobacco and alcohol use that is associated with increased HNSCC risk so that a meaningful NSND definition can be adopted. Although many studies measure tobacco and alcohol, they often fail to report data for NSND, limiting the information for this population. HNSCC in NSND is associated with an array of nontraditional risk factors, and increased awareness is needed to stimulate the routine stratification of NSND results in research studies. Risk factors for HNSCC in NSND have not been adequately explored, and further research is needed.

ACKNOWLEDGMENTS

The authors thank Dr. Wayne M. Koch for helpful comments on the manuscript. Maura Gillison is a Damon Runyon-Lilly Clinical Investigator supported (in part) by the Damon Runyon Cancer Research Foundation.

REFERENCES

1. Franceschi S, Levi F, La Vecchia C, et al. Comparison of the effect of smoking and alcohol drinking between oral and pharyngeal cancer. Int J Cancer 1999; 83:1–4.
2. Lewin F, Norell SE, Johansson H, et al. Smoking tobacco, oral snuff, and alcohol in the etiology of squamous cell carcinoma of the head and neck: a population-based case-referent study in Sweden. Cancer 1998; 82:1367–1375.
3. Day GL, Blot WJ, Austin DF, et al. Racial differences in risk of oral and pharyngeal cancer: alcohol, tobacco, and other determinants. J Natl Cancer Inst 1993; 85:465–473.
4. Jaber MA, Porter SR, Scully C, Gilthorpe MS, Bedi R. The role of alcohol in non-smokers and tobacco in non-drinkers in the aetiology of oral epithelial dysplasia. Int J Cancer 1998; 77:333–336.
5. Talamini R, La Vecchia C, Levi F, Conti E, Favero A, Franceschi S. Cancer of the oral cavity and pharynx in nonsmokers who drink alcohol and in nondrinkers who smoke tobacco. J Natl Cancer Inst 1998; 90:1901–1903.
6. Castellsague X, Quintana MJ, Martinez MC, et al. The role of type of tobacco and type of alcoholic beverage in oral carcinogenesis. Int J Cancer 2004; 108:741–749.

7. Inagaki S, Esaka Y, Deyashiki Y, Sako M, Goto M. Analysis of DNA adducts of acetaldehyde by liquid chromatography-mass spectrometry. J Chromatogr A 2003; 987:341–347.

8. Edenberg HJ, Brown CJ. Regulation of human alcohol dehydrogenase genes. Pharmacogenetics 1992; 2:185–196.

9. Harty LC, Caporaso NE, Hayes RB, et al. Alcohol dehydrogenase 3 genotype and risk of oral cavity and pharyngeal cancers. J Natl Cancer Inst 1997; 89:1698–1705.

10. Bouchardy C, Hirvonen A, Coutelle C, Ward PJ, Dayer P, Benhamou S. Role of alcohol dehydrogenase 3 and cytochrome P-4502E1 genotypes in susceptibility to cancers of the upper aerodigestive tract. Int J Cancer 2000; 87:734–740.

11. Coutelle C, Ward PJ, Fleury B, et al. Laryngeal and oropharyngeal cancer, and alcohol dehydrogenase 3 and glutathione S-transferase M1 polymorphisms. Hum Genet 1997; 99:319–325.

12. Mashberg A, Boffetta P, Winkelman R, Garfinkel L. Tobacco smoking, alcohol drinking, and cancer of the oral cavity and oropharynx among U.S. veterans. Cancer 1993; 72:1369–1375.

13. Balaram P, Sridhar H, Rajkumar T, et al. Oral cancer in southern India: the influence of smoking, drinking, paan-chewing and oral hygiene. Int J Cancer 2002; 98:440–445.

14. Garrote LF, Herrero R, Reyes RM, et al. Risk factors for cancer of the oral cavity and oro-pharynx in Cuba. Br J Cancer 2001; 85:46–54.

15. Salaspuro V, Salaspuro M. Synergistic effect of alcohol drinking and smoking on in vivo acetaldehyde concentration in saliva. Int J Cancer 2004; 111:480–483.

16. Brugere J, Guenel P, Leclerc A, Rodriguez J. Differential effects of tobacco and alcohol in cancer of the larynx, pharynx, and mouth. Cancer 1986; 57:391–395.

17. Boffetta P, Mashberg A, Winkelmann R, Garfinkel L. Carcinogenic effect of tobacco smoking and alcohol drinking on anatomic sites of the oral cavity and oropharynx. Int J Cancer 1992; 52:530–533.

18. Franceschi S, Talamini R, Barra S, et al. Smoking and drinking in relation to cancers of the oral cavity, pharynx, larynx, and esophagus in northern Italy. Cancer Res 1990; 50:6502–6507.

19. De Stefani E, Boffetta P, Oreggia F, Mendilaharsu M, Deneo-Pellegrini H. Smoking patterns and cancer of the oral cavity and pharynx: a case-control study in Uruguay. Oral Oncol 1998; 34:340–346.

20. Znaor A, Brennan P, Gajalakshmi V, et al. Independent and combined effects of tobacco smoking, chewing and alcohol drinking on the risk of oral, pharyngeal and esophageal cancers in Indian men. Int J Cancer 2003; 105:681–686.

21. Zheng TZ, Boyle P, Hu HF, et al. Tobacco smoking, alcohol consumption, and risk of oral cancer: a case-control study in Beijing, People's Republic of China. Cancer Causes Control 1990; 1:173–179.

22. Talamini R, Bosetti C, La Vecchia C, et al. Combined effect of tobacco and alcohol on laryngeal cancer risk: a case-control study. Cancer Causes Control 2002; 13:957–964.

23. Castelletto R, Castellsague X, Munoz N, Iscovich J, Chopita N, Jmelnitsky A. Alcohol, tobacco, diet, mate drinking, and esophageal cancer in Argentina. Cancer Epidemiol Biomarkers Prev 1994; 3:557–564.

24. Sankaranarayanan R, Duffy SW, Day NE, Nair MK, Padmakumary G. A case-control investigation of cancer of the oral tongue and the floor of the mouth in southern India. Int J Cancer 1989; 44:617–621.

25. Hodge KM, Flynn MB, Drury T. Squamous cell carcinoma of the upper aerodigestive tract in nonusers of tobacco. Cancer 1985; 55:1232–1235.

26. Sorensen DM, Lewark TM, Haney JL, Meyers AD, Krause G, Franklin WA. Absence of p53 mutations in squamous carcinomas of the tongue in nonsmoking and nondrinking patients younger than 40 years. Arch Otolaryngol Head Neck Surg 1997; 123:503–506.

27. Koch WM, McQuone S. Clinical and molecular aspects of squamous cell carcinoma of the head and neck in the nonsmoker and nondrinker. Curr Opin Oncol 1997; 9:257–261.

28. Lazarus P, Garewal HS, Sciubba J, et al. A low incidence of p53 mutations in pre-malignant lesions of the oral cavity from non-tobacco users. Int J Cancer 1995; 60:458–463.

29. Schantz SP, Byers RM, Goepfert H, Shallenberger RC, Beddingfield N. The implication of tobacco use in the young adult with head and neck cancer. Cancer 1988; 62:1374–1380.

30. de Boer MF, Sanderson RJ, Damhuis RA, Meeuwis CA, Knegt PP. The effects of alcohol and smoking upon the age, anatomic sites and stage in the development of cancer of the oral cavity and oropharynx in females in the south west Netherlands. Eur Arch Otorhinolaryngol 1997; 254:177–179.

31. Freije JE, Beatty TW, Campbell BH, Woodson BT, Schultz CJ, Toohill RJ. Carcinoma of the larynx in patients with gastroesophageal reflux. Am J Otolaryngol 1996; 17:386–390.

32. Constantinides MS, Rothstein SG, Persky MS. Squamous cell carcinoma in older patients without risk factors. Otolaryngol Head Neck Surg 1992; 106:275–277.

33. Agudelo D, Quer M, Leon X, Diez S, Burgues J. Laryngeal carcinoma in patients without a history of tobacco and alcohol use. Head Neck 1997; 19:200–204.

34. Fouret P, Monceaux G, Temam S, Lacourreye L, St Guily JL. Human papillomavirus in head and neck squamous cell carcinomas in nonsmokers. Arch Otolaryngol Head Neck Surg 1997; 123:513–516.
35. Rodriguez T, Altieri A, Chatenoud L, et al. Risk factors for oral and pharyngeal cancer in young adults. Oral Oncol 2004; 40:207–213.
36. Brennan JA, Boyle JO, Koch WM, et al. Association between cigarette smoking and mutation of the p53 gene in squamous-cell carcinoma of the head and neck. N Engl J Med 1995; 332:712–717.
37. Muscat JE, Richie JP, Jr., Thompson S, Wynder EL. Gender differences in smoking and risk for oral cancer. Cancer Res 1996; 56:5192–5197.
38. Dahlstrom KR, Adler-Storthz K, Etzel CJ, et al. Human papillomavirus type 16 infection and squamous cell carcinoma of the head and neck in never-smokers: a matched pair analysis. Clin Cancer Res 2003; 9:2620–2626.
39. Wiseman SM, Swede H, Stoler DL, et al. Squamous cell carcinoma of the head and neck in nonsmokers and nondrinkers: an analysis of clinicopathologic characteristics and treatment outcomes. Ann Surg Oncol 2003; 10:551–557.
40. Lazarus P, Stern J, Zwiebel N, Fair A, Richie JP, Jr., Schantz S. Relationship between p53 mutation incidence in oral cavity squamous cell carcinomas and patient tobacco use. Carcinogenesis 1996; 17:733–739.
41. Kreimer AR, Alberg AJ, Daniel R, et al. Oral human papillomavirus infection in adults is associated with sexual behavior and HIV serostatus. J Infect Dis 2004; 189:686–698.
42. Maden C, Beckmann AM, Thomas DB, et al. Human papillomaviruses, herpes simplex viruses, and the risk of oral cancer in men. Am J Epidemiol 1992; 135:1093–1102.
43. Schwartz SM, Daling JR, Doody DR, et al. Oral cancer risk in relation to sexual history and evidence of human papillomavirus infection. J Natl Cancer Inst 1998; 90:1626–1636.
44. Doll R, Peto R, Wheatley K, Gray R, Sutherland I. Mortality in relation to smoking: 40 years' observations on male British doctors. Bmj 1994; 309:901–911.
45. Gillison ML, Koch WM, Capone RB, et al. Evidence for a causal association between human papillomavirus and a subset of head and neck cancers. J Natl Cancer Inst 2000; 92:709–720.
46. Smith EM, Hoffman HT, Summersgill KS, Kirchner HL, Turek LP, Haugen TH. Human papillomavirus and risk of oral cancer. Laryngoscope 1998; 108:1098–1103.
47. Koch WM, Lango M, Sewell D, Zahurak M, Sidransky D. Head and neck cancer in nonsmokers: a distinct clinical and molecular entity. Laryngoscope 1999; 109:1544–1551.
48. Snijders PJ, Scholes AG, Hart CA, et al. Prevalence of mucosotropic human papillomaviruses in squamous-cell carcinoma of the head and neck. Int J Cancer 1996; 66:464–469.
49. Herrero R, Castellsague X, Pawlita M, et al. Human papillomavirus and oral cancer: the International Agency for Research on Cancer multicenter study. J Natl Cancer Inst 2003; 95:1772–1783.
50. Smith EM, Ritchie JM, Summersgill KF, et al. Human papillomavirus in oral exfoliated cells and risk of head and neck cancer. J Natl Cancer Inst 2004; 96:449–455.
51. Zhang ZF, Morgenstern H, Spitz MR, et al. Environmental tobacco smoking, mutagen sensitivity, and head and neck squamous cell carcinoma. Cancer Epidemiol Biomarkers Prev 2000; 9:1043–1049.
52. Tan EH, Adelstein DJ, Droughton ML, Van Kirk MA, Lavertu P. Squamous cell head and neck cancer in nonsmokers. Am J Clin Oncol 1997; 20:146–150.
53. Yuan JM, Wang XL, Xiang YB, Gao YT, Ross RK, Yu MC. Non-dietary risk factors for nasopharyngeal carcinoma in Shanghai, China. Int J Cancer 2000; 85:364–369.
54. Rajkumar T, Sridhar H, Balaram P, et al. Oral cancer in Southern India: the influence of body size, diet, infections and sexual practices. Eur J Cancer Prev 2003; 12:135–143.
55. Sanchez MJ, Martinez C, Nieto A, et al. Oral and oropharyngeal cancer in Spain: influence of dietary patterns. Eur J Cancer Prev 2003; 12:49–56.
56. Fioretti F, Bosetti C, Tavani A, Franceschi S, La Vecchia C. Risk factors for oral and pharyngeal cancer in never smokers. Oral Oncol 1999; 35:375–378.
57. Tavani A, Gallus S, La Vecchia C, et al. Diet and risk of oral and pharyngeal cancer. An Italian case-control study. Eur J Cancer Prev 2001; 10:191–195.
58. Mackerras D, Buffler PA, Randall DE, Nichaman MZ, Pickle LW, Mason TJ. Carotene intake and the risk of laryngeal cancer in coastal Texas. Am J Epidemiol 1988; 128:980–988.
59. Tavani A, Negri E, Franceschi S, Barbone F, La Vecchia C. Attributable risk for laryngeal cancer in northern Italy. Cancer Epidemiol Biomarkers Prev 1994; 3:121–125.
60. Farrow DC, Vaughan TL, Berwick M, Lynch CF, Swanson GM, Lyon JL. Diet and nasopharyngeal cancer in a low-risk population. Int J Cancer 1998; 78:675–679.
61. Hsu TC, Johnston DA, Cherry LM, et al. Sensitivity to genotoxic effects of bleomycin in humans: possible relationship to environmental carcinogenesis. Int J Cancer 1989; 43:403–409.

62. Schantz SP, Zhang ZF, Spitz MS, Sun M, Hsu TC. Genetic susceptibility to head and neck cancer: interaction between nutrition and mutagen sensitivity. Laryngoscope 1997; 107:765–781.
63. Cloos J, Spitz MR, Schantz SP, et al. Genetic susceptibility to head and neck squamous cell carcinoma. J Natl Cancer Inst 1996; 88:530–535.
64. Yu GP, Zhang ZF, Hsu TC, Spitz MR, Schantz SP. Family history of cancer, mutagen sensitivity, and increased risk of head and neck cancer. Cancer Lett 1999; 146:93–101.
65. Llewellyn CD, Johnson NW, Warnakulasuriya KA. Risk factors for squamous cell carcinoma of the oral cavity in young people—a comprehensive literature review. Oral Oncol 2001; 37:401–418.
66. La Vecchia C, Negri E. The role of alcohol in oesophageal cancer in non-smokers, and of tobacco in non-drinkers. Int J Cancer 1989; 43:784,785.
67. Talamini R, Franceschi S, Barra S, La Vecchia C. The role of alcohol in oral and pharyngeal cancer in non-smokers, and of tobacco in non-drinkers. Int J Cancer 1990; 46:391–393.
68. Mackenzie J, Ah-See K, Thakker N, et al. Increasing incidence of oral cancer amongst young persons: what is the aetiology? Oral Oncol 2000; 36:387–389.
69. Verschuur HP, Irish JC, O'Sullivan B, Goh C, Gullane PJ, Pintilie M. A matched control study of treatment outcome in young patients with squamous cell carcinoma of the head and neck. Laryngoscope 1999; 109:249–258.
70. Lipkin A, Miller RH, Woodson GE. Squamous cell carcinoma of the oral cavity, pharynx, and larynx in young adults. Laryngoscope 1985; 95:790–793.
71. Hart AK, Karakla DW, Pitman KT, Adams JF. Oral and oropharyngeal squamous cell carcinoma in young adults: a report on 13 cases and review of the literature. Otolaryngol Head Neck Surg 1999; 120:828–833.
72. Khuri FR, Kim ES, Lee JJ, et al. The impact of smoking status, disease stage, and index tumor site on second primary tumor incidence and tumor recurrence in the head and neck retinoid chemoprevention trial. Cancer Epidemiol Biomarkers Prev 2001; 10:823–829.
73. Sisk EA, Soltys SG, Zhu S, Fisher SG, Carey TE, Bradford CR. Human papillomavirus and p53 mutational status as prognostic factors in head and neck carcinoma. Head Neck 2002; 24:841–849.
74. Ritchie JM, Smith EM, Summersgill KF, et al. Human papillomavirus infection as a prognostic factor in carcinomas of the oral cavity and oropharynx. Int J Cancer 2003; 104:336–344.
75. Brandwein M, Zeitlin J, Nuovo GJ, et al. HPV detection using "hot start" polymerase chain reaction in patients with oral cancer: a clinicopathological study of 64 patients. Mod Pathol 1994; 7:720–727.
76. Haraf DJ, Nodzenski E, Brachman D, et al. Human papilloma virus and p53 in head and neck cancer: clinical correlates and survival. Clin Cancer Res 1996; 2:755–762.
77. Paz IB, Cook N, Odom-Maryon T, Xie Y, Wilczynski SP. Human papillomavirus (HPV) in head and neck cancer. An association of HPV 16 with squamous cell carcinoma of Waldeyer's tonsillar ring. Cancer 1997; 79:595–604.
78. Balz V, Scheckenbach K, Gotte K, Bockmuhl U, Petersen I, Bier H. Is the p53 inactivation frequency in squamous cell carcinomas of the head and neck underestimated? Analysis of p53 exons 2-11 and human papillomavirus 16/18 E6 transcripts in 123 unselected tumor specimens. Cancer Res 2003; 63:1188–1191.
79. Hafkamp HC, Speel EJ, Haesevoets A, et al. A subset of head and neck squamous cell carcinomas exhibits integration of HPV 16/18 DNA and overexpression of p16INK4A and p53 in the absence of mutations in p53 exons 5-8. Int J Cancer 2003; 107:394–400.
80. Niedobitek G, Pitteroff S, Herbst H, et al. Detection of human papillomavirus type 16 DNA in carcinomas of the palatine tonsil. J Clin Pathol 1990; 43:918–921.
81. Snijders PJ, Meijer CJ, van den Brule AJ, Schrijnemakers HF, Snow GB, Walboomers JM. Human papillomavirus (HPV) type 16 and 33 E6/E7 region transcripts in tonsillar carcinomas can originate from integrated and episomal HPV DNA. J Gen Virol 1992; 73:2059–2066.
82. Wilczynski SP, Lin BT, Xie Y, Paz IB. Detection of human papillomavirus DNA and oncoprotein overexpression are associated with distinct morphological patterns of tonsillar squamous cell carcinoma. Am J Pathol 1998; 152:145–156.
83. Mellin H, Friesland S, Lewensohn R, Dalianis T, Munck-Wikland E. Human papillomavirus (HPV) DNA in tonsillar cancer: clinical correlates, risk of relapse, and survival. Int J Cancer 2000; 89:300–304.
84. Strome SE, Savva A, Brissett AE, et al. Squamous cell carcinoma of the tonsils: a molecular analysis of HPV associations. Clin Cancer Res 2002; 8:1093–1100.
85. Klussmann JP, Weissenborn SJ, Wieland U, et al. Human papillomavirus-positive tonsillar carcinomas: a different tumor entity? Med Microbiol Immunol (Berl) 2003; 192:129–132.
86. Schwartz SR, Yueh B, McDougall JK, Daling JR, Schwartz SM. Human papillomavirus infection and survival in oral squamous cell cancer: a population-based study. Otolaryngol Head Neck Surg 2001; 125:1–9.
87. Ringstrom E, Peters E, Hasegawa M, Posner M, Liu M, Kelsey KT. Human papillomavirus type 16 and squamous cell carcinoma of the head and neck. Clin Cancer Res 2002; 8:3187–3192.

88. Braakhuis BJ, Snijders PJ, Keune WJ, et al. Genetic patterns in head and neck cancers that contain or lack transcriptionally active human papillomavirus. J Natl Cancer Inst 2004; 96:998–1006.

89. Mellin H, Dahlgren L, Munck-Wikland E, et al. Human papillomavirus type 16 is episomal and a high viral load may be correlated to better prognosis in tonsillar cancer. Int J Cancer 2002; 102:152–158.

90. Klussmann JP, Weissenborn SJ, Wieland U, et al. Prevalence, distribution, and viral load of human papillomavirus 16 DNA in tonsillar carcinomas. Cancer 2001; 92:2875–2884.

91. Klussmann JP, Gultekin E, Weissenborn SJ, et al. Expression of p16 protein identifies a distinct entity of tonsillar carcinomas associated with human papillomavirus. Am J Pathol 2003; 162:747–753.

92. Ha PK, Pai SI, Westra WH, et al. Real-time quantitative PCR demonstrates low prevalence of human papillomavirus type 16 in premalignant and malignant lesions of the oral cavity. Clin Cancer Res 2002; 8:1203–1209.

93. Steenbergen RD, Hermsen MA, Walboomers JM, et al. Integrated human papillomavirus type 16 and loss of heterozygosity at 11q22 and 18q21 in an oral carcinoma and its derivative cell line. Cancer Res 1995; 55:5465–5471.

94. Lindel K, Beer KT, Laissue J, Greiner RH, Aebersold DM. Human papillomavirus positive squamous cell carcinoma of the oropharynx: a radiosensitive subgroup of head and neck carcinoma. Cancer 2001; 92:805–813.

95. Wiest T, Schwarz E, Enders C, Flechtenmacher C, Bosch FX. Involvement of intact HPV16 E6/E7 gene expression in head and neck cancers with unaltered p53 status and perturbed pRb cell cycle control. Oncogene 2002; 21:1510–1517.

96. Koskinen WJ, Chen RW, Leivo I, et al. Prevalence and physical status of human papillomavirus in squamous cell carcinomas of the head and neck. Int J Cancer 2003; 107:401–406.

97. Ke LD, Adler-Storthz K, Mitchell MF, Clayman GL, Chen Z. Expression of human papillomavirus E7 mRNA in human oral and cervical neoplasia and cell lines. Oral Oncol 1999; 35:415–420.

98. van Houten VM, Snijders PJ, van den Brekel MW, et al. Biological evidence that human papillomaviruses are etiologically involved in a subgroup of head and neck squamous cell carcinomas. Int J Cancer 2001; 93:232–235.

99. Zumbach K, Kisseljov F, Sacharova O, et al. Antibodies against oncoproteins E6 and E7 of human papillomavirus types 16 and 18 in cervical-carcinoma patients from Russia. Int J Cancer 2000; 85:313–318.

100. Mork J, Lie AK, Glattre E, et al. Human papillomavirus infection as a risk factor for squamous-cell carcinoma of the head and neck. N Engl J Med 2001; 344:1125–1131.

101. Yu MC, Yuan JM. Epidemiology of nasopharyngeal carcinoma. Semin Cancer Biol 2002; 12:421–429.

102. Nicholls JM, Agathanggelou A, Fung K, Zeng X, Niedobitek G. The association of squamous cell carcinomas of the nasopharynx with Epstein-Barr virus shows geographical variation reminiscent of Burkitt's lymphoma. J Pathol 1997; 183:164–168.

103. Akao I, Sato Y, Mukai K, et al. Localization of Epstein-Barr virus in lymph node metastasis with nasopharyngeal carcinoma. Acta Otolaryngol Suppl 1996; 522:86–68.

104. Raab-Traub N, Rajadurai P, Flynn K, Lanier AP. Epstein-Barr virus infection in carcinoma of the salivary gland. J Virol 1991; 65:7032–7036.

105. zur Hausen H, Schulte-Holthausen H, Klein G, et al. EBV DNA in biopsies of Burkitt tumours and anaplastic carcinomas of the nasopharynx. Nature 1970; 228:1056–1058.

106. Nam JM, McLaughlin JK, Blot WJ. Cigarette smoking, alcohol, and nasopharyngeal carcinoma: a case-control study among U.S. whites. J Natl Cancer Inst 1992; 84:619–622.

107. Zhu K, Levine RS, Brann EA, Gnepp DR, Baum MK. A population-based case-control study of the relationship between cigarette smoking and nasopharyngeal cancer (United States). Cancer Causes Control 1995; 6:507–512.

108. Cheng YJ, Hildesheim A, Hsu MM, et al. Cigarette smoking, alcohol consumption and risk of nasopharyngeal carcinoma in Taiwan. Cancer Causes Control 1999; 10:201–207.

109. Vaughan TL, Shapiro JA, Burt RD, et al. Nasopharyngeal cancer in a low-risk population: defining risk factors by histological type. Cancer Epidemiol Biomarkers Prev 1996; 5:587–593.

110. Goodman M, Morgan RW, Ray R, Malloy CD, Zhao K. Cancer in asbestos-exposed occupational cohorts: a meta-analysis. Cancer Causes Control 1999; 10:453–465.

111. Browne K, Gee JB. Asbestos exposure and laryngeal cancer. Ann Occup Hyg 2000; 44:239–250.

112. Gustavsson P, Jakobsson R, Johansson H, Lewin F, Norell S, Rutkvist LE. Occupational exposures and squamous cell carcinoma of the oral cavity, pharynx, larynx, and oesophagus: a case-control study in Sweden. Occup Environ Med 1998; 55:393–400.

113. Berrino F, Richiardi L, Boffetta P, et al. Occupation and larynx and hypopharynx cancer: a job-exposure matrix approach in an international case-control study in France, Italy, Spain and Switzerland. Cancer Causes Control 2003; 14:213–223.

114. Marchand JL, Luce D, Leclerc A, et al. Laryngeal and hypopharyngeal cancer and occupational exposure to asbestos and man-made vitreous fibers: results of a case-control study. Am J Ind Med 2000; 37:581–589.

115. De Stefani E, Boffetta P, Oreggia F, Ronco A, Kogevinas M, Mendilaharsu M. Occupation and the risk of laryngeal cancer in Uruguay. Am J Ind Med 1998; 33:537–542.

116. Ahrens W, Jockel KH, Patzak W, Elsner G. Alcohol, smoking, and occupational factors in cancer of the larynx: a case-control study. Am J Ind Med 1991; 20:477–493.

117. Dietz A, Ramroth H, Urban T, Ahrens W, Becher H. Exposure to cement dust, related occupational groups and laryngeal cancer risk: results of a population based case-control study. Int J Cancer 2004; 108:907–911.

118. Maier H, Dietz A, Gewelke U, Heller WD. [Occupational exposure to hazardous substances and risk of cancer in the area of the mouth cavity, oropharynx, hypopharynx and larynx. A case-control study]. Laryngorhinootologie 1991; 70:93–98.

119. Cauvin JM, Guenel P, Luce D, Brugere J, Leclerc A. Occupational exposure and head and neck carcinoma. Clin Otolaryngol 1990; 15:439–445.

120. IARC. Wood dust and formaldehyde. IARC Monographs on the Evaluation of the Carcinogenic Risks to Humans 1995; 62:94–215.

121. Blot WJ, Chow WH, McLaughlin JK. Wood dust and nasal cancer risk. A review of the evidence from North America. J Occup Environ Med 1997; 39:148–156.

122. Demers PA, Boffetta P, Kogevinas M, et al. Pooled reanalysis of cancer mortality among five cohorts of workers in wood-related industries. Scand J Work Environ Health 1995; 21:179–190.

123. Stellman SD, Demers PA, Colin D, Boffetta P. Cancer mortality and wood dust exposure among participants in the American Cancer Society Cancer Prevention Study-II (CPS-II). Am J Ind Med 1998; 34:229–237.

124. t Mannetje A, Kogevinas M, Luce D, et al. Sinonasal cancer, occupation, and tobacco smoking in European women and men. Am J Ind Med 1999; 36:101–107.

125. Demers PA, Kogevinas M, Boffetta P, et al. Wood dust and sino-nasal cancer: pooled reanalysis of twelve case-control studies. Am J Ind Med 1995; 28:151–166.

126. Muscat JE, Wynder EL. Tobacco, alcohol, asbestos, and occupational risk factors for laryngeal cancer. Cancer 1992; 69:2244–2251.

127. Zagraniski RT, Kelsey JL, Walter SD. Occupational risk factors for laryngeal carcinoma: Connecticut, 1975-1980. Am J Epidemiol 1986; 124:67–76.

128. Coble JB, Brown LM, Hayes RB, et al. Sugarcane farming, occupational solvent exposures, and the risk of oral cancer in Puerto Rico. J Occup Environ Med 2003; 45:869–874.

129. Brown LM, Moradi T, Gridley G, Plato N, Dosemeci M, Fraumeni JF, Jr. Exposures in the painting trades and paint manufacturing industry and risk of cancer among men and women in Sweden. J Occup Environ Med 2002; 44:258–264.

130. Maier H, Tisch M, Enderle G, Dietz A, Weidauer H. [Occupational exposure to paint, lacquer and solvents, and cancer risk in the area of the upper aero-digestive tract]. HNO 1997; 45:905–908.

131. Goldberg P, Leclerc A, Luce D, Morcet JF, Brugere J. Laryngeal and hypopharyngeal cancer and occupation: results of a case control-study. Occup Environ Med 1997; 54:477–482.

132. Pogoda JM, Preston-Martin S. Solar radiation, lip protection, and lip cancer risk in Los Angeles County women (California, United States). Cancer Causes Control 1996; 7:458–463.

133. Wiklund K, Holm LE. Trends in cancer risks among Swedish agricultural workers. J Natl Cancer Inst 1986; 77:657–664.

134. Dardanoni L, Gafa L, Paterno R, Pavone G. A case-control study on lip cancer risk factors in Ragusa (Sicily). Int J Cancer 1984; 34:335–337.

135. Perea-Milla Lopez E, Minarro-Del Moral RM, Martinez-Garcia C, et al. Lifestyles, environmental and phenotypic factors associated with lip cancer: a case-control study in southern Spain. Br J Cancer 2003; 88:1702–1707.

136. Lissowska J, Pilarska A, Pilarski P, et al. Smoking, alcohol, diet, dentition and sexual practices in the epidemiology of oral cancer in Poland. Eur J Cancer Prev 2003; 12:25–33.

137. Maier H, Tisch M, Kyrberg H, Conradt C, Weidauer H. [Occupational hazardous substance exposure and nutrition. Risk factors for mouth, pharyngeal and laryngeal carcinomas?]. HNO 2002; 50:743–752.

138. Winn DM, Ziegler RG, Pickle LW, Gridley G, Blot WJ, Hoover RN. Diet in the etiology of oral and pharyngeal cancer among women from the southern United States. Cancer Res 1984; 44:1216–1222.

139. Zheng W, Blot WJ, Shu XO, et al. Risk factors for oral and pharyngeal cancer in Shanghai, with emphasis on diet. Cancer Epidemiol Biomarkers Prev 1992; 1:441–448.

140. Zheng W, Blot WJ, Diamond EL, et al. Serum micronutrients and the subsequent risk of oral and pharyngeal cancer. Cancer Res 1993; 53:795–798.

141. Kucuk O, Pung A, Franke AA, et al. Correlations between mutagen sensitivity and plasma nutrient levels of healthy individuals. Cancer Epidemiol Biomarkers Prev 1995; 4:217–221.

142. Brady WE, Mares-Perlman JA, Bowen P, Stacewicz-Sapuntzakis M. Human serum carotenoid concentrations are related to physiologic and lifestyle factors. J Nutr 1996; 126:129–137.

143. Ross MA, Crosley LK, Brown KM, et al. Plasma concentrations of carotenoids and antioxidant vitamins in Scottish males: influences of smoking. Eur J Clin Nutr 1995; 49:861–865.

144. Faruque MO, Khan MR, Rahman MM, Ahmed F. Relationship between smoking and antioxidant nutrient status. Br J Nutr 1995; 73:625–632.

145. Kucuk O, Prasad A. Chapter 14: Nutrients, phytochemicals, and squamous cell carcinoma of the head and neck. In: Ensley JF, Gutkind JS, Jacobs JR, Lippman SM, eds. Head and Neck Cancer: Emerging Perspectives: Academic Press; San Diego CA, 2003, pp. 201–211.

146. Albanes D, Heinonen OP, Taylor PR, et al. Alpha-Tocopherol and beta-carotene supplements and lung cancer incidence in the alpha-tocopherol, beta-carotene cancer prevention study: effects of base-line characteristics and study compliance. J Natl Cancer Inst 1996; 88:1560–1570.

147. Gagari E, Kabani S. Adverse effects of mouthwash use. A review. Oral Surg Oral Med Oral Pathol Oral Radiol Endod 1995; 80:432–439.

148. Morse DE, Katz RV, Pendrys DG, et al. Mouthwash use and dentures in relation to oral epithelial dysplasia. Oral Oncol 1997; 33:338–343.

149. Mashberg A, Barsa P, Grossman ML. A study of the relationship between mouthwash use and oral and pharyngeal cancer. J Am Dent Assoc 1985; 110:731–734.

150. Wynder EL, Kabat G, Rosenberg S, Levenstein M. Oral cancer and mouthwash use. J Natl Cancer Inst 1983; 70:255–260.

151. Elmore JG, Horwitz RI. Oral cancer and mouthwash use: evaluation of the epidemiologic evidence. Otolaryngol Head Neck Surg 1995; 113:253–261.

152. Young TB, Ford CN, Brandenburg JH. An epidemiologic study of oral cancer in a statewide network. Am J Otolaryngol 1986; 7:200–208.

153. Winn DM, Blot WJ, McLaughlin JK, et al. Mouthwash use and oral conditions in the risk of oral and pharyngeal cancer. Cancer Res 1991; 51:3044–3047.

154. Blot WJ, Winn DM, Fraumeni JF, Jr. Oral cancer and mouthwash. J Natl Cancer Inst 1983; 70:251–253.

155. Winn DM, Diehl SR, Brown LM, et al. Mouthwash in the etiology of oral cancer in Puerto Rico. Cancer Causes Control 2001; 12:419–429.

156. Bundgaard T, Wildt J, Frydenberg M, Elbrond O, Nielsen JE. Case-control study of squamous cell cancer of the oral cavity in Denmark. Cancer Causes Control 1995; 6:57–67.

157. Zheng TZ, Boyle P, Hu HF, et al. Dentition, oral hygiene, and risk of oral cancer: a case-control study in Beijing, People's Republic of China. Cancer Causes Control 1990; 1:235–241.

158. Marshall JR, Graham S, Haughey BP, et al. Smoking, alcohol, dentition and diet in the epidemiology of oral cancer. Eur J Cancer B Oral Oncol 1992; 28B:9–15.

159. Franco EL, Kowalski LP, Oliveira BV, et al. Risk factors for oral cancer in Brazil: a case-control study. Int J Cancer 1989; 43:992–1000.

160. Maier H, Zoller J, Herrmann A, Kreiss M, Heller WD. Dental status and oral hygiene in patients with head and neck cancer. Otolaryngol Head Neck Surg 1993; 108:655–661.

161. Moreno-Lopez LA, Esparza-Gomez GC, Gonzalez-Navarro A, Cerero-Lapiedra R, Gonzalez-Hernandez MJ, Dominguez-Rojas V. Risk of oral cancer associated with tobacco smoking, alcohol consumption and oral hygiene: a case-control study in Madrid, Spain. Oral Oncol 2000; 36:170–174.

162. Talamini R, Vaccarella S, Barbone F, et al. Oral hygiene, dentition, sexual habits and risk of oral cancer. Br J Cancer 2000; 83:1238–1242.

163. Ward PH, Hanson DG. Reflux as an etiological factor of carcinoma of the laryngopharynx. Laryngoscope 1988; 98:1195–1199.

164. Morrison MD. Is chronic gastroesophageal reflux a causative factor in glottic carcinoma? Otolaryngol Head Neck Surg 1988; 99:370–373.

165. Koufman JA. The otolaryngologic manifestations of gastroesophageal reflux disease (GERD): a clinical investigation of 225 patients using ambulatory 24-hour pH monitoring and an experimental investigation of the role of acid and pepsin in the development of laryngeal injury. Laryngoscope 1991; 101:1–78.

166. Biacabe B, Gleich LL, Laccourreye O, Hartl DM, Bouchoucha M, Brasnu D. Silent gastroesophageal reflux disease in patients with pharyngolaryngeal cancer: further results. Head Neck 1998; 20:510–514.

167. El-Serag HB, Hepworth EJ, Lee P, Sonnenberg A. Gastroesophageal reflux disease is a risk factor for laryngeal and pharyngeal cancer. Am J Gastroenterol 2001; 96:2013–2018.

168. Singh B, Sabin S, Rofim O, Shaha A, Har-El G, Lucente FE. Alterations in head and neck cancer occurring in HIV-infected patients—results of a pilot, longitudinal, prospective study. Acta Oncol 1999; 38:1047–1050.

169. Barry B, Gehanno P. [Squamous cell carcinoma of the ENT organs in the course of the HIV infection]. Ann Otolaryngol Chir Cervicofac 1999; 116:149–153.

170. Frisch M, Biggar RJ, Goedert JJ. Human papillomavirus-associated cancers in patients with human immunodeficiency virus infection and acquired immunodeficiency syndrome. J Natl Cancer Inst 2000; 92:1500–1510.

171. Bradford CR, Hoffman HT, Wolf GT, Carey TE, Baker SR, McClatchey KD. Squamous carcinoma of the head and neck in organ transplant recipients: possible role of oncogenic viruses. Laryngoscope 1990; 100:190–194.

172. Duvoux C, Delacroix I, Richardet JP, et al. Increased incidence of oropharyngeal squamous cell carcinomas after liver transplantation for alcoholic cirrhosis. Transplantation 1999; 67:418–421.

173. Zhang L, Epstein JB, Poh CF, et al. Comparison of HPV infection, p53 mutation and allelic losses in posttransplant and non-posttransplant oral squamous cell carcinomas. J Oral Pathol Med 2002; 31:134–141.

174. Silverman S, Jr., Bahl S. Oral lichen planus update: clinical characteristics, treatment responses, and malignant transformation. Am J Dent 1997; 10:259–263.

175. van der Meij EH, Schepman KP, Smeele LE, van der Wal JE, Bezemer PD, van der Waal I. A review of the recent literature regarding malignant transformation of oral lichen planus. Oral Surg Oral Med Oral Pathol Oral Radiol Endod 1999; 88:307–310.

176. Hietanen J, Paasonen MR, Kuhlefelt M, Malmstrom M. A retrospective study of oral lichen planus patients with concurrent or subsequent development of malignancy. Oral Oncol 1999; 35:278–282.

177. Epstein JB, Wan LS, Gorsky M, Zhang L. Oral lichen planus: progress in understanding its malignant potential and the implications for clinical management. Oral Surg Oral Med Oral Pathol Oral Radiol Endod 2003; 96:32–37.

178. Zhang L, Cheng X, Li Y, et al. High frequency of allelic loss in dysplastic lichenoid lesions. Lab Invest 2000; 80:233–237.

179. Zhang L, Michelsen C, Cheng X, Zeng T, Priddy R, Rosin MP. Molecular analysis of oral lichen planus. A premalignant lesion? Am J Pathol 1997; 151:323–327.

180. Foulkes WD, Brunet JS, Kowalski LP, Narod SA, Franco EL. Family history of cancer is a risk factor for squamous cell carcinoma of the head and neck in Brazil: a case-control study. Int J Cancer 1995; 63:769–773.

181. Brown LM, Gridley G, Diehl SR, et al. Family cancer history and susceptibility to oral carcinoma in Puerto Rico. Cancer 2001; 92:2102–2108.

182. Foulkes WD, Brunet JS, Sieh W, Black MJ, Shenouda G, Narod SA. Familial risks of squamous cell carcinoma of the head and neck: retrospective case-control study. BMJ 1996; 313:716–721.

183. Copper MP, Jovanovic A, Nauta JJ, et al. Role of genetic factors in the etiology of squamous cell carcinoma of the head and neck. Arch Otolaryngol Head Neck Surg 1995; 121:157–160.

184. Mork J, Moller B, Glattre E. Familial risk in head and neck squamous cell carcinoma diagnosed before the age of 45: a population-based study. Oral Oncol 1999; 35:360–367.

185. Goldstein AM, Blot WJ, Greenberg RS, et al. Familial risk in oral and pharyngeal cancer. Eur J Cancer B Oral Oncol 1994; 30B(5):319-22.

186. Li X, Hemminki K. Familial upper aerodigestive tract cancers: incidence trends, familial clustering and subsequent cancers. Oral Oncol 2003; 39:232–239.

187. Hemminki K, Li X. Familial risks of cancer as a guide to gene identification and mode of inheritance. Int J Cancer 2004; 110:291–294.

188. Bongers V, Braakhuis BJ, Tobi H, Lubsen H, Snow GB. The relation between cancer incidence among relatives and the occurrence of multiple primary carcinomas following head and neck cancer. Cancer Epidemiol Biomarkers Prev 1996; 5:595–598.

189. Dong YJ, Peng TK, Yin SJ. Expression and activities of class IV alcohol dehydrogenase and class III aldehyde dehydrogenase in human mouth. Alcohol 1996; 13:257–262.

190. Bosron WF, Li TK. Genetic polymorphism of human liver alcohol and aldehyde dehydrogenases, and their relationship to alcohol metabolism and alcoholism. Hepatology 1986; 6:502–510.

191. Olshan AF, Weissler MC, Watson MA, Bell DA. Risk of head and neck cancer and the alcohol dehydrogenase 3 genotype. Carcinogenesis 2001; 22:57–61.

192. Zavras AI, Wu T, Laskaris G, et al. Interaction between a single nucleotide polymorphism in the alcohol dehydrogenase 3 gene, alcohol consumption and oral cancer risk. Int J Cancer 2002; 97:526–530.

193. Geisler SA, Olshan AF. GSTM1, GSTT1, and the risk of squamous cell carcinoma of the head and neck: a mini-HuGE review. Am J Epidemiol 2001; 154:95–105.

194. Cheng L, Sturgis EM, Eicher SA, Char D, Spitz MR, Wei Q. Glutathione-S-transferase polymorphisms and risk of squamous-cell carcinoma of the head and neck. Int J Cancer 1999; 84:220–224.

195. Olshan AF, Weissler MC, Watson MA, Bell DA. GSTM1, GSTT1, GSTP1, CYP1A1, and NAT1 polymorphisms, tobacco use, and the risk of head and neck cancer. Cancer Epidemiol Biomarkers Prev 2000; 9:185–191.

196. Kutler DI, Auerbach AD, Satagopan J, et al. High incidence of head and neck squamous cell carcinoma in patients with Fanconi anemia. Arch Otolaryngol Head Neck Surg 2003; 129:106–112.

197. Alter BP. Cancer in Fanconi anemia, 1927-2001. Cancer 2003; 97:425–440.

198. Rosenberg PS, Greene MH, Alter BP. Cancer incidence in persons with Fanconi anemia. Blood 2003; 101:822–826.

199. Kutler DI, Wreesmann VB, Goberdhan A, et al. Human papillomavirus DNA and p53 polymorphisms in squamous cell carcinomas from Fanconi anemia patients. J Natl Cancer Inst 2003; 95:1718–1721.

200. Lowy DR, Gillison ML. A new link between Fanconi anemia and human papillomavirus-associated malignancies. J Natl Cancer Inst 2003; 95:1648–1650.

201. Kutler DI, Singh B, Satagopan J, et al. A 20-year perspective on the International Fanconi Anemia Registry (IFAR). Blood 2003; 101:1249–1256.

202. Singh B, Wreesmann VB, Phister, et al. Chromosomal aberrations in patients with head and neck squamous cell carcinoma do not vary based on severity of tobacco/alcohol exposure. BMC Genet 2002;3:22.

2

Laryngeal Preservation Surgery

Joseph Scharpf, MD *and Robert R. Lorenz,* MD

1. INTRODUCTION

Patients afflicted with selected laryngeal and hypopharyngeal cancers have garnered benefit from laryngeal preservation procedures for more than a century. Billroth performed the first hemilaryngectomy for malignancy in 1874 *(1)*. Over the ensuing decades numerous procedures evolved to afford patients the maintenance of speech and swallowing without permanent tracheostomy. In 1947, Alonso *(2,3)* first described the open supraglottic laryngectomy to spare the true vocal cords and arytenoids by resecting the upper portion of the thyroid cartilage with the supraglottic structures. The procedure was popularized in Europe by Bocca and in the United States by Ogura, Som, and Kirchner *(4)*. The boundaries of resection were pushed further by Majer and Reider *(5)* in 1959 with the introduction of the supracricoid partial laryngectomy, which provided an alternative to total laryngectomy for patients with selected glottic and supraglottic cancers. Critical review has provided refinements in these procedures. Specific indications have been established based on an improved understanding of surgical anatomy and patterns of tumor spread that have allowed for selected ablation of laryngeal components without the need for total laryngectomy and its associated morbidity.

2. ANATOMY AND PATTERNS OF TUMOR SPREAD

The larynx, which is situated in front of the fourth to sixth cervical vertebrae in an adult, consists of a framework of cartilages held in position by an intrinsic and extrinsic musculature and lined by epithelium that is arranged in characteristic folds *(6–8)*. The skeletal framework and connective tissues create barriers to prevent the spread of tumor growth. Spaces containing fat, musculature, blood vessels, nerves, and adnexa are created by these tissue barriers. Organ preservation surgery is predicated on a thorough understanding of these spaces and the implications surrounding the compromise of the integrity of these barriers by disease.

The larynx is clinically divided into three areas—the supraglottis, the glottis, and the subglottis. This subdivision reflects the unique embryologic development of the larynx. The supraglottis develops from the buccopharyngeal anlage, and the glottis and subglottis organize around the pulmonary diverticulum *(9)*. The intervening embryologic fusion plane does appear to form a barrier to the spread of early-stage cancers. However, more advanced cancers will traverse from one compartment to the next *(10)*. The supraglottis extends from the tip of the epiglottis to the junction between the lateral wall and the floor of the ventricle. The subsites of the supraglottis consist of the arytenoid cartilages, the aryepiglottic folds, the false vocal folds, and the infrahyoid and suprahyoid epiglottis. The glottis is comprised of the true vocal

From: *Current Clinical Oncology: Squamous Cell Head and Neck Cancer*
Edited by: D. J. Adelstein © Humana Press Inc., Totowa, NJ

cords, the posterior commissure between the two cords, and the anterior commissure. Finally, the subglottis extends from the junction of the squamous and respiratory epithelium on the undersurface of the true cords to the inferior edge of the cricoid cartilage. The superior margin has been arbitrarily assigned to the point 5 mm below the free edge of the true vocal cords (11).

The thyroid cartilage maintains a dominant presence in the laryngeal skeleton and encloses the larynx anteriorly and laterally. The hyoid bone is located superior to the thyroid cartilage and is connected to the thyroid cartilage by the thyrohyoid membrane. This bony landmark forms the upper boundary of the laryngeal framework and serves as an important point for extrinsic laryngeal muscular attachments. The thyroid cartilage articulates posterolaterally with the cricoid cartilage, which is shaped like a signet ring and lies inferior to the thyroid cartilage. The cricoid cartilage is required for maintenance of the enclosed airway because it is the only complete annular support of the laryngeal skeleton (11). The cricoid cartilage also provides support for the two arytenoid cartilages on its posterosuperior aspect.

The epiglottis, containing numerous fenestrations, extends from a tendenous attachment on the thyroid cartilage to project superiorly and posteriorly above the laryngeal opening. It is attached also at the superior aspect of the thyroid cartilage just below the thyroid notch by the thyroepiglottic ligament. The pre-epiglottic space, which is a common location for supraglottic tumor spread, is bounded by the epiglottis, the thyroid cartilage, the thyrohyoid membrane, and the vallecular mucosa. Kirchner has shown through whole organ sections that supraglottic cancers overlying the epiglottic cartilage extend into the preepiglottic space through the epiglottic cartilage fenestrations (12).

Fibrous tissue connections contribute to the 3D construct of the larynx. The quadrangular membrane is the upper part of the elastic membrane of the larynx. It extends from the lateral margin of the epiglottis to the arytenoids and to the false vocal cord. The conus elasticus forms the lower part of the elastic membrane of the larynx. It attaches from each vocal cord down to the cricoid cartilage. The vocal ligament is the free upper edge of the conus elasticus. The anterior condensation of the ligament inserts at the anterior commissure as Broyle's ligament, which is recognized as a pathway for direct tumor extension into cartilage. The paraglottic space, a common route for transglottic tumor spread, is bounded by the thyroid cartilage lamina, conus elasticus, and quadrangular membrane.

In addition to the local routes of tumor spread, regional and distant patterns of spread must be considered. Because of the sparse lymphatics of the glottis, true vocal cord lesions rarely present with cervical metastases. Supraglottic cancer, on the other hand, has a propensity for early neck metastasis, which occurs in nearly half of all cases (13). Occult bilateral metastases have been reported to occur in more than 25% of patients (14).

Only 5% of patients with laryngeal squamous cell carcinoma will have distant metastatic spread. Supraglottic cancers have higher distant metastatic rates than glottic tumors (15). The most common site of distant spread is to the lung; the liver and bone must also be considered.

3. HISTOLOGY

The normal histology of the larynx varies between the compartments. The glottis is comprised of nonkeratinizing stratified squamous epithelium. There is a transition to ciliated pseudostratified columnar epithelium as the subglottis and trachea are approached. The supraglottis is lined by ciliated columnar cells and contains multiple minor salivory glands. More than 90% of malignant tumors of the larynx are caused by squamous cell carcinoma.

Salivary gland lesions of the larynx account for only 1% of laryngeal malignancies *(16)*. Tumors can also rarely arise from the soft tissue and supporting structures of the larynx and include chondrosarcoma, fibrosarcoma, fibrous histiocytoma, carcinoid tumor, liposarcoma, and lymphoma *(16–18)*.

4. ASSESSMENT

4.1. Clinical Examination

The clinical presentation of the patient will be a reflection of the laryngeal site involved with tumor. Cancers of the supraglottis often cause a muffled voice. Impairment of the arytenoid cartilages or extension to the glottis will cause vocal cord mobility impairment and subsequent hoarseness.

Clinical examination focuses on evaluation of the neck for nodal involvement and potential preepiglottic space involvement as evidenced by bulging through the thyrohyoid membrane. Indirect mirror or fiberoptic laryngoscopy allows for visualization of endolaryngeal structures. Assessment of the endolarynx consists of general airway patency, gross pathologic characteristics of the disease, delineation of tumor extent, and both arytenoid and vocal cord mobility status. Direct laryngoscopy is then performed under general anesthesia to gain a more thorough understanding of tumor extent and to obtain biopsies of the lesion.

Glottic cancers present with hoarseness necessitating the aforementioned clinical examination. In contrast to supraglottic cancers, the impaired mobility from glottic cancers often results from superficial thyroarytenoid muscle invasion or bulk on the surface of an exophytic lesion *(19)*. Primary tumors of the subglottis are rare; however, glottic tumors may extend into the subglottis, with resulting fixation to the cricoid cartilage, fixation of the cord, and invasion of the lateral cricoarytenoid musculature and cricoarytenoid joint *(20)*.

In addition to primary site and neck evaluation, the overall condition of the patient must be taken into account. This includes appropriate workup for any systemic disease that will impair wound healing or otherwise adversely affect the patient's postoperative course. Of particular interest to the surgeon performing conservative laryngeal surgery is the pulmonary reserve of the patient. The patient will probably need to tolerate a certain degree of aspiration during the postoperative period *(21)*. The amount of postoperative aspiration will be determined by the nature and extent of the conservative laryngeal surgery procedure performed. There is no general consensus on the criteria that constitute adequate pulmonary function. Formal pulmonary function tests are used routinely by some physicians, whereas others take a more pragmatic approach and test the patient's ability to walk up two flights of stairs without becoming short of breath *(21)*.

4.2. Radiology

The clinical assessment can be complemented by imaging studies of the primary site and neck. Both magnetic resonance imaging (MRI) and computed tomography (CT) provide valuable information that is contingent on the clinical scenario. For example, MRI can demonstrate submucosal transglottic spread and is highly sensitive to cartilage invasion *(22)*. It is also both sensitive and specific for determining preepiglottic space invastion *(23)*. CT scanning, on the other hand, would be best suited for evaluating cricoarytenoid area involvement. Sclerotic changes indicate perichondrial or direct cartilage invasion *(24)*. It is important to note that both modalities are insensitive to superficial mucosal masses, which underscores the importance of the endoscopic examination.

4.3. Staging

The clinical and radiographic examinations culminate in the assignment of a tumor stage for the patient. The T staging system of the larynx is performed by dividing the larynx into its three discrete parts (supraglottis, glottis, and subglottis). Although the system allows for treatment comparison and prognostication for modalities addressing the entire larynx, it does not address the feasibility of conservative laryngeal surgery for any individual patient *(25)*. In other words, within each of the four T stages at each site, organ preservation surgery may performed. The extent of mucosal involvement, invasion depth, and vocal fold and arytenoid mobilities will be the determining factors that may preclude conservative laryngeal surgery *(4)*.

5. SURGICAL PROCEDURES

The numerous conservative laryngeal procedures have evolved over time with many modifications. It is not the intent of this section to convey the nuances of surgical technique necessary for the extirpation of these tumors, but instead to provide an overview of the available procedures, their indications, contraindications, oncologic results, and functional outcomes. Procedures will be presented based on the site and extent of the tumor.

5.1. Glottic Carcinoma

Early glottic carcinoma may be surgically treated with endoscopic procedures utilizing phonomicrosurgical instruments for removal or increasingly popular endoscopic laser techniques as described elsewhere in this text. Vertical partial laryngectomies are open procedures approached transcutaneously and employed for the removal of glottic cancers. This category involves a vertical transection through the thyroid cartilage and paraglottic space. The point of transection is based on the extent of tumor, which has been both preoperatively and intraoperatively determined. The disadvantage of this approach is a "blind" entry into the larynx through a narrow exposure *(26)*.

5.2. Cordectomy

Within the category of vertical partial laryngectomies with open approaches is the minimal surgical resection termed laryngofissure with cordectomy. This procedure allows for removal of the vocal cord after visualization of the cancer through a midline thyrotomy incision. It is indicated for early lesions that do not extend to the anterior commissure or involve the arytenoid cartilage region. Tracheotomies may be performed for postoperative airway management. The procedure has excellent oncologic results, particularly for midcord lesions of the mobile true vocal cord. In a study of 182 patients, Neel et al. *(27)* reported a 2.3% local recurrence rate for lesions limited to the true vocal cords, which was consistent with reports by other authors *(28,29)*. Patients generally have good functional outcomes. Swallowing is adequate, with persistent dysphagia rarely extending beyond the acute postoperative period *(4)*. If the overlying thyroid cartilage is resected (Fig. 1), the remaining cartilage is pulled together or "imbricated" to shorten the vertical height of the hemilarynx. The false vocal cords can be elevated as a flap and sewn inferiorly to reconstruct the glottis. Speech results with this reconstruction strategy have been studied. Brasnu et al. *(30)* found that 82% of patients without reconstructed larynges had severe postoperative voice alteration compared with the 18% of those with reconstruction.

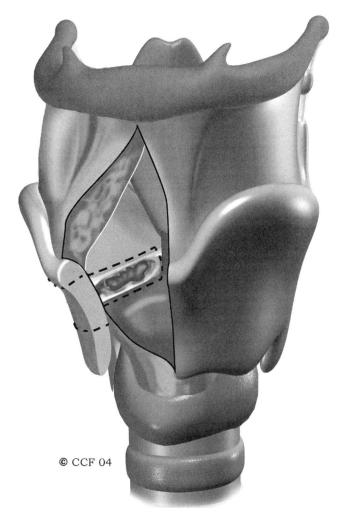

© CCF 04

Fig. 1. Laryngofissure with cordectomy and resection of overlying thyroid cartilage. (Reprinted with permission from the Cleveland Clinic Foundation [http://www.clevelandclinic.org/heartcenter].)

5.3. Vertical Hemilaryngectomy

For larger glottic carcinomas with extension to the vocal process or involvement of the ventricle, or for transglottic lesions without cord fixation, a vertical hemilaryngectomy is used (Fig. 2). In standard hemilaryngectomies, the thyroid cartilage is cut in the center to allow entry into the laryngeal lumen at the anterior commissure. The resection specimen includes most of the true vocal cord, the overlying thyroid cartilage, and the involved false vocal cord. Subglottic extension of more than 10 mm anteriorly or 5 mm posteriorly is a contraindication for vertical partial laryngectomy. In addition, lesions with invasion of the cricoarytenoid joint, interarytenoid region, thyroid cartilage, or both arytenoids should not be removed via this method. Vocal cord fixation is a relative contraindication, depending on the cause of the fixation and tumor size. Extended procedures to the vertical hemilaryngectomy include the frontolateral, posterolateral, and extended vertical hemilaryngectomies. In cases of bilateral lesions in which the tumor involves the anterior commissure, the frontolateral vertical partial

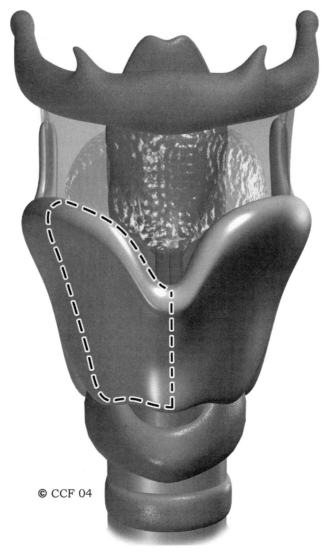

© CCF 04

Fig. 2. Vertical hemilaryngectomy. (Reprinted with permission from the Cleveland Clinic Foundation [http://www.clevelandclinic.org/heartcenter].)

laryngectomy can provide an increased extent of resection by moving the vertical thyrotomy from the midline toward the less involved side. In the posterolateral vertical hemilaryngectomy, all the endolaryngeal circumference except for one arytenoid region and the posterior commissure can be removed. The extended vertical hemilaryngectomy removes the superior aspect of the cricoid cartilage *(31)*.

A variety of reconstructions have been proposed. Common to all reconstructions is the reapproximation of overlying thyroid perichondrium. Many surgeons prefer to include some muscle in the repair to increase the bulk of the neocord. A popular strategy is the utilization of bilateral bipedicle strap muscle flaps to reconstruct the defect. Reconstruction can also be undertaken with the preserved epiglottis. Epiglottic laryngoplasty is performed by advancing the epiglottis inferiorly and laterally to reconstruct the larynx after vertical hemilaryngectomy or anteroinferiorly to reconstruct after a frontolateral vertical laryngectomy *(4)*.

Many authors have reported excellent survival results with their vertical partial laryngectomy experiences. Olsen and DeSanto report that their use of vertical partial laryngectomies produces better patient survival and fewer total laryngectomies for salvage in comparison with radiation therapy *(32)*. Several series have reported local control rates for T1 lesions of greater than 90%. Factors that portend a worse prognosis are involvement at the anterior commissure and extension beyond the confines of the glottis. The challenge of managing higher grade T2 glottic carcinomas with vertical hemilaryngectomy is evidenced by several series in which there were local failure rates greater than 20% *(33,34)*. There is great variability in local control of T3 glottic cancers managed with vertical partial laryngectomy with reported local failure rates ranging from 0 to 46% *(4)*. Because of the higher failure rates for more advanced T2 lesions, as well as T3 and T4 lesions, vertical partial laryngectomies are often not recommended for these lesions.

5.4. Supracricoid Laryngectomy With Cricohyoidoepiglottopexy

Supracricoid partial laryngectomy with cricohyoidoepiglottopexy (SCPL-CHEP) is a horizontal partial laryngectomy operation for glottic cancer management in selected patients. It provides an alternative to total laryngectomy, while offering better local control for selected lesions than extended partial laryngectomies. There is preservation of speech and swallowing without a permanent stoma. The operation encompasses removal of both the true and false vocal cords, both paraglottic spaces, the petiole of the epiglottis, and the thyroid cartilage (Fig. 3). The cricohyoidoepiglottopexy refers to the reconstruction that is performed by suturing the cricoid to the hyoid and the remnant of epiglottis (Fig. 4). In contrast to other partial laryngectomies that require variable types of reconstruction, the supracricoid partial laryngectomy with cricohyoidoepiglottopexy has a single method of reconstruction, thus ensuring reliable functional outcomes *(35)*.

The indications for the SCPL-CHEP are bilateral true vocal cord involvement, T3 glottic lesions with true vocal cord fixation but mobile arytenoid motion, impaired true vocal cord mobility with limited subglottic extension, and unilateral true vocal cord mobility with anterior commissure involvement *(36)*. Patients must have adequate pulmonary reserve to withstand anticipated postoperative aspiration. Furthermore, there are oncologic contraindications that would preclude this procedure. Glottic tumors that cause arytenoid fixation or invade the posterior commissure are not amenable to SCPL-CHEP. Preepiglottic space invasion and subglottic extension of more than 1 cm anteriorly or 5 mm posteriorly are contraindications to this approach *(35)*. Thyroid cartilage invasion is a relative contraindication depending on the presence of extralaryngeal spread.

Postoperative rehabilitation regimens vary from institution to institution. Dysphagia is expected postoperatively, but it is rare to have long-term dysphagia. We perform a cricopharyngeal myotomy at the time of sugery, which assists postoperative swallowing. Patients work with the speech pathology team as outpatients to improve and "relearn" speech and swallowing techniques. Patients will often go home with a tracheostomy, which is removed in the outpatient setting after the edema from surgery has resolved. In a study by Nadou et al. *(37)*, the postoperative mortality and morbidity rates, 1 and 11.7%, respectively, were low compared with other partial laryngectomy procedures.

Oncologic outcomes are excellent. Local control rates for T2 and T3 glottic cancers have been reported to be greater than 90% *(38–40)*. In a series of 9 patients with T1 glottic lesions, eight of which were classified as T1b, Laccourreye et al. *(41)* reported no recurrences. Further studies analyzing T2 lesions revealed a 4.5% recurrence rate in 67 patients *(38)*, and a 10%

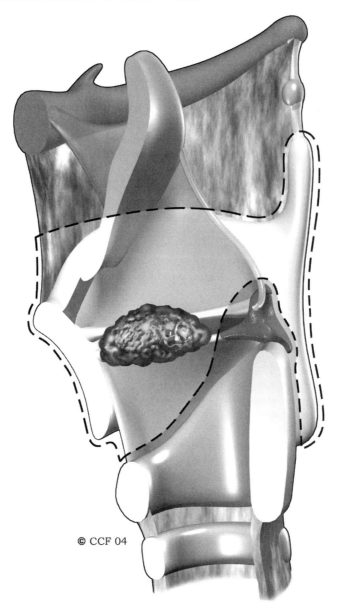

© CCF 04

Fig. 3. Supracricoid laryngectomy with cricohyoidoepiglottopexy (SCPL-CHEP). (Reprinted with permission from the Cleveland Clinic Foundation [http://www.clevelandclinic.org/heartcenter].)

recurrence rate in a group of patients afflicted with selected T3 glottic carcinomas *(42)*. The authors felt that excellent control rates were achieved because of the nature of the procedure, which entails a complete bilateral resection of the paraglottic spaces and removal of the entire thyroid cartilage. SCPL-CHEP thus achieves local control rates comparable to those of total laryngectomy for selected laryngeal cancers while still preserving the functions of deglutition and speech.

5.5. Supraglottic Carcinoma

Supraglottic cancers behave in a different fashion than primary glottic tumors. Because the supraglottis has a distinctly different embryologic origin from the glottis, it was a widely held

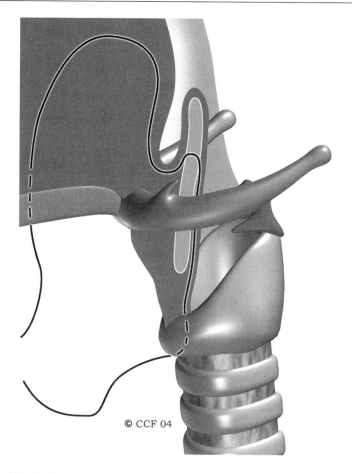

© CCF 04

Fig. 4. Cricohyoidoepiglottopexy reconstruction after SCPL. (Reprinted with permission from the Cleveland Clinic Foundation [http://www.clevelandclinic.org/heartcenter].)

belief for many years that supraglottic cancers remain confined to the supraglottis. This has proved not to be the case. Supraglottic cancers do tend to remain supraglottic until late in their course when paraglottic spread or ventricular mucosa provide a route for extension out of the supraglottis with subsequent cord fixation. Most cancers of the epiglottis tend to have pushing rather than infiltrating borders, and this characteristic allows for narrow resection margins.

5.6. Supraglottic Laryngectomy

The standard open supraglottic laryngectomy is designed for ablation of tumors confined to the supraglottis. In this procedure, there is sparing of both true vocal cords, both arytenoids, and the tongue base (Fig. 5). T1 or T2 lesions of the epiglottis, false vocal cords, AE folds, and T3 lesions owing to preepiglottic space involvement are well addressed by this approach. It is not used to address lesions that extend to the glottic level, an important contraindication. Lesions within 5 mm of the anterior commisure are contraindications to supraglottic laryngectomies. Supraglottic laryngectomies must be avoided when there is decreased vocal cord mobility or ventricle involvement. A supracricoid partial laryngectomy with cricohyoidopexy (SCPL-CHP) as described in Subheading 5.7. would be a viable alternative for such lesions. Other contraindications to the supraglottic laryngectomy are tongue base involvement causing impairment of mobility or tumor that approaches within 1 cm of the circumvallate papilla

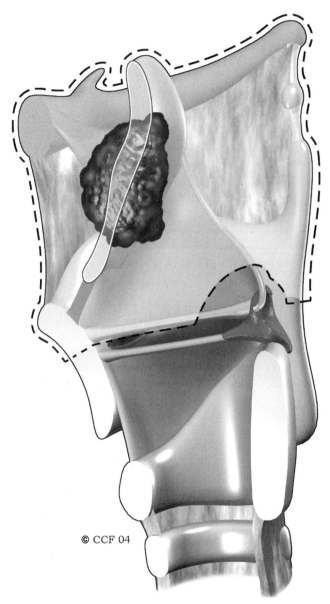

© CCF 04

Fig. 5. Supraglottic laryngectomy. (Reprinted with permission from the Cleveland Clinic Foundation [http://www.clevelandclinic.org/heartcenter].)

and thyroid cartilage invasion. Reconstruction is accomplished via a laryngoplasty that brings the inferior half of the thyroid cartilage in contact with the tongue (Fig. 6). The external thyroid cartilage perichondrium is sutured up to the tongue base; mucosa-to-mucosa closure is not attempted. The procedure has excellent results in regard to oncologic control; the main caveat is proper patient selection, a recurring theme in all conservative laryngeal procedures.

T1 and T2 local control rates range from 85 to 100% *(43,44)*. The local control of T3 and T4 lesions with supraglottic laryngectomy alone has been reported at 70 to 85% *(45)*. However, the success rate for those patients with T3 and T4 lesions has been extremely variable. The literature does not make clear which patients with specific T3 or T4 lesions are at highest risk for recurrence *(4)*. It is postulated that there is a failure to appreciate fully the extent of

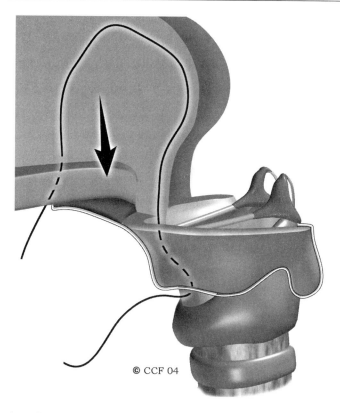

Fig. 6. Reconstruction after a supraglottic laryngectomy. (Reprinted with permission from the Cleveland Clinic Foundation [http://www.clevelandclinic.org/heartcenter].)

tumor before treatment as the reason for such variability. Supraglottic laryngectomy should therefore be performed with caution for those patients with highly selected T3 and T4 lesions. It remains an important treatment modality, though, for patients with T1 and T2 lesions by providing consistently excellent oncologic results.

After supraglottic laryngectomy, many surgeons advocate the use of a percutaneous gastrostomy tube to allow for outpatient swallowing rehabilitation with removal after nutritional demands are met via an oral diet, which may be delayed if postoperative radiation is required. Thick liquid purées are first introduced followed by solids and then thin liquids. The patient must adapt to the altered anatomy to expedite swallowing, and this may be accelerated by early removal of the tracheostomy tube once the operative edema has resolved. The need for postoperative radiation therapy will result in a higher incidence of tracheostomy and gastrostomy dependence. The reported complication of tracheostomy dependence ranges from 2.1 to 29% *(46,47)*. Other complications include pneumonia from aspiration. This incidence ranges from 2.1 to 19.5%, and recurrent episodes may necessitate a secondary conversion to a total laryngectomy.

5.7. Supracricoid Laryngectomy With Cricohyoidopexy

As previously mentioned, glottic extension of supraglottic carcinoma precludes a supraglottic laryngectomy. The other open partial surgical alternative is SCPL-CHP. It is similar to cricohyoidoepiglottopexy, but it is a more extensive resection that additionally removes the

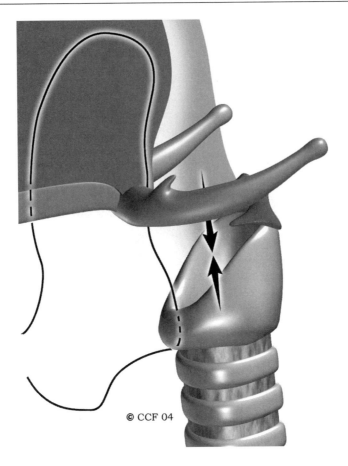

Fig. 7. Cricohyoidopexy reconstruction after SCPL. (Reprinted with permission from the Cleveland Clinic Foundation [http://www.clevelandclinic.org/heartcenter].)

whole epiglottis and preepiglottic space. Preservation of the cricoid cartilage and hyoid bone are necessary for the reconstruction, which places these structures in apposition to one another through suturing techniques (Fig. 7). Therefore, compromise of these two structures by subglottic extension, arytenoid fixation, massive preepiglottic extension, or extension to the pharyngeal wall, vallecula, base of tongue, postcricoid area, or interarytenoid region would serve as contraindications and necessitate a different strategy *(46)*.

Tumor control rates with SCPL-CHP have been reported by Lacourreye et al. *(46)*, who found no local recurrences in 68 patients; most of the carefully selected patients were staged T2 and T3. Further reporting by Laccourreye et al. *(47)* on patients with preepiglottic invasion displayed a 94% local control rate in 19 patients. Chevalier et al. *(48)* have reported similar excellent results for local control (3.3% recurrence) of supraglottic cancer managed with supracricoid laryngectomy with cricohyoidopexy. The procedure achieves successful results in selected patients because it addresses potential pathways of tumor spread such as the paraglottic spaces, which may harbor occult disease. In regard to functional outcome, many patients will experience temporary dysphagia and a tracheostomy. Long-term dysphagia is rare, but patients will most commonly experience hoarseness as a long-term functional sequela.

5.8. Near Total Laryngectomy

An uncommon procedure that has proven oncologic efficacy for supraglottic cancer with a fixed cord or glottic cancer with significant subglottic extension is the near total laryngectomy, which was introduced by Pearson *(49)*. The procedure entails the preservation of the posterior half of the uninvolved hemilarynx and is dependent on a long-term tracheotomy. Using the preserved tissue, an internal shunt is created with a superiorly based pharyngeal flap. This allows for an adequate voice by leaving an innervated arytenoid that will permit the air to pass into the pharynx and guard against aspiration. It is not classified as a true conservation operation because neither the voice nor the airway is "conserved." It resects a much larger specimen and is indicated when the aforementioned conservation operations are inadequate. The main advantages of the procedure are the persistence of voice without the replacement of synthetic prostheses *(50)* and the fact that air enters the pharynx around the tracheotomy directly rather than starting as a bolus in the esophagus. The latter advantage is important because cricopharyngeal dysfunction can have an adverse impact on the voice *(51)*.

In regard to oncologic results, the local recurrence rate was 7% in a series of 225 patients undergoing near total laryngectomies for intermediate and advanced cancer of the larynx or pharynx *(52)*. Near total laryngectomy for supraglottic or pyriform carcinoma after failed radiotherapy was associated with a shunt recurrence rate of 20%, and surgical salvage was 0%. Therefore it is not used as a salvage procedure after radiation failure. Speech acquisition rate was 85% overall.

5.9. Radiation Salvage

It is often difficult to identify patients readily who have failed radiotherapy because the early sequelae of treatment include edema, erythema, and changes in laryngeal mobility, which all act to obfuscate the clinical diagnosis. As a result, the delayed diagnosis of recurrent disease often relegates patients to the option of a total laryngectomy despite their prior eligibility for conservative laryngeal surgery. Surgical salvage after nonsurgical therapy failure was examined by Barthel and Esclamado *(53)*, who analyzed primary radiation therapy results in glottic cancer. In their retrospective series of 45 patients, the local control rate after radiation therapy alone was 80% overall, 87.5% for initially T1 lesions, and 75% for T2 lesions. Of the nine patients with recurrences, only four were candidates for and underwent vertical hemilaryngectomy; salvage without recurrence was successful in only one. Salvage without recurrence was successful in all six patients who underwent total laryngectomy. This finding of poor laryngeal preservation for recurrent early glottic cancer after radiation was supported by DeSanto et al. *(54)*, who reported similar radiation cure rates. They found that only 30% of their 86 patients were candidates for conservation procedures when disease recurred. A supracricoid laryngectomy with cricohyoidopexy or cricohyoidoepiglottopexy has been used as a salvage procedure for larger lesions. Excellent local control rates, 83% in 12 patients, in a small series have been reported *(55)*.

5.10. Partial Pharyngectomy

Because of the anatomic proximity of the pharynx to the larynx, situations arise in which a tumor will involve the medial wall of the pyriform sinus. These lesions may be amenable to conservative surgery via a partial laryngopharyngectomy, as described initially by Ogura et al. *(56)*. An important characteristic of the medial wall lesions is their propensity for laryngeal infiltration and contralateral lymphatic spread, as high as 64% *(57)*.

Partial laryngopharyngectomy for tumors of the medial pyriform sinus is contraindicated when there is involvement to within 1.5 cm of the apex of the pyriform sinus, extensive submucosal spread, and deep invasion of the lateral pyriform sinus wall. Ipsilateral arytenoidectomy is often necessary when tumor involves the pyriform. Reconstruction requires that the vocal ligament be sutured directly to the cricoid cartilage.

In conclusion, total laryngectomy continues to maintain an important role in the treatment of head and neck cancer patients, but the introduction and development of conservation laryngeal procedures has augmented the quality of life for appropriately selected candidates. It is paramount that patients be accurately examined to determine their candidacy for these procedures. Partial laryngeal surgery provides important options for consideration in the context of a multidisciplinary approach to the treatment of head and neck cancer patients.

REFERENCES

1. Tucker HM. Conservation laryngeal surgery in the elderly patient. Laryngoscope 1977; 87:1995.
2. Alonso JM. Conservative surgery of the larynx. Trans Am Acad Ophthalmol Otolaryngol 1947; 51:633–642.
3. Alonso CM, Jackson CL. Conservation of function in surgery of cancer of the larynx bases, techniques and results. Trans Am Acad Ophthalmol Otolaryngol 1952; 56:722.
4. Weinstein GS, Laccourreye O, Rassekh C. Conservation laryngeal surgery. In: Cummings et al., eds. Otolaryngology—Head and Neck Surgery, 2nd ed. St. Louis, Mosby, 1993.
5. Majer H, Reider W: Technique de laryngectomie permettant de conserver la permeabilité respiratoire de la cricohyoido-pexie. Ann Otolarygol Chir Cervicofac 76:677-683, 1959.
6. Bailey BJ, Johnson JT, Kohut RI, et al. Head and Neck Surgery-Otolaryngology. Philadelphia, JB Lippincott, 1993.
7. Cummings CW, Frederickson JM, Harker LA, et al. (eds.). Otolaryngology—Head and Neck Surgery, 2nd ed. St. Louis, Mosby, 1993.
8. Fried MP. The Larynx—A Multidisciplinary Approach, 2nd ed. St. Louis, Mosby, 1996.
9. Tucker HM. Developmental anatomy. In: Tucker HM, ed. The Larynx. New York, Thieme, 1987:18.
10. Johnson J, Curtin H. Carcinoma of the Supraglottic Larynx. Alexandria, VA, American Academy of Otolaryngology—Head and Neck Surgery Foundation, 2000:17.
11. Lee KJ. Essential Otolaryngology, 8th ed. New York, McGraw Hill, 2003:724.
12. Kirchner JA. One hundred laryngeal cancers studied by serial section. Laryngoscope 1969; 78:689.
13. Kirschner JA, Owens JR. Five hundred cancers of the larynx and pyriform sinus: results of treatment by radiation and surgery. Laryngoscope 1977; 87:1288–1303.
14. Byers RM, Wolf PF, Ballantyne AJ. Rationale for elective modified neck dissection. Head Neck Surg 1988; 10:160–167.
15. Probert JC, Thompson RW, Bagshaw MA. Patterns of spread of distant metastases in head and neck cancer. Cancer 1974; 33:127–133.
16. Hyams VS, Batsakis JG, Michaels L. Tumors of the upper respiratory tract and ear. In: Hartman WH, Sobin LH, eds. An Atlas of Tumor Pathology. Bethesda, MD, Armed Forces Institute of Pathology, 1988 pp. 256–298.
17. Nicolai P, Ferlito A, Sasaki CT. Laryngeal chondrosarcoma: incidence, pathology, biological behavior and treatment. Ann Otol Rhinol Laryngol 1990; 99:515–523.
18. Snyderman C, Johnson JT, Barnes L. Carcinoid tumor of the larynx: case report and review of the world literature. Otolaryngol Head Neck Surg 1986; 95:158–164.
19. Kirchner JA. Two hundred laryngeal cancers: patterns of growth and spread as seen in serial section. Laryngoscope 1977; 87:474.
20. Olofsson J, Lord IJ, van Nostrand AWP. Vocal cord fixation in laryngeal carcinoma, Acta Otolaryngol 1973; 75:496.
21. Lutz CK, et al. Supraglottic carcinoma: patterns of recurrence, Ann Otol Rhinol Laryngol 99:12, 1990.
22. Kikinis R, et al. Larynx: MR imaging at 2.35 T. Radiology 1989; 171:165.
23. Loevner L, et al. Can MR accurately predict pre-epiglottic fat invasion, 81st Scientific Assembly and Annual Meeting of the Radiologic Society of North America, Chicago, 1995.
24. Becker M, et al. Neoplastic invasion of the laryngeal cartilage: comparison of MR imaging and CT with histopathologic correlation. Radiology 1995; 194:661.
25. Cancer AJCO. Manual for staging of cancer. Philadelphia, JB Lippincott, 1988.
26. Laccourreye H, et al. Vertical partial laryngectomy: a critical analysis of local recurrence, Ann Otol Rhinol Laryngol 1991; 100:68.

27. Neel B, Devine DD, Desanto LW, Laryngofissure and cordectomy for early cordal carcinoma: outcome in 182 patients. Otolaryngol Head Neck Surg 1980; 88:79.
28. Daly JF, Kwok FN. Laryngofissure and cordectomy. Laryngoscope 1975; 85:1290.
29. Thomas JV, et al. Early glottic carcinoma treated with open laryngeal procedures. Arch Otolaryngol Head Neck Surg 1994; 120:264.
30. Brasnu D, et al. False vocal cord reconstruction of the glottis following vertical partial laryngectomy: a preliminary analysis. Laryngoscope 1992; 102:717.
31. Bailey BJ, Johnson JT, Kohut RI, et al. Head and Neck Surgery—Otolaryngology, vol 2, 3rd ed, vol 2., Philadelphia, JB Lippincott, 2001:1476.
32. Olsen KD, DeSanto LW. Partial laryngectomy—indications and surgical technique. Am J Otolaryngol 1990; 11:153.
33. Johnson JT, et al. Outcome of open surgical therapy for glottic carcinoma. Ann Otol Rhinol Laryngol 1993; 102:752.
34. Laccourreye O, et al. Vertical partial laryngectomy: a critical analysis of local recurrence, Ann Otol Rhinol Laryngol 1991; 100:68.
35. Lai SY, Laccourreye O, Weinstein GS. Supracricoid partial larygectomy with cricohyoidopexy. In: Friedman M, ed. Operative Techniques in Otolaryngology Head and Neck Surgery, vol 14, Orlando, WB Saunders, 2003:34–39.
36. Laccourreye H, Laccourreye O, Weinstein, GS, et al. Supracricoid laryngectomy with cricohyoidoepiglottopexy: a partial laryngeal procedure for glottic carcinoma. Ann Otol Rhinol Laryngol 1990; 99:421–426.
37. Nadou P, Laccourreye O, Weinstein GS, et al. Functional outcome and prognosis factors after supracricoid partial laryngectomy with cricohyoidopexy. Ann Otol Rhinol Laryngol 1997; 106:291–295.
38. Laccourreye O, Weinstein GS, Brasnu, et al. A clinical trial of continuous cisplatin-fluorouracil induction chemotherapy and supracricoid partial laryngectomy for glottic carcinoma classified as T2. Cancer 1994; 74:2781–2790.
39. Laccourreye O, Weinstein GS, Brasnu D, et al. Glottic carcinoma with a fixed true vocal cord: outcomes after neoadjuvant chemotherapy and supracricoid partial laryngectomy with cricohyoidoepiglottopexy. Otol Head Neck Surg 1996; 114:440–446.
40. Piquet JJ, Cevalier D. Subtotal laryngectomy with crico-hyoido-epiglottopexy for the treatment of extended glottic carcinomas. Am J Surg 1991; 162:357–361.
41. Laccourreye H, et al. Supracricoid laryngectomy with cricohyoidoepiglottopexy: a partial laryngeal procedure for glottic carcinoma. Ann Otol Rhinol Laryngol 1990; 99:421.
42. Laccourreye O, et al. Glottic carcinoma with a fixed true vocal cord: outcomes after neoadjuvant chemotherapy and supracricoid partial laryngectomy with cricohyoidoepiglottopexy, Otolaryngol Head Neck Surg 1996; 114:400.
43. Bocca E, Pignataro O, Oldini C. Supraglottic laryngectomy: 30 years experience. Ann Otol Rhinol Laryngol 1983; 92:14–18.
44. DeSanto LW. Early supraglottic carcinoma. Ann Otol Rhinol Laryngol 1990; 99:593–597.
45. DeSanto LW. Cancer of the supraglottic larynx: a review of 260 patients. Otolaryngol Head Neck Surg 1985; 93:705–711.
46. Laccourreye H, et al. Supracricoid laryngectomy with cricohyoidopexy: a partial laryngeal procedure for selected supraglottic and transglottic carcinomas. Laryngoscope 1990; 100:735.
47. Laccourreye O, et al. Cricohyoidopexy in selected infrahyoid epiglottic carcinomas presenting with pathologic preepiglottic space invasion. Arch Otolaryngol Head Neck Surg 1993; 119:881.
48. Chevalier D, Piquet JJ. Subtotal laryngectomy with cricohyoidopexy for supraglottic carcinoma: review of 61 cases. Am J Surg 1994; 168(5):472,473.
49. Pearson B. Near-total laryngectomy. In: Silver CE, ed. Atlas of Head and Neck Surgery. New York, Churchill Livingstone, 1986:235–252.
50. Hoasjoe DK, Martin GF, Doyle PC, Wong FS. A comparative acoustic analysis of voice production by near-total laryngectomy and normal laryngeal speakers. J Otolaryngol 1992; 21:39–43.
51. Weinberg B, Horii Y, Blom E, Singer M. Airway resistance during esophageal phonation. J Speech Hear Disord 1982; 47:194–199.
52. Pearson BW, DeSanto LW, Olsen KD, et al. Results of near-total laryngectomy. Ann Oto Rhinol Laryngol 1998; 107:820–825.
53. Barthel SW, Esclamado RM. Primary radiation therapy for early glottic cancer. Otolaryngol Head Neck Surg 2001; 124:35–39.
54. DeSanto LW, Lillie JC, Devine KD. Surgical Salvage after radiation for laryngeal cancer. Laryngoscope 1975; 85:649-56.

55. Laccourreye O, et al. Supracricoid partial laryngectomy after failed laryngeal radiation therapy. Laryngoscope 1996; 106:495.
56. Ogura JH, Marks JE, Freemant RB. Results of conservation surgery for cancers of the supraglottic and pyriform sinus. Laryngoscope YEAR; 90:591–600.
57. Zbaren P, Egger C. Growth patterns of pyriform sinus carcinomas. Laryngoscope 1999; 107:511–519.

3

Laser Surgery for Head and Neck Cancer

Lee M. Akst, MD and Marshall Strome, MD

1. INTRODUCTION

Lasers have broad applications in otolaryngology. The myriad possible uses result from the combination of many different anatomic subsites, different types of pathology (both benign and malignant), and several different types of available lasers. A comparison of the KTP laser for hemorrhagic hereditary telangectasias of the nasal cavity, for instance, with photodynamic therapy for esophageal lesions reveals the wide range of applications for laser technology in the head and neck region. It is difficult, however, to make generalizations about laser use when one considers such disparate functions, sites, and pathology. This chapter, then, is limited to a discussion of lasers in the management of squamous cell carcinoma of the oral cavity, oropharynx, hypopharynx, and larynx.

The term *laser* is an acronym for light amplification by stimulated emission of radiation. The first laser was built by Maiman in 1960 *(1)*, and its first documented medical use occurred only 6 mo later: this ruby laser was directed towards the destruction of a retinal tumor *(2)*. Further medical applications were limited by imprecision secondary to the handheld nature of this laser, as well as its variable tissue effects. When Jako *(3)* and Polanyi et al. *(4)* coupled the carbon dioxide (CO_2) laser to the operating microscope, they were able to use the laser with laryngoscopic precision and thus introduced the use of lasers to otolaryngology. From those beginnings, the laser was popularized for management of laryngeal lesions by Jako *(3)*, Strong *(5)*, Vaughan et al. *(6)*, and the remainder of the Boston University group *(7)*. After its introduction, the CO_2 laser became more popular for use in benign rather than malignant conditions *(8)*. However, this trend was reversed as the use of the CO_2 laser for the management of laryngeal malignancies was popularized by Steiner and Ambrosoh starting in the 1980s *(9)*.

The CO2 laser has several properties that make it suitable for use in the management of squamous cell cancers of the head and neck. First, the ability to couple the laser to an operating microscope has increased the degree of surgical precision available with laser resection. Because the CO_2 laser itself is invisible, a coaxial helium-neon laser mounted on the micromanipulator allows precise targeting along the line of vision provided by the operating microscope. The 10.6-μm wavelength of CO_2 lasers has a high coefficient of absorption for water, so the laser rapidly heats tissue. At 65°C proteins begin to denature, and at 100°C intracellular water vaporizes. Therefore, the tissue effects of a CO_2 laser depend on the rate at which thermal energy dissipates into the surrounding tissue. The center of a lesion experiences vaporization, the next 100-μm rim of tissue experiences thermal necrosis, and an even wider range of 300–500 μm undergoes temporary injury with subsequent thermal repair *(10)*. One side effect of this thermal energy is the coagulative property of a laser, which allows the

From: *Current Clinical Oncology: Squamous Cell Head and Neck Cancer*
Edited by: D. J. Adelstein © Humana Press Inc., Totowa, NJ

surgical field to remain relatively bloodless during laser dissection. Less well known is whether surrounding thermal damage slows tissue healing following laser surgery relative to nonlaser surgery. Many of the studies investigating these issues have methodological limitations, and the controversy continues *(11)*. At any rate, because markedly different reconstructive needs are associated with traditional open surgery and transoral laser surgery, any comparison of mucosal healing times following laser vs nonlaser injury is inconsequential.

2. BENEFITS

Advocates of transoral laser surgery for resection of head and neck malignancies offer several arguments as to why laser surgery is beneficial *(12)*. The true benefits of laser surgery relative to the alternatives of traditional therapy or radiation depend on the location and extent of tumor involvement for each particular patient, so generalizations are difficult. Broadly, however, some advantages of transoral laser resection over traditional surgery may include avoidance of tracheotomy *(13)*, decreased length of hospitalization *(12,14)*, and best chance for recovery of normal swallowing *(15)*. Other advantages of laser surgery include the possibility of tailoring surgery to the boundaries of an individual tumor, without the need to sacrifice predetermined anatomic subunits, as often occurs with traditional resection. In this fashion, laser surgery functions as Moh's surgery of the aerodigestive tract and avoids the overtreatment associated with removal of uninvolved tissue *(9)*.

Laser surgery is thought to have some benefits compared with radiation therapy as well. The course of treatment is shorter with laser surgery than with radiation, and laser surgery provides pathologic staging information that may not be available from nonsurgical approaches. Again, treatment with the laser can be limited to resection of the disease itself, whereas radiation necessarily affects adjacent but uninvolved tissue within the treatment ports. Finally, the long-term consequences of radiation such as xerostomia and the risk of osteoradionecrosis are not seen with laser therapy.

Importantly, these benefits of laser surgery do not occur at the expense of local control. Oncologic results will be discussed in the next section, but as a generalization, available data concerning laser resection show that it to offers local control rates that are at least equivalent to radiation or traditional resection *(9,12)*. Additionally, in the event that local recurrence or persistence does occur following laser therapy, all subsequent treatment options are preserved—patients may go on to receive further laser resection, traditional open resection, or radiation therapy. Similarly, laser therapy for a first primary preserves all available treatment modalities should the patient later develop a second primary malignancy of the head and neck. By contrast, patients typically may receive only one course of radiation therapy to any single anatomic area within their lifetime. Therefore, one of the greatest benefits of transoral laser resection may be that it does not burn any bridges with respect to other therapies.

Unfortunately, many of these functional benefits of transoral laser resection of head and neck malignancies are not as statistically well documented as the survival rates that accompany these surgeries. As seen in the following sections, data concerning survival and recurrence rates following transoral laser surgery for head and neck malignancy are readily available and allow comparison of laser surgery vs traditional surgery or radiation. However, claims of improved function and quicker recovery with laser surgery seem to be made more often on the basis of accumulated experience instead of statistical comparison *(8,9,12,13)*. Some of these perceived advantages are certainly justified based on differences in surgical technique alone; for instance, traditional supraglottic laryngectomy requires tracheotomy whereas transoral laser resection of supraglottic tumors does not, and a claim about reduced tracheotomy rates with laser resection is undoubtedly true. Unfortunately, other functional issues are less clear. For example, although proponents of laser surgery claim that it allows more rapid return of swallowing and removal of feeding tubes than traditional surgery, these claims are offered as anecdotal judgments in the absence of statistical analysis. Therefore, further controlled studies remain necessary to demonstrate some benefits that laser surgery may have over its alternatives.

3. TECHNIQUE

3.1. Proper Setup

Although the laser is a safe instrument when used properly, certain precautions are necessary to minimize the risk of complications. Several of these precautions involve proper setup of the operating room even before the laser is activated. All personnel in the operating room should wear eye protection at all times during a laser case, in order to prevent retinal injury. Once the patient is properly positioned, moist eye pads and moist towels should be placed to protect the patient as well. Particular care should be taken to prevent inadvertent laser injury to exposed skin of the face that might be adjacent to the laryngoscope. In setting up the laryngoscope, appropriate suction tubing should be established to ensure adequate evacuation of smoke once the surgery begins.

The next choice that the surgeon must make is one of intubation vs jet ventilation. Although jet ventilation avoids the introduction of an endotracheal tube into the operating field, the need to maintain an axis of jet ventilation parallel with the airway itself can limit the ability of the surgeon to reposition the laryngoscope to visualize more peripheral portions of the larynx. Also, jet ventilation causes passive motion of the vocal cords, which means that laser applications must often be limited to apneic periods during the jet ventilation cycle. An endotracheal tube has the advantages of continuous ventilation, regardless of laryngoscope position or laser use. Additionally, it does not introduce passive motion of the vocal cords. However, use of an endotracheal tube does introduce the risk of endotracheal tube ignition, which is the most feared complication of laser surgery (16–18). For this reason, care should always be taken to intubate using a 'laser' tube, which is meant to resist combustion. Also, moist sponges placed within the operative field between the area of intended resection and the tube can decrease the risk of fire. With proper precautions such as these, the complication rate of CO_2 laser surgery can be reduced to as low as 0.2% (19).

3.2. Operative Principles

Once the case is appropriately setup, careful operative technique with use of the laser itself can also promote safety. For instance, exposure during surgery is crucial, and choice for the appropriate laryngoscope can maximize the chance for a successful resection. Experience has shown that for the larynx, the largest bore laryngoscope that fits into the laryngeal lumen without distorting anatomic relationships is the one which should be used (9). In the case of supraglottic tumors, however, a distending laryngoscope is preferred so that one blade may be placed into the vallecula while the other is placed beneath the epiglottis (9). It should be expected that patients with narrow dental arches, large tongue bases, and/or anteriorly placed larynges may be difficult or impossible to expose adequately; in these cases, transoral laser surgery should be abandoned in favor of traditional open techniques (20).

Whichever scope is chosen, proper technique next involves stabilizing the scope through either true gallows suspension or a Lewy arm suspended from a Mayo stand overlying the patient's chest. Proponents of gallows suspension claim that it improves exposure *(21)*. Meanwhile, among those surgeons who use a Lewy arm, it should be realized that the impact of ventilatory chest rise on the stability of the operating field can be minimized if the laryngoscope is suspended from a Mayo stand rather than the patient's chest. Once the laryngoscope is positioned and the laser is turned on, care is taken to operate at the highest magnification possible, and muscle relaxant can be used to limit vocal cord motion. The laser is kept in the center of the field, and binocular vision is maintained as much as possible. Although frequent repositioning of the laryngoscope might be necessary, maintenance of the laser in the center of the field lessens the risk for scatter artifact caused by the sides of the laryngoscope. As the case progresses, any char that accumulates at the margins of excision should be periodically removed with a cottonoid pledget. Not only does removal of char promote better visualization of the tissue, but because the char itself is flammable, its removal also decreases the possibility of an airway fire.

Lastly, it needs to be stated that transoral laser resection only addresses the primary tumor. Depending on tumor burden and cervical lymph node involvement, appropriate neck management might be necessary. This management can occur either at the same time as laser resection or as a staged procedure. Steiner *(9)*, who stages neck dissection 4–8 d after transoral laser resection, uses this second trip to the operating room as a chance to reinspect the primary site with an operating microscope as necessary in order to evaluate completeness of resection. Endoscopy can also be repeated several weeks after primary tumor resection in order to assess healing and evaluate for persistent disease *(9)*. Appropriate techniques for neck management are discussed elsewhere in this book.

3.3. En Bloc *vs Piecemeal Resection*

The principle guiding *en bloc* laser resection of tumors through the laryngoscope parallels the traditional doctrine of open oncologic resection. The goal is to identify tumor margins and, with an appropriate margin of uninvolved tissue, resect the lesion in one piece. Use of increased magnification through the operating microscope may aid in the discrimination of involved from uninvolved tissue. An essential difference between transoral and open *en bloc* resection depends on the amount of uninvolved adjacent tissue that is taken as part of the resection specimen. Whereas open techniques typically predetermine what the boundaries of dissection will be, endoscopic resections may be individually tailored to the extent of the tumor. Because reconstructive needs do not dictate operative margins, no "extra" normal tissue needs to be removed endoscopically, in comparison with open techniques. Unfortunately, given the size of the laryngoscope used in the resection, *en bloc* endoscopic techniques are limited to small lesions.

Therefore, endoscopic resection of larger lesions depends on the technique of piecemeal resection—removing the tumor piece by piece. Such a technique greatly expands the role for endoscopic resection, but cutting across the tumor itself while it remains *in situ* violates traditional oncologic principles. These principles were based on the belief that a scalpel that had violated the tumor itself could transfer viable tumor cells to other sites within the operative field *(12)*. With laser resection, there is no physical conduit for such tumor transfer—use of a laser in one place cannot spread cells to an adjacent location with later use. Despite this essential difference between the scalpel and the laser, initial concerns about tumor spillage and local recurrence led to slow acceptance of transoral laser resection *(7)*.

The first surgeon to have the insight that infiltrative cancer could be safely removed from the larynx in pieces with the CO_2 laser was Wolfgang Steiner, in the early 1980s *(22,23)*. Later reports documented that laser transection of a tumor (in order to determine tumor depth) did not increase local recurrence rates *(24,25)*. As reports of the safety of laser resection mounted, acceptance of the technique gradually improved, and numerous clinical studies have since substantiated the safety of piecemeal resection with regard to local recurrence *(9,14,26–28)*. These same studies also suggest that transection of the tumor does not increase regional or distant metastases; it has been hypothesized that use of the CO_2 laser seals lymphatic channels as it cuts across them, therefore limiting this route of tumor escape during resection *(29)*. Now many surgeons regard transoral laser resection as Moh's surgery of the upper airway—not only is piecemeal transection accepted as oncologically safe, but transection of the tumor has also been embraced as a technique for optimizing resection by improving visualization and enabling determination of tumor depth.

4. RESULTS BY SUBSITE

4.1. Oral Cavity

Transoral laser resection of oral cavity lesions is different from resection of lesions in other anatomic subsites. Either a CO_2 laser mounted on a micromanipulator of an operating microscope *(8)* or a hand-held neodymium:yttrium-aluminum-garnet (Nd:YAG) *(30)* laser may be used for tumor resection. Rather than using a laryngoscope for exposure, resection of oral cavity lesions typically involves placement of mouth gags and tongue blades (such as might be used for open resection). Nasotracheal intubation removes the endotracheal tube from the field, improving visualization and decreasing the fire hazard if laser resection is to be performed. Once exposure has been obtained, the laser can be brought into the field and used for wide local excision of most T1 and T2 oral cavity tumors *(31)*. Large tumors that are deeply invasive or that involve the mandible are not generally well suited for laser excision *(32)*. A laser can, however, be used to resect lesions that extend to, but do not invade, the mandible; in these cases, the mandibular periosteum can be taken as a tumor margin *(9)*.

In 1979, Strong et al. *(32)* were the first to describe use of the CO_2 laser for resection of tongue lesions. Since then, several studies have demonstrated that the local control rate for previously untreated T1–T2 lesions of the oral cavity with local resection ranges between 80 and 100% with 2–5 yr follow-up *(33–35)*. As with other subsites, small tumors may be removed *en bloc* with a uniform deep margin determined without tumor transection; alternatively, the tumor may be transected in order to identify the deep margin and limit dissection to involved tissue alone. In either case, one advantage of the laser in this setting is the hemostasis that it provides relative to "cold" instruments in this highly vascular field.

4.2. Tongue Base and Oropharynx

Reports suggest that even though laser resection of tongue base malignancies may be technically demanding, oncologic results have been sound. Anatomically, the tongue base presents challenges to both exposure of the tumor and recognition of boundaries between tumor and uninvolved tissue *(8)*. Submucosal spread of tumor is common in this area, and differentiation between cancerous and noncancerous tissue is more difficult here than in the larynx *(8)*. For this reason, even small tumors may best be removed with piecemeal resection, so that submucosal extent can be analyzed and tumor boundaries more clearly seen *(36)*. Also, use of a bivalved laryngoscope can expand the size of the operating field, helping to expose both the tumor itself and relevant anatomic landmarks simultaneously and therefore improving surgical orientation.

Using these techniques, the use of the laser in the tongue base has been efficacious from both an oncologic and a functional point of view. In their report of 48 patients with tongue base primary tumors, Steiner et al. *(36)* describe no local recurrences among T1–T2 lesions, and a 20% recurrence rate for T3–T4 lesions at 5 yr. In a patient population that was skewed toward more advanced tumors, overall Kaplan-Meier 5-yr local control rate was 85%. Of course, many of these patients received radiation therapy in addition to laser resection, and neck dissection was performed as necessary as well. Complications were rare, with only five instances of postoperative hemorrhage and no incidence of orocutaneous fistula. By description, most patients had good postoperative functional results, with mean performance status for diet and speech equal to or better than those rates achieved for similar lesions with open resection, radiotherapy, or chemoradiotherapy *(36)*. The authors, however, caution that to prevent poor functional outcomes, laser resection should bot be performed for tongue base tumors that infiltrate the soft tissues of the neck or have extensive spread to adjacent structures.

Other areas of the oropharynx aside from the tongue base are also amenable to laser resection. For instance, tonsillar and soft palate tumors can be excised with transoral application of the CO_2 laser, again with good functional results *(9)*. Even in this area, Steiner et al. *(9)* find that reconstruction is rarely necessary—even soft palate defects that result in velopharyngeal insufficiency typically heal with scar contraction that corrects the difficulty spontaneously. By description, none of the patients with soft palate tumors that Steiner has treated with CO_2 laser have had posttreatment swallowing difficulty, and even the use of a palatal prosthesis to correct hypernasal speech is rare *(9)*.

4.3. Hypopharynx

Like tongue base tumors, hypopharyngeal tumors show a tendency toward submucosal spread that makes their resection technically demanding. Tumor extension seen on the mucosal surface itself rarely reflects overall tumor burden *(8)*, so preoperative imaging studies are necessary adjuncts to direct endoscopic visualization in planning tumor resection. For instance, pyriform sinus lesions might extend deeply into the paraglottic space, preepiglottic space, arytenoid cartilage, thyroid cartilage, or deep neck itself with any evidence for such spread on endoscopy. Preoperative imaging can help define tumor extent, as well as identify those lateral pyriform tumors that may directly extend to the great vessels. In this case, endoscopic resection should be performed only with great caution, and open neck exploration in order to "control" these vessels preoperatively might be warranted *(9)*.

With these caveats in mind, hypopharyngeal tumors are rarely removed *en bloc*, and tumor transection with definition of tumor depth becomes necessary. Piecemeal resection proceeds in a craniocaudal fashion, with tumor removal occurring layer by layer. Orthogonal cuts across the tumor can divide a large tumor into a grid, with each "square" being removed in turn. Removal of the superior portions of the tumor in this way can aid visualization of the inferior and deep portions of the lesion. It is crucial, however, that proper orientation and labeling of each specimen be maintained, so that an accurate intraoperative tumor map can be created to aid pathologic evaluation. Once negative margins are confirmed with intraoperative pathology, a 5–10-mm margin of normal tissue can typically be taken without adding much functional morbidity. Healing occurs by secondary intent, with generally good functional results being obtained within the first several weeks postoperatively.

Among published series of CO_2 laser resection for hypopharyngeal cancer, two of the largest series belong to Rudert et al. *(37)* and Steiner et al. *(38)*. Rudert et al. studied 29 patients following laser resection of hypopharyngeal lesions; 26 of these patients received adjuvant radiation therapy, but no patients required either tracheotomy or free flap reconstruction as part of their surgical approach. Among disease-free survivors, 94% had "no functional deficit" at 3 yr post therapy and this number increased to 100% at 4- and 5-yr follow-up. Overall 5-yr survival was 71% for patients with stage I/II disease, and 47% for patients with stage III/IV disease *(37)*.

Steiner et al. *(38)* published a larger series of 129 patients who received laser resection of hypopharyngeal lesions, with similar results. In this series, 75% of patients had advanced (stage III or IV disease), and 58% of patients received adjuvant radiation therapy. Five-year disease-specific recurrence-free survival was 95% for patients with stage I/II disease, and 69% for patients with stage III/IV disease. Hemorrhage was a rare postoperative complication (3.9%), and only one patient in the entire series required tracheotomy. Overall, Steiner et al. concluded that transoral laser resection provided local control rates that were better than those obtained by radiation therapy, with decreased morbidity, decreased complications, and similar functional outcomes. Relative to survival, many patients with hypopharyngeal tumors will fail with regional or distant disease rather than local recurrence. In view of these trends, proponents of laser resection find it judicious to consider the possible organ preservation and improved quality of life possible with transoral laser surgery rather than proceeding to open resection of advanced hypopharyngeal lesions *(39)*.

4.4. Supraglottic Larynx

The possibility of using the CO_2 laser for resection of supraglottic lesions was first reported by Vaughan in 1978 *(40)*. The growth of laser use in this subsite, however, was somewhat slowed by the popularity of radiation therapy for early supraglottic tumors—owing to the rich lymphatic drainage of this area and the risk for bilateral cervical metastases, traditional thinking favored radiation therapy over surgical therapy because radiation could address the bilateral necks at the same time it treated the primary lesion. As the morbidity from neck dissections has decreased over time and surgery has reclaimed its role in the treatment of supraglottic tumors, however, the laser has become increasingly popular. As experience with laser supraglottic resection increases, the indications have been expanding to include more advanced supraglottic disease as well as early lesions.

The technique for laser supraglottic resection depends on the extent of the lesion. A distending laryngoscope is suspended in the supraglottis, positioned so that one blade is in the vallecula and the other is in the glottis, with the supraglottic structures displayed between them. For limited suprahyoid lesions, the tumor can generally be removed *en bloc* without functional compromise. Tumors that extend beneath the level of the hyoid, however, typically require piecemeal resection. The first laser incision in these cases should be made in the sagittal plane, splitting the epiglottis and cutting straight through the tumor if necessary. This sagittal cut aids evaluation of tumor depth, and allows for assessment of preepiglottic space involvement. When the tumor is bulky, the initial sagittal cut can be followed by horizontal cuts and removal of the superior portions of the tumor, permitting improved visualization of the inferior tumor extent. As the resection proceeds in a superior-to-inferior stepwise fashion, the laryngoscope can be progressively repositioned more distally to maintain optimal exposure. Laser release of the bilateral pharyngoepiglottic folds and medial glossoepiglottic fold mobilizes the tumor and allows for improved access as well. If required, dissection can include removal of the preepiglottic space transorally, down to the level of the thyroid cartilage *(9,28)*. In this fashion, even large supraglottic tumors can be removed through transoral laser resection.

Some of the advantages of laser resection for supraglottic lesions relative to traditional open supraglottic laryngectomy include preservation of the thyroid cartilage and superior laryngeal neurovascular bundles. Other benefits include a decreased incidence of clinically relevant aspiration events following laser resection as well as decreased length of feeding tube use following surgery (41). These benefits may be secondary to the protection of pharyngeal and tongue base musculature possible with laser resection; even if open resection preserves these structures, it violates them as part of the resection and reconstruction. This violation of the pharyngeal mucosa, in association with external skin incisions and violation of the neck, also makes open approaches susceptible to the complication of pharyngocutaneous fistula. This risk is avoided in transoral approaches (27). Finally, transoral laser resection can be performed without tracheotomy, whereas open approaches cannot.

Several studies have documented the oncologic efficacy of laser resection for supraglottic malignancies. In 1994, Zeitels et al. (42) demonstrated the feasibility of the technique by showing that there were no local recurrences among 19 patients with T1 or T2 supraglottic lesions who underwent complete laser resection. By 1997, Eckels et al. (14) published mature data for 46 patients with T1 or T2 supraglottic cancer who received laser resection, with or without adjuvant radiation therapy. A 5-yr disease-specific survival rate of 72% was documented (14). Later series by Ambrosch et al. (41) and Rudert et al. (43) explored laser resection for T1, T2, and early T3 lesions. Both series found 3-yr survival rates for early lesions to be 87 to 89%, with 5-yr local control rates for pathologically staged T1 lesions reaching 100% in the Ambrosch et al. study—both groups conclude that the oncologic results achieved by laser resection equal those attained by traditional open resection.

Experience with more advanced tumors reveals, as expected, that survival rates decrease as tumor stage increases. When Rudert et al. (43) analyzed their patients with stage III or stage IV disease, 3-yr survival fell to 50% (compared with 88% for stage I or stage II disease). The largest series of patients with laser resection of supraglottic tumors shows a similar trend, although the results are somewhat paradoxical (27). In this study by Iro et al. (27) of 141 consecutive patients with supraglottic cancers treated with the laser, 5-yr recurrence free survival rates were 85% for stage I, 63% for stage II, 74% for stage III, and 45% for stage IV disease. The unexpected increase in survival between stage II and stage III may be attributed to a proportional increase in patients receiving elective neck dissections or postoperative radiation therapy among the stage III group. Among all groups, the most important predictor of clinical success with laser resection was achieving pathologically negative margins; if negative margins cannot be obtained transorally, then transcervical approaches must be considered.

4.5. Glottic Larynx

Much has been written about transoral laser resection for glottic malignancies. Laser surgery was first used in the larynx for benign conditions, although the technique was quickly adapted for use in early malignancies as well (3,5,6). Since its introduction, laser surgery has established its role in the management of early glottic malignancies with good functional and oncologic results. The role of laser surgery for more advanced lesions continues to evolve. This section addresses some techniques of transoral laser resection that are particular to the glottic larynx, including the role of laser resection for anterior commissure disease. The oncologic results achieved with laser resection for glottic lesions will be summarized.

The technique of transoral laser resection for laryngeal lesions, just as in other subsites, is dictated by the extent of tumor involvement. Traditionally, laser resection was limited to small, minimally invasive lesions localized to the mid or anterior portion of the true vocal cord, without anterior commissure, arytenoid, subglottic, or supraglottic extent; some surgeons still advocate this conservative view *(20)*. It was thought that laser resection of lesions that were not localized in this fashion ran higher risks of failure. Steiner et al. were the first group to expand beyond T1a lesions, and their 1993 paper included 34 patients with small T2 laryngeal lesions treated with definitive laser therapy only *(24)*. This report also included 5-yr data on patients with more advanced T2, T3, and T4 lesions who were treated between 1979 and 1985. Based on their results, including a recurrence rate of only 6% among the patients with early disease treated with laser resection only, the group concluded that laser microsurgery was useful for laryngeal carcinoma. As experience treating larger laryngeal lesions accumulates, more aggressive surgeons have realized that it is unimportant whether the tumor is unilateral or bilateral, has supraglottic or subglottic extent, or involves the anterior commissure *(24)*. Instead, the limit to laryngeal laser surgery depends primarily on exposure—if the tumor can be adequately exposed, it can be resected transorally *(8)*.

The techniques for transoral laser resection of glottic carcinoma closely follow the principles elucidated for resection of tumor from other anatomic subsites. Small tumors are removed *en bloc*, whereas larger tumors are again removed through piecemeal resection. Surgery is continued until negative margins are achieved, just as with Moh's surgery of other anatomic sites. Sometimes, paraglottic space involvement necessitates dissection to the level of the thyroid cartilage and removal of the perichondrium itself as a tumor margin. In experienced hands, this has been accomplished with the laser transorally with good results *(9)*. Some surgeons have even removed portions of the cartilage itself if it is involved by tumor, taking prelaryngeal soft tissue as a tumor margin *(8)*. When there is any uncertainty as to the completeness of tumor resection, repeat microlaryngoscopy can be performed at a later date; Steiner routinely brings patients back to the operating room 4–6 wk following initial surgery in order to debride eschar and obtain a second look at the operative site *(9)*. There are some anatomic limits, however, to laser resection. For instance, resection of the bilateral arytenoid cartilages, although technically possible, often creates intractable problems with aspiration and therefore might be better managed with traditional open total laryngectomy. Also, removal of such advanced lesions requires both a surgeon and a pathologist who have appropriate experience and comfort levels with laser surgery.

Using the above techniques, the oncologic safety of laser resection for glottic malignancies has been demonstrated in several large case series *(15,24,44,45)*. In 2000, Moreau *(44)* published results of laser resection for 98 patients with infiltrative glottic cancer, as well as 27 patients with *in situ* carcinoma. By observing strict selection criteria (such as avoiding cases with "significant involvement of the anterior commissure"), Moreau was able to achieve a local control rate of 100%. Eckel *(15)* published a larger data series, including 161 patients with T1 lesions and 91 patients with T2 lesions, with local recurrence rates of 13 and 15%, respectively; statistically, there was no difference in recurrence rates depending on stage. Overall, Eckel concluded that transoral laser surgery accomplishes local control rates that are comparable to those achieved with radiotherapy for T1 lesions and that laser therapy provided improved control rates over radiotherapy for T2 lesions. Additionally, for patients who did experience local recurrence following laser therapy, Eckel stated that initial laser therapy preserved more retreatment options than either open surgery or radiotherapy might have.

Despite the safety documented with laser resection of early glottic carcinoma, indications for laser resection of advanced disease continue to evolve. As described earlier, some surgeons use laser resection even for T3 and T4 lesions *(24)*, and techniques have been described for transoral resection of the thyroid cartilage *(8,9)*. However, resection of such advanced lesions entails additional risk of recurrence. As Peretti et al. *(45)* demonstrated among 140 patients who were treated with laser alone for Tcis, T1, or T2 glottic carcinoma, disease-free survival was negatively impacted by involvement of the anterior third of the vocal cord, involvement of the false vocal cord, and infiltration of the vocalis muscle. Among authors who describe laser excision of both early and advanced glottic lesions, both Steiner's original report in 1993 *(24)* and Pearson and Salass's report in 2003 *(12)* found higher local recurrence rates among patients with more progressive disease. Unfortunately, limited sample size and the confounding impact of additional (nonlaser) therapies impede meaningful extrapolation and comparison with traditional open resection. Therefore, although it is generally agreed that early glottic lesions may be safely resected transorally, the role of laser for advanced lesions continues to evolve.

The debate concerning treatment of glottic carcinoma with anterior commissure involvement highlights the continuing evolution of transoral laser resection. Initial concerns concerning functional results and oncologic safety led many surgeons to believe that anterior commissure involvement was a contraindication to transoral laser resection. In particular, it was thought that anterior commissure involvement made determination of subglottic or supraglottic extension anteriorly difficult *(7)*. Furthermore, possible tumor extension along Broyle's ligament with subsequent cartilage involvement was thought to limit transoral resection of anterior commissure lesions. Careful consideration of existing evidence, however, led some surgeons to question this supposed risk of cartilage involvement with anterior commissure lesions. Kirchner's tumor studies, for instance, had demonstrated that relatively few anterior commissure lesions actually spread along Broyle's ligament *(46,47)*. Also, the success rates of radiotherapy, even with anterior T1 lesions, were taken as indirect evidence that cartilage involvement was rare—with true cartilage involvement, radiotherapy success rates for anterior lesions would have been lower. Therefore, based on these arguments that anterior lesions did not necessarily mean that a lesion was unresectable, some surgeons began to attempt transoral laser resection of anterior commissure lesions.

At present, the debate concerning the safety of laser resection for such lesions continues. Some surgeons maintain that anterior commissure lesions do poorly with laser excision *(48–50)* and therefore use such involvement as a relative contraindication to laser therapy. For other surgeons, anterior commissure lesions are routinely resected by CO_2 laser *(9,12,28,51)*. As experience with resection of anterior lesion accumulates, even laser frontolateral vertical hemilaryngectomy has been described *(52)*. Overall, however, those surgeons who use the laser for treatment of anterior commissure lesions do so with the knowledge that given the intrinsic limitations of anterior exposure, recurrence rates may be higher in this area *(8,15,45,53)*. Again, laser resection for early glottic lesions seems to be well accepted, but a role for the use of laser in treatment of more advanced lesions continues to evolve.

5. CONTROVERSIES

Evolving indications (and contraindications) are not the only controversies involving transoral laser resection of head and neck malignancies. Even in situations in which laser resection is clearly oncologically safe, debate persists over the choice of laser surgery, traditional surgery, or radiotherapy based on functional issues and cost. Given voice concerns, this issue has been addressed most extensively regarding early glottic carcinoma. Additionally, some surgeons have begun to use laser surgery for salvage treatment of recurrent disease. Each of these issues is discussed more fully below.

5.1. Radiation vs "Cold" Microsurgery vs Laser Surgery for Early Glottic Cancer

The treatment of choice for early glottic cancer is subject to great debate. Depending on the preference of the treating physician, an isolated T1 or small T2 lesion of the vocal folds can be treated with radiation therapy, "cold instrument" laryngeal microsurgery, or transoral laser resection. In general, all three of these treatments are equally efficacious, with the proper application of any of these modalities yielding cure rates ranging from 85 to 95% *(7,15,20)*. With equal oncologic efficacy, the debate over which technique to use depends largely on issues of voice outcomes, cost, surgeon experience, and patient preference.

In choosing between laser surgery or "cold instrument" surgery, the chief concern is one of vocal outcome, as cost of surgery, time of surgery, and other similar factors are comparable. The chief concern about laser surgery is that unintended transmission of heat to tissue within the superficial lamina propria might lead to fibrosis of the regenerating epithelium, with subsequent compromise of vocal cord vibration and voice *(54)*. The injudicious use of "cold instruments," however, can also lead to vocal fold scarring. Therefore, the decision about choice of instrument often depends on which tool is thought to yield the best precision *(7)*. Although this is a preference which may vary from one surgeon to another, there are some intrinsic differences between the two techniques. For instance, the laser provides hemostasis as it dissects, which can become especially important if surgery involves deeper, more vascular, structures such as the vocalis muscle. Additionally, the micromanipulator may improve precision among surgeons who are not experienced with microlaryngeal surgery, particularly with use of the nondominant hand. In choosing between laser or cold instruments, then, the surgeon must weigh these perceived benefits of laser against the risk of unintended thermal damage to normal adjacent superficial lamina propria. The balance may change depending on the type of lesion. For instance, superficial lesions may favor resection by cold instrument given the concern of protecting adjacent tissue. Deeper lesions that reach the vocalis muscle, however, may be better resected by laser given the increased need for hemostasis and the fact that preservation of superficial lamina propria is less of a concern for these lesions *(55)*.

With either technique, the degree of resection impacts on the voice. Knowledge of lesion size, then, can provide a pretreatment estimate of posttreatment voice, which can inform decisions concerning surgery or radiation for early glottic lesions. With resection of unilateral lesions limited to the superficial lamina propria, skilled surgery can typically yield a perceptually normal voice *(7)*. When dissection must be carried down the vocal ligament, healing generally results in a neocord that is straight, with a limited mucosal wave; although the voice may be perceptually normal to an untrained listener, a skilled voice professional will typically be aware of subtle deficiencies. When dissection is carried even further, down to the vocalis muscle, healing may result in a concave neocord with subsequent glottic insufficiency and breathy dysphonia, which may be obvious to even an untrained observer. Studies that have examined this issue have correlated the degree of resection with voice outcome following surgery for early glottic lesions *(56–58)*. The relationship between tissue resection and voice outcome, however, may not be linear. Instead, the mechanism of voice production that follows surgery may be a more important determinant. If healing following transoral resection yields a larynx that produces voice at the glottic level, voice will be better than if voice is produced at a supraglottic level *(9,59)*. For dissection at any depth, it is the experience of the senior author that the addition of cryotherapy following laser resection may help improve posttreatment voice *(60)*; the mechanism through which this voice improvement occurs is under active investigation.

At any rate, decisions between laser surgery and radiotherapy concerning voice outcome depend on a pretreatment estimate of the expected posttreatment voice. Additionally, it must be realized that radiotherapy affects an entire field and is not limited only to the area of disease. For instance, radiation will be received by both vocal cords, even in a unilateral lesion, whereas surgery can be restricted only to the affected site. Studies of voice quality following CO_2 laser excision compared with radiotherapy are rare. One study by Rydell et al. (61) found that voice was significantly better following radiotherapy than it was following laser excision of T1a lesions. Other studies, however, have concluded that there is no significant difference between the two treatments (56,62,63). None of these studies separated surgical groups based on the depth of resection, and none of these studies accounted for postablative reconstruction techniques (64), which might help improve voices in the surgical group. It may be that more sophisticated analyses will be necessary in the future to help determine which lesions might best be treated by which therapy.

Having acknowledged that the controversy surrounding voice outcomes is not yet settled, some general differences exist between laser surgery (or cold surgery) and radiotherapy, which may help guide surgeon and patient preference. First, surgery is generally accomplished in a single session, whereas a course of radiotherapy requires multiple treatments stretching over several weeks. Additionally, although exact estimates vary, there is a general consensus that may be more cost effective than radiotherapy (15,59,65,66). Finally, transoral surgery has the advantages of obtaining tissue for diagnosis, preventing treatment morbidity to uninvolved tissue, and being repeatable over several sessions (compared with radiation, which cannot be repeated).

With these differences in mind, and with knowledge of similar oncologic efficacy, the choice between surgery or radiotherapy for early glottic lesions largely depends on surgeon and patient preference. The general teaching that earlier lesions favor surgery whereas the expected decreased voice outcomes following resection of deeper lesions might favor radiotherapy may be true, but such generalizations disregard the potential for vocal reconstruction that may improve postsurgical voices. Also, this teaching presupposes that voice outcomes following radiotherapy are the same for all lesions, regardless of depth; however, because pathologic staging is unavailable with radiotherapy, this assumption cannot be accurately tested. Until more data are available, the controversy concerning the choice of transoral laser resection, cold instrument resection, or radiotherapy for early glottic lesions will continue.

5.2. Laser for Oncologic Salvage

Another controversy includes the use of laser surgery for the treatment of recurrent disease. The role of any conservation surgery in this situation is itself controversial, and more information concerning this debate is available in Chapter 5, on oncologic salvage. When this argument is extended to the relatively new field of laser surgery, few data are available. The first attempts at using laser surgery to salvage radiation failures dates to 1992 (67), but the use of laser surgery is this fashion is still thought to remain both difficult and risky (20). Compared with the initial presentation of primary tumors, recurrent tumors may present in a multifocal fashion or with advanced submucosal extension. Additionally, the radiation fibrosis present in the "skip" areas between foci of recurrent cancer may make pathologic diagnosis less reliable, which in turn makes transoral laser resection more difficult. Still, laser resection allows voice preservation, and as long as the area is amenable to close follow-up, total laryngectomy remains a possibility in the future should laser salvage fail. On this basis, surgeons have begun to offer laser surgery for treatment of recurrent cancer *(68,69)*. Quer et al. *(67)* found that laser successfully salvaged 18/24 patients with recurrent glottic or supraglottic carcinoma, with the remaining 6 patients proceeding to total laryngectomy. In a larger study of 40 patients, de Gier et al. *(68)* found that with a mean follow-up extending beyond 5 yr, 17 patients were salvaged with a single laser surgery, and 3 more patients were salvaged with repeated laser therapy without the need for traditional resection. Overall, then, the rate of successful laser salvage was 50%. Such treatment, however, remains at the forefront of transoral laser surgery, and much depends on both the surgeon's and the patient's willingness to balance possible functional preservation with an increased risk of further recurrence. As experience with the laser as a tool for surgical salvage grows, the indications for transoral laser resection may expand.

6. CONCLUSIONS

Overall, then, transoral laser resection for head and neck malignancies is a growing field. Initially applied to the *en bloc* resection of relatively small lesions, the development of piece-meal resection techniques has led to transoral laser resection of increasingly advanced tumors in many different anatomic subsites. The most appropriate comparison for laser surgery of early lesions might be radiation therapy; here the decision probably depends on surgeon and patient preference. For those larger lesions that are not amenable to radiation alone, the appropriate comparison is between laser surgery and traditional open resection. In this case, there are many perceived advantages to laser surgery in terms of both function and recovery. Despite case series documenting the oncologic efficacy and functional results possible with laser surgery, however, direct comparisons between laser and traditional surgery remain scarce. As those at the forefront of laser surgery accumulate experience with increasingly advanced lesions, however, the indications for laser surgery are likely to continue to grow. As more understanding of the risks and benefits of laser surgery is gained in this fashion, the role of transoral laser resection for head and neck malignancy will be further delineated.

REFERENCES

1. Maiman TH. Stimulated optical radiation in ruby. Nature 1960; 187:493–494.
2. Koester CJ, Snitzer E, Campbell CJ, Rittler MC. Experimental laser retina photocoagulation. J Opt Soc Am 1962; 52:607.
3. Jako GJ. Laser surgery of the vocal cords. Laryngoscope 1972; 82:2204–2215.
4. Polanyi T, Bredermeier HC, Davis TW Jr. CO_2 laser for surgical research. Med Biol Eng Comput 1970; 8:548–558.
5. Strong MS. Laser excision of carcinoma of the larynx. Laryngoscope 1975; 85:1286–1289.
6. Vaughan CW, Strong MS, Jako GJ. Laryngeal carcinoma: transoral treatment using the CO_2 laser. Am J Surg 1978; 136:490–493.
7. Zeitels SM. Endoscopic treatment of glottic atypia and carcinoma. In: Ossoff R, Shapshay SM, Woodson GE, Netterville JL, eds. The Larynx. Philadelphia, Lipincott Williams & Wilkins, 2003:519–528.
8. Werner JA, Dunne AA, Folz BJ, Lippert BM. Transoral laser microsurgery in carcinomas of the oral cavity, pharynx, and larynx. Cancer Control 9:379–386.
9. Steiner W, Ambrosch P. Endoscopic laser surgery of the upper aerodigestive tract with special emphasis on cancer surgery. Stuttgart: Thieme Medical, 2000.
10. Ossoff RH, Coleman JA, Courey MS, Duncavage JA, Werkhaven JA, Reinisch L. Clinical applications of lasers in otolaryngology-head and neck surgery. Lasers Surg Med 1994; 15:217–248.
11. Lippert BM, Teymoortash A, Folz BJ, Werner JA. Wound healing after laser treatment of oral and oropharyngeal cancer. Lasers Med Sci 2003; 18:36–42.
12. Pearson BW, Salassa JR. Transoral laser micoresection for cancer of the larynx involving the anterior commissure. Laryngoscope 2003; 113:1104–1112.

13. Motta G, Esposito E, Cassiano B, Motta S. T1-T2-T3 glottic tumors: fifteen years experience with the CO_2 laser. Acta Otolaryngol Suppl (Stockh) 1997; Suppl 527:155–159.

14. Eckel HE. Endoscopic laser resection of supraglottic carcinoma. Otolaryngol Head Neck Surg 1997; 117:681–687.

15. Eckel HE. Local recurrences following transoral laser surgery for early glottic carcinoma: frequency, management, and outcome. Ann Otol Rhinol Laryngol 2001; 110:7–15.

16. Fried MP. Limitations of laser laryngoscopy. Otolaryngol Clin N Am 1984; 17:199–207.

17. Hirshman CA, Smith J. Indirect ingnition of the endotracheal tube during carbon dioxide laser surgery. Arch Otolaryngol 1980; 106:639–641.

18. Meyers A. Complication of CO_2 laser surgery of the larynx. Ann Otol Rhinol Laryngol 1981; 90:132–134.

19. Healy GB, Strong MS, Shapshay S, Vaughan C, Jako G. Complication of CO_2 laser surgery of the aerodigestive tract: experience of 4416 cases. Otolaryngol Head Neck Surg 1984; 92:13–18.

20. Rebeiz EE, Shapshay SM. Laser surgery of the larynx. In: Cummings CW, Fredrickson JM, Harker LA, Krause CJ, Richardson MA, Schuller DE, eds. Otolaryngology Head & Neck Surgery, 3rd ed., vol. 3. St. Louis: Mosby, 1998:2176–2186.

21. Zeitels SM. Universal modular glottiscope system: the evolution of a century of design and technique for direct laryngoscopy. Ann Otol Rhinol Laryngol Suppl 1999;179:2–24.

22. Steiner W. Endoscopic therapy of early laryngeal cancer. In: Wigand M, Steiner W, Snell PM, eds. Functional Partial Laryngectomy. Berlin: Springer-Verlag, 1984:163–170.

23. Steiner W. Transoral microsurgical CO_2-laser resection of laryngeal carcinoma. In: Wigand M, Steiner W, Snell PM, eds. Functional Partial Laryngectomy. Berlin: Springer-Verlag, 1984:121–125.

24. Steiner W. Results of curative laser microsurgery of laryngeal carcinomas. Am J Otolaryngol 1993; 14:116–121.

25. Rudert HH. Transoral CO_2-laser surgery in advanced supraglottic cancer. In: Smee R, Bridger GP, eds. Laryngeal Cancer: Proceedings of the 2nd World Congress on Laryngeal Cancer. Amsterdam: Elsevier, 1994:457–461.

26. Rudert H. Laser surgery for carcinomas of the larynx and hypopharynx. In: Panje WR, Herberhold C, eds. Neck, 2nd ed., vol. 3. Stuttgart: Thieme Medical, 1998:355–370.

27. Iro H, Waldfahrer F, Altendorf-Hofmann A, Weidenbacher M, Sauer R, Steiner W. Transoral laser surgery of supraglottic cancer: follow-up of 141 patients. Arch Otolaryngol Head Neck Surg 1998; 124:1245–1250.

28. Zeitels SM. Infrapetiole exploration of the supraglottis for exposure of the anterior glottal commissure. J Voice 1998; 12:117–122.

29. Werner JA, Lippert BM, Schunke M, et al. Animal experiment studies of laser effects on luymphatic vessels: a contribution to the discussion of laser surgery segmental resection of carcinomas [German]. Laryngorhinootologie 1995; 74:748–755.

30. Luukkaa M, Aitasalo K, Pulkkinen J, Lindholm P, Valavaara R, Grenman R. Neodymium YAG contact laser in the treatment of cancer of the mobile tongue. Acta Otolaryngol 2002; 122:318–322.

31. Burkey BB, Garrett G. Use of the laser in the oral cavity. Otolaryngol Clin N Am 1996; 29:949–962.

32. Strong MS, Vaughan CW, Healy GB, Shapshay SM, Jako GT. Transoral management of localized carcinoma of the oral cavity using the CO_2 laser. Laryngoscope 1979; 89:897–905.

33. Guerry TL, Silverman S, Dedo HH. Carbon dioxide laser resections of superficial oral carcinoma: indications, technique, and results. Ann Otol Rhinol Laryngol 1986; 95:547–555.

34. Bier-Laning C, Adams G. Patterns of recurrence after carbon dioxide laser excision of intraoral squamous cell carcinoma. Arch Otolaryngol Head Neck Surg 1995; 121:1239–1244.

35. Williams SR, Carruth JAS. The role of the carbon dioxide laser in treatment of carcinoma of the tongue. J Laryngol Otol 1988; 102:1122–1123.

36. Steiner W, Fierek O, Ambrosch P, Hommerich CP, Kron M. Transoral laser microsurgery for squamous cell carcinoma of the base of the tongue. Arch Otolaryngol Head Neck Surg 2003; 129:36–43.

37. Rudert HH, Hoft S. Transoral carbon-dioxide laser resection of hypopharyngeal carcinoma. Eur Arch Otorhinolaryngol 2003; 260:198–206.

38. Steiner W, Ambrosch P, Hess CF, Kron M. Organ preservation by transoral laser microsurgery in piriform sinus carcinoma. Otolaryngol Head Neck Surg 2001; 124:58–67.

39. Allal AS. Cancer of the pyriform sinus: the trend towards conservative treatment. Bull Cancer 1997; 84:757–762.

40. Vaughan CW. Transoral laryngeal surgery using the CO_2 laser: laboratory experiments and clinical experience. Laryngoscope 1978; 88:1399–1420.

41. Ambrosch P, Kron M, Steiner W. Carbon dioxide laser microsurgery for early supraglottic carcinoma. Ann Otol Rhinol Laryngol 1998; 107:680–688.

42. Zeitels SM, Koufman JA, Davis K, Vaughan CW. Endoscopic treatment of supraglottic and hypopharynx cancer. Laryngoscope 1994; 104:71–78.

43. Rudert HH, Werner JA, Hoft S. Transoral carbon dioxide laser resection of supraglottic carcinoma. Ann Otol Rhinol Laryngol 1999; 108:819–827.

44. Moreau PR. Treatment of laryngeal carcinomas by laser endoscopic microsurgery. Laryngoscope 2000; 110:1000–1006.

45. Peretti G, Nicolai P, de Zinis LOR, et al. Endoscopic CO_2 lase excision for Tis, T1, and T2 glottic carcinomas: cure rate and prognostic factors. Otolaryngol Head Neck Surg 2000; 123:124–131.

46. Kirchner JA, Carter D. Intralaryngeal barriers to the spread of cancer. Acta Otolaryngol 1987; 103:503–513.

47. Kirchner JA. What have whole organ sections contributed to the treatment of laryngeal cancer? Ann Otol Rhinol Laryngol 1989; 98:661–667.

48. Wolfensberger M, Dort JC. Endoscopic laser surgery for early glottic carcinoma: a clinical and experimental study. Laryngoscope 1990; 100:1100–1105.

49. Krespi Y, Meltzer CJ. Laser surgery for vocal cord carcinoma involving the anterior commissure. Ann Otol Rhinol Laryngol 1989; 98:105–109.

50. Casiano R, Cooper JD, Lundy DS, et al. Laser cordectomy for T1 glottic carcinoma: a 10-year experience and videostroboscopic findings. Otolaryngol Head Neck Surg 1991; 104:831–837.

51. Desloge RB, Zeitels SM. Endolaryngeal microsurgery at the anterior glottal commissure: controversies and observations. Ann Otol Rhinol Laryngol 2000; 109:385–392.

52. Zeitels SM. Technique of en bloc laser endoscopic frontolateral laryngectomy for glottic cancer. Laryngoscope 2004; 114:175–180.

53. Puxeddu R, Argiolas F, Bielamowicz, et al. Surgical therapy of T1 and selected cases of T2 glottic carcinoma: cordectomy, horizontal glottectomy, and CO_2 laserendoscopic resection. Tumori 2000; 86:277–282.

54. Zeitels SM. Laser versus cold instruments for microlaryngoscopic surgery. Laryngoscope 1996; 106:545–552.

55. Zeitels SM. Premalignant epithelium and microinvasive cancer of the vocal fold: the evolution of phonomicrosurgical management. Laryngoscope 1995; 105:1–51.

56. McGuirt WF, Blalock D, Koufman JA, et al. Comparative voice results after laser resection or irradiation for T1 vocal cord carcinoma. Arch Otolaryngol Head Neck Surg 1994; 120:951–955.

57. Remacle M, Lawson G, Jamart J, et al. CO_2 laser in the diagnosis and treatment of early cancer of the vocal fold. Eur Arch Otorhinolaryngol 1997; 254:169–276.

58. Flint PW. Minimally invasive techniques for management of early glottic cancer. Otolaryngol Clin N Am 2002; 35:1055–1066.

59. Sittel C, Eckel HE, Eschenburg C. Phonatory results after laser surgery for glottic carcinoma. Otolaryngol Head Neck Surg 1998; 119:418–424.

60. Milstein CF, Hicks D, Abelson T, Strome M. Voice quality and laryngeal function outcomes after endoscopic laser therapy and cryoablation for treatment of early stage glottic carcinoma. presentation, 33rd Annual Symposium of The Voice Foundation, Philadelphia, June 2004.

61. Rydell R, Schalen L, Fex S, Elner A. Voice evaluation before and after laser excision vs. radiotherapy of T1A glottic carcinoma. Acta Otolaryngol (Stock) 1995; 115:560–565.

62. Cragle SP, Brandenburg JH. Laser cordectomy or radiotherapy: cure rates, communication, and cost. Otolaryngol Head Neck Surg 1993; 108:648–654.

63. Delsupehe KG, Zink I, Lejaegere M, Bastian RW. Voice quality after narrow-margin laser cordectomy compared with laryngeal irradiation. Otolaryngol Head Neck Surg 1999; 121:528-533.

64. Zeitels SM. Glottic reconstruction and voice rehabilitation. In: Atlas of Phonomicrosurgery and Other Endolaryngeal Procedures for Benign and Malignany Disease. San Diego: Singular Publishing Group, 2001:219–221.

65. Myers EN, Wagner RL, Johnson JT. Microlaryngoscopic surgery for T1 glottic lesions: a cost-effective option. Ann Otol Rhinol Laryngol 1994; 103:28–30.

66. Brandenburg JH. Laser cordotomy versus radiotherapy: an objective cost analysis. Ann Otol Rhinol Laryngol 2001; 110:312–318.

67. Kerrebijn JDF, de Boar MF, Knegt PPM. CO_2-laser treatment of recurrent glottic carcinoma. Clin Otolaryngol 1992; 17:430–432.

68. Quer M, Leon X, Orus C, Venegas P, Lopez M, Burgues J. Endoscopic laser surgery in the treatment of radiation failure of early laryngeal carcinoma. Head Neck 2000; 22:520–523.

69. de Gier HHW, Knegt PPM, de Boer MF, Meeuwis CA, van der Velden L-A, Kerrebijn JDF. CO_2-laser treatment of recurrent glottic carcinoma. Head Neck 2001; 23:177–180.

4

The Evolving Role of Neck Dissection in the Era of Organ Preservation Therapy for Head and Neck Squamous Cell Carcinoma

Tung T. Trang, MD and Pierre Lavertu, MD

1. INTRODUCTION

Chemotherapy in combination with radiation therapy has evolved over the last several decades as an important modality in the treatment of head and neck squamous cell carcinoma. Because of the effectiveness of chemoradiation therapy at controlling disease at the primary site, ablative surgery is generally reserved for surgical salvage if chemoradiation fails to control primary site disease. However, the role of surgery in the treatment of regional neck metastases remains controversial. At the core of this controversy is whether chemoradiation alone is adequate to control neck metastases or whether adjunctive neck dissection should be added for effective control.

2. NECK DISSECTION WITH RADIATION THERAPY ALONE

The history of neck dissection in organ preservation therapy of head and neck cancer can be traced to early reports of the role of neck dissection after definitive radiation treatment. In 1982 Parsons et al. reported better control of regional metastases from base of tongue cancer treated with definitive radiation therapy with the addition of planned neck dissection. Of their patients with N2 and N3 pretreatment disease, those who had planned neck dissections failed 25% of the time, whereas those who did not receive neck dissection failed 49% of the time. No failures were seen among patients with N0 or N1 disease in either group, suggesting that radiation alone was sufficient to control N0 or N1 disease *(1)*. In a later report from the same group, the authors found that adding planned neck dissection after definitive radiation therapy for patients who had incisional biopsy of their neck disease prior to treatment resulted in significantly better control of neck metastases compared with those who did not receive planned neck dissection *(2)*.

Mendenhall et al. *(3)* also compared radiation alone with radiation followed by planned neck dissection in the control of regional neck metastases. They also found that for N1 disease, both modalities were equal with respect to their ability to control neck disease. However, for patients with multiple nodes, nodes greater than 3 cm, or fixed nodes, the addition of a neck dissection resulted in greater control of metastases to the neck *(3)*. In a later study, this group

From: *Current Clinical Oncology: Squamous Cell Head and Neck Cancer*
Edited by: D. J. Adelstein © Humana Press Inc., Totowa, NJ

showed that the combination of radiation and planned neck dissection was vastly superior to radiation only for control of neck disease *(4)*. In 1989 Parsons et al. *(5)* reiterated the same findings.

From these early studies, it is clear that the addition of a planned neck dissection after definitive radiation therapy for head and neck cancer resulted in better control of regional metastatic disease. Another finding that arose from these early studies was that patients who harbored viable tumor cells in their planned neck dissection specimens had a worse prognosis than those who had no viable tumor cells *(3,5)*. This finding would ultimately also hold true for later patients treated with chemoradiation.

3. NECK DISSECTION WITH INDUCTION CHEMOTHERAPY AND RADIATION

With the addition of chemotherapy as adjuvant therapy in the treatment of head and neck cancer, different authors suggested different roles for neck dissection. Some authors argued that if a complete response was obtained after chemotherapy and radiation therapy, a neck dissection could be omitted given a low probability of residual disease. It is important to note that these authors often defined a complete response in different ways. Other authors recommended that planned neck dissections continue to be performed on all N2–N3 necks based on their institutional experience.

The early experiences with chemotherapy involved induction chemotherapy. In 1992 Wolf and Fisher *(6)* reviewed the subset of patients in the Veterans Affairs cooperative laryngeal cancer study who had N2 or N3 disease and were treated with induction chemotherapy followed by definitive radiation therapy. In this study, a complete response was defined as complete disappearance of all clinically evident tumor on physical exam. A partial response was defined as at least a 50% reduction in the sum of the products of the longest tumor dimensions multiplied by their perpendicular compared with initial tumor dimensions on physical exam. In this arm of the study, neck partial responders to induction chemotherapy had a neck dissection 12 wk after radiotherapy, whereas complete responders did not have neck surgery. They found that patients who achieved a complete response in the neck after induction chemotherapy had a statistically significant $(p = 0.008)$ lower need for subsequent salvage surgery than patients with a less than complete response. In these patients the overall death rate was also statistically lower $(p = 0.014)$, and they survived longer $(p = 0.0476)$ compared with patients with a less than complete response. Specifically, of the 18 patients who achieved a complete response, 5 had salvage neck surgery and 1 died of neck recurrence without surgery. This was contrasted to the 19 partial responders who underwent neck dissection for persistent disease; 13 of these died with 5 dying because of to uncontrolled neck disease. Given the high recurrence rate among partial responders in this study and the lack of effectiveness of neck surgery, the authors suggested earlier neck dissection among patients with less than a complete response *(6)*. It is important to point out that even among complete responders to induction chemotherapy in this study, 6/18 (33%) still needed neck surgery.

Norris et al. *(7)* also found that initial response to induction chemotherapy could forecast the rate on neck control. That is, patients achieving a complete response to induction chemotherapy had an 85% 3-yr regional control rate without surgery. This was contrasted to patients with less than a complete response who had a 33% control rate with radiation therapy only and 71% control rate with surgery and radiation. The high rate of regional disease control among complete responders to induction chemotherapy led these authors to suggest that neck dissection could be omitted in this subgroup *(7)*.

Similarly, Armstrong et al. *(8)* recommended that for complete responders to induction chemotherapy, a neck dissection might not be needed. A complete response was defined as the absence of palpable metastases for a minimum of 4 wk. A partial response in the neck required a 50% or greater decrease in the sum of the product of the diameters of each measurable lesion for 4 wk or longer. In this study, there were 54 patients with metastatic nodal disease among whom 35 achieved either a complete or a partial response to induction chemotherapy. In 22 of these 35 patients with a major response, radiation only was then given as sole definitive therapy. In another 10 patients, a neck dissection was performed prior to receiving radiation therapy. Of the radiation therapy only group, 2/22 (9%) failed compared with 3/10 (30%) that failed in the surgery and radiation group. In a further analysis of the two failures in the radiation only group, they found that 1/17 (6%) failed who had a complete response and 1/5 (20%) failed who had a partial response to induction chemotherapy. They also report no difference in overall survival between those who received adjunctive surgery and those who did not. Given the above results, the authors conclude that complete responders to induction chemotherapy have an excellent neck control rate with radiation alone and thus may not need a neck dissection *(8)*. Their conclusion must be tempered by the fact that many patients in the radiation only group had N1 disease (41%) compared with none in the surgery group.

Giovana et al. *(9)* also did not perform neck dissection on their patients with neck metastases who attained a complete response after induction chemotherapy. Instead, they used neck dissection for patients with a less than complete response to induction chemotherapy prior to radiation therapy. For these authors, a complete response was defined as no measurable or palpable tumor or induration in the neck on clinical examination. Patients achieving a partial response in the neck had a 50% decrease in the product of the longest diameter multiplied by its perpendicular diameter of the largest reference neck node compared with initial size. Using neck dissection in this manner, the authors compared the group of complete responders with partial responders and found that the recurrence rates (53 vs 40% respectively) were similar. They further found that disease-free survival ($p = 0.48$) and overall survival ($p = 0.75$) rates did not differ significantly among complete and partial responders *(9)*. These findings are in contrast to those of Wolf and Fisher *(6)* who showed that having a less than complete response to induction chemotherapy was associated with a significantly worse survival. They thus suggest that the role of neck dissection is to improve regional control in those patients who have a less than complete response to induction chemotherapy. One shortcoming of this study lies in the fact that only 6/58 (10%) of their patients had N3 disease compared with 30/46 (65%) of patients who had N3 disease in the study by Wolf and Fisher. Another concern about this study is the high recurrence rate in both groups.

From these early studies using induction chemotherapy, it becomes clear that patients with a complete response to induction chemotherapy generally had better regional control of metastatic disease than patients with less than a complete response. The above studies suggest that neck dissection may be saved for patients with a less than complete response to induction chemotherapy. However, without neck dissection, regional recurrences are seen in 10–35% of these complete responders.

4. NECK DISSECTION WITH CONCURRENT CHEMORADIATION THERAPY

Most recent studies focused on concomitant chemotherapy and radiation therapy (chemoradiation) because it decreased treatment time, did not delay curative therapy, increased locoregional control, and decreased distant metastases. Among studies using concurrent chemoradiation, neck dissection was suggested in either of two settings. One group of authors suggested that neck dissection should be considered after assessing response to chemoradiation and should be applied to patients who did not achieve a complete response in the neck. Another group of authors suggested that the need for a neck dissection should be based not only on response but also on all pretreatment neck staging.

Dagum et al. *(10)* recommended that neck dissection be performed only on patients who fail to achieve a clinical complete response after chemoradiation. Clinical examination and computed tomography (CT) or magnetic resonance imaging (MRI) imaging were used to assess for neck response. A clinical complete response was defined as the absence of clinically evident tumor, and a clinical partial response as a 50% or more decrease in the sum of the products of the major and minor diameters of all tumor masses. In their study, induction chemotherapy was followed by concurrent chemoradiation on 41 patients with neck metastases, and a neck dissection was reserved for less than complete responders after chemoradiation therapy. They found no difference in overall survival between patients who achieved a complete response after induction chemotherapy (11 patients) and patients who achieved a complete response after chemoradiation (7 patients). Thus, 18/41 (44%) eventually achieved a complete response after definitive treatment. Among 23 patients with a less than complete response to treatment, 22 went on to have a neck dissection. Of these 22 patients, 11 had a pathologic negative neck dissection. The overall survival of these 11 pathologic complete responders did not differ in survival from the above clinical complete responder group. However, among the other 11 patients who achieved less than a complete response that had positive neck dissection specimens, the overall survival was significantly worse compared with clinical or pathologic complete responders ($p = 0.03$). The 5-yr actuarial survival of clinical and pathologic complete responders was 66% compared with 41% for pathologic partial responders *(10)*. These observations led the authors to recommend that neck dissection should be saved for less than clinical complete responders after chemoradiation.

Sanguineti et al. *(11)* also recommended assessment of response to chemoradiation in order to assess the need for neck surgery. Both physical examination and CT scanning were used to assess for response. A complete response was defined as disappearance of all palpable neck disease at physical examination or a greater than 75% reduction in node size (product of the greatest diameter by its perpendicular diameter) on CT scans. Partial responders had a greater than 50% reduction in node size as measured on both physical exam and CT scans. In their study of 43 patients who received chemoradiation, 25 (58%) had a clinical complete response and therefore did not have follow-up neck surgery as per study protocol. Of these 25 clinical complete responders, 3 (12%) eventually had recurrence. Of the other 18 patients with less than a complete response, 5 had neck dissection, with 2 (40%) of these 5 having residual positive disease on pathology. In these 18 patients with a less than complete response, 15 eventually recurred in the neck. The authors more closely examined the 25 complete responders and found that the 2-yr neck control probability was 100% and 90% for patients with N1 and N2 disease, respectively. This was in marked contrast to 0% neck control probability among N3 patients. In conclusion, they recommend neck dissection for clinically less than complete responders. However, these authors also go on to recommend planned neck dissection for all N3 patients as they found that these patients were unlikely to have controlled neck disease with chemoradiation treatment alone even if they achieved a clinical complete response *(11)*.

In 1997, Lavertu et al. *(12)* reviewed 100 patients treated with either radiation therapy or chemoradiation for head and neck cancer. In this study, patients with N2 or higher disease were offered a planned neck dissection regardless of response to treatment. Overall, this study showed that adding concurrent chemotherapy to radiation therapy increased the rate of clinical complete response at the primary site ($p = 0.007$) and regionally ($p = 0.09$), although the disease-specific survival was not statistically improved.

In this study, patients with no palpable neck disease on physical examination were considered complete responders. Partial responders had greater than 50% reduction in nodal size (product of greatest diameter by its perpendicular diameter). Among the 53 patients in this study with N2 or N3 disease, 35 had neck dissection and 18 did not. Among the 35 dissected necks, 18 had achieved a clinical complete response prior to surgery. However, in 4 of these 18 (22%) patients, viable tumor was found within the neck dissection specimens. Of the 17 less than complete responders in the neck dissection group, 8 patients (47%) had viable tumor cells on pathologic examination. Only one patient had neck recurrence in the neck dissection group, and this patient had residual tumor after a less than complete response to initial therapy. There were 18 patients with no neck surgery after initial treatment, and 12 achieved a clinical complete response. Three of these 12, however, eventually recurred in the neck. Although the authors found that achieving a clinical complete response in the neck was associated with significantly improved disease specific survival ($p = 0.002$), the addition of neck dissection did not significantly improve disease-specific survival ($p = 0.40$). Neck dissection, however, did significantly decrease the risk of neck recurrence ($p = 0.05$).

Like other authors, they found that having a positive neck dissection specimen was associated with a significantly worse survival ($p = 0.03$). Also, because 22% of clinical complete responders had residual disease on pathologic examination, the presence of a complete response could not reliably be used to predict the absence of disease in the neck. The recommendation for planned neck dissection was still made in spite of the finding that neck dissection did not improve disease-specific survival: of the 12 patients who had residual disease on pathology, 6 were still alive who would have otherwise died of neck disease without surgery. They recommend that a planned neck dissection be performed for N2 and N3 pretreatment necks because of a 22% rate of occult disease after achieving a complete response. It was further recommended that planned neck surgery be performed on N2 and N3 necks because of the low morbidity of neck dissection compared with the high morbidity associated with dying of neck recurrence *(12)*.

In 1999 Robbins et al. *(13)* also used the strategy of planned neck dissection after a targeted chemoradiation protocol (RADPLAT). Although the authors used both physical examination and CT scans to determine response to treatment, they do not mention the specific criteria used to define a complete or partial response. In their study, 56 hemi-necks with N2–N3 disease were evaluated, with 33 achieving a clinical complete response and 21 a less than complete response. Of the 33 complete responders, 16 had planned neck dissection with no specimens revealing residual disease. In keeping with this finding, all 17 patients with a complete response who did not have surgery did not have recurrances in the neck. Of the 21 less than complete responders, 18 had neck dissection with 14 showing positive residual tumor. Of these 14 patients with residual tumor, only 1 recurred in the neck and this recurrence was successfully salvaged. They report a 3-yr locoregional control rate of 77%. Because no patient with a complete response in the neck had recurrence whether or not neck dissection was performed, the authors suggest that planned neck dissection may not be necessary if a clinical complete response is achieved after using targeted intraarterial chemotherapy with concurrent radiation therapy *(13)*.

Puc et al. *(14)* also report that the addition of neck dissection did not result in improved survival. In their report, of 71 patients treated with chemoradiation, 47 (66%) had a clinical complete response whereas 24 (34%) had less than a complete response. Response was measured by manual palpation after therapy, but the authors did not elaborate on the specific criteria used to determine a complete or partial response. Among complete responders, 41 had a neck dissection yielding 17 (41%) patients with residual disease. Of the 24 less than complete responders, only 7 had neck dissection. Thus 47 patients had neck dissection whereas 23 did not. The difference in survival between surgical (52%) and nonsurgical (39%) patients was not significant ($p = 0.40$). In the same study, the percentage of neck complete responders that died of disease was similar whether or not a neck dissection was performed ($p > 0.99$). This finding led the authors to question the role of routine planned neck dissection in the treatment of regionally metastatic disease *(14)*.

In 2003 Grabenbauer et al. *(15)* also questioned the role of routine neck dissection after they examined the effect of neck dissection among the primary site complete responders to their chemoradiation treatments. Of 142 total patients, 97 were found to be complete responders at the primary site to chemoradiation, although they did not detail how they defined a complete response. Neck dissection was offered to all of these 97 patients, but only 56 went on to have neck dissection, leaving 41 who refused neck dissection. The regional control rate among neck dissection and nondissected patients was 80 and 85%, respectively ($p = 0.47$). For the complete responders who had neck dissection, the 5-yr overall and disease specific survival rates were 44 and 55%, respectively, compared with 42 and 47%, respectively, in the nondissected complete responders. These differences were not statistically significant ($p = 0.9$) Based on these findings, the authors conclude that there was no clear evidence for routine use of neck dissection after chemoradiation in advanced head and neck cancer. They also found a statistical trend toward higher morbidity as measured by pain, dysphagia, and hoarseness among neck-dissected patients compared with their nondissected counterparts *(15)*.

McHam et al. *(16)* have recently reviewed their data regarding the effect of chemoradiation on metastatic neck disease. Out of 109 total patients with N2–N3 disease, 65 had a complete response to chemoradiation in the neck. Disappearance of palpable neck disease confirmed by a negative CT scan defined a complete response. Partial response was defined as any residual palpable disease. Of the 65 complete responders, 32 eventually had neck dissection of which 8 (25%) still had residual disease on pathology. Only one of these eight patients had regional recurrence. Of the remaining 33 patients who had a complete response but did not receive neck dissection, 4 (12%) had regional failure. All 44 less than complete responders had neck dissection, with 17 (39%) neck dissection specimens positive for residual disease. Four of these 17 patients eventually went on to have regional failure, whereas none of the pathologically negative patients failed regionally. The authors found that the establishment of a complete response in the neck compared with a less than a complete response did not predict a pathologic complete response in neck dissection specimens ($p = 0.21$) or regional failure ($p = 0.80$). They thus suggest that planned neck dissection be considered for all N2–N3 patients because even a clinical complete response to treatment does not predict a pathologic complete response. Even though the authors found no difference in disease-specific or overall survival, they again echo the recommendation that planned neck dissection should be performed because dying of uncontrolled neck disease is highly possible but potentially avoidable if neck dissection is performed. Additionally, like many previous authors, they also found that regional failure was statistically more likely among patients whose neck dissection specimens showed residual disease compared with their disease free counterparts ($p \leq 0.001$) *(16)*.

From these studies, it becomes apparent that neck dissection plays an important role in the management of regional metastases in less than complete responders to chemoradiation. For patients with a complete response after treatment of an N1 neck, there is no need for a neck dissection. For more advanced neck disease on presentation, the addition of a neck dissection after a complete response is controversial. Although no survival benefit may be derived from the addition of a neck dissection, it results in a lesser incidence of neck failure.

5. COMPLICATIONS

As stated above, dying of metastatic neck disease is very possible. Neck dissection can reduce this morbidity if the surgery itself does not carry significant morbidity. Taylor et al. *(17)* reviewed 27 patients treated with definitive radiation therapy who suffered postoperative complications and performed logistic regression on these data to identify factors that were more common among these patients. They found that the use of flaps in the closure of the wound was associated with increased wound complications. They further found a trend that higher total doses and treatment times were associated with wound complications and that lower fraction sizes were associated with lower complication rates *(17)*. In 1997, Newman et al. *(18)* described their complication rate for surgery after induction followed by concurrent chemoradiation. In this study, the protocol was to offer surgery for less than complete responders after induction or concurrent chemoradiation and for progressive disease. Thus, patients did not have planned neck dissections. They report that of 17 patients who received surgery, 6 (35%) patients had eight complications within the first 30 postoperative days. There were three major complications, which were pharyngocutaneous fistula, carotid rupture, and tracheocutaneous fistula, as well as five minor wound complications. When they compared these patients with a similar group of patients who underwent similar surgery over the same time, they found no statistical difference between complication rates and thus conclude that surgery after chemoradiation does not carry an increased complication rate compared with nonchemoradiated patients *(18)*.

Similarly, in 1998 Lavertu et al. *(19)* reported a complication rate of 33% for planned neck dissection after concurrent chemoradiation. This complication rate was found not to be significantly different from that of patients who had planned neck dissections after radiation therapy alone (29%). From these data, one can conclude that post-chemoradiation neck surgery carries an acceptable complication rate that does not vary significantly from neck surgery in other settings. Obviously the addition of a neck dissection to the therapeutic regimen should be carefully weighed as it may cause a higher incidence of morbidity in the form of residual pain, dysphagia, and hoarseness, as suggested by Grabenbauer et al. *(15)*.

6. EXTENT OF NECK DISSECTION

Another important issue in neck dissection is the extent of surgery. Early authors mostly used the classic radical neck dissection. Some later studies have suggested that less radical procedures may be performed safely. For instance, in the study by Robbins et al. *(13)* selective neck dissections were used in 33 of the 35 patients undergoing neck dissection. The selective nature of the surgery mostly entailed omitting either level I or level V from the neck dissection. The impressive results obtained in this trial suggested that selective neck dissection might be used in planned neck dissections in place of the classic radical neck dissection *(13)*. Stenson et al. *(20)* also suggest that selective neck dissection may be feasible in post-chemoradiotherapy neck dissection. In their study, 69 patients had neck dissections 5–17 wk after chemoradiotherapy. Fifty-six of these patients had selective neck dissections, and 13 patients had modified radical or classic radical neck dissections. The selective neck dissections consisted of preserving the sternocleidomastoid muscle, internal jugular vein, and spinal accessory nerve when removing levels I–III, II–IV, or rarely II–V lymph nodes. They report 24/69 (35%) patients with residual pathologically positive nodes after dissection, yet only one of these patients failed in the neck. They thus conclude that neck dissection is important in obtaining control of metastatic neck disease and that selective neck dissection can be performed in many cases *(20)*.

7. SALVAGE NECK DISSECTION

Many authors have explored the role of neck dissection as a salvage procedure for recurrence after definitive treatment. Most of these authors conclude that salvage neck dissection is generally not effective at controlling neck disease. Mendenhall et al. *(4)* found that successful salvage surgery was achieved in only 50 to 60% of patients initially treated with definitive radiation therapy. They postulate that salvage surgery is often unsuccessful because the increased fibrosis in the neck after radiation therapy makes detecting neck recurrence very difficult *(4)*. Mabanta et al. *(21)* also looked at the issue of postradiation therapy salvage neck dissection and similarly conclude that it is rarely successful. From their population of 51 patients who had neck recurrence after definitive radiation therapy for head and neck cancer, 33 (65%) could not undergo salvage because of either unresectable disease at recurrence, medical instability, distant metastatic disease, or patient refusal of further treatment. Of the remaining 18 patients who had salvage treatment, 14 received neck dissection as part of their salvage therapy. Locoregional and/or metastatic disease developed in all of these patients. They report that the rate of neck control at 5 yr post treatment for all 18 patients undergoing salvage treatment was only 9%. They thus conclude that the likelihood of successful salvage treatment after a neck recurrence is remote *(21)*.

In addition, Lavertu et al. *(19)* also report that salvage neck surgery is associated with a significantly increased rate of surgical complications. They report that salvage procedures had an overall complication rate of 60%, which differed significantly from the 31% rate for planned neck dissections. They further report that the rate of major complications (20%) was also significantly increased among salvage neck dissection patients compared with planned neck dissection patients (3.4%) *(19)*. These data show that salvage treatment for recurrence in the neck is rarely successful and can be associated with a high morbidity from operative complications.

8. ROLE OF IMAGING

In evaluating patients after chemoradiation, many authors had elected to obtain CT scans as an adjunct to physical exam to look for evidence of recurrent neck disease. In 2004, Velazquez et al. *(22)* examined the records of 43 patients who underwent 53 neck dissections who also had preoperative CT scans. The CT scans were read as positive or negative for residual disease, and this reading was then correlated to the pathologic findings in the neck dissection specimens. The criteria used for a positive CT scan included node less than 1 cm, the presence of multiple nodes or confluent nodes (> 8 mm), central necrosis, and extracapsular spread. All of these 43 patients had chemotherapy and radiation therapy as definitive treatment for their head and neck cancer. They report that CT scans after definitive chemoradiation treatment had an 85% sensitivity but only a 24% specificity in predicting residual metastatic neck disease. Furthermore, CT scan in this setting yielded a positive predictive value of 40% and a negative predictive value of 73%. From these data, the authors conclude that "the negative predictive value of 73% and low specificity of 24% found in [this] study preclude the use of CT scans as the sole indicator for determining the need for posttreatment neck dissection in patients with advanced head and neck squamous cell carcinoma" *(22)*.

In the future, if postchemoradiation residual metastatic disease in the neck could be predicted, the use of planned neck dissection could potentially be eliminated. In this regard, the role of fluoro-1-deoxy-*d*-glucose positron emission tomography (FDG-PET) in head and neck cancer is being defined. Greven et al. *(23)* evaluated 45 head and neck cancer patients using FDG-PET scans before and serially after radiotherapy. They report that at 1 mo post radiotherapy, the false-positive rate was 28%. At 4 mo, the FDG-PET scans were more accurate *(23)*. Wong et al. *(24)* report that the sensitivity and specificity for recurrent head and neck cancer are 96 and 74%, respectively. More studies using FDG-PET scans in head and neck cancer need to be done before this tool can be routinely used to determine the need for neck dissection after therapy.

9. CONCLUSION

From the data presented, it is clear that for patients who achieve a less than complete response to chemotherapy and radiation therapy, there is a role for planned neck dissection. The role for neck dissection for complete responders to chemotherapy and radiation therapy is more controversial. It is likely to remain controversial until a tool to identify residual disease accurately is identified. Robbins et al. *(16)* are the only authors who have shown that a complete response to chemoradiation (using the RADPLAT protocol) translates into complete sterilization of disease in the neck. All other authors have shown that a certain percentage of complete responders still harbor viable cancer cells in the neck. Excluding the results of Robbins et al., the percentages of patients whose necks still harbor disease in the neck dissection specimen despite a complete response to chemoradiation therapy were 22% *(12)*, 41% *(14)*, and 25% *(16)*. Although this does not necessarily translate into a subsequent neck recurrence, the addition of a neck dissection may be reasonable in these cases, especially with more advanced neck disease on presentation.

Although no study to date has shown that the addition of a neck dissection improves survival, it does reduce the rate of regional failure and improves the quality of life in the patients who would otherwise have failed in the neck.

REFERENCES

1. Parsons JT, Million RR, Cassisi NJ. Carcinoma of the base of tongue: results of radical irradiation with surgery reserved for irradiation failure. Laryngoscope 1982; 92:689–696.
2. Parsons JT, Million RR, Cassisi NJ. The influence of excisional or incisional biopsy of metastatic neck nodes on the management of head and neck cancer. Int J Radiat Oncol Biol Phys 1985; 11:1447–1454.
3. Mendenhall WM, Million RR Cassisi NJ. Squamous cell carcinoma of the head and neck treated with radiation therapy: the role of neck dissection for clinically positive neck nodes. Int J Radiat Oncol Biol Phys 1986; 12:733–740.
4. Mendenhall WM, Parsons JT, Stringer SP, Cassisi NJ, Million RR. Squamous cell carcinoma of the head and neck treated with irradiation: management of the neck. Semin Radiat Oncol 1992; 2:163–170.
5. Parsons JT, Mendenhall WM, Cassisi NJ, Stringer SP, Million RR. Neck dissection after twice-a-day radiotherapy: morbidity and recurrence rates. Head Neck 1989; 11:400–404.
6. Wolf GT, Fisher SG Effectiveness of salvage neck dissection for advanced regional metastases when induction chemotherapy and radiation are used for organ preservation. Laryngoscope 1992; 102:934–939.
7. Norris CM, Busse PM, Clark JR. Evolving role of surgery after induction chemotherapy and primary site radiation in head and neck cancer. Semin Surg Oncol 1993; 9:3–13.
8. Armstrong J, Pfister D, Strong E, et al. The management of the clinically positive neck as part of a larynx preservation approach. Int J Radiat Oncol Biol Phys 1993; 26:759–765.

9. Giovana RT, Greenberg J, Wu KT, et al. Planned early neck dissection before radiation for persistent neck nodes after induction chemotherapy. Laryngoscope 1997; 107:1129–1137.

10. Dagum P, Pinto HA, Newman JP, et al. Management of the clinically positive neck in organ preservation for advanced head and neck cancer. Am J Surg 1998; 176:448–452.

11. Sanguineti G, Corvo R, Benasso M, et al. Management of the neck after alternating chemoradiotherapy for advanced head and neck cancer. Head Neck 1999; 21:223–228.

12. Lavertu P, Adelstein DJ, Saxton JP, et al. Management of the neck in a randomized trial comparing concurrent chemotherapy and radiotherapy with radiotherapy alone in resectable stage III and IV squamous cell head and neck cancer. Head Neck 1997; 19:559–566.

13. Robbins KT, Wong FSH, Kumar P, et al. Efficacy of targeted chemoradiation and planned selective neck dissection to control bulky nodal disease in advanced head and neck cancer. Arch Otolaryngol Head Neck Surg 1999; 125:670-675.

14. Puc MM, Chrzanowski FA, Hoang ST, et al. Preoperative chemotherapy-sensitized radiation therapy for cervical metastases in head and neck cancer. Arch Otolaryngol Head Neck Surg 2000; 126:337–342.

15. Grabenbauer GG, Rodel C, Ernst-Stecken A, et al. Neck dissection following radiochemotherapy of advanced head and neck cancer—for selected cases only? Radiother Oncol 2003; 66:57–63.

16. McHam SA, Adelstein DJ, Rybicki LA, et al. Who merits a neck dissection after definitive chemoradiotherpy for N2-N3 squamous cell head and neck cancer? Head Neck 2003; 25:791–798.

17. Taylor JMG, Mendenhall WM, Parsons JT, Lavey RS. The influence of dose and time on wound complications following post-radiation neck dissection. Int J Radiat Oncol Biol Phys 1992; 23:41–46.

18. Newman JP, Terris DJ, Pinto HA, et al. Surgical morbidity of neck dissection after chemoradiotherapy in advanced head and neck cancer. Ann Oto Rhinol Laryngol 1997; 106:117–122.

19. Lavertu P, Bonafede JP, Adelstein DJ, et al. Comparison of surgical complications after organ-preservation therapy in patients with stage III or IV squamous cell head and neck cancer. Arch Otolaryngol Head Neck Surg 1998; 124:401–406.

20. Stenson KM, Haraf DJ, Pelzer H, et al. The role of cervical lymphadenectomy after aggressive concomitant chemoradiotherapy. Arch Otolaryngol Head Neck Surg 2000; 126:950–956.

21. Mabanta SR, Mendenhall WM, Stringer SP, Cassisi NJ. Salvage treatment for neck recurrence after irradiation alone for head and neck squamous cell carcinoma with clinically positive nodes. Head Neck 1999; 21:591–594.

22. Velazquez RA, McGuff S, Sycamore D, Miller FR. The role of computed tomographic scans in the management of the N-positive neck in head and neck squamous cell carcinoma after chemoradiotherapy. Arch Otolaryngol Head Neck Surg 2004; 130:74–77.

23. Greven KM, Williams DW, McGuirt F. Serial positron emission tomography scans after radiation therapy of patients with head and neck cancer. Head Neck 2001; 23:942–946.

24. Wong RJ, Lin DT, Schoder H. Diagnostic and prognostic value of fluorodeoxyglucose positron emission tomography for recurrent head and neck squamous cell carcinoma. J Clin Oncol 2002; 20:4199–4208.

5

Salvage Surgery
After Chemoradiation Therapy

Walter T. Lee, MD and Ramon M. Esclamado, MD

1. INTRODUCTION

The past two decades have seen significant advances in the efficacy of combined chemotherapy and radiation in the management of advanced stage squamous cell carcinoma (SCC) of the head and neck. This is especially true for SCC of the oropharynx, hypopharynx, and larynx. Primary surgery for advanced T-stage tumors, despite sophisticated reconstruction of the surgical defect, may result in a significant impact on speech, swallowing, and respiration. Organ preservation protocols using definitive radiation with or without chemotherapy may provide an effective primary treatment while avoiding the functional and cosmetic morbidity associated with surgery.

Recent reports have described impressive results using this treatment approach. Organ preservation protocols are successful in nearly 40 to 50% of cases (1–3). Forastiere et al. (4) demonstrated that in patients with concurrent chemoradiation therapy for advanced laryngeal cancer, there was a 43% absolute reduction in total laryngectomy rates. We have been able to demonstrate similar results at our institution. Lavertu et al. (5) reported that only 30% of patients with stage III or IV head and neck SCC required salvage surgery of the primary site after organ preservation therapy. In another study, concurrent chemoradiation was given to 105 patients with SCC with most having the primary site in either the oropharynx, larynx, or hypopharynx. Local control was seen in 87% of patients, and salvage was successful in 64% of the recurrences. The overall 4-yr projected survival was 60% (6). Adelstein et al. (7) reported a local control rate of stage IV squamous cell head and neck cancer patients of 91% with concurrent chemoradiation therapy. With salvage surgery, this local control rate was increased to 97%.

Surgery in these circumstances is then reserved for salvage in patients with persistent or recurrent disease and is a critical component of managing regional nodal metastases. The importance of effective and appropriate surgery in these situations cannot be understated, as this remains the patient's only hope for cure. With more patients being entered into organ preservation protocols, surgical salvage will form an increasingly important part of the multidisciplinary care of patients with head and neck cancer. The purpose of this chapter is to review the surgical considerations and strategy in the multidisciplinary management of patients with advanced SCC of the head and neck.

From: *Current Clinical Oncology: Squamous Cell Head and Neck Cancer*
Edited by: D. J. Adelstein © Humana Press Inc., Totowa, NJ

2. PRETREATMENT EVALUATION

A multidisciplinary team approach is paramount for the successful management of these challenging patients. This team includes head and neck oncologic surgeons, medical oncologists, radiation oncologists, dentists, speech pathologists, and dedicated nursing support. The role of the surgeon at this stage of the patient's management is to help provide the most accurate clinical staging of the primary tumor, neck disease, and possible distant metastases. Accurate clinical staging and documentation of the primary tumor and regional disease is critical for two reasons: (1) to determine the most appropriate treatment approach given the extent of the disease, patient comorbidities, patient biases, and psychosocial factors that influence the decision-making process; and (2) to provide critical information that guides decision making as to the appropriate extent of salvage surgery, should the patient fail initial nonsurgical management. The importance of this is highlighted by our experience that patients who are initially evaluated and undergo chemoradiation treatment at the Cleveland Clinic Foundation have excellent surgical salvage rates when they have persistent or recurrent disease *(6)*. In contrast, patients who are referred to a tertiary care institution for surgical salvage after receiving their initial treatment at a different institution have an overall 5-yr survival rate of approx 25 to 35% *(8–10)*.

Pretreatment evaluation includes an appropriate history and complete head and neck physical examination. Particular attention is given to symptoms and signs of advanced disease, such as dysarthria from impaired tongue mobility, dysphagia resulting in weight loss, trimus, otalgia, stridor, vocal fold immobility, cranial nerve involvement, or massive neck nodes with fixation to the carotid sheath or deep neck musculature. Radiologic evaluation routinely includes a computed tomography (CT) scan of the neck with contrast, a chest radiograph, or chest CT to rule out lung metastasis or a synchronous lung cancer. We also utilize flurodeoxyglucose position emission tomography (FDG-PET) scans in patients with unknown primary cancers and in patients who may be treated with chemoradiation therapy to help assess response to treatment.

It is imperative that cancer patients presenting for initial tumor treatment undergo examination under general anesthesia to map the tumor extent accurately and to exclude synchronous primary cancers of the lung and esophagus. The examination under anesthesia provides vital information through direct inspection and bimanual palpation as to the deep extent of tumor involvement of the tongue, floor of mouth, and preepiglottic space; whether the mandible is involved; and determination of the size and extent of mucosal subsite involvement in the larynx, hypopharynx, and oropharynx that cannot be obtained with radiographic imaging. Examination of a primary laryngeal tumor with the operating microscope or a rigid fiberoptic telescope gives an accurate assessment of tumor extent and the appropriateness and feasibility of conservation laryngeal surgery as a primary treatment option. We routinely document the extent of the tumor by mapping the extent of the carcinoma with descriptions of involved structures on standardized anatomical diagrams after a thorough examination with palpation and direct laryngoscopy. These maps become part of the permanent chart and provide a schematic record of the initial presenting tumor.

The patients' clinical history and tumor maps are then presented at a regularly held meeting of the multidisciplinary treatment team, or tumor board. This tumor board not only provides a forum for coordination of patient care but also affords the opportunity to formulate the optimal treatment plan. At this time, management of the primary site is considered separately from management of the neck. If a complete response is obtained at the primary site, it is important to make a decision at this time regarding incorporation of a planned neck dissection 2–3 mo after treatment. If a neck dissection is not planned and the patient has clinically palpable regional disease, the radiation dose to the neck is adequately boosted to maximize regional control in the involved neck.

3. ASSESSMENT OF TREATMENT RESPONSE

Early detection of persistent disease is critical for successful surgical salvage and requires analyzing response of the primary site separately from the response in the involved regional nodes. Patients are reevaluated in the fifth week of treatment (after completing the second cycle of chemotherapy) to ensure that there is an appropriate disease response at the primary site. In the rare situations in which there is no response or progressive disease at the primary site, immediate surgical salvage is warranted. If there is an appropriate response, treatment is completed, and patients are reevaluated 8–10 wk later. At this time, response at the primary site and neck are determined separately. This can be difficult owing to the mucositis, skin reaction, and dysphagia that result from treatment. This can persist for 2–6 mo and must be distinguished from the patient's pretreatment tumor-related symptoms *(7,11)*. Careful clinical evaluation requires an attempt to determine whether the patient's pretreatment symptoms from the tumor have resolved and affords the opportunity for both visualization and palpation of the primary site and necks. Posttreatment CT and FDG-PET scans are helpful in determining treatment response if performed 2–3 mo after completion of treatment. If the outpatient clinical exam is suboptimal and/or radiographic studies suggest residual/persistent disease, patients are routinely brought to the operating room for examination under anesthesia and biopsy as indicated.

Patients who successfully complete initial treatment and are rendered disease free are carefully followed according to the Society of Head and Neck Surgery recommendations. Regular follow-up appointments occur every 1–3 mo for the first year, every 2–4 mo during the second year, every 3–6 mo during the third year, every 4–6 mo during the fourth year, and then every year afterwards. Chest radiographs are be performed yearly and more frequently if clinically indicated. Any suspicious lesions are evaluated with a chest CT and subsequent biopsy if warranted. Thyroid-stimulating hormone (TSH) levels are checked every 3 mo for the first year and then yearly because chemoradiation-induced hypothyroidism occurs early and in nearly 50% of patients *(12)*. Additional follow-up, laboratory tests (or imaging) should be performed as clinically indicated.

The long-term evaluation of patients who have undergone radiation with or without chemotherapy can be challenging. Organ preservation protocols are not without their own morbidity. The long-term effects of radiation may include edema, chronic fibrosis, tissue necrosis, dysphagia, and chondro- or osteoradionecrosis. Postradiation edema and scarring distort anatomy and can hinder examination of mucosal surfaces. Postradiation fibrosis can make palpation of lymphadenopathy challenging. Symptoms and signs that may indicate possible recurrences (such as otalgia, neck pain, unilateral headache, worsening dysphagia, or odynophagia) need to be carefully elicited and evaluated, especially in the background of posttreatment changes. The goal of frequent and careful follow-up visits, particularly in the first 2 yr after treatment, is to diagnose recurrent disease or a metachronous tumor early so that surgical salvage can be attempted.

When suspicious clinical findings or symptoms warrant further radiographic investigation, a neck CT with contrast should be performed to evaluate the primary site, regional lymph nodes, cartilage involvement, carotid sheath involvement, and deep neck muscle infiltration. Magnetic resonance imaging may assist in further evaluation of soft tissue involvement. When recurrence is suspected, an examination in the operating room with biopsy needs to be performed. Direct laryngoscopy and biopsy remain the primary means of establishing treatment failure or recurrence. Patients who have persistent postradiation edema at 3 mo after completion of the organ preservation regimens are often brought to the operating room for examination under anesthesia and directed biopsies, as this edema may be a sign of residual carcinoma. Other patients who should be routinely evaluated in the operating room after organ preservation are those with tumors in areas that are not adequately examined in an outpatient setting, such as hypopharyngeal tumors or laryngeal tumors with subglottic extension.

Patients who are referred from outside our institution after tumor recurrence may present unique hurdles that can make successful salvage more difficult. If the original tumor maps are not done or available, the original tumor stage cannot be accurately correlated with the actual anatomic sites of involvement. These recurrences are often advanced stage and are referred to a tertiary care center because of complexities in ablation, reconstruction, or rehabilitation. It can also be difficult to ascertain whether the carcinoma as seen represents focal recurrence or persistent tumor. This affects surgical planning, as persistent tumor requires surgical excision of the original tumor-bearing area compared with a focal recurrence, which may need a less extensive resection. Furthermore, physical findings are seen without a prior reference point for comparison. In light of these issues, successful salvage surgery as reflected in overall 5-yr survival is 20 to 35%.

If cancer is confirmed, detailed tumor mapping and thorough examination of surrounding structures should be done. Complete restaging of the tumor should be done at this time, as this was found to be more predictive of survival following surgical salvage *(13)*. We recommend that staging procedures be performed as a separate procedure from the salvage surgery. This allows pathologic confirmation of recurrent disease, which can be difficult to make on frozen sections, for accurate surgical planning, presentation at the tumor board, and an opportunity for the patient and their family to have questions answered and give informed consent.

4. EVALUATION FOR SURGICAL SALVAGE

Basic planning and preparation steps occur in all patients considered for surgical salvage, irrespective of the initial treatment situation. First, a thorough metastatic workup must be done. A chest CT is obtained to evaluate for pulmonary metastasis, but the indications for CT of the abdomen and pelvis as well as a bone scan are clinically driven. FDG-PET scan shows promise as a screening tool for distant metastases, but its role has yet to be defined.

A patient's nutritional and metabolic status must be carefully evaluated, as recovery from chemotherapy and radiation can be prolonged. Tumors in the upper aerodigestive tract may also impede the patient's ability to swallow. Weight loss and nutritional deficits are often seen secondary to poor oral intake. These patients may need nutritional supplements or tube feedings prior to surgery. Many head and neck cancer patients have a significant history of alcohol and tobacco abuse. Consideration should be given to detoxification to prevent postoperative alcohol withdrawal and delirium tremens. Laboratory tests such as albumin, pre-albumin, and liver function tests are important to assess the overall nutritional status and a complete blood count (CBC) to determine adequate bone marrow recovery from chemotherapy. Preoperative arterial blood gas as a baseline in patients with a significant pulmonary disease such as chronic obstructive pulmmonary disease is helpful information that facilitates postoperative care.

Furthermore, thyroid function (serum TSH) should be evaluated early in this process in order to correct biochemical or clinical hypothyroidism, which can result in poor wound healing.

Once the head and neck oncologic surgeon has determined the extent for the resection of the primary site and appropriate neck dissections, consideration is then given to what type of reconstruction should be performed. There are numerous options for reconstruction. They range in complexity and include primary closure, rotational flaps, pedicled flaps, and revascularized "free" flaps. Free flaps involve harvesting tissue with a defined arterial and venous blood supply from various donor sites away from the head and neck and reconnecting the blood supply to recipient vessels in the neck near the surgical resection via microvascular techniques. The use of free flap reconstruction has revolutionized the once disfiguring head and neck surgical ablative procedures. Currently, patients not only can achieve oncological resection but also have socially acceptable cosmetic appearance and function. Free flap reconstruction requires a surgeon with advanced training in microvascular techniques, but it carries the advantage of incorporating abundant, healthy, composite tissue such as skin, muscle, fascia, viscera, or bone into the surgical defect. This improves wound healing by providing a tension-free closure with healthy, vascularized, nonirradiated tissue. There is an increase in meaningful function and improvement in cosmetic appearance with free flap reconstruction *(14,15)*. Evaluation by a reconstructive surgeon should be done prior to salvage surgery.

Finally, an in-depth discussion with the patient and family needs to be undertaken. They must be aware of the morbidity and mortality associated with salvage surgery. It is important to remember the emotional toll that being diagnosed with a recurrence can have on a patient and family. It can be both disappointing and frustrating for a patient to be told of persistent or recurrent cancer despite enduring weeks of radiation and chemotherapy. An open and honest discussion with them as to the risks, expectations, morbidity, and chance for cure is imperative prior to any definitive salvage surgery. The impact of surgery on speech, swallowing, voice, and cosmesis must be anticipated and explained by the surgeon, particularly when surgery may result in dysphagia with G-tube dependence, the loss of laryngeal voice, or both, which is especially devastating to a patient.

5. SURGERY

The primary treatment goals of salvage surgery should be discussed and defined with the patient and family. In order of priority, these goals are: (1) to achieve oncological cure; (2) to preserve function, particularly speech and swallowing but also vision, hearing, taste, olfaction, facial and shoulder motion, and sensory innervation to the head and neck: and (3) to preserve or restore cosmesis. At times, the surgical morbidity may be unacceptable to the patient, which may compromise the adequacy of the resection and ultimately the chance for cure. For example, a patient may refuse a total laryngectomy and insist on a subtotal conservation laryngeal procedure when it is contraindicated by the extent of the tumor. Another patient may agree to a total laryngectomy but refuse an extended total laryngectomy that requires significant resection of the tongue, preventing restoration of swallowing and speech.

The patient must understand the implications of such a decision, and the surgeon must make the difficult decision of whether to proceed with surgery that may be inadequate for the disease.

The surgical procedure itself requires one to address the disease in the primary site, necks, and appropriate reconstruction. Appropriate surgery of the primary site for persistent disease requires considerable surgical judgment. Generally, if the persistence or recurrence is larger than the original tumor, resection of this tumor with 1–2 cm of normal surrounding tissue is necessary. If the primary site tumor is persistent disease that is no larger than the original tumor, resection of the original volume of tumor with 1–2 cm of normal tissue surrounding the tumor is done to achieve negative margins. Appropriate resection of a recurrent primary site tumor is more controversial. We generally consider these as tumors that had an initial complete clinical response to nonsurgical therapy and then recur 6 mo or more after completion of treatment. These tumors may theoretically be a solitary clonal population of resistant cells, rather than multifocal polyclonal disease scattered throughout the original tumor volume. Therefore, if the recurrence is smaller than the original tumor, we attempt resection of the recurrence with 1–2-cm margins, rather than resecting the original tumor volume with margins. The surgeon and patient should be prepared, however, for a more extensive resection if intraoperative findings or frozen section margins reveal that there are microscopic nests of tumor throughout the original tumor volume. These considerations again highlight the importance of accurate pretreatment evaluation and mapping of the tumor, ideally by the surgeon who will be responsible for performing the salvage procedure if it is needed.

Surgical management of the neck is considered after appropriate surgery for the primary site is determined. Neck dissection is indicated if: (1) there is clinical or radiographic evidence of disease in the neck; (2) the neck is clinically negative but carries a more than 20% incidence of occult disease; (3) resection of the primary site requires access through the neck; (4) free tissue reconstruction is needed; and (5) the patient is poorly compliant for follow-up. It is our bias to be more aggressive in electively dissecting necks, even bilaterally, in the patient who has failed chemoradiation at the primary site because the neck becomes quite fibrotic and it can be difficult to detect a recurrence early enough to salvage the patient successfully. The disadvantage to this approach is that the fibrosis that results from neck dissection after chemoradiation can be significant and bothersome, negatively impacting the pateint's overall quality of life (16).

Patients who have a complete response at the primary site are recommended to undergo neck dissection if they have persistent palpable disease in the neck 2 mo after completing treatment, or if at the time of the original staging, the largest lymph node in the neck was more than 3 cm. This recommendation is based on our experience that 60% of patients with persistent palpable disease in the neck have histologically proven disease at neck dissection. In addition, those patients with more than 3 cm nodes at initial diagnosis and a complete response in the neck have a 25% incidence of histologically positive disease at the time of neck dissection (17). Others have also agreed with this approach in treating the neck disease (18–21). The appropriate management of patients with advanced (> 3 cm) bilateral adenopathy who undergo a complete clinical response is more problematic. This is because of the fibrosis after bilateral neck dissection and the difficulties in managing the dissected neck should the patient developed a primary site recurrence or second primary tumor at a later date. We are currently evaluating the role of pre- and posttreatment CT/PET imaging to predict response in the neck, with the premise that a negative CT/PET 2–3 mo posttreatment will be highly predictive of a pathologic complete response, thereby reducing the frequency that neck dissections are performed in patients with advanced regional disease who have a complete response in the neck.

The surgeon's decision regarding the type of neck dissection performed for regional salvage should be tempered by the realization that excision of the disease should be complete since radiation therapy post neck dissection is not an option. The regional control rate should be greater than 90–95% in an appropriately treated neck when the primary site is controlled. A radical neck dissection removes lymph node levels I–V and the sternocleidomastoid muscle, the internal jugular vein, the spinal accessory nerve, and the cervical sensory nerves. This results in neck numbness and deformity, inability to raise the humerus from the horizontal to vertical plane, and possible chronic shoulder discomfort. A radical neck dissection is indicated in advanced persistent regional disease (>3 cm), particularly when there is involvement of the aforementioned structures. A modified radical neck dissection removes all five nodal groups but preserves one or more of either the sternocleidomastoid muscle, the internal jugular vein, or the spinal accessory nerve. This results in less shoulder impairment if the spinal accessory nerve can be preserved *(16)*. Modified neck dissection is indicated for patients who have palpable residual disease in the neck that is freely mobile from the surrounding structures. A selective neck dissection removes only the lymph node groups in the neck that drain the specific primary site and does not remove level V, which preserves sensory and motor function of the neck and shoulder. This has been shown to be effective in managing a neck previously treated with chemoradiation or radiation therapy alone that is clinically and radiographically negative when there is persistent or recurrent primary site disease. In these patients, the incidence of occult disease in the neck was 25% and the nodal drainage was not altered by the previous radiation therapy *(22)*.

5.1. Surgical Complications

The initial experience with surgical salvage after chemotherapy and radiation therapy was associated with a high complication rate, particularly with wound healing and postoperative pharyngocutaneous fistulas *(23)*. This resulted in prolonged hospitalization and a significant delay in the restoration of speech and swallowing in laryngectomized patients. What was not appreciated in this early experience was the high incidence of early unrecognized hypothyroidism and its detrimental impact upon wound healing. In addition, careful attention to gentle tissue handling, the avoidance of electrocautery in making mucosal incisions, and the importance of wound closure under minimum tension, often with the liberal use of revascularized tissue transfer, have reduced the rate of complications to a rate equal to that seen in nonirradiated patients *(1,2,13,23,24)*. Hall et al. *(25)* compared 147 patients who had undergone laryngectomy for advanced laryngopharyngeal cancer. Thirty of these patients had persistent or recurrent disease after initial radiotherapy. History of prior radiation treatment was not a significant factor in pharyngocutaneous fistula formation *(25)*. Davidson et al. *(26)* did not demonstrate a significant difference in surgical complications between standard vs hyperfractionated radiation therapy groups.

Chemotherapy has not been shown to cause an increase in surgical complications. Agra et al. *(27)* reported an increased incidence, but not a statistically significant one ($p = 0.08$), of minor complications. There was no difference in major complications. Lavertu et al. *(5)* also reported no significant difference in salvage surgery complications in patients who had concurrent chemotherapy compared with radiation therapy alone. However, most patients in this series underwent salvage neck dissection alone without resection of the primary site, which prevented salivary contamination of the wound and eliminated the risk of pharyngocutaneous fistula because of the absence of a mucosal repair.

5.2. Results of Salvage Surgery

The outcomes of salvage surgery are site specific because of the different patterns of tumor spread and risk of nodal metastases. Cancer of the larynx has the most favorable outcome with salvage surgery because the pattern of tumor spread in the larynx is compartmentalized, well defined, and generally contained within the larynx except for very advanced T-stage tumors.

Total laryngectomy for recurrent or persistent tumors of the larynx has been routinely used because of the wide margins that can be achieved. Furthermore, the laryngeal complex is readily surgically accessible, and closure can be done primarily. In many cases, this surgery provides the best chance for cure. Parsons et al. *(28)* were able to salvage over half of the patients with advanced laryngeal cancer by total laryngectomy. Yuen et al. *(29)* achieved a 5-yr survival rate of 45% in patients with advanced laryngeal carcinoma salvaged with laryngectomy.

Early T-stage laryngeal cancers that recur after initial organ preservation protocols may be amenable to conservation laryngeal surgery. These include vertical partial and supracricoid laryngectomies. These surgeries should only be used in tumors that meet established criteria. Contraindications to vertical partial laryngectomy include any of the following: 5-mm subglottic extension posteriorly, 10-mm subglottic extension anteriorly, extension beyond one-third of the contralateral cord, extension to the arytenoid, and cricoid or thyroid cartilage involvement.

Supracricoid laryngectomy may also be used for salvage. This operation allows resection of the thyroid cartilage and endolaryngeal tissues above the cricoid. At least one cricoarytenoid unit must be preserved. Respiration, deglutition, and voice functions are possible without the need for a permanent tracheostomy. Reconstruction is done with either a cricohyoido-epiglottopexy (CHEP) or cricohyoidopexy (CHP). Any patient considered for conservation laryngeal surgery should have good pulmonary function, limited comorbidity, and ability to undergo postoperative rehabilitation. Prior treatment with radiation with or without chemotherapy is not a contraindication for these procedures.

In contrast to laryngeal tumors, tumors of the oropharynx are especially notorious for rampant invasion. There are no true anatomical barriers in this region that can help control its spread. For example, tongue base lesions often spread laterally and superiorly to involve the tonsil, lateral pharyngeal wall, and soft palate; inferiorly to involve the extrinsic tongue muscles and the larynx; and anteriorly to involve the mobile tongue, mandible, and floor of mouth. Surgery of a recurrent tongue base cancer may be extended to include any of these structures to encompass the tumor adequately. This results in increased functional morbidity.

There are also important factors to consider in surgery of hypopharyngeal carcinomas. When the carcinoma is located on the posterior hypopharyngeal wall, the prevertebral fascia provides a barrier to further posterior spread. Thus, the tumor tends to grow in a vertical fashion. Initally, tumors of the posterior cricoid area tend to grow vertically and horizontally since the cricoid cartilage is a barrier to anterior progression. Partial or complete pharyngectomy may also have to include total laryngectomy to obtain adequate tumor margins. Finally, with hypopharyngeal tumors, one crucial question is the proximity to the cricopharyngeus muscle. If the resection cannot leave an adequate margin to provide for anastomosis, then a gastric pull-up is performed. This is done to avoid an intrathoracic anastomosis and the potentially life-threatening complication of mediastinitis.

Krause et al. *(24)* reported a statistically significant local control difference of 86% in laryngeal primaries compared with local control of nonlaryngeal primaries at 53%. Two-year disease-specific survival was 56% for laryngeal primaries vs 24% in oropharyngeal and hypopharyngeal primaries after failed organ preservation protocol and surgery for salvage *(24)*. Weber et al. *(2)* reported an overall disease-free survival of 82% in patients who had undergone organ preservation protocols and total laryngectomy surgical salvage for advanced laryngeal carcinoma. Stoeckli et al. *(30)* reported a 5-yr disease survival rate of 63% in 39 patients after salvage surgery for laryngeal SCC. Most of these patients had advanced TNM tumor staging compared with initial TNM stages. Salvage of the primary site consisted of total laryngectomy in 92% of these patients, and 8% underwent partial laryngectomy. All underwent bilateral neck dissections of levels II–IV.

Furthermore, Stoeckli et al. *(30)* reported a worse survival for hypopharyngeal SCC that fail primary radiation therapy. Their found a 5-yr survival rate of 20% in 15 patients after salvage for hypopharyngeal SCC *(30)*. Jones *(31)* reported a similar survival rate (25%) for hypopharyngeal SCC after failed radiation therapy. There was also a significant number of major complications (42%) in these salvage patients. These included tissue necrosis of free flaps and carotid artery rupture *(31)*.

Success rates in surgical salvage of the neck are different for a planned neck dissection, compared with salvage for recurrence after previous neck radiation. When neck dissections are performed after radiation therapy in patients who have persistent palpable disease, local regional control is improved. Chan et al. *(32)* reported a 3-yr regional control rate of 75% in patients. Isolated neck failures were found to be 8%. This is in contrast to having neck disease appear after initial treatment. Salvage surgery for neck disease after radiation in these cases is dismal. In a series of 51 patients who failed initial radiotherapy, 18 were found to be unresectable. Eighteen other patients underwent salvage treatment with either chemotherapy, radiation, and/or surgery. Only one patient was alive at 5 yr *(33)*.

Salvage surgery after radiation with or without chemotherapy is a vital part of the multidisciplinary care of a head and neck cancer patient. The challenges lie first in the decision to treat a newly diagnosed head and neck cancer patient with chemoradiation therapy or primary surgery and then recognizing that salvage surgery can be successful in improving survival when nonsurgical management fails. Salvage surgery demands careful evaluation prior to initiation of treatment, careful follow-up for early detection of recurrences, surgical judgment and skill in both the ablative and reconstructive components of the operation, meticulous postoperative care, and rehabilitation.

REFERENCES

1. Jorgensen K, Godballe C, Olfred H, et al. Cancer of the larynx: treatment results after primary radiotherapy with salvage surgery in a series of 1005 patients. Acta Oncol 2002; 41:69–72.
2. MacKenzie RG, Franssen E, Balogh JM, et al. Comparing treatment outcomes of radiotherapy and surgery in locally advanced carcinoma of the larynx: a comparison limited to patients eligible for surgery. Int J Radiat Oncol Biol Phys 2000; 47:65–71.
3. Weber RS, Berkey BA, Forastiere AA, et al. Outcome of salvage total laryngectomy following organ preservation therapy. Arch Otolaryngol Head Neck Surg 2003; 129:44–49.
4. Forastiere AA, Goepfert H, Maor M, et al. Concurrent chemotherapy and radiotherapy for organ preservation in advanced laryngeal cancer. N Engl J Med 2003; 349:2091–2098.
5. Lavertu P, Bonafede JP, Adelstein DJ, et al. Comparison of surgical complications after organ-preservation therapy in patients with stage III or IV squamous cell head and neck cancer. Arch Otolaryngol Head Neck Surg 1998; 124:401–406.
6. Lavertu P, Adelstein DJ, Saxton JP, et al. Aggressive concurrent chemoradiotherapy for squamous cell head and neck cancer: an 8-year single-institution experience. Arch Otolaryngol Head Neck Surg 1999; 125:142–148.
7. Adelstein DJ, Saxton JP, Lavertu P, et al. Maximizing local control and organ preservation in stage IV squamous cell head and neck cancer with hyperfractionated radiation and concurrent chemotherapy. J Clin Oncol 2002; 20:1405–1410.
8. Laccourreye O, Laccourreye L, Muscatello L, et al. Local failure after supracricoid partial laryngectomy: symptoms, management, and outcome. Laryngoscope 1998; 108:339–344.
9. Gehanno P, Depondt J, Guedon C, et al. Primary and salvage surgery for cancer of the tonsillar region: a retrospective study of 120 patients. Head Neck 1993; 15:185–189.
10. Yuen APW, Wei WI, Ho CM. Results of surgical salvage for radiation failures of laryngeal carcinoma. Otolaryngol Head Neck Surg 1995; 112:405–409.

11. Adelstein DJ, Li Y, Adams GL, et al. An intergroup phase III comparison of standard radiation therapy and two schedules of concurrent chemoradiotherapy in patients with unresectable squamous cell head and neck cancer. J Clin Oncol 2003; 21:92–98.

12. Mercado G, Adelstein DJ, Saxton JP, et al. Hypothyroidism: a frequent event after radiotherapy and after radiotherapy with chemotherapy for patients with head and neck carcinoma. Cancer 2001; 92:2892–2897.

13. Davidson J, Briant D, Gullane P, et al. The role of surgery following radiotherapy failure for advanced laryngopharyngeal cancer: a prospective study. Arch Otolaryngol Head Neck Surg 1994; 120:269–276.

14. Teknos TN, Myers LL, Bradford CR, et al. Free tissue reconstruction of the hypopharynx after organ preservation therapy: analysis of wound complications. Laryngoscope 2001; 111:1192–1196.

15. Wei F, Celik N, Yang W, et al. Complications after reconstruction by plate and soft-tissue free flap in composite mandibular defects and secondary salvage reconstruction with osteocutaneous flap. Plast Reconstr Surg 2003; 112:37–42.

16. Terrell JE, Ronis DL, Fowler KE, et al. Clinical predictors of quality of life in patients with head and neck cancer. Arch Otolaryngol Head Neck Surg 2004; 130:401–408.

17. Lavertu P, Adelstein DJ, Saxton JP, et al. Management of the neck in a randomized trial comparing concurrent chemotherapy and radiotherapy with radiotherapy alone in respectable stage III and IV squamous cell head and neck cancer. Head Neck 1997; 19:559–566.

18. Peters LJ, Weber RS, Morrison WH, et al. Neck surgery in patients with primary oropharyngeal cancer treated by radiotherapy. Head Neck 1996; 18:552–559.

19. Narayan K, Crane CH, Kleid S, et al. Planned neck dissection as an adjunct to the management of patients with advanced neck disease treated with definitive radiotherapy: for some or for all? Head Neck 1999; 21:606–613.

20. Mendenhall WM, Villaret DB, Amdur RJ, et al. Planned neck dissection after definitive radiotherapy for squamous cell carcinoma of the head and neck. Head Neck 2002; 24:1012–1018.

21. Hoffman HT. Planned neck dissection after definitive radiotherapy for squamous cell carcinoma of the head and neck. Head Neck 2002; 24:1012–1018.

22. Fritz MA, Esclamado RM, Lorenz RR, et al. Recurrent rates after selective neck dissection in the N0 irradiated neck. Arch Otolaryngol Head Neck Surg 2002; 128:292-5.

23. Sassler AM, Esclamado RM, Wolf GT. Surgery after organ preservation therapy: analysis of wound complications. Arch Otolaryngol Head Neck Surg 1995; 121:162–165.

24. Krause DH, Pfister DG, Harrison LB, et al. Salvage laryngectomy for unsuccessful larynx preservation therapy. Otol Rhino Laryngol 1995; 104:936–941.

25. Hall FT, O'Brien CJ, Clifford AR, et al. Clinical outcome following total laryngectomy for cancer. ANZ J Surg 2003; 73:300–305.

26. Davidson J, Keane T, Brown D, et al. Surgical salvage after radiotherapy for advanced laryngopharyngeal carcinoma. Arch Otolaryngol Head Neck Surg 1997; 123:420–424.

27. Agra IM, Carvalho AL, Pontes E, et al. Postoperative complications after en bloc salvage surgery for head and neck cancer. Arch Otolaryngol Head Neck Surg 2003; 129:1317–1321.

28. Parsons JT, Mendelhall WM, Stringer SP, et al. Salvage surgery following radiation failure in squamous cell carcinoma of the supraglottic larynx. Int J Radiat Oncol Biol Phys 1995; 32:605–609.

29. Yuen AP, Ho CM, Wei WI, et al. Prognosis of recurrent laryngeal carcinoma after laryngectomy. Head Neck 1995; 17:526–530.

30. Stoeckli SJ, Pawlik AB, Lipp M, et al. Salvage surgery after failure of nonsurgical therapy for carcinoma of the larynx and hypopharynx. Arch Otolaryngol Head Neck Surg 2000; 126:1473–1477.

31. Jones AS. The management of early hypopharyngeal cancer: Primary radiotherapy and salvage surgery. Clin Otolaryngol 1992; 17:545–549.

32. Chan AW, Ancukeiwicz M, Carballo N, et al. The role of postradiotherapy neck dissection in supraglottic carcinoma. Int J Radiat Oncol Biol Phys 2001; 50:367–375.

33. Mabanta SR, Mendenhall WM, Stringer SP, et al. Salvage treatment for neck recurrence after irradiation alone for head and neck squamous cell carcinoma with clinically positive neck nodes. Head Neck 1999; 21:591–594.

6

T3–T4 Squamous Cell Carcinoma of the Larynx Treated With Radiation Therapy Alone or Combined With Adjuvant Chemotherapy

William M. Mendenhall, MD

1. INTRODUCTION

Depending on the site and extent of disease, treatment alternatives for T3–T4 cancers include partial laryngectomy, total laryngectomy, and radiation therapy (RT) alone or combined with adjuvant chemotherapy. The prevailing treatment philosophy varies significantly from one country to another *(1)*. Patients in the United States and Australia are usually treated surgically, which often necessitates total laryngectomy *(1)*. In contrast, patients in Canada and Great Britain are often treated with RT alone, with surgery reserved as salvage treatment for those who experience recurrent disease. Patients treated with RT in the United States sometimes receive induction chemotherapy before RT *(2)*. The rationale for this strategy is based on the Veterans Affairs Laryngeal Cancer Study Group trial which compared induction chemotherapy and RT (in the subset of patients who responded to chemotherapy) with initial laryngectomy and postoperative RT; survival rates were similar, and patients randomized to the induction chemotherapy arm had a higher rate of laryngeal voice preservation *(3)*. A similar trial conducted by the European Organization for Research and Treatment of Cancer (EORTC) evaluated induction chemotherapy followed by RT for patients who had a complete response to treatment for advanced pyriform sinus and aryepiglottic fold malignancies *(4)*. Patients randomized to receive induction chemotherapy had 5-yr survival rates similar to those for patients randomized to undergo initial surgery. Approximately one-third of patients who received induction chemotherapy retained their larynx. More recently, concomitant chemoradiation has gained popularity because it has been shown to improve survival compared with RT alone for patients with local-regionally advanced head and neck cancer.

The purpose of this chapter is to review the results of RT alone or combined with adjuvant chemotherapy for T3 and T4 squamous cell carcinoma of the larynx.

From: *Current Clinical Oncology: Squamous Cell Head and Neck Cancer*
Edited by: D. J. Adelstein © Humana Press Inc., Totowa, NJ

2. SELECTION FOR TREATMENT

2.1. Glottic Carcinoma

Fixed-cord cancers (T3) may be stratified into relatively favorable and unfavorable lesions. Patients with favorable tumors have disease that is low volume, mostly confined to one side of the larynx, have a good airway, and are reliable for close follow-up (5,6). Unfavorable cancers are usually high volume, have extensive bilateral disease, and are often associated with airway compromise. In addition to physical findings, primary tumor volume calculated on pretreatment computed tomography (CT) or magnetic resonance imaging (MRI) is a useful predictor of local control after RT (5–7). Patients with tumors 3.5 cm^3 or smaller have a higher likelihood of local control after irradiation than those with higher volume cancers. The choice of CT vs MRI is dependent on the diagnostic radiologist; CT is the preferred modality used to image the larynx at the University of Florida. The "threshold" volume at which the likelihood of local control after RT diminishes may vary with the observer and/or the imaging modality.

Patients with favorable tumors may be treated with RT or conservation surgery, which would necessitate an extended hemilaryngectomy or a near-total laryngectomy. The major disadvantage of partial laryngectomy is that a relatively small subset of patients (probably less than 10%) is suitable for the procedure (8). In contrast, 36 of 54 patients (67%) treated at the University of Florida between 1980 and 1988 for T3 glottic cancer received RT alone (6). Additionally, the functional outcome after partial laryngectomy may vary considerably, from that of a classical hemilaryngectomy to a controlled fistula for speaking with a permanent tracheostomy. Therefore, the preferred conservation treatment for patients with favorable T3 tumors is RT alone. Recent data suggest that altered fractionation schedules may offer improved local-regional control rates compared with conventional fractionation (9,10). Two alternatives shown to be efficacious include the University of Florida hyperfractionation schedule and the M.D. Anderson Cancer Center concomitant boost technique (10).

Patients with unfavorable T3 cancers may be treated either with total laryngectomy and neck dissection, which is usually followed by postoperative RT, or with two to three cycles of induction chemotherapy followed by RT for those patients who have a partial (≥50% response) or complete response to the chemotherapy. Recent data suggest that although induction chemotherapy may be used to select patients who are more likely to be cured by RT, it does not improve local-regional control or survival (11). In contrast, concomitant RT and chemotherapy appear to offer improved local-regional control and survival rates for patients with advanced head and neck cancers (11–15). In addition to the high primary tumor volume that defines the unfavorable cancer, pretreatment CT of the larynx may be used to detect cartilage sclerosis, which is also significantly related to the likelihood of tumor control with RT (5,7).

Patients with T4 glottic carcinoma may be treated with either total laryngectomy and neck dissection combined with adjuvant RT or RT combined with adjuvant chemotherapy. Conservation surgery is not a realistic option, and RT alone is feasible only for the small subset of patients with low-volume disease who are staged as having T4 tumors based on minimal cartilage involvement or minimal extension into the soft tissues of the neck (usually through the cricothyroid membrane). Our philosophy is to treat patients with advanced T4 cancers with total laryngectomy and to treat patients who have relatively low-volume tumors with RT and concomitant chemotherapy. Although patients who undergo a total laryngectomy may be rehabilitated with a tracheoesophageal puncture, the majority use an artificial ("electric") larynx *(16)*. Adjuvant chemotherapy regimens usually include cisplatin, carboplatin, and/or fluorouracil. The optimal combination of RT and concomitant chemotherapy is currently unclear. Our current preference is to use hyperfractionated RT and weekly cisplatin (30 mg/m^2). Another option is RT and concomitant weekly carboplatin and paclitaxel *(9,17)*.

2.2. Supraglottic Carcinoma

Favorable T3 cancers are low-volume, exophytic lesions with involvement of the preepiglottic space *(18,19)*. Unfavorable T3 tumors are high-volume, endophytic lesions that are often associated with vocal cord fixation and airway compromise *(18)*. Volume of the primary tumor on pretreatment CT or MRI is a useful predictor of local control after RT; patients with tumors 6 cm^3 or less have a significantly higher likelihood of local control than those with higher volume cancers *(7,19)*. Patients with favorable T3 cancers are treated with either supraglottic laryngectomy or RT. Our preference is to use a hyperfractionated RT schedule if patients are treated with a conventional portal arrangement. The M.D. Anderson Cancer Center concomitant boost technique is used because of logistical considerations if the patient is treated with intensity-modulated radiation therapy (IMRT) *(9)*. Compared with RT alone, supraglottic laryngectomy results in a better local control rate but is associated with an increased risk of complications; in approximately 5% of surgery patients, the procedure is converted to a total laryngectomy because of the anatomic extent of the lesion *(18)*. However, most patients with T3 lesions are unsuitable for conservation surgery because of their medical condition (cardiac and/or pulmonary disease) or anatomic extent of the primary tumor. Approximately 15 to 20% are suitable for supraglottic laryngectomy; the remaining patients are treated with RT.

Patients with unfavorable T3 cancers are treated with total laryngectomy and neck dissection followed by postoperative RT or RT and concomitant chemotherapy. Few such patients are suitable for conservation surgery.

T4 supraglottic cancers are treated with total laryngectomy and dissection followed by postoperative RT. Patients with low-volume T4 tumors, usually owing to modest involvement of the base of tongue or pharyngeal wall, are treated with RT and concomitant chemotherapy.

3. RADIATION THERAPY TECHNIQUE

3.1. Glottic Carcinoma

Patients are treated with parallel-opposed fields that include the primary lesion and internal jugular lymph nodes (levels II, III, and IV) *(20)*. Most patients have a clinically negative neck so that it is not necessary to electively irradiate the lateral retropharyngeal nodes that are usually located anterolateral to the C1 and C2 vertebral bodies *(21)*. Thus, a significant amount of salivary tissue is excluded from the initial portals so there is no clear advantage associated with IMRT. The anterior aspect of the neck is tangentially irradiated because of the proximity of the anterior commissure to the anterior skin surface (usually approx 1 cm); the inferior border is 2 cm below the inferior extent of the primary tumor (usually 1–2 cm below the bottom of the cricoid cartilage) (Fig. 1) *(22)*. Patients receive 1.2 Gy per fraction twice daily with a minimum 6-h interfraction interval in a continuous course to a total dose of 74.4 Gy; the dose is usually specified to an isodose line that includes the tumor with minimal if any margin (usually the 95% isodose line, normalized to D_{max} at the central axis of the fields). The fields are weighted 3:2 to the side of the lesion (if it is lateralized) and reduced at 45.6 and 60 Gy. The low neck receives 50 Gy in 25 fractions, once-daily fractionation with a thin midline trachea block (Fig. 2) *(23)*.

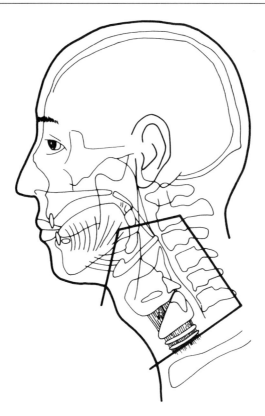

Fig. 1. Radiation treatment technique for carcinoma of glottic larynx, stage T3–T4N0. The patient is treated supine, and the field is shaped with Lipowitz's metal. Anteriorly, the field is allowed to fall off. The entire preepiglottic space is included by encompassing the hyoid bone and epiglottis. The superior border (just above the angle of the mandible) includes the jugulodigastric lymph nodes. Posteriorly, a portion of the spinal cord must be included within the field to ensure adequate coverage of the midjugular lymph nodes: spinal accessory lymph nodes themselves are at little risk of involvement. The lower border is slanted (1) to facilitate matching with the low neck field and (2) to reduce the length of the spinal cord in the high-dose field. The inferior border is placed at the bottom of the cricoid cartilage if the patient has no subglottic spread; in the presence of subglottic extension, the inferior border must be lowered according to the disease extent. (Reprinted from ref. *22*, with permission from Elsevier.)

3.2. Supraglottic Carcinoma

The portals for supraglottic carcinoma are similar to those used for advanced glottic cancer except that the anterior neck skin may sometimes be spared, and the inferior border is usually at the bottom of the cricoid cartilage (Fig. 3) *(23)*. The likelihood of positive retropharyngeal lymph nodes is low; however, if clinically positive neck nodes are present, the risk is increased, and the superior border of the field is placed at the jugular foramen *(21)*. The dose fractionation schedule is the same as that described for T3–T4 glottic cancers. Patients with ipsilateral positive nodes may benefit from IMRT to reduce the dose to the contralateral parotid and, thus, long-term xerostomia. The M.D. Anderson Cancer Center concomitant boost technique, consisting of 72 Gy in 42 fractions over 6 wk, is employed for patients who receive IMRT *(9)*.

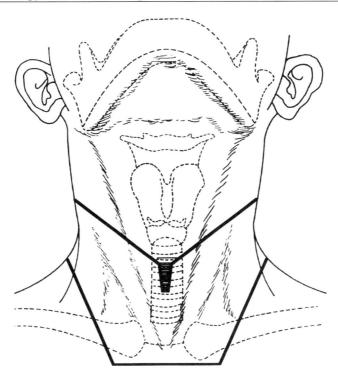

Fig. 2. Example of a portal for T3N0 glottic carcinoma. Low neck portal. The main nodes at risk are the low jugular and lateral paratracheal. The delphian node would be in the primary portal. A very narrow and short midline shield is used. (Reprinted from ref. *23*, with permission from Lippincott Williams & Wilkins.)

3.3. Treatment of the Neck

The risk of subclinical disease in the cervical lymph nodes exceeds 20% for patients with T3–T4 laryngeal cancer. Therefore, the internal lymph nodes (levels II, III, and IV) are electively irradiated bilaterally. Patients with N1 or early N2B neck disease with the positive nodes located within the high-dose fields are treated with RT alone *(24)*. Patients with more advanced neck disease usually undergo a planned neck dissection after RT *(24,25)*. Recent data suggest that for patients who have experienced a complete response of the neck disease after RT, the likelihood of an isolated recurrence in the neck is low regardless of the initial N stage *(26–28)*. Therefore, it is our current practice to evaluate the response in the neck 1 mo after completion of RT with CT scan and to proceed with a planned neck dissection if the probability of residual disease is thought to be 5% or higher *(28,29)*. Patients who are thought to have less than a 5% risk of persistent neck disease undergo a second CT scan in 3–4 mo after the first posttreatment scan.

4. TREATMENT RESULTS

4.1. Glottic Carcinoma

Seventy-five patients were treated with RT alone for T3 squamous cell carcinoma of the glottic larynx at the University of Florida between 1966 and 1994; no patient received adjuvant chemotherapy *(30)*. The local control and ultimate local control rates at 5 yr were 63 and 86%, respectively. A recent multivariate analysis of 55 patients with glottic carcinoma treated

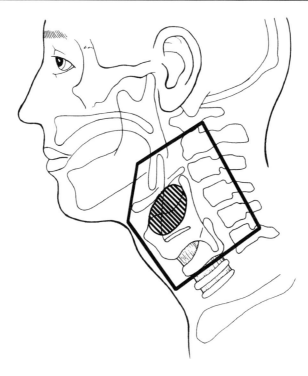

Fig. 3. Example of a portal for a lesion of the lower epiglottis or false vocal cord and a clinically negative neck. The subdigastric nodes are included but not the junctional nodes. Depending on the anatomy and tumor extent, the anterior border may fall off (i.e., "flash"), or a small strip of skin may be shielded. (Reprinted from ref. *23*, with permission from Lippincott Williams & Wilkins.)

with definitive RT revealed that tumor volume ($p = 0.0042$) had a more significant impact on local control than T stage ($p = 0.0629$) *(7)*. Pameijer et al. *(5)* found that cartilage sclerosis, in addition to tumor volume, is a useful determinant of local control after RT (Table 1) *(5)*. The relationship of vocal cord mobility, at various points during and after radiotherapy, to local control after RT has been evaluated. Whether the vocal cord becomes mobile or remains fixed does not appear to affect the probability of local control *(30)*.

The local control rates after RT and ultimate local control rates from several institutions, including the University of Florida, are summarized in Table 2 *(22,30–36)*. Wang *(32)* reported a 67% rate of local control after radiotherapy for 41 patients treated with twice-daily fractionation, compared with 42% in 24 patients treated with once-daily RT.

The 5-yr local-regional control and ultimate local-regional control rates for patients treated at the University of Florida were 61 and 86%, respectively. The 5-yr absolute and cause-specific survival rates were 54 and 78%, respectively. Foote et al. *(8)* reported on 81 patients treated with surgery alone for previously untreated T3 glottic carcinoma at the Mayo Clinic between 1979 and 1981; 6 patients (7%) underwent a near-total laryngectomy, and the remainder underwent total laryngectomy. The investigators observed a 74% 5-yr local-regional control rate and 5-yr absolute and cause-specific survival rates of 54 and 78%, respectively. A review of the literature indicates that primary RT and laryngectomy result in similar rates of ultimate local-regional control, survival, and severe complications *(30)*. This is true even for patients treated at institutions at which the policy is to treat essentially all patients with T3 cancers with primary RT. The major reason to select patients unlikely to be cured by RT alone

Table 1
Computed Tomography Risk Profiles for Patients With T3 Glottic Larynx Carcinoma (N = 42)

Risk groups (for local recurrance)	Criteria	No. of patients	Local control
Low risk (n = 21)	Volume < 3.5 cm^3 No cartilage sclerosis	13	19/21 (90%)
	Volume < 3.5 cm^3 Single cartilage sclerosis	8	
Moderate risk (n = 14)	Volume < 3.5 cm^3 >1 cartilage sclerosis	5	
	Volume > 3.5 cm^3 No cartilage sclerosis	3	6/14 (43%)
	Volume > 3.5 cm^3 Single cartilage sclerosis	6	
High risk (n = 7)[a]	Volume > 3.5 cm^3 >1 cartilage sclerosis	7	1/7 (14%)

[a]Two of these patients had focal cartilage erosion.
Reprinted from ref. 5.

Table 2
Stage T3 Glottic Carcinoma Treated With Radiation

Investigator	Institution	No. of patients	Minimum follow-up (yr)	Local control (%)	Ultimate control after salvage surgery (%)
Harwood et al. *(31)*	Princess Margaret, Toronto	112	3	51	77
Wang *(32)*	Massachusetts General, Boston	65	Not stated	57	—
Fletcher et al. *(33)*	M. D. Anderson, Houston	17	2	77	—
Skolyszewski and Reinfuss *(34)*	15 European centers	91	3	50	—
Wylie et al. *(35)*	Christie Hospital, Manchester, England	114	1.9	68	80
Mills *(36)*	Capetown, South Africa	18	2	44	78
Mendenhall et al. *(30)*	University of Florida, Gainesville	75	2	63	86

Adapted from ref. 22.

is the morbidity and expense associated with a course of unsuccessful RT and the approximately one-in-three risk of a major complication associated with salvage surgery, such as an orocutaneous fistula. The major difference between RT and surgery is that RT is associated with a significantly increased likelihood of laryngeal voice preservation *(8,30)*.

Nine patients with T4 glottic carcinomas were treated with radical RT at the University of Florida between 1964 and 1994; in 8 of 9 patients, the disease was locally controlled after RT *(37)*. The results of radiation treatment from the University of Florida and several other institutions are summarized in Table 3 *(37–44)*; the tumor was locally controlled after RT for

Table 3
Literature Review: Treatment of T4 Laryngeal Cancer
With Radical Radiotherapy

	No. of patients	Local control
Glottis		
Parsons et al. *(37)*	9	8
Sagerman et al. *(38)*	1	0
Karim et al. *(39)*	38	24
Harwood et al. *(40)*	39	22
Total	87	54 (62%)
Supraglottis		
Parsons et al. *(37)*	21	8
Karim et al. *(39)*	79	55
Bataini et al. *(41)*	61	20
Issa *(42)*	20	6
Fletcher et al. *(43)*	26	14
Harwood et al. *(44)*	168	81
Sagerman et al. *(38)*	11	3
Total	386	187 (48%)

Adapted from ref. *37.*

Table 4
Treatment of Stage T4 Glottic Carcinoma

Investigator	Tumor stage	No. of patients	Method of treatment	Results (NED) (%)
Jesse *(45)*	T4 N0–N+	48	Laryngectomy	54 at 4 yr
Ogura et al. *(46)*	T4 N0	11	Laryngectomy	45 at 3 yr
Skolnick et al. *(47)*	T4 N0	7	Laryngectomy	30 at 5 yr
Vermund *(48)*	T4 N0	31	Laryngectomy	35 at 5 yr
Stewart and Jackson *(49)*	T4 N0	13	RT with surgery for salvage	38 at 5 yr
Harwood et al. *(40)*	T4 N0	56	RT with surgery for salvage	49 at 5 yr[a]

Abbreviations: NED, no evidence of disease; RT, radiotherapy.
[a]Life-table method: uncorrected for deaths from intercurrent disease.
Reprinted from ref. *40*, with permission.

almost two-thirds of patients *(37)*. The cure rates after surgery or RT for T4 glottic cancers are summarized in Table 4 *(40,45–49)*.

4.2. Supraglottic Larynx

One hundred ten patients were treated with radical RT for T3 (89 patients) and T4 (21 patients) supraglottic carcinoma at the University of Florida between 1964 and 1992; 1 patient received induction chemotherapy, and the remainder underwent RT alone or combined with a planned neck dissection *(50)*. Fifty-six patients had American Joint Committee on Cancer (AJCC) stage III disease (T3N0–N1), and 54 patients had stage IV disease (T3–T4; N2–N3). The 5-yr rate of local control after RT for 89 patients with T3 cancers was 68%. Excluding 19 patients who died less than 2 yr from treatment with the primary site continuously disease free,

Table 5
T3 Supraglottic Carcinoma Treated With Irradiation

Investigator	Institution	No. of patients	Local control (%)
Mendenhall et al. (51)	University of Florida, Gainesville	89	68
Fletcher and Hamberger (52)	M.D. Anderson, Houston	29	62
Ghossein et al. (53)	Institut Curie, Paris	35	46
Wang et al. (54)	Massachusetts General, Boston	51	76

Reprinted from ref. 50, with permission.

the local control, and ultimate local control rates were 45 of 70 (64%) and 57 of 70 (81%), respectively. Local control after RT vs subsite within the supraglottis revealed the following: suprahyoid epiglottis, 2 of 3 (67%); infrahyoid epiglottis, 23 of 32 (72%); false vocal cord, 8 of 18 (44%); aryepiglottic fold, 11 of 16 (69%); and arytenoid, 1 of 1 (100%). Local control vs vocal cord mobility revealed the following: normal mobility, 34 of 48 (71%); impaired mobility, 6 of 11 (55%); and fixation, 4 of 9 (44%). False vocal cord tumors are probably more likely to be high-volume, endophytic lesions associated with reduced or absent vocal cord mobility and a lower probability of cure after RT.

Local control after RT was inversely related to tumor volume as calculated on pretreatment CT scans: < 6 cm^3, 11 of 13 (85%) vs ≥6 cm^3 or more, 9 of 19 (47%; $p = 0.04$). High tumor volume is also associated with a lower rate of local control with a functional larynx compared with low-volume primary tumor (19). Multivariate analysis of local control results revealed the following ranking of possible prognostic factors: twice-daily vs once-daily fractionation ($p = 0.0677$), site within the supraglottis ($p = 0.1033$), N stage ($p = 0.0756$), sex ($p = 0.1812$), T stage ($p = 0.6290$), vocal cord mobility ($p = 0.6817$), suitability for conservation surgery ($p = 0.6650$), and pretreatment CT scan obtained ($p = 0.7738$). A recent multivariate analysis of 114 patients treated with definitive RT for supraglottic carcinoma revealed that tumor volume ($p = 0.0220$) had a more significant impact on local control compared with T stage ($p = 0.2791$) (7).

Local control after RT at several institutions is illustrated in Table 5 (50–54). The application of the 1998 AJCC (55) staging has led to a "negative stage migration" whereby some T3–T4 cancers are categorized into earlier T stages. Hinerman et al. (56) reported on 99 patients with 1998 AJCC T3 cancers treated with RT at the University of Florida and observed a 5-yr local control rate of 62%.

Twenty-one patients with T4 supraglottic carcinomas had a 5-yr local control rate of 56% after RT (50). In a recent update of the University of Florida experience, Hinerman et al. (56) reported a 62%, 5-year local control rate for 28 patients treated with RT for 1998 AJCC T4 carcinomas. RT local control rates from a variety of institutions are summarized in Table 3. Overall, the disease was locally controlled in approx 50% of patients, which is somewhat less than observed after treatment of T4 glottic cancer (50).

Local-regional control rates at 5 yr for 110 patients with T3–T4 cancers treated at the University of Florida were as follows: stage III, 68%; stage IV, 51%; and overall, 60%. The 5-yr cause-specific and absolute survival rates were as follows: stage III, 83 and 52%; stage IV, 48 and 28%; and overall, 66 and 40%, respectively.

Comparison of local-regional control and survival rates for patients treated with primary RT vs surgery is difficult because surgical series tend to contain a higher proportion of patients with early N-stage disease that is significantly related to long-term control of neck disease and the likelihood of distant metastases *(51,56,57)*. If any differences exist, they are probably modest.

4.3. Chemoradiation

Almost all the data pertaining to efficacy of adjuvant chemotherapy for patients with head and neck cancer include patients with a variety of primary sites, including the larynx. The Radiation Therapy Oncology Group (RTOG) recently reported on the results of their 91–11 trial whereby patients with laryngeal squamous cell carcinoma were randomized to three cycles of induction fluorouracil and cisplatin chemotherapy followed by RT in complete and partial responders, three cycles of cisplatin and concomitant RT, and RT alone *(15)*. The RT consisted of 70 Gy in 35 once-daily fractions in all three arms. There were no significant differences in survival or laryngectomy-free survival between the three arms. However, time to laryngectomy for patients who received concomitant cisplatin and RT was significantly improved compared with those who received induction chemotherapy ($p = 0.009$) or RT alone ($p = 0.0004$).

5. COMPLICATIONS

5.1. Glottic Carcinoma

Severe complications are defined as those that necessitate an operation or hospitalization and/or result in death. Five of 75 patients (7%) treated with RT alone for T3 glottic cancer at the University of Florida experienced severe complications including the following: laryngeal edema necessitating a temporary (1 patient) or permanent (1 patient) tracheostomy, chondronecrosis that necessitated total laryngectomy (1 patient), total laryngectomy for a suspected local recurrence with a pathologically negative specimen (1 patient), and fatal airway obstruction (1 patient) *(30)*. Severe complications developed in 7 of 21 patients (33%) who underwent a salvage laryngectomy: wound dehiscence that necessitated a split-thickness skin graft (1 patient) and pharyngocutaneous fistula (6 patients). Therefore, 11 patients (15%) experienced severe complications after RT and/or salvage surgery.

Foote et al. *(8)* reported that 13 of 81 patients (16%) treated surgically at the Mayo Clinic experienced significant postoperative complications; 1 patient (1%) died postoperatively of a myocardial infarction. Ten of 65 patients (15%) treated with surgery alone or combined with adjuvant RT at the University of Florida experienced a severe complication; 1 (1%) died postoperatively of upper gastrointestinal bleeding and sepsis *(6)*.

One of 9 patients (11%) irradiated at the University of Florida for T4 vocal cord cancer experienced a severe treatment complication *(37)*.

5.2. Supraglottic Carcinoma

Eight of 110 patients irradiated for T3 (3 of 89, 3%) and T4 (5 of 21, 24%) carcinomas of the supraglottic larynx experienced severe complication *(50)*. The risk of major complications after RT is lower than for patients undergoing a supraglottic laryngectomy, particularly for those with T3 cancers.

6. FOLLOW-UP

Patients return to report an interim history and undergo a head and neck examination every 4–8 wk for the first 2 yr, every 3 mo for the third year, every 6 mo for the fourth and fifth years, and annually thereafter. Chest radiographs and thyroid function tests are obtained yearly.

CT may be used for follow-up examination of patients after RT and may detect local recurrences earlier than physical examination would (58). Fluorodeoxyglucose (FDG)–positron emission tomography (PET) may be used to detect local recurrence in patients with findings on CT that are highly suspicious for local recurrence. Patients with increased uptake on the FDG-PET scan would undergo biopsy and salvage surgery (if positive), whereas those with a negative scan would have follow-up observation and would not be subjected to the risk of chondronecrosis precipitated by the biopsy procedure. Salvage laryngectomy may be indicated for the occasional patient with findings that are very suspicious for a local recurrence in the absence of a positive biopsy.

7. CONCLUSIONS

Pretreatment CT of the larynx can be used to select patients with favorable lesions for treatment with radiotherapy alone with a high likelihood of cure with larynx preservation (59). Those with unfavorable cancers are probably best treated by surgery and postoperative RT or induction chemotherapy followed by RT in those patients whose tumors respond (9,60). Because pretreatment CT of the larynx is routinely part of the workup for patients with advanced laryngeal cancer, it has the obvious advantages of no additional cost or morbidity, compared with induction chemotherapy. The major disadvantage of pretreatment CT is that it is operator dependent and information pertaining to tumor volume and cartilage sclerosis may not be obtained if the quality of the scan and/or diagnostic radiologist is suboptimal.

Recent data suggest that some altered fractionation schedules result in improved local-regional control rates compared with conventionally fractionated RT (9). Additionally, concomitant RT and chemotherapy appear to result in improved local-regional control and survival compared with RT alone (11,15). The major disadvantage of concomitant RT and chemotherapy is increased acute toxicity. The optimal combination of the two modalities is unclear and under investigation.

REFERENCES

1. O'Sullivan B, Mackillop W, Gilbert R, et al. Controversies in the management of laryngeal cancer: results of an international survey of patterns of care. Radiother Oncol 1994; 31:23–32.
2. Harari PM. Why has induction chemotherapy for advanced head and neck cancer become a United States community standard of practice? J Clin Oncol 1997; 15:2050–2055.
3. Department of Veterans Affairs Laryngeal Cancer Study Group. Induction chemotherapy plus radiation compared with surgery plus radiation in patients with advanced laryngeal cancer. N Engl J Med 1991; 324:1685–1690.
4. Lefebvre JL, Chevalier D, Luboinski B, et al. Larynx preservation in pyriform sinus cancer: preliminary results of a European Organization for Research and Treatment of Cancer phase III trial. EORTC Head and Neck Cancer Cooperative Group. J Natl Cancer Inst 1996; 88:890–899.
5. Pameijer FA, Mancuso AA, Mendenhall WM, et al. Can pretreatment computed tomography predict local control in T3 squamous cell carcinoma of the glottic larynx treated with definitive radiotherapy? Int J Radiat Oncol Biol Phys 1997; 37:1011–1021.
6. Mendenhall WM, Parsons JT, Stringer SP, et al. Stage T3 squamous cell carcinoma of the glottic larynx: a comparison of laryngectomy and irradiation. Int J Radiat Oncol Biol Phys 1992; 23:725–732.

7. Mendenhall WM, Morris CG, Amdur RJ, et al. Parameters that predict local control after definitive radiotherapy for squamous cell carcinoma of the head and neck. Head Neck 2003; 25:535–542.

8. Foote RL, Olsen KD, Buskirk SJ, et al. Laryngectomy alone for T3 glottic cancer. Head Neck 1994; 16:406–412.

9. Mendenhall WM, Riggs CE, Amdur RJ, et al. Altered fractionation and/or adjuvant chemotherapy in definitive irradiation of squamous cell carcinoma of the head and neck. Laryngoscope 2003; 113:546–551.

10. Fu KK, Pajak TF, Trotti A, et al. A Radiation Therapy Oncology Group (RTOG) phase III randomized study to compare hyperfractionation and two variants of accelerated fractionation to standard fractionation radiotherapy for head and neck squamous cell carcinomas: first report of RTOG 9003. Int J Radiat Oncol Biol Phys 2000; 48:7–16.

11. Pignon JP, Bourhis J, Domenge C, et al. Chemotherapy added to locoregional treatment for head and neck squamous-cell carcinoma: three meta-analyses of updated individual data. Lancet 2000; 355:949–955.

12. Brizel DM, Albers ME, Fisher SR, et al. Hyperfractionated irradiation with or without concurrent chemotherapy for locally advanced head and neck cancer. N Engl J Med 1998; 338:1798–1804.

13. Adelstein DJ, Lavertu P, Saxton JP, et al. Mature results of a phase III randomized trial comparing concurrent chemoradiotherapy with radiation therapy alone in patients with stage III and IV squamous cell carcinoma of the head and neck. Cancer 2000; 88:876–883.

14. Jeremic B, Shibamoto Y, Milicic B, et al. Hyperfractionated radiation therapy with or without concurrent low-dose daily cisplatin in locally advanced squamous cell carcinoma of the head and neck: a prospective randomized trial. J Clin Oncol 2000; 18:1458–1464.

15. Forastiere AA, Berkey B, Maor M, et al. Phase III trial to preserve the larynx: Induction chemotherapy and radiotherapy versus concomitant chemoradiotherapy versus radiotherapy alone, Intergroup Trial R91-11. [Abstr.] Proc Annu Meet Am Soc Clin Oncol 2001; 20:2a.

16. Mendenhall WM, Morris CG, Stringer SP, et al. Voice rehabilitation after total laryngectomy and postoperative radiotherapy. J Clin Oncol 2002; 20:2500–2505.

17. Suntharalingam M, Haas ML, Conley BA, et al. The use of carboplatin and paclitaxel with daily radiotherapy in patients with locally advanced squamous cell carcinoma of the head and neck. Int J Radiat Oncol Biol Phys 2000; 47:49–56.

18. Mendenhall WM, Parsons JT, Mancuso AA, Stringer SP, Cassisi NJ. Larynx. In: Perez CA, Brady LW, eds. Principles and Practice of Radiation Oncology, 3rd ed. Philadelphia: Lippincott-Raven, 1997:1075–1099.

19. Mancuso AA, Mukherji SK, Schmalfuss I, et al. Preradiotherapy computed tomography as a predictor of local control in supraglottic carcinoma. J Clin Oncol 1999; 17:631–637.

20. Mendenhall WM, Million RR. Elective neck irradiation for squamous cell carcinoma of the head and neck: analysis of time-dose factors and causes of failure. Int J Radiat Oncol Biol Phys 1986; 12:741–746.

21. McLaughlin MP, Mendenhall WM, Mancuso AA, et al. Retropharyngeal adenopathy as a predictor of outcome in squamous cell carcinoma of the head and neck. Head Neck 1995; 17:190–198.

22. Parsons JT, Mendenhall WM, Mancuso AA, et al. Twice-a-day radiotherapy for T3 squamous cell carcinoma of the glottic larynx. Head Neck 1989; 11:123–128.

23. Million RR, Cassisi NJ, Mancuso AA, Stringer SP, Mendenhall WM, Parsons JT. Management of the neck for squamous cell carcinoma. In: Million RR, Cassisi NJ, eds. Management of Head and Neck Cancer: A Multidisciplinary Approach, 2nd ed. Philadelphia: JB Lippincott, 1994:75–142.

24. Mendenhall WM, Million RR, Cassisi NJ. Squamous cell carcinoma of the head and neck treated with radiation therapy: the role of neck dissection for clinically positive neck nodes. Int J Radiat Oncol Biol Phys 1986; 12:733-740.

25. Ellis ER, Mendenhall WM, Rao PV, et al. Incisional or excisional neck-node biopsy before definitive radiotherapy, alone or followed by neck dissection. Head Neck 1991; 13:177–183.

26. Johnson CR, Silverman LN, Clay LB, et al. Radiotherapeutic management of bulky cervical lymphadenopathy in squamous cell carcinoma of the head and neck: is postradiotherapy neck dissection necessary? Radiat Oncol Invest 1998; 6:52–57.

27. Peters LJ, Weber RS, Morrison WH, et al. Neck surgery in patients with primary oropharyngeal cancer treated by radiotherapy. Head Neck 1996; 18:552–559.

28. Mendenhall WM, Villaret DB, Amdur RJ, et al. Planned neck dissection after definitive radiotherapy for squamous cell carcinoma of the head and neck. Head Neck 2002; 24:1012–1018.

29. Ojiri H, Mendenhall WM, Stringer SP, et al. Post-RT CT results as a predictive model for the necessity of planned post-RT neck dissection in patients with cervical metastatic disease from squamous cell carcinoma. Int J Radiat Oncol Biol Phys 2002; 52:420–428.

30. Mendenhall WM, Parsons JT, Mancuso AA, et al. Definitive radiotherapy for T3 squamous cell carcinoma of the glottic larynx. J Clin Oncol 1997; 15:2394–2402.

31. Harwood AR, Beale FA, Cummings BJ, et al. T3 glottic cancer: an analysis of dose-time-volume factors. Int J Radiat Oncol Biol Phys 1980; 6:675–680.
32. Wang CC. Carcinoma of the larynx. In: Wang CC, ed. Radiation Therapy for Head and Neck Neoplasms, 3rd ed. New York: Wiley-Liss, 1997:221–255.
33. Fletcher GH, Lindberg RD, Jesse RH. Radiation therapy for cancer of the larynx and pyriform sinus. Eye Ear Nose Throat Digest 1969; 31:58–67.
34. Skolyszewski J, Reinfuss M. The results of radiotherapy of cancer of the larynx in six European countries. Radiobiol Radiother (Berl) 1981; 22:32–43.
35. Wylie JP, Sen M, Swindell R, et al. Definitive radiotherapy for 114 cases of T3N0 glottic carcinoma: influence of dose-volume parameters on outcome. Radiother Oncol 1999; 53:15–21.
36. Mills EE. Early glottic carcinoma: factors affecting radiation failure, results of treatment and sequelae. Int J Radiat Oncol Biol Phys 1979; 5:811–817.
37. Parsons JT, Mendenhall WM, Stringer SP, et al. T4 laryngeal carcinoma: radiotherapy alone with surgery reserved for salvage. Int J Radiat Oncol Biol Phys 1998; 40:549–552.
38. Sagerman RH, Chung CT, King GA, et al. High dose preoperative irradiation for advanced laryngeal-hypopharyngeal cancer. Ann Otol Rhinol Laryngol 1979; 88:178–182.
39. Karim AB, Kralendonk JH, Njo KH, et al. Radiation therapy for advanced (T3T4N0-N3M0) laryngeal carcinoma: the need for a change of strategy: A radiotherapeutic viewpoint. Int J Radiat Oncol Biol Phys 1987; 13:1625–1633.
40. Harwood AR, Beale FA, Cummings BJ, et al. T4N0M0 glottic cancer: an analysis of dose-time-volume factors. Int J Radiat Oncol Biol Phys 1981; 7:1507–1512.
41. Bataini JP, Brugere J, Jaulerry CH, et al. Radiation treatment of lateral epilaryngeal cancer. Prognostic factors and results. Am J Clin Oncol 1984; 7:641–645.
42. Issa PY. Cancer of the supraglottic larynx treated by radiotherapy exclusively. Int J Radiat Oncol Biol Phys 1988; 15:843–850.
43. Fletcher GH, Lindberg RD, Hamberger A, et al. Reasons for irradiation failure in squamous cell carcinoma of the larynx. Laryngoscope 1975; 85:987–1003.
44. Harwood AR, Beale FA, Cummings BJ, et al. Supraglottic laryngeal carcinoma: an analysis of dose-time-volume factors in 410 patients. Int J Radiat Oncol Biol Phys 1983; 9:311–319.
45. Jesse RH. The evaluation of treatment of patients with extensive squamous cancer of the vocal cords. Laryngoscope 1975; 85:1424–1429.
46. Ogura JH, Sessions DG, Spector GJ. Analysis of surgical therapy for epidermoid carcinoma of the laryngeal glottis. Laryngoscope 1975; 85:1522–1530.
47. Skolnik EM, Yee KF, Wheatley MA, et al. Carcinoma of the laryngeal glottis: therapy and end results. Laryngoscope 1975; 85:1453–1466.
48. Vermund H. Role of radiotherapy in cancer of the larynx as related to the TNM system of staging. A review. Cancer 1970; 25:485–504.
49. Stewart JG, Jackson AW. The steepness of the dose response curve both for tumor cure and normal tissue injury. Laryngoscope 1975; 85:1107–1111.
50. Mendenhall WM. T3-4 squamous cell carcinoma of the larynx treated with radiation therapy alone. Semin Radiat Oncol 1998; 8:262–269.
51. Mendenhall WM, Parsons JT, Mancuso AA, et al. Radiotherapy for squamous cell carcinoma of the supraglottic larynx: an alternative to surgery. Head Neck 1996; 18:24–35.
52. Fletcher GH, Hamberger AD. Causes of failure in irradiation of squamous-cell carcinoma of the supraglottic larynx. Radiology 1974; 111:697–700.
53. Ghossein NA, Bataini JP, Ennuyer A, et al. Local control and site of failure in radically irradiated supraglottic laryngeal cancer. Radiology 1974; 112:187–192.
54. Wang CC, Nakfoor BM, Spiro IJ, et al. Role of accelerated fractionated irradiation for supraglottic carcinoma: assessment of results. Cancer J Sci Am 1997; 3:88–91.
55. American Joint Committee on Cancer, American Cancer Society, American College of Surgeons, Fleming ID. AJCC Cancer Staging Handbook From the AJCC Cancer Staging Manual, 5th ed. Philadelphia: Lippincott-Raven, 1998.
56. Hinerman RW, Mendenhall WM, Amdur RJ, et al. Carcinoma of the supraglottic larynx: treatment results with radiotherapy alone or with planned neck dissection. Head Neck 2002; 24:456–467.
57. Ellis ER, Mendenhall WM, Rao PV, et al. Does node location affect the incidence of distant metastases in head and neck squamous cell carcinoma? Int J Radiat Oncol Biol Phys 1989; 17:293–297.
58. Pameijer FA, Hermans R, Mancuso AA, et al. Pre- and post-radiotherapy computed tomography in laryngeal cancer: imaging-based prediction of local failure. Int J Radiat Oncol Biol Phys 1999; 45:359–366.

59. Mendenhall WM, Mancuso AA, Morris CG, et al. Influence of tumour volume on the probability of local control after radiotherapy for squamous cell carcinoma of the head and neck. J Hong Kong Coll Radiol 2003; 6:119–125.

60. Mendenhall WM, Amdur RJ, Hinerman RW, et al. Postoperative radiation therapy for squamous cell carcinoma of the head and neck. Am J Otolaryngol 2003; 24:41–50.

7

Role of Brachytherapy in Treatment of Head and Neck Malignancy

Ravi A. Shankar, MD, Kenneth S. Hu, MD, and Louis B. Harrison, MD

1. INTRODUCTION

Brachytherapy is an important armament available to the radiation oncologist treating cancers occurring in the head and neck region. It is all the more important in this era of organ preservation and improving quality of life *(1,2)*. There are very few sites in the body where locoregional control is so vital to ultimate quality of life, organ function, and survival as in head and neck cancer. Brachytherapy permits dose intensification specifically to the tumor site while minimizing damage to the surrounding normal tissue and organs *(3,4)*. This leads to an increased therapeutic ratio, while the patient also stands to gain functionally, psychologically, and cosmetically.

Brachytherapy can be used as a single modality of treatment in early-stage malignancies *(5)*. Occasionally in early-stage malignancies, brachytherapy has been used in combination with external radiation. It can also be employed in the adjuvant setting following surgery *(6)*. Brachytherapy is a good boost technique for treating tumors with high-grade malignancy, lymphovascular or perineural invasion, and cases in which positive or close margins result following surgery *(7–9)*. In advanced cancers, brachytherapy may be used with external beam radiation, surgery, and chemotherapy, in varying combinations *(10)*. Overwhelmingly, the role of brachytherapy in head and neck cancer is limited to tumors with squamous cell pathology.

Another important role of brachytherapy is in the treatment of second and third malignancies of the aerodigestive tract, seen commonly in head and neck cancer patients treated previously with radiation. Conversely, in early stage malignancy, brachytherapy may be utilized as a single modality, reserving other forms of radiation for lesions that may develop at a later date.

However, it important to mention that there have been no prospective double-blind randomized studies comparing brachytherapy with conformal fractionated external radiation in any select group of patients with malignancies of the head and neck region. Given the complex anatomy of the head and neck region, the superior results obtained with brachytherapy can be attributed to the training, skill, technique, and experience of the brachytherapist. These techniques are ideally performed by radiation oncologists in centers with large patient volume, well-trained physicists, a highly functioning multidisciplinary team of head and neck surgeons, plastic surgeons, radiologists, dental surgeons, a pain management team, speech and

From: *Current Clinical Oncology: Squamous Cell Head and Neck Cancer*
Edited by: D. J. Adelstein © Humana Press Inc., Totowa, NJ

swallowing rehabilitation specialists, social workers, and dedicated and knowledgeable nursing staff.

This review will discuss the general principles of brachytherapy in the treatment and management of cancers of the head and neck. Criteria with respect to patient selection, choice of radionuclides, permanent versus temporary implants, low dose rate (LDR) vs high dose rate (HDR) and other multidisciplinary issues will be addressed. For simplicity of presentation, the chapter is subdivided into primary sites.

2. HISTORY

Brachytherapy as a mode of cancer treatment is as old as the history of radiation therapy itself (11). Soon after the discovery of radium in 1898, both radium and radon implants were performed, primarily in France (12) and the United States (13). The earliest applicators were crude devices of capsules of radioactive material placed over the skin. In 1904 Wickham and Derais (14) used sharpened goose quills to perform intratumoral implantations. Abbe (15) and Morton (16) have reported anecdotal reports of cure for cancers in the head and neck. In the 1930s Paterson and Parker (17), in Manchester, devised a method for implantation of radioactive sources, to permit a uniform dose distribution throughout the target volume. Quimby, at Memorial Sloane Kettering (18,19), developed a system of tables and rules in relation to placement of sources in a uniform grid thereby achieving higher doses at the center compared with the periphery of the tumor (18,19).

The discovery of artificial radionuclides in the 1950s opened a new era in brachytherapy. These new radioactive sources could be molded and fashioned to be accommodated in pragmatic ways. Iridium-192 (Ir-192) seeds and ribbons in plastic catheters were used for implanting tumors. In the 1960s, Henschke et al. (20) introduced the ingenious technique of afterloading into tubes/catheters placed within the tumor. Remote afterloading techniques further minimized the medical personnel's risk of radiation exposure. Over the years, dedicated physicians, greater sophistication in application techniques, improvement in dosimetry planning, and stringent quality control measures have made brachytherapy "the ultimate conformal radiation therapy" technique. These scientific advances have enabled brachytherapy to become an effective and important part of the radiation oncologist's arsenal for combating head and neck cancer.

3. BASIC PRINCIPLES

3.1. Patient Selection

The optimal delivery of radiation using brachytherapy begins with selection of the appropriate patient. Patients with alcohol dependency, major neurological deficits, decompensated cardiorespiratory status, memory disorders, and hematological diseases, as well as patients who have contraindications to surgical procedure; are poor candidates for brachytherapy. The presence of multiple comorbid factors may preclude the use of brachytherapy (21); however, age by itself is not a contraindication. Patients must be able to comprehend the brachytherapy procedure so as to provide baseline self-care needs. During the delivery of radiation, the patient must be able to impart care to the tracheostomy site, self-administer feeds via a previously placed nasogastric tube or percutaneous endoscopic gastrostomy (PEG) tube, and operate the patient-controlled anesthesia (PCA) pump, if necessary. A visit to a dentist, familiar with radiation and its risks, prior to initiation of radiation is imperative in this subset of patients. The patient must be able to tolerate the placement of a mandibular shield in the oral cavity to protect against osteoradionecrosis *(22)*.

3.2. Radioisotopes Used in Head and Neck Brachytherapy

Almost all radioactive sources used nowadays are artificially manufactured. The decision to use temporary or permanent implants requires thoughtful decision making and depends on many factors, such as site of tumor, size, organ motion, geometry of target volume, experience of the brachytherapist in the use of the radioisotope, dosimetry, presence of surrounding critical structures, and so on.

Currently the most commonly used removable radioactive source is Ir-192. This γ-emitting isotope undergoes beta decay with a half-life of 73.9 d, and produces polyenergetic γ rays (201–884 Kev), with an average energy of 380 Kev, having a half-value layer of 0.03 cm in lead. Ir-192 is produced in the form of seeds that are encapsulated in steel or platinum. Ir-192 seeds are assembled for clinical application in the form of "ribbons" in nylon tubes, with seeds placed at 1-cm, center-to-center intervals. Usual strengths of Ir-192 seeds are in the range of 0.3–1.0 mg Ra Eq.

Another radioactive source used in temporary implants is iodine 125 (I-125). This isotope decays by electron capture with a half-life of 59.6 d. It emits a polyenergetic beam (27–35 Kev) with an average energy of 23 Kev. Although I-125 is mainly used in permanent implants, it may be an ideal temporary source when rapid fall-off of dose is required *(23)*. This may be the case when critical structures are in close proximity to the target volume. I-125 has a half-value layer of 0.002 cm in lead. In the past, Cesium 137 (Cs-137) in the form of seeds has been used. Radionuclides such as radon 222, radium 226, and tantalum 182 are no longer used *(24)*.

Permanent implants may be advantageous when the target volume is irregular, catheter placement is impractical, and kinking of the nylon tubes is highly probable. I-125 is the most commonly used radioisotope in permanent implants. Other radioisotopes used in permanent implants include palladium 103 and gold 198.

3.3. Techniques

Successful brachytherapy requires meticulous placement of radioactive sources in a tumor volume. In fact, palpation of the tumor and its boundaries, awareness of adjacent critical structures, and the relationship of the tumor to the surrounding structures are of utmost importance for optimal placement of radioactive sources. The main techniques used in photon-emitting implants will be mentioned briefly *(28)*. Many modifications of these techniques have evolved over the years. The main techniques that have been utilized in the placement of radioactive sources in the head and neck are described below.

3.3.1. PIERQUIN AND CHASSAGNE GUIDE GUTTER OR HAIRPIN TECHNIQUE

In this technique, hairpins consisting of two parallel branches with the top shaped like the letter M are implanted into tumors with the help of rigid guides. The guide materials are either twin or single guide gutters made of stainless steel. This technique is used in most anatomical sites within the head and neck region and can be useful when the tumor volumes are small to moderate.

3.3.2. PLASTIC TUBE TECHNIQUE OF HENSCHKE

Rigid metal guide needles are implanted in the target volume. The placement and spacing can be verified by visualization, ultrasound guidance, or under fluoroscopy. Plastic tubes are then threaded into these rigid hollow needles to cover the entire target volume and are left in place over the entire duration of treatment. The rigid metal needles are removed. The plastic tubes are secured in close proximity to the skin with metallic buttons. Radioactive sources are then afterloaded into these plastic wires following dosimetry planning. This is one of the most popular techniques, and many alterations exist, such as the pushing method of substitution and Raynal's pulling method of substitution. The latter is an excellent technical method for making loops within the tumor volume and is commonly used in base of tongue brachytherapy implants. Large tumors can be effectively treated.

3.3.3. HYPODERMIC NEEDLE TECHNIQUE OF PIERQUIN

Hypodermic needles, beveled at both ends, are introduced into the tumor and transfixed to the skin at either end. Ir-192 wires are introduced into the hollow needles until only a small segment protrudes on both ends. Spacing material is then slipped into the ends, and lead caps are crushed into place. This technique is especially useful in tumors of the lip.

3.3.4. THREAD TECHNIQUE

Radioactive sources are braided onto suture materials and then directly sewn into desired positions within the target volume. Modifications of this technique exist whereby threaded radioactive sources are initially evenly sutured onto a mesh, which is then secured onto the tumor bed.

3.3.5. DIRECT IMPLANTATION METHOD

Radioactive seeds are directly placed into the planned target volume, permanently. This requires meticulous planning and radiological guidance for accurate placement of the seeds to achieve good geometry and dose distribution.

A full description of the techniques of brachytherapy, appropriate for each individual site in the head and neck region, is beyond the scope of this chapter, and interested readers are referred to standard publications (25–29).

3.4. High-Dose Rate vs Low-Dose Rate Brachytherapy

The miniaturization of high-activity radioisotopes is one of the many technological advances in radiation oncology. Moreover the progress in computer technology has led to the establishment of remote afterloading high-dose rate (HDR) brachytherapy. HDR brachytherapy is now considered a safe and efficient technique. The advantages of HDR compared with low-dose rate (LDR) are enhanced ability to conform to target volume more precisely, decreased risk of radiation exposure for medical personnel, better dose distribution and increased homogeneity within the target volume, less radiation dose to normal tissue, decreased delivery time (thus potentially sparing the patient a hospital admission), and less effect of organ motion on dose delivery. The debatable point of HDR vs LDR is related to the radiobiological effects on tissue and cancer cells being exposed to LDR or HDR radiation. Advantages of LDR are continuous exposure of cancer cells to radiation during the entire cell cycle, reduced effects owing to hypoxia in the cells, decreased risk of late normal tissue injury, and the increased repair capacity of normal tissue.

A large number of patients with head and neck malignancies have been treated by HDR brachytherapy (25,49,57,58). Local control rates are as good as those obtained by LDR therapy. Data are continuing to accumulate, given the promising nature of this technique.

Pulsed dose rate (PDR) brachytherapy and fractionated HDR brachytherapy are being investigated whereby the advantages of both HDR and LDR can be achieved advantageously

(30,31). In this remote afterloading technique, the patient receives radiation from a medium dose rate radioisotope. Typically the radiation dose is given for about 10–20 min (pulse dose), every hour, over a period of days. Between pulses, the patient does not receive any radiation and is free to ambulate.

3.5. Team Approach

To perform a successful implant, a radiation oncologist needs the coordinated support of an experienced and well-informed team of anesthesiologists, head and neck surgeons, plastic surgeons, dental surgeons, and physicists. Placement of the surgical incision, grafts, drains, and tracheostomy and wound closure techniques need to be meticulously planned and discussed prior to surgery.

In the postoperative period, well-trained nursing staff should care for the tracheostomy as well as provide appropriate nutrition. During the treatment the patient should receive adequate analgesia. The implantation site is inspected at least twice a day.

Following completion of brachytherapy, removal of the tubes should be carried out in coordination with the ear, nose, and throat surgeons. Prior to removal of the tubes, patients must have intravenous access along with suction and bandage material. A known complication during removal of brachytherapy catheters is arterial hemorrhage, which can be controlled effectively by bidigital compression.

In the postimplant period, the expected side effects such as mucositis, pain, and decreased intake of food and water, need to be addressed with analgesics, mouthwashes, and adequate alimentation.

4. SITES

4.1. Nasopharynx

Cancer of the nasopharynx is surrounded by critical structures such as the brainstem, cochlea, pituitary, optic chaisma, temporal lobes, and salivary glands. Therefore brachytherapy with either permanent or temporary implants *(32)* is often integral and important in the management of nasopharyngeal cancer. Nasopharyngeal tumors are highly radiosensitive and are usually treated with chemoradiation *(33)*. Brachytherapy is more commonly used in the treatment of locally recurrent disease, given its steep dose fall-off with distance and dose optimization potential.

When the entire nasopharyngeal mucosa requires irradiation, temporary intracavitary implants are optimal *(34)*. However, in situations in which the lesion is discrete and localized, permanent implants have been more successful *(35–37)*. Permanent implants can be done via a transoral *(36)*, transnasal *(37)*, or transpalatal *(38)* approach.

Vikram et al. *(37)* using the transnasal approach reported a 2-yr local control rate of 100% in primary nasopharyngeal cancers. Harrison et al. *(38)* used the transpalatal approach in the treatment of recurrent nasopharyngeal tumor, especially for tumors located in the posteriosuperior wall of the nasopharynx. Harrison et al. *(36)* have also applied the transoral technique with equally good control rates.

In the setting of recurrent *(39–43)* nasopharyngeal carcinoma, using brachytherapy, several institutions have reported local control rates of 20–60%. Fu et al. *(44)* treated patients with a combination of limited external radiation and brachytherapy. They obtained a 5-yr survival of 41%. Teo et al. *(45)* utilized brachytherapy alone and obtained 5-yr local control rates of 69% with a 5-yr disease-free survival of 58%. Choy et al. *(46)* treated 43 patients with interstitial implant using Au-198 and obtained a 5-yr local control of 44 to 81% with a 5-yr overall survival of 25 to 65%.

Brachytherapy can also be given as a boost in primary nasopharyngeal tumors or for residual localized disease. Syed et al. *(47)* reported on 15 patients with primary nasopharyngeal cancer who were treated with external radiation and intracavitary boost. The 5- and 10-yr overall rate was 61% for both, whereas the local control rates at 5 and 10 yr were 93 and 77%, respectively. Similarly Wang *(48)* also achieved a markedly improved 5-yr local control rate of 93% by giving a 7–10-Gy intracavitary boost following external radiation of 64 Gy.

Levendag et al. *(49)* reported their experience wherein 91 patients received fractionated intracavitary HDR boost after 60–70 Gy to a cumulative dose of 78–82 Gy. Twenty-one of these patients, who were stage II–IVB, also received chemotherapy. They concluded that for stage I–IIB patients, external beam radiation therapy with intracavitary radiation remains their standard of care with local control and overall survival rates of 97 and 67%, respectively. For the higher stage tumors, which were additionally treated with chemotherapy, local control was 86% and overall survival was 72%.

4.2. Oral Cavity

Structures within the oral cavity are essential for speech, deglutition, airway protection, good dentition, and taste, apart from cosmesis. Preservation of this complex functioning system is of paramount importance in the patient's quality of life. The overwhelming majority of cancers of the oral cavity are squamous cell in origin.

4.3. LIP

Surgical excision is recommended for small lesions that can be primarily closed without cosmetic or functional deficit. However, most of the other lesions, especially of the upper lip, commissure lesions, and large malignant ulcers can be effectively treated with definitive brachytherapy. The European Group of Brachytherapy reported results of over 1800 cases of lip cancer treated with implants *(50)*. Local control for T1, T2, and T3 tumors were 98.4, 96.6, and 89.9%, respectively. Jorgensen et al. *(51)*, in their study of more than 800 patients, reported local control of 93, 87, and 75% for T, T2, and T3 tumors, respectively. The vast majority of studies have utilized single-plane Ir-192 temporary implants, to deliver a dose of approx 60 Gy over a period of 6 d (Fig. 1). T3 tumors and thicker lesions can be treated to slightly higher doses.

4.4. Oral Tongue

There are several reports of improved local control in patients with tumors of the oral tongue following treatment with brachytherapy, either alone or in combination with external bean radiation *(52–58)*. The largest study (more than 600 patients) is from the Curie Institute in Paris *(56)*. Most patients, who had T1 and T2 disease, were treated with implant alone, to a dose of 70 Gy over 6–9 d. Large T2 and T3 lesions received a combination of external beam and interstitial implant. Local control for T1, T2, and T3 lesions were 86, 80, and 68%, respectively. Similarly Mazeron et al. *(52)* also treated 166 patients with Ir-192 implants for stage T1 and T2 patients. Five-year local control in 153 of these patients, who were node negative, was 87%. These results are similar to those obtained by Spiro et al. *(59)*: all patients with T1, T2, and T3 lesions were treated with partial glossectomy alone. Local control was 85% for T1, 77% for T2, and 50% for T3 cancers.

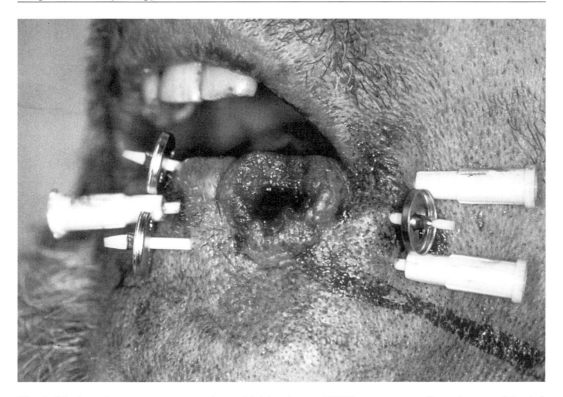

Fig. 1. Lip low-dose rate temporary interstitial implant: a T2N0 squamous cell carcinoma of the left lower lip near the commissure. Catheters (14 gage) were percutaneously introduced through the lesion and spaced 8–10 mm apart. Ir-192 ribbons were afterloaded to deliver a dose of 60 Gy in 6 d. The patient had a complete response and is without recurrence at 10-yr follow-up.

Another subgroup of patients who benefit from brachytherapy includes those who have undergone surgery for small lesions, yet are found to have close pathologic margins, deep muscle involvement, perineural invasion, or lymphovascular invasion *(60–63)*. Without additional treatment, these patients have a high rate of local recurrence. Ange et al. *(62)* reviewed the records of 23 patients, who after excision biopsies of oral tongue and floor of mouth lesions underwent primary radium implants. Local control was 100%, with good preservation of function. They suggested doses between 5500 and 6000 cGy. Hu and Harrison *(63)* reported the results of 13 patients with oral tongue and floor of mouth cancers treated with Ir-192 implants after excision of T1 or T2 tumors with close or positive margins. All patients had pathologically negative neck dissections except one patient who had a N1 neck. A median dose of 50 Gy (range, 45–57 Gy) was delivered at LDR, with a surgery-to-brachytherapy interval of about 8 wk (range, 15–77 d). No patients received external beam radiation therapy. At a median follow-up of 25 mo, no local failures occurred; two patients developed neck failure, one of which was salvaged by additional surgery and external beam radiation. Overall survival was 92%, with no patients developing distant metastases. A soft tissue ulcer occurred in one patient and healed with conservative medical management. Thirty-one percent developed a RTOG grade 3 mucositis and 23% developed a grade 2 xerostomia (3/13).

Mendenhall et al. *(64)* also analyzed the results of 16 patients (9 oral tongue and 7 floor of mouth) who were treated with radiation therapy following excision biopsy. While eight of these patients were treated with interstitial implants alone, and the others were treated with a combination of external radiation and brachytherapy. All patients had at least a 2-yr follow-up, and 81% had a 5-yr follow-up. One patient developed intercurrent disease and succumbed. Of the remaining 15 patients, local control was obtained in 7 of the 8 oral tongue patients and in all 7 floor of mouth patients. These results show that brachytherapy alone leads to an exceedingly high rate of local control and can be used as the primary treatment of choice in this subset of patients. As minimal volume of tissue has been irradiated, the chance for further use of radiation is available in the unlikely scenario of a second malignancy developing within or close to a previously radiated field.

In clinically T2N0 oral tongue patients, risk of occult nodal disease warrants treatment to the neck. Hence a combination of external beam and brachytherapy boost is recommended. Chu and Fletcher (65) obtained excellent local control with interstitial boost of 30 Gy. They treated T1 and T2 oral tongue cancers with this method and achieved local controls of 94.3 and 83%, respectively. However, the proportion of the dose given by brachytherapy compared with external beam dose is subject to debate. Benk et al. (66) compared 110 T2N0 patients who were treated with either brachytherapy implant (85 patients) or a combination of external radiation to the primary and neck followed by a brachytherapy boost (25 patients). Local control in those patients subjected to interstitial implant alone was 88% compared with 36% in the other group. Pernot et al. (53) reviewed the results of 147 T2N0 patients in similar settings. Seventy patients were treated with interstitial implant alone and compared with 77 patients who had been treated with external beam and implant. The 5-yr local control was 89.8% in those treated with implant alone and 50.6% in those treated with external irradiation and brachytherapy implant.

Two studies also support the concept that in early-stage oral tongue cancer patients, the greater the proportion of dose by brachytherapy, the higher the probability of local control. Wendt et al. (67) showed that the 2-yr local control was 92% for patients treated with brachytherapy plus external radiation less than 40 Gy, compared with 65% for patients who received brachytherapy plus external radiation more than 40 Gy. Similarly, Mendenhall et al. (68) reported a local control rate of 75% for an implant plus ≤30 Gy external beam radiotherapy compared with 40% for an implant plus >30 Gy external beam radiotherapy.

To achieve optimal dosimetry and decrease incidence of side effects, certain factors need to be considered. Multivariate analysis have revealed that dose, dose rate, and tumor size are strongly correlative of local control, while only size and location are prognostic for necrosis. Intersource spacing has also been studied. Simon et al. (69) treated 131 T1 and 142 T2 oral tongue and floor of mouth cancer patients with Ir-192 implant alone. They were grouped into 2 sets based on the spacing between the sources, 9–14 mm, group 1 and 15–20 mm, group 2. Results revealed 5-yr local control of 86% in group 1 and 76% in group 2. There was no statistical difference based on the source distance, but it was for dose and dose rate.

Mazeron et al. (70) retrospectively analyzed 134 T1 and 145 T2 oral tongue cancers for influence of dose and dose rate on local control and necrosis. They concluded that to achieve maximum local tumor control and decrease the incidence of necrosis, the tumor dose of 65–70 Gy should be given at a rate of 0.3–0.5 Gy/h. At the Henri Mondor hospital, results of 121 patients were reviewed to look for predictors of local control and necrosis (54). Age, sex, total dose, dose rate, linear activity, and inter-source spacing were examined. Minimum follow-up was 2 yr. They found that local control increased with increasing dose of radiation. However, the risk of necrosis also increased with increasing dose. Pernot et al. (71) undertook a similar study, reporting that smaller size correlated with improved local control. The ratio of treated surface to tumoral surface appeared to be important in predicting better control (if <1.2 the local control was 75 vs 52% if >1.2).

Results following treatment with HDR brachytherapy for early oral tongue cancers have been analyzed (57,58). Inoue et al. (57) conducted a phase III trial wherein patients with T1T2N0 squamous cell carcinoma of the oral tongue were treated with either LDR brachytherapy (15 patients) or HDR brachytherapy (14 patients). Two-year local control rates in the LDR and HDR groups were 86 and 100%, respectively. Leung et al. (58) treated 19 T1T2N0 patients with HDR brachytherapy. They achieved a local control rate of 94.7% with acceptable morbidity. Yamazaki et al. (72) compared 341 patients (T1T2N0) who had been treated by LDR brachytherapy with a group of 58 patients who received HDR brachytherapy. In their analysis, the 3- and 5-yr local control rates in patients treated with LDR brachytherapy were 85 and 80%, respectively. The local control rate in the HDR group was 84% for both 3- and 5-yr follow-up.

Placement of a custom-built, lead-coated mandibular shield markedly reduces the incidence of mandibular osteoradionecrosis (ORN). Miura et al. (73) performed retrospective analysis on 103 patients with T1 and T2 oral cancers, treated with Ir-192 implants. The incidence of ORN of mandible was only 2.1% in the presence of a mandibular shield; the incidence rose to 40% without a mandibular shield. Pernot et al. (74) also showed that routine use of the mandibular shield reduced the incidence of osteoradionecrosis from 10.5 to 5.5%.

4.5. Floor of Mouth

Early floor of mouth cancers can be successfully managed with either radiation or surgery, with similar outcomes. When radiation therapy is considered, improved outcomes are noted with the addition of brachytherapy. However, certain floor of mouth cancers can be in close proximity to the mandible; hence one must be cautious and cognizant of the risk of ORN of that bone. Pernot et al. (75) analyzed 207 patients who presented with cancer of the floor of mouth. Brachytherapy alone was used in the treatment of 102 patients. Results revealed a 5-yr local control rate of 97, 72, and 51% for T1, T2, and T3 patients, respectively. They also concluded that brachytherapy alone is more advantageous than a combination of external radiation plus implant in T1T2N0 lesions. Chu et al. (65) treated T1 and T2 floor of mouth cancers with a combination of external beam radiation (50 Gy) and brachytherapy boost (30 Gy). The local control was 98 and 88.5% for T1 and T2 cancers, respectively. As in oral tongue cancer, certain factors can influence local control. Most important among them is the presence of gingival extension.

Mazeron et al. (76) reviewed data on 117 T1 and T2 floor of mouth cancer patients who were treated with brachytherapy alone. The local control was 86% for tumors without gingival extension; those with gingival extension had a local control of only 50%. Another predictive factor that correlates with local control is size of tumor. Matsumoto et al. (77) analyzed 90 patients with T1 and T2 floor of mouth lesions who had undergone Au-198 implants. Local control was 89, 76, and 56% for lesions 0-2 cm, 2–3 cm, and >3 cm, respectively. In this population, local control with gingival extension was 55%; in the absence of gingival extension, it was 82%.

The risk of ORN of the mandible is clearly the major disadvantage of brachytherapy procedures on floor of mouth cancer patients. As mentioned previously (73,74), placement of a leaded mandibular shield markedly decreases the radiation dose to the mandible and in turn decreases incidence of ORN.

4.6. Buccal Mucosa

Buccal mucosa cancers are relatively uncommon in the western world. They are more commonly seen in Southeast Asian countries, owing to the habitual use of chewing tobacco either alone or mixed with areca nut, lime, and flavoring agents. This leads to oral submucous fibrosis *(78)*, a precursor to oral cancer.

One of the largest reviews on buccal mucosa cancers is by the European Group of Curietherapy *(79)*. Seven hundred and forty-eight patients who had undergone either brachytherapy alone (226 patients), or brachytherapy with external radiation (80 patients), or external radiation (273 patients) alone were followed up for a minimum of 3 yr. Brachytherapy alone was carried out if the lesion was less than 5 cm. Local control rates were 81% for brachytherapy alone, 65% for combined treatment, and 66% for external radiation alone.

Nair et al. *(80)* performed another large retrospective analysis. In their series of 234 patients with T1, T2, and T3 buccal mucosa cancer, interstitial implant was undertaken to deliver a dose of 65 Gy over a period of 6 d. Stage-specific disease free survival rates were 75, 65, and 46% for T1, T2, and T3 tumors, respectively. Large tumors also require radiation treatment to the neck.

4.7. Oropharynx

Surveillance, Epidemiology, and End Results (SEER) results estimate that more than 8000 new cases of oropharyngeal cancer will be diagnosed in the United States in 2004 *(81)*. There will be approx 2000 deaths *(81)*, many of which will probably be attributable to locoregional failure. Brachytherapy plays an important role in the local control of malignancies in the oropharynx. The combined use of external irradiation and brachytherapy has led to an increase in organ preservation that in turn improved the quality of life in these patients.

4.8. Faucial Arch and Tonsil

Squamous cell carcinoma of the faucial arch and tonsil are relatively rare in the United States. Generally speaking, squamous cell cancers arising in the anterior tonsillar pillars and soft palate have a better prognosis compared with tonsillar fossa lesions *(82)*. Tumors limited to the posterior tonsillar pillar are rare.

One of the largest studies on T1–3 squamous cell carcinomas of the velotonsillar region was by Pernot et al. *(83)*. They evaluated the results of 361 patients who received either brachytherapy alone (18 patients) or a combination of external beam and brachytherapy (343 patients) using an Ir-192 radioactive source. The patient distribution with respect to cancer site was as follows: tonsils 128, soft palate 134, posterior tonsillar pillar 9, anterior tonsillar pillar 63, and glossotonsillar sulcus 27. The 5- and 10-yr local control rates were 80 and 74%, and the overall survival rates were 53 and 27%, respectively. The study also showed that 5-yr local control for T1–2 tumors was 87%, compared with T3 tumors, which was 67%. The local control for N0 was 80%; for N+ it was 55%.

Mazeron et al. *(84)* reviewed the outcome of 165 T1–2 faucial arch squamous cell cancer patients who were treated with either external irradiation, or brachytherapy alone, or a combination of both. In this study 5-yr local control was 58, 100, and 91%, with 5-yr overall survival being 21, 50.5, and 60%, respectively. As both local control and overall survival improved with brachytherapy as part of treatment, they recommend that T1–2 tumors of the faucial arch be treated with external radiation of 45 Gy followed by a brachytherapy boost of 30 Gy. If neck nodes are clinically positive, they should receive an additional 25–30 Gy, or an elective node dissection should be performed.

Similar results were duplicated in studies by Puthawala et al. *(85)*, Behar et al. *(86)*, and Amornmarn et al. *(87)*. The integrated therapy of external beam radiation and interstitial implant for tonsillar cancers resulted in improved local control and overall survival with good function and quality of life.

Levendag et al. *(30)* retrospectively analyzed the results of 38 patients with squamous cell carcinomas of the tonsil and soft palate who received treatment using PDR or fractionated HDR brachytherapy alone or combined with external irradiation. These results were compared with those obtained in 72 patients treated with external beam radiation alone. Their analysis indicates that there was no difference in the local relapse-free survival or overall survival between the two groups, at 3 yr of follow-up.

4.9. Base of Tongue

Cancers of the base of tongue are silent in the early stages owing to the lack of pain fibers in the region as well as difficulty in visualizing them on routine physical examination *(88)*. However, owing to the rich lymphatics in the region, following an insidious period, many of them present as locally advanced lesions. The incidence of ipsilateral neck nodes at presentation is approx 70%; bilateral neck nodes are present in 20%.

Early-stage cancers can be effectively managed by either surgery or radiation. Radiation is usually a combination of external beam radiation with a brachytherapy boost or external beam radiation alone. Comparative analysis has also been carried out in patients with early-stage base of tongue cancer who were treated with either surgery followed by postoperative external radiation or primary external radiation with an interstitial implant. Houssett et al. *(91)* retrospectively studied three treatment options in T1–2 base of tongue cancer patients: surgery followed by external irradiation (arm 1), external radiation plus interstitial implant (arm 2), and external radiation alone (arm 3). With a median follow-up of 8 yr and a minimum follow-up of 4 yr, they found that local failure was twice as common in the external radiation alone (arm 3 = 43%) compared with the other two (arm 1 = 18.5% and arm 2 = 20.5%). In their opinion, external radiation followed by interstitial implantation is the best of the three therapeutic options. Analyses by Regueiro et al. *(92)* and Goffinet et al. *(29)* also validate the concept that addition of a brachytherapy implant improves local control and preserves function in early-stage base of tongue cancer patients.

The surgical treatment for locally advanced base of tongue cancers consists of partial glossectomy, neck dissection, and reconstruction with a myocutaneous flap. Occasionally surgery may also entail supraglottic laryngectomy or even a total pharyngolaryngectomy with reconstruction. Apart from the associated morbidity (prolonged anesthesia, increased hospital stay, infection, ventilator dependency, intensive nursing care) of such surgery, this also can lead to serious functional deficits such as difficulty in speech and swallowing causing inability to work, communicate with others, and eat in public. Moreover, patients undergoing surgery for locally advanced base of tongue cancer do require postoperative radiation.

Current literature data *(29,89,93–95)* strongly support external beam radiation to the primary and neck combined with a brachytherapy boost to the primary. This has resulted in excellent locoregional control along with highly desired minimal functional deficit. This is turn has noticeably led to organ preservation and improved quality of life in this set of patients.

Harrison et al. *(93)* have published long-term results of base of tongue cancer patients who were primarily treated with radiation, with neck dissection added for those initially seen with palpable neck nodes. Initially, patients received external beam radiation to the primary site and upper neck (54 Gy) and to the low neck (50 Gy). Clinically node-positive necks received

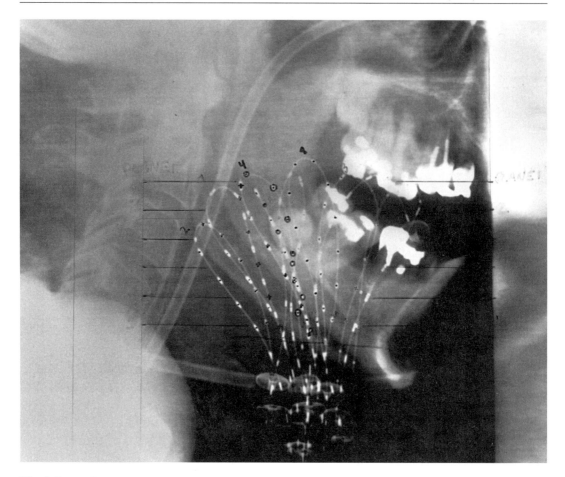

Fig. 2. Base of tongue low-dose rate implant. Patient is a 57-yr-old male who presented with a T4N0M0 squamous cell carcinoma of the tongue base. He received a course of external beam radiation to a dose of 54 Gy to the tongue base and 54 Gy electively to both sides of the neck. Within 3 wk of completion he underwent base of tongue implant. The implant was done via the looping technique, introducing the catheters in the submental area using curved metal trochars. A dose of 30Gy was delivered to complete treatment.

an additional 6 Gy with external beam radiation. An Ir-192 boost of 20–30 Gy was given 3 wk later, at the same time as the neck dissection (Fig. 2). In their analysis of 68 patients, the actuarial 5- and 10-yr local control was 89 and 89%, with overall survival of 86 and 52%, respectively. The actuarial 5- and 10-yr neck control was 96% overall, 86% after radiation alone, and 100% after radiation plus neck dissection.

Harrison et al. *(96,97)* also performed detailed quality of life assessments on long-term survivors of locally advanced base of tongue cancer patients who had undergone primary radiation treatment. Patients completed (1) the Memorial Symptom Assessment scale (MSAS), (2) the Functional Assessment of Cancer Therapy (FACT), (3) the Performance Status Scale for Head and Neck cancer (PSS) *(98)*, and a sociodemographic and economic questionnaire. The PSS scoring revealed that 83% were able to eat in public comfortably, 75% could tolerate a normal diet, and 93% were able to communicate effectively. FACT results revealed that 72% were able to maintain their full-time employment status. Of those who were working part-time prior to their diagnosis, 83% were able to continue to do so after radiation treatment.

Other investigators *(29,89,94,95)* have also demonstrated effective local control rates when patients with locally advanced base of tongue lesions are treated primarily with external beam radiation and brachytherapy boost. Crook et al. *(89)* analyzed the results of T1 and T2 patients treated by external radiation and interstitial implant. Few of these patients were treated exclusively with implant alone. Five-year local control rates were 85% for T1 lesions and 71% for T2 lesions. Horwitz et al. *(94)* treated 20 base of tongue cancer patients with a combination of external beam radiation and interstitial boost of I-125 seeds. The 5-yr actuarial local control and overall survival rates were 88 and 72%, respectively. Puthawala et al. *(95)* published their 10-yr experience on the treatment of 70 patients with base of tongue cancer. Following a minimum follow-up of 2 yr, the overall local control was 83%, and the absolute 3-yr disease-free survival for the entire group was 67%. Goffinet et al. *(29)* also evaluated 28 base of tongue cancer patients 29. They received combined external radiation and brachytherapy boost using an Ir-192 radioactive source; 71% of the patients remained disease free at a mean follow-up of 32 mo. The authors conclude that base of tongue cancers can be effectively treated with a combination of external beam and interstitial radiation.

4.10. Neck Nodes

Prognosis in patients with large nodal recurrence following failure of primary treatment is dismal. Aside from failure of treatment, these patients have a very poor quality of life owing to severe pain, wound breakdown, infection, fistula formation, bleeding, and necrosis within the cervical lymph nodes. These terminally ill patients are also prone to receive limited medical attention, given their poor prognosis. Brachytherapy can be a useful last option in these patients

Inoperable neck nodes in locally advanced or recurrent head and neck cancer may be managed by either temporary or permanent implantation of radioactive seeds. Cornes et al. *(99)* reported their analysis of 39 patients who underwent maximal surgical resection and reirradiation with implantation of Ir-192 seeds. Thirteen patients underwent salvage surgery and brachytherapy without reconstruction. The local control at 1 yr was 68%. However, 46% also experienced severe radiation induced fibrosis and neck contracture. In the remaining 26 patients, who underwent salvage surgery and brachytherapy with a reconstruction flap, local control at 1 yr was 63%, with severe side effects in 12%.

Choo et al. *(100)*, at the Ottawa regional cancer center, treated 20 patients with recurrent or persistent neck metastases with Ir-192 implants. Of the 20 patients, 9 also underwent salvage surgery, 3 other patients received additional external beam radiation, and 8 were treated with brachytherapy as the sole modality of treatment. They reported that in 15 patients, immediate local control was 100%. At 27 mo of follow up, 25% were alive.

Goffinet et al. *(101)* reported a neck implant technique using I-125 seeds braided onto a vicryl suture. After maximal surgical debulking, the braided seeds are sutured in regular rows, according to a preplan whereby a dose of 80–120 Gy is delivered. The higher dose is given if the patient has not received any radiation previously. In 53 nonirradiated patients treated with this technique, effective local control in the head and neck region was obtained in 71%. In 38 patients who had been irradiated previously, local control was 59%. Goffinet et al. *(102)* also placed afterloading tubes in the neck. Ir-192 or I-125 radioactive sources were afterloaded to deliver a dose of 20–30 Gy. They obtained local control of 80% in 13 patients who were treated with this technique.

4.11. Skull Base Tumors

Skull base tumors, as the name implies, are critically close to such vital structures as cranial nerves, brain parenchyma, spinal cord, and major blood vessels. Radiation dose by external beam may be limited, unless given by stereotactic technique, owing to the tolerance of the surrounding normal structures. Kumar et al. *(103,104)* treated 15 patients with skull base meningioma, by placement of permanent radioactive I-125 seeds, under local anesthesia. The dose administered was 100–500 Gy, at a dose rate of 0.05–0.25 Gy/h. At a median follow-up of 15 mo all patients were alive. The authors also note that there were no early or late complications in their patients. Gutin et al. *(105)* treated 13 patients with recurrent and locally advanced skull base and spine tumors with placement of I-125 seeds. All 13 patients had been previously treated with radiation. In their analysis, the tumor regressed or stabilized in three patients, and two other patients had long-term remission.

5. RECURRENT HEAD AND NECK CANCER

Retreatment of locally recurrent head and neck cancer is a technical challenge to the head and neck oncologist. The use of a single modality of treatment, be it surgery or radiation or chemotherapy, is rarely curative. Prior to initiating treatment, a complete restaging workup is essential. This will help in formulating a treatment plan for the individual. The risk–benefit ratio of intensive therapy to the site of failure in the head and neck is taken into account. Results of retrospective analysis are further complicated the heterogenous population of patients in these studies. Nevertheless, most studies show that optimal locoregional control can be achieved with the inclusion of brachytherapy as a component of the treatment.

Goffinet et al. *(101)* reported their series of 34 patients with recurrent head and neck cancer. They underwent intraoperative placement of permanent implantation of I-125 seeds impregnated on a vicryl suture at the time of salvage surgery (Fig. 3). A local control rate of 59% was obtained. Mazeron et al. *(106)* treated 70 recurrent head and neck cancer patients, who had been previously irradiated, with an Ir-192 implant. The actuarial local control at 5 yr was 69%. In patients with recurrences in the faucial arch and posterior pharyngeal arch, the local control was 100%. Syed et al. *(107)* treated 29 persistent or recurrent head and neck cancer patients who had had a full course of radiation previously. A dose of 50–70 Gy was administered over a period of 3–5 d. Sixty-three percent of patients had complete local control at 18–36 mo.

Peiffert et al. *(108)* treated 73 patients with recurrent velotonsillar carcinomas who had been previously irradiated. Ir-192 radioactive sources were implanted to deliver a dose of approximately 60 Gy. Grade 2, soft tissue necrosis, was seen in 10 patients in whom the implanted dose was greater than 60 Gy. The 5-yr specific survival was 64%; however, the overall survival was only 30%. It was commented that 42% of the patient succumbed to another malignancy, and all but two of these patients continued to abuse tobacco and alcohol products. Lee et al. *(109)* analyzed the results of 41 patients who underwent salvage surgery with I-125 implant, for a diagnosis of extensive recurrent head and neck carcinoma. Reconstruction using myocutaneous flaps was done in 18 patients. The average I-125 dose was approximately 80 Gy. The 5-yr local control and actuarial overall survival rates were 44 and 40%, respectively. Major complications were transient wound infection (32%), flap necrosis (24%), fistula formation (10%), and carotid rupture (5%).

Because of the increased potential for morbidity and mortality (carotid rupture is inevitability fatal), a surgical reconstruction using free tissue transfer flaps or myocutaneous flaps have been performed to reduce complications in this setting.

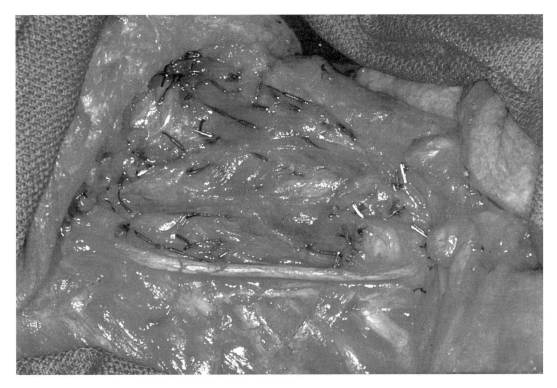

Fig. 3. I-125 permanent implant. The patient was previously treated with external beams radiation for a supraglottic larynx carcinoma. He did well until a neck recurrence developed 18 mo later. He underwent neck dissection, and a permanent I-125 seed implant embedded in a vicryl suture was sewn into the soft tissues of the neck.

6. INTRAOPERATIVE RADIATION THERAPY

Intraoperative radiation therapy (IORT) is a special type of brachytherapy technique that delivers, in a single session, a radiation dose to the tumor bed under direct visualization with normal tissues shielded or displaced from the irradiated area. Thus, a single large dose of radiation (10–20 Gy) can be delivered to the tumor bed after surgical resection with even further protection of adjacent normal tissue, particularly the skin and suture line, which can decrease the risk of postoperative complications. Also, direct visualization and placement of the applicator over the tumor site for a short period insures greater accuracy of delivery. This results in an improved therapeutic ratio of local control vs complications. The biologic effectiveness of a single-dose IORT is considered equivalent to 1.5–2.5 times the same total dose of fractionated electron beam radiotherapy *(110)*, which allows dose escalation.

Intraoperative brachytherapy can be given by placement of a sterile flaccid applicator over the tumor bed that acts as a conduit, allowing a high-dose radioactive source (IORT-HDR) to deliver radiation to the tumor bed (Fig. 4). Alternatively, it can be delivered via electrons (IOERT) using special cones that are placed in direct contact with the tumor bed. In the United States, both modalities of IORT are restricted to institutions with experience in the technique.

Hu et al. *(111)* have evaluated the use of IORT-HDR in 15 patients with locally advanced or recurrent head and neck cancer. A median dose of 12 Gy was delivered to the tumor bed, using the Harrison-Anderson-Mick (HAM) applicator. At a median follow-up of 10 mo, the crude local control was 80%, with a disease-free survival of 74%. Nag et al. *(112)* analyzed

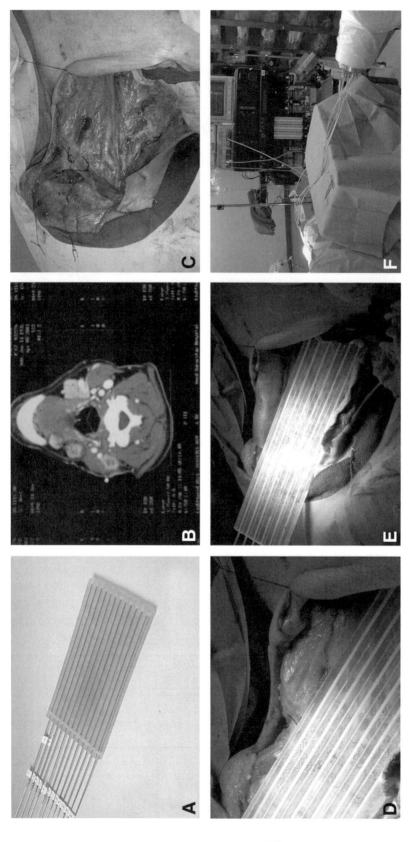

Fig. 4. High-dose rate intraoperative radiation (HDR-IORT) using the Harrison–Anderson–Mick (HAM) applicator. (**A**) The HAM applicator is composed of a transparent flexible material that is precut to specific sizes and thicknesses. Its flexibility allows it to bend and contour to virtually any surface in the neck. (**B**) Patient treated with HDR-IORT. The patient is a 68-yr-old male who had a recurrent mucoepeidermoid carcinoma of the right parotid gland 4 yr after undergoing resection and postoperative external beam radiation to 60 Gy. Computed tomography of the neck shows a nodal recurrence with extracapsular extension to the undersurface of the sternocleiodomastoid muscle. It was located within the previous radiation field at the margin. (**C**) The patient underwent resection. Tumor bed outline. (**D,E**) An appropriately sized applicator was placed, and normal tissues such as the larynx were protected with lead shield or packing. (**F**) The final setup is illustrated with the applicator connected to the Ir-192 Remote Afterloader (Nucelotron, Columbia, MD).

the results of 29 patients with base of skull involvement. Following maximal surgical resection, patients received 7.5–15 Gy via IORT-HDR. Twenty-one percent had received external radiation previously. Overall local control and survival rates were 66 and 72%, respectively.

Garrett et al. *(113)* treated 28 patients with IOERT, 61% of who had previously received external radiation. Local control and overall survival rates were 66 and 67%, respectively. In this group of patients, 23% had gross residual disease following maximal surgery. Rate et al. *(114)* delivered a median dose of 20 Gy using IOERT to 47 patients with recurrent head and neck cancer. All had received external radiation previously. The local control rate was 62%. Even in this series, 23% of patients had residual tumor after surgery. A study by Coleman et al. *(115)* yielded similar results.

These studies reveal that in the setting of locally advanced or recurrent head and neck cancer, the best results using IORT are obtained following maximal surgical resection combined with external beam radiation *(116)*.

7. CONCLUSIONS

In head and neck cancer patients, curative treatment and quality of life are inextricably linked. Minimizing toxicity in the planned treatment protocol will help to preserve organs and decrease treatment-related morbidity. Brachytherapy provides curative doses to the tumor while minimizing dose to the surrounding normal tissue. Most importantly, the improved therapeutic ratio increases the chance of organ preservation, leading to improved quality of life with respect to function, emotion, and cosmesis. Brachytherapy has been proved to be effective either as a single modality of treatment or in combination with external beam radiation, surgery, and chemotherapy. It has a proven role in the setting of recurrent or persistent disease. Retrospective studies have shown that both LDR and HDR brachytherapy are effective in head and neck cancers. PDR is a promising approach that is under active investigation.

Proper patient selection, a radiation oncologist skilled in brachytherapy, and good dosimetry planning can minimize risks and complications. A coordinated team approach, with personnel well versed in brachytherapy, maximizes the potential to perform a high-quality brachytherapy implant. All these factors are pivotal in making brachytherapy a successful and essential component in the treatment of head and neck malignancies.

REFERENCES

1. Harrison LB, Zelefsky MJ, Pfister DG, et al. Detailed quality of life assessment in patients treated with primary radiotherapy for squamous cell cancer of the base of the tongue. Head Neck 1997; 19:169–175.
2. Barrett WL, Gleich L, Wilson K, et al. Organ preservation with interstitial radiation for base of tongue cancer. Am J Clin Oncol 2002; 25:485–488.
3. Mazeron JJ, Noel G, Simon JM. Head and neck brachytherapy. Semin Radiat Oncol 2002; 12:95–108.
4. Levendag P, Nijdam W, Noever I, et al. Brachytherapy versus surgery in carcinoma of tonsillar fossa and/or soft palate: late adverse sequelae and performance status: can we be more selective and obtain better tissue sparing? Int J Radiat Oncol Biol Phys 2004; 59:713–724.
5. Pigneux J, Richaud PM, Lagarge C. The placement of interstitial therapy using Ir-192 in the management of cancer of the lip. Cancer 1979; 43:1073–1077.
6. Lapeyre M, Bollet MA, Racodot S, et al. Postoperative brachytherapy alone and combined postoperative radiotherapy and brachytherapy boost for squamous cell carcinoma of the oral cavity, with positive or close margins. Head Neck 2004; 26:216–223.
7. Beitler JJ, Smith RV, Silver CE, et al. Close or positive margins after surgical resection for the head and neck cancer patient: the addition of brachytherapy improves local control. Int. J Radiat Oncol Biol Phys 1998; 40:313–317.
8. Vikram B, Mishra S. Permanent iodine-125 implants in postoperative radiotherapy for head and neck cancer with positive surgical margins. Head Neck 1994; 16:155–157.

9. Looser KG, Shah JP, Strong EW. The significance of positive margins in surgically resected epidermoid carcinoma. Head Neck 1978; 1:107.

10. Fu K, Ray JW, Chan EK et al. External and interstitial radiation therapy of carcinomas of the oral tongue: a review of 32 years of experience. Am J Roentgenol 1976; 127:107–115.

11. Brucer M. Brachytherapy. Am J Roentgenol 1968; 79:1080–1090.

12. Mazeron JJ, Gerbaulet A. The centenary of the discovery of radium. Cancer Radiother 1999; 3:19–29.

13. Failla G. The development of filtered radon implants 1926; 16:507–525.

14. Wickham L, Degrais P. Radiumtherapie. Paris: Bailliere, 1909 (English ed: Radiumtherapy. London: Cassell, 1910; Radiumtherapy. New York: Funk and Wagnals, 1910.

15. Abbe R. Radium in surgery. JAMA 1906; 47:103.

16. Morton R. Treatment by roentgen and radium rays. Br. Med J 1904; 166:941–944.

17. Paterson R, Parker HMA. A dosage system for gamma ray therapy. Br J Radiol 1934; 7:592–612.

18. Quimby EQ. Dosage tables for linear radium sources. Radiology 1944; 43:572.

19. Quimby EQ. The grouping of radium tubes in packs on plaques to produce the desired distribution of radiation. Am J Roentgenol 1932; 27:18.

20. Henschke U, Hilaris BS, Mahan GD. Afterloading in interstitial and intracavitary radiation therapy. Am J Roentgenol 1963; 90:386–395.

21. Pernot M, Luporsi E, Hoffstetter S, et al. Complications following definitive irradiation for cancers of the oral cavity and the oropharynx (in a series of 1134 patients). Int J Radiat Oncol Biol Phys 1997; 37:577–585.

22. Piro JD, Battle LW, Harrison LB. Conversion of complete dentures to a radiation shield prosthesis. J Prosthetic Dentistry 1991; 65:731–732.

23. Clarke DH, Edmundson GK, Martinez A, et al. The utilization of I-125 seeds as a substitute for Ir-192 seeds in temporary interstitial implants: an overview and a description of the William Beaumont Hospital technique. Int J Radiat Oncol Biol Phys 1988; 15:1027–1033.

24. Nath R. New directions in radionuclide sources for brachytherapy. Semin Radiat Oncol 1993; 3:278.

25. Nag S. Principles and Practice of Brachytherapy. Blackwell Futura, July 1997.

26. Joslin CAF, Flynn A, Hall EJ. Principles and Practice of Brachytherapy: Using Afterloading Systems. Hodder Arnold, June 2001.

27. Harrison LB, Zelefsky M, Armstrong JG, et al. Performance status after treatment for squamous cell cancer of the base of tongue—a comparison of primary radiation versus primary surgery. Int J Radiat Oncol Biol Phys 1994; 30:953–957.

28. Pierquin B, Chassagne DJ, Chahbazian CM, et al. Brachytherapy. Warren H. Green, 1978.

29. Goffinet DR, Fee WE Jr, Wells J, et al. [192]Ir pharyngoepiglottic fold interstitial implants. The key to successful treatment of base tongue carcinoma by radiation therapy. Cancer 1985; 55:941–948.

30. Levendag PC, Schmitz PIM, Jansen PP, et al. Fractionated high dose rate and pulsed dose rate brachytherapy: first clinical experience in squamous cell carcinoma of the tonsillar fossa and soft palate. Int J Radiat Oncol Biol Phys 1997; 38:497–506.

31. Strnad V, Lotter M, Grabenbauer G, et al. Early results of pulsed-dose-rate interstitial brachytherapy for head and neck malignancies after limited surgery. Int J Radiat Oncol Biol Phys 2000; 46:27–30.

32. Erickson BA, Wilson JF. Nasopharyngeal brachytherapy. Am J Clin Oncol 1993; 16:424–443.

33. Al-Sarraf M, LeBlanc M, Giri PG, et al. Chemoradiotherapy versus radiotherapy in patients with advanced naospharyngeal cancer: phase III randomized Intergroup study 0099. J Clin Oncol 1998; 16:1310–1317.

34. Wang CC, Busse J, Gitterman M. A simple afterloading applicator for intracavitary irradiation of carcinoma of the nasopharynx. Radiology 1975; 115:737–738.

35. Harrison LB, Nori D, Hilaris B, et al. Nasopharynx. in: The Interstitial Collaborative Working Group, ed. Interstitial Brachytherapy. New York: Raven, 1990:95–109.

36. Harrison LB, Weissberg JB. A technique for interstitial nasopharyngeal brachytherapy. Int J Radiat Oncol Biol Phys 1987; 13:451–453.

37. Vikram B, Hilaris B. Transnasal permanent interstitial implantation of carcinoma of the nasopharynx. Int J Radiat Oncol Biol Phys 1984; 10:153–155.

38. Harrison LB, Sessions RB, Fass DE, et al. Nasopharyngeal brachytherapy with access via a transpalatal flap. Am J Surg 1992; 164:173–175.

39. Syed AM, Puthawala AA, Damore SJ, et al. Brachytherapy for primary and recurrent nasopharyngeal carcinoma: 20 years' experience at Long Beach Memorial. Int J Radiat Oncol Biol Phys 2000; 47:1311–1321.

40. Pryzant RM, Wendt CD, Delclos L, et al. Re-treatment of nasopharyngeal carcinoma in 53 patients. Int J Radiat Oncol Biol Phys 1992; 22:941–947.

41. Lee AW, Law SC, Foo W, et al. Retrospective analysis of patients with nasopharyngeal carcinoma treated during 1976–1985: survival after local recurrence. Int J Radiat Oncol Biol Phys 1993; 26:773–782.

42. Kwong DL, Wei WI, Cheng AC, et al. Long term results of radioactive gold grain implantation for treatment of persistent and recurrent nasopharyngeal carcinoma. Cancer 2001; 91:1105–1113.

43. Wang CC. Re-irradiation of recurrent nasopharyngeal carcinoma-treatment techniques and results. Int J Radiat Oncol Biol Phys 1987; 13:953–956.

44. Fu KK, Newman H, Phillips TL. Treatment of locally recurrent carcinoma of the nasopharynx. Radiology 1975; 117:425–431.

45. Teo P, Leung SF, Choi P, et al. Afterloading radiotherapy for local persistence of nasopharyngeal carcinoma. Br J Radiol 1994; 67:181–185.

46. Choy D, Sham JST, Wei WI, et al. Transpalatal insertion of radioactive gold grain for the treatment of persistent and recurrent nasopharyngeal carcinoma. Int J Radiat Oncol Biol Phys 1993; 25:505–512.

47. Syed AMN, Puthawala AA, Damore SJ, et al. Brachytherapy for primary and recurrent nasopharyngeal carcinoma: 20 years experience at Long Beach Memorial. Int J Radiat Oncol Biol Phys 2000; 47:1311–1321.

48. Wang CC. Improved local control of nasopharyngeal carcinoma after intracavitary brachytherapy boost. Am J Clin Oncol 1998; 14:5–8.

49. Levendag PC, Lagerwaard FJ, Noever I, et al. Role of endocavitary brachytherapy with or without chemotherapy in cancer of the nasopharynx. Int J Radiat Oncol Biol Phys 2002; 52:755–768.

50. Mazeron JJ, Richaud P: Lip cancer. Report of the 18th annual meeting of the European Curietherapy Group. J Eur Radiother 1984; 5:50–56.

51. Jorgensen K, Elbrond O, Anderson AP. Carcinoma of the lip: a series of 869 cases. Acta Radiol Ther Phys Biol 1973; 12:177–190.

52. Mazeron JJ, Crook JM Benck V et al. Iridium 192 implantation of T1 and T2 carcinomas of the mobile tongue. Int J Radiat Oncol Biol Phys 1990; 19:1369–1376.

53. Pernot M, Malissard L, Aletti P, et al. Iridium 192 brachytherapy in the management of 147 T2N0 oral tongue carcinomas treated with irradiation alone: comparison of two treatment techniques. Radiother Oncol 1992; 23:223–228.

54. Mazeron JJ, Crook JM, Marinello G, et al. Prognostic factors of local outcome for T1, T2 carcinomas or oral tongue treated by iridium 192 implantation. Int J Radiat Oncol Biol Phys 1990; 19:281–285.

55. Puthawala A, Syed A, Neblett D, et al. The role of afterloading iridium implant in the management of carcinoma of the tongue. Int J Radiat Oncol Biol Phys 1981; 7:407–412.

56. Decroix Y, Ghossein NA. Experience of the Curie Institute in treatment of cancer of the mobile tongue: treatment policies and results. Cancer 1981; 47:496–502.

57. Inoue T, Inoue T, Teshima T, et al. Phase III trial of high and low dose rate interstitial radiotherapy for early oral tongue cancer. Int J Radiat Oncol Biol Phys 1996; 36:1201–1204.

58. Leung TW, Wong VY, Kwan KH, et al. High dose brachytherapy for early stage oral tongue cancer. Head Neck 2002; 24:274–281.

59. Spiro RH, Strong EW. Epidermoid carcinoma of the mobile tongue. Treatment by partial glossectomy alone. Am J Surg 1971; 122:707–710.

60. Lapeyre M, Bollet MA, Racadot S, et al. Postoperative brachytherapy alone and combined postoperative radiotherapy and brachytherapy boost for squamous cell carcinoma of the oral cavity, with positive or close margins. Head Neck 2004; 26:216–223.

61. Lapeyre M, Hoffstetter S, Peiffert D, et al. Postoperative brachytherapy alone for T1-2 N0 squamous cell carcinomas of the oral tongue and floor of mouth with close or positive margins. Int J Radiat Oncol Biol Phys 2000; 48:37–42.

62. Ange DW, Lindberg RD, Guillamondegui OM. Management of squamous cell carcinoma of the oral tongue and floor of mouth after excisional biopsy. Radiology 1975; 116:143–146.

63. Hu KS, Sachdeva G, Harrison LB. Adjuvant interstitial iridium 192 brachytherapy for resected T1 and T2 cancers of the oral cavity with close or positive margins. Presented at the 6th International Head and Neck Conference, Washington DC, August, 2004.

64. Mendenhall WM, Parsons JT, Stringer SP, et al. Radiotherapy after excisional biopsy of carcinoma of the oral tongue/floor of mouth. Head Neck 1989; 11:129–131.

65. Chu A, Fletcher GH. Incidences and causes of failure to control by irradiation the primary lesion in squamous cell carcinomas of the anterior two thirds of the tongue and floor of mouth. Am J Roentgenol 1973; 117:502–508.

66. Benk V, Mazeron JJ, Grimard L, et al. Comparison of curietherapy versus external irradiation combined with curietherapy in stage II squamous cell carcinomas of the mobile tongue. Radiother Oncol 1990; 18:339–347.

67. Wendt CD, Peters LJ, Delclos L, et al. Primary radiotherapy in the treatment of stage I and II oral tongue cancers: importance of the proportion of therapy delivered with interstitial therapy. Int J Radiat Oncol Biol Phys 1995; 18:1287–1298.

68. Mendenhall WM, Parsons JM, Stringer SP, et al. T2 oral tongue carcinoma treated with radiotherapy; analysis of local control and complications. Radiother Oncol 1989; 16:275–281.

69. Simon JM, Mazeron JJ, Pohar S, et al. Effect of intersource spacing on local control and complications in brachytherapy of mobile tongue and floor of mouth. Radiother Oncol 1993; 26:19–25.

70. Mazeron JJ, Simon JM, Le Péchoux C, et al. Effect of dose rate on local control and complications in definitive irradiation of T1-2 squamous cell carcinoma of mobile tongue and floor of mouth with interstitial iridium 192. Radiother Oncol 1991; 21:39–47.

71. Pernot M, Malissard L, Hoffstetter S, et al. The study of tumoral, radiobiological and general health factors that influence results and complications is a series of 448 oral oral tongue carcinomas treated exclusively by irradiation. Int J Radiat Oncol Biol Phys 1994; 29:673–679.

72. Yamazaki H, Inoue T, Yoshida K, and et al. Brachytherapy for early oral tongue cancer: low dose rate to high dose rate. J Radiat Res 2003; 44:37–40.

73. Miura M, Takeda M, Sasaki T, et al. Factors affecting mandibular complications in low dose rate brachytherapy for oral tongue carcinoma with special reference to spacer. Int J Radiat Oncol Biol Phys 1998; 41:763–770.

74. Pernot M, Luporsi E, Hoffsteitter S, et al. Complications following definitive irradiation of the oral cavity and the oropharynx (in a series of 1134 patients). Int J Radiat Oncol Biol 1997; 37:577–585.

75. Pernot M, Hoffstetter S, Peiffert D, et al. Epidermoid carcinomas of the floor of mouth treated by exclusive irradiation: statistical study of a series of 207 cases. Radiother Oncol 1995; 35:177–185.

76. Mazeron JJ, Grimard L, Raynal M, et al. Iridium 192 for T1 and T2 epidermoid carcinomas of the floor of mouth. Int J Radiat Oncol Biol Phys 1990; 18:1299–1306.

77. Matsumoto S, Takeda M, Shibuya H, et al. T1 and T2 squamous cell carcinomas of the floor of the mouth: results of brachytherapy mainly using [198]Au grains. Int J Radiat Oncol Biol Phys 1996; 34:833–841.

78. Jeng JH, Chang MC, Hahn LJ. Role of areca nut in betel quid-associated chemical carcinogenesis: current awareness and future perspectives. Oral Oncol 2001; 37:477–492.

79. Gerbaulet A, Pernot A. Cancer of the buccal mucosa. In: Proceedings of the 20th Annual Meeting of the European Curietherapy Group. J Eur Radiother 1985; 6:1–4.

80. Nair MK, Sankaranarayanan R, Padmanabhan TK. Evaluation of the role of radiotherapy in the management of carcinoma of the buccal mucosa. Cancer 1988; 61:1326–1331.

81. Jemal A, Tiwari RC, Murray T, et al. Cancer statistics, 2004. CA Cancer J Clin 2004; 54:8–29.

82. Jesse RH Jr, Fletcher GH. Metastases in cervical lymph nodes from oropharyngeal cancer: treatment and results. Am J Roentgenol 1963; 90:990–996.

83. Pernot M, Malissard L, Hoffstetter S, et al. Influence of tumoral, radiobiological and general health factors on local control and survival of a series of 361 tumors of the velotonsillar area treated by exclusive irradiation (external beam + brachytherapy or brachytherapy alone). Int J Radiat Oncol Biol Phys 1994; 30:1021–1027.

84. Mazeron JJ, Belkacemi Y, Simon JM, et al. Place of iridium 192 implantation in definitive irradiation of faucial arch squamous cell carcinomas. Int J Radiat Oncol Biol Phys 1993; 27:251–257.

85. Puthawala AA, Syed AM, Eads DL, et al. Limited external irradiation and interstitial 192 iridium implant in the treatment of squamous cell carcinoma of the tonsillar region. Int J Radiat Oncol Biol Phys 1985; 11:1595–1602.

86. Behar RA, Martin PJ, Fee WE Jr, et al. Iridium-192 interstitial implant and external beam radiation therapy in the management of squamous cell carcinomas of the tonsil and soft palate. Int J Radiat Oncol Biol Phys 1994; 28:221–227.

87. Amornmarn R, Prempree T, Jaiwatana J, et al. Radiation management of carcinoma of the tonsillar region. Cancer 1984; 54:1293–1299.

88. Shugar MA, Nosal P, Gavron JP. Technique for routine screening for carcinoma of the base of tongue. J Am Dent Assoc 1982; 104:646–647.

89. Crook J, Mazeron JJ, Marinello G, et al. Combined external irradiation and interstitial implantation for T1 and T2 epidermoid carcinomas of base of tongue: the Criteil experience (1971–1981). Int J Radiat Oncol Biol Phys 1988; 15:105–114.

90. Simon JM, Mazeron JJ, Pohar S, et al. Effect of intersource spacing on local control and complications in brachytherapy of mobile tongue and floor of mouth. Radiother Oncol 1993; 26:19–25.

91. Housset M, Baillet F, Dessard-Diana B, et al. A retrospective study of three treatment techniques for T1-T2 base of tongue lesions: surgery plus postoperative radiation, external radiation plus interstitial implant and external irradiation alone. Int J Radiat Oncol Biol Phys 1987; 13:511–516.

92. Regueiro CA, Millan I, de la Torre A, et al. Influence of boost technique (external beam radiotherapy or brachytherapy) on the outcome of patients with carcinoma of the base of tongue. Acta Oncol 1995; 34:225–233.

93. Harrison LB, Lee HJ, Pfister DG, et al. Long-term results of primary radiotherapy with/without neck dissection for squamous cell carcinoma of the base of tongue. Head Neck 1998; 20:668–673.

94. Horowitz EM, Frazier AJ, Martinez AA, et al. Excellent functional outcome in patients with squamous cell carcinoma of the base of tongue with external irradiation and interstitial iodine 125 boost. Cancer 1996; 78:948–957.

95. Puthawala AA, Syed AM, Eads DL, et al. Limited external beam and interstitial 192 iridium irradiation in the treatment of carcinoma of the base of tongue: a ten-year experience. Int J Radiat Oncol Biol Phys 1988; 14:839–848.

96. Harrison LB, Zelefsky M, Pfister D, et al. Detailed quality of life assessment on long term survivors of primary radiation therapy for cancers of the base of tongue (abstract). Int J Radiat Oncol Biol Phys 1995; 32(suppl 1):180.

97. Harrison LB, Zelefsky MJ, Sessions RB, et al. Base of tongue cancer treated with external beam irradiation plus brachytherapy: oncologic and functional outcome. Radiology 1992; 184:267–270.

98. List MA, Ritter-Sterr C, Lansky SB. A performance status scale for head and neck cancer patients. Cancer 1990; 66:564–569.

99. Cornes PG, Cox HJ, Rhys-Evans PR, et al. Salvage treatment for inoperable neck nodes in head and neck cancer using combined iridium-192 brachytherapy and surgical reconstruction. Br J Surg 1996; 83:1620–1622.

100. Choo R, Grimard L, Esche B, et al. Brachytherapy of neck metastases. J Otolaryngol 1993; 1:54–57.

101. Goffinet DR, Martinez A, Fee WE. I-125 vicryl suture implants as a surgical adjuvant in cancer of the head and neck. Int J Radiat Oncol Biol Phys 1985; 11:399–402.

102. Goffinet DR. Brachytherapy for head and neck cancer. Semin Radiat Oncol 1993; 3:250–259.

103. Kumar PP, Good RR, Leibrock LG, et al. High activity Iodine 125 endocurietherapy for recurrent skull base tumors. Cancer 1988; 61:1518–1527.

104. Kumar PP, Good RR, Leibrock LG, et al. Tissue tolerance and tumor response following high activity iodine 125 endocurietherapy for skull base tumors. Endo Hyper Oncol 1990; 6:223–230.

105. Gutin PH, Leibel SA, Hosobuchi Y, et al. Brachytherapy of recurrent tumors of the skull base and spine with iodine-125 sources. Neurosurgery 1987; 20:938–945.

106. Mazeron JJ, Langlois D, Glaubiger D, et al. Salvage irradiation of oropharyngeal cancers using Iridium 192 wire implants: 5-year results of 70 cases. Int J Radiat Oncol Biol Phys 1987; 13:957–962.

107. Syed AMN, Feder BH, George FW, et al. Iridium 192 afterloaded implant in the retreatment of head and neck cancers. Br J Radiol 1978; 51:814–820.

108. Peiffert D, Pernot M, Malissard L, et al. Salvage irradiation by brachytherapy of velotonsillar squamous cell carcinoma in a previously irradiated field: results in 73 cases. Int J Radiat Oncol Biol Phys 1994; 29:681–686.

109. Lee DJ, Liberman FZ, Park RI, et al. Intra-operative I-125 seed implantation for extensive recurrent head and neck carcinomas. Radiology 1991; 178:879–882.

110. Okuneiff P, Sundararaman S, Chen Y. Biology—IORT dose. In: Gunderson LL, Willet CG, Harrison LB, eds. Intraoperative Irradiation. Humana, Totowa, NJ: 1999:25–46.

111. Hu K, White C, Sachdeva G, et al. High Dose-Rate Intraoperative (HDR-IORT) iridium-192 radiation for head and neck cancer. In: American Brachytherapy Society, New York, May 2003.

112. Nag S, Schuller D, Pak V, et al. Pilot study of intraoperative high dose rate brachytherapy for head and neck cancer. Radiother Oncol 1996; 41:125–130.

113. Garrett P, Pugh N, Ross D, et al. Intra-operative radiation therapy for advanced or recurrent head and neck cancer. Int J Radiat Oncol Biol Phys 1987; 13:785–788.

114. Rate WR, Garrett P, Hamaker R, et al. Intra-operative radiation therapy for recurrent head and neck cancer. Cancer 1991; 67:2738–2740.

115. Coleman CW, Roach M 3rd, Ling SM, et al. Adjuvant electron-beam IORT in high-risk head and neck cancer patients. Front Radiat Ther Oncol 1997; 31:105–111.

116. Hu KS, Enker WE, Harrison LB. High-dose-rate intraoperative irradiation: current status and future directions. Semin Radiat Oncol 2002; 12:62–80.

8

Intensity-Modulated Radiation Therapy in the Management of Head and Neck Cancer

Theodore S. Hong, MD, Wolfgang A. Tomé, PhD, and Paul M. Harari, MD

1. INTRODUCTION

Head and neck cancer represents a complex collection of tumors involving mucosal surfaces of the upper aerodigestive tract. Approximately 43,000 cases are diagnosed each year in the United States, representing 3 to 4% of all cancers *(1)*. Worldwide, head and neck cancer represents a much broader oncology problem (~500,000 annual cases), with tumor development strongly associated with chronic tobacco and alcohol use.

Radiation plays a central role in the treatment of head and neck cancer. New radiation delivery techniques offer a powerful potential to diminish the spectrum and severity of radiation toxicities for head and neck cancer patients. For many decades, conventional head and neck radiation techniques have involved treatment with generous opposed lateral beams to encompass the known primary tumor and upper cervical lymphatics. This classical technique produces a relatively homogeneous dose distribution that allows excellent target dosing while minimizing hot and cold spots. However, owing to the tight proximity of tumor targets and normal tissue in the head and neck region, many uninvolved structures including salivary glands, spinal cord, auditory apparatus, optic apparatus, mandible, and vocal cords can unnecessarily receive high doses of radiation.

Intensity-modulated radiation therapy (IMRT) represents an advance in technology that allows the radiation oncologist to "shape" radiation dose profiles around normal structures while fully dosing the tumor and at-risk nodal regions. This capacity for improved dose distribution affords considerable opportunity to reduce the overall toxicity profile associated with head and neck radiation. However, despite high promise, IMRT use remains in its early stages, and must be delivered with strict attention to quality assurance, as relatively few long-term clinical data exist. Furthermore, IMRT is quite labor intensive for the practitioner, with a strong dependence on physics and quality assurance support, thus leaving open the possibility for significant heterogeneity across practitioners and institutions.

1.2. What is Intensity-Modulated Radiation Therapy?

IMRT refers to a specific technique of linear accelerator-based radiation therapy whereby radiation beams are modulated in such a manner as to produce highly conformal dose distri-

From: *Current Clinical Oncology: Squamous Cell Head and Neck Cancer*
Edited by: D. J. Adelstein © Humana Press Inc., Totowa, NJ

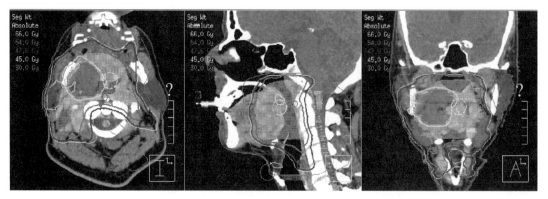

Fig. 1. Transverse, sagittal, and coronal images of head and neck IMRT plan for a patient with squamous cell carcinoma of the right tonsil. The left parotid gland (arrow) is specifically spared from high-dose radiation (mean dose of approx 22 Gy for left parotid).

butions. A primary objective of IMRT is to reduce dose to selected normal tissue structures in an effort to preserve function, while maintaining full dose delivery to tumor targets. In conventional head and neck radiotherapy, the fields are shaped by blocks and potentially modulated by wedges or custom tissues compensators *(2)*. In contrast, IMRT is delivered by either multiple modulated static fields (step and shoot) or by a continuously rotating gantry (serial tomotherapy). As the radiation is delivered, specific subsections of each field, known as beamlets, are delivered at different intensities to produce highly conformal dose distribution around irregular shapes (Fig. 1).

IMRT planning is conceptually distinct from conventional radiotherapy planning. With conventional head and neck planning, the radiation oncologist will shape beams by viewing anteroposterior (AP) and lateral radiographs of the head and neck. A generous field margin is used to account for setup variation and physical characteristics of the beam itself. The radiation dose and profile are then calculated using broad and simple beams in a process known as *forward planning*. In contrast, IMRT planning requires the up-front designation of specific targets (gross tumor, elective nodal regions) and avoidance structures (spinal cord, salivary glands, optic apparatus, and so on). Dose specifications are then defined for each of the targets and avoidance structures. The computer planning software then creates a series of beam angles with modulation patterns that strive to achieve the physician's dose prescription goals. This process is known as *inverse planning*.

1.3. History

IMRT was first conceptualized in the 1960s. However, it was not until the 1980s and 1990s that the computing capability needed for the complex inverse planning algorithms became commercially available *(3)*. In 1994, the NOMOS Peacock system was introduced as the first commercial IMRT delivery unit. The Peacock system required that an existing linac be retrofitted with a beam modulation device known as a dynamic multivane intensity-modulating collimator (MIMiC). The MIMiC allowed a radiation beam to be continuously modulated as the gantry rotated. This particular form of IMRT is called serial tomotherapy, as "slices" could be treated by a continually rotating gantry. More recently, other forms of IMRT have come into common use. Step and shoot IMRT represents another commonly used technique whereby multiple static beams are subdivided into "beamlets." Each individual beamlet is then modulated. Helical tomotherapy is similar to the Peacock system but has the added features of a

Table 1
Principal Stages of IMRT Treatment Planning

1. Image acquisition
2. Target delineation
3. Inverse planning

moving treatment table, allowing large fields to be treated in a single spiral, with a computed tomography (CT) array diametrically opposed to the energy source allowing for imaging capability during the time of treatment. Each of these systems shares the commonality of need for intensive physics support, precise anatomical target definition, and rigorous quality assurance processes.

2. TREATMENT PLANNING

IMRT treatment planning involves three principal stages. These general stages include image acquisition from the patient for treatment planning, target and avoidance structure delineation by the physician, and inverse planning by physics and dosimetry (Table 1).

In the first step (image acquisition), a CT scan of the head and neck region is performed. This scan is similar to that performed for standard 3D conformal radiation therapy (3D-CRT). Initially, some form of head and neck immobilization mask is created for patient positioning. Selected institutions will engage additional immobilization measures such as reinforced thermoplastic masking *(4)*, shoulder immobilization, or maxillofacial biteblocks for optical guidance *(5)*. A thin-sliced CT scan or CT-positron emission tomography (PET) fusion scan is then acquired in the treatment position. Despite these additional measures for enhanced setup reproducibility, from the patient's perspective, the preplanning process is not substantially different from conventional radiation planning.

Once high-quality imaging is acquired, primary tumor and elective nodal targets are defined by the physician on serial CT scan images (target delineation). The primary tumor target (gross tumor volume [GTV]), represents the radiographically visible tumor as seen on the CT scan and complemented by physical exam findings. Thereafter, elective or "at-risk" nodal regions are contoured on a slice-by-slice basis for establishment of a clinical target volume (CTV). One common approach involves the designation of a high-risk CTV (CTV-1) encompassing soft tissue and nodal regions adjacent to the GTV *(6)*. A lower risk CTV-2 may also be designated, which commonly represents nodal regions contralateral to the primary tumor. Selected avoidance structures are then defined such as parotid glands, spinal cord, mandible, and optic apparatus/chiasm (if applicable).

Despite emerging publications with suggested guidelines to standardize and simplify the process of elective nodal coverage, target definition remains a highly labor-intensive process *(7–14)*. Furthermore, significant target-delineation heterogeneity exists across institutions. Publications regarding head and neck IMRT from institutions with significant expertise can demonstrate significant variation in the design of coverage volumes *(15)*.

Once the tumor targets and avoidance structures are defined, the physician prescribes actual doses that each target should receive. Commonly, the GTV may receive doses of approx 70 Gy, whereas CTV-1 may receive 54–66 Gy, and CTV-2 may receive 50–54 Gy in the definitive treatment setting *(6)*. Final doses for grossly involved nodes may depend on whether or not the patient is scheduled for a planned postradiation (or chemoradiation) neck dissection as well as the overall volume of the involved nodes *(16)*. Avoidance structures may have specific dose limitations assigned to them based on accepted tolerances. For example, dose to the contralateral parotid gland may be limited to a mean dose of 20–26 Gy *(17)* in an effort to preserve long term salivary function.

In the final phase of IMRT treatment planning, physics and dosimetry develop a deliverable IMRT plan using an inverse planning process. During this process, a specific beam arrangement and modulation pattern are created. The physician then reviews the plan to ensure that target coverage is adequate while striving to achieve the normal tissue avoidance goals successfully. Once the plan is physician approved, physics performs further quality assurance at the treatment machine prior to the first treatment to ensure that radiation is delivered as planned.

3. TREATMENT DELIVERY

From the patient's perspective, IMRT treatments are quite similar to conventional treatments, as the treatments are delivered daily with a linear accelerator. However, the treatments can differ for the patient in certain ways. First, the daily treatment time is somewhat longer, as more individual treatment fields are used. The increased beam modulation necessitates longer "beam-on" times to deliver the same dose. A conventional head and neck radiation treatment is delivered in approx 5–10 min. In contrast, an IMRT head and neck treatment may be delivered over approx 25–30 min.

With a goal to diminish toxicities, IMRT dose profiles commonly reveal steep dose gradients between tumor and adjacent normal structures. Therefore, quality head and neck IMRT requires highly reproducible patient setup and positioning on a daily basis. For conventional head and neck radiotherapy, patients are aligned with simple laser and mask marks using weekly position check films for quality assurance. This setup method safely allows 3–8-mm variations in daily setup *(18)*. Conventional radiotherapy design with large lateral fields readily accounts for this daily setup variation. High-quality IMRT demands more rigorous setup verification and immobilization. A number of techniques can be used, such as optical guidance *(5)*, daily portal filming, or the use of linac/imaging machine hybrids. These techniques may require patients to use an additional apparatus like a maxillary bite tray for optical guidance or have their treatment time extended slightly for daily imaging. Nonetheless, most patients appear to accept IMRI readily, particularly if the goal of normal tissue protection is appreciated.

4. CLINICAL DATA

Several reports have described early clinical promise with head and neck IMRT, for both tumor control and reduction of xerostomia. These data generally represent limited single-institution experience, often with a heterogeneous group of patients (postoperative vs definitive, chemotherapy vs no chemotherapy, varying dose/fractionation schemes). Prospective, multiinstitutional protocols that incorporate IMRT for head and neck cancer patients remain in the early stages.

Mature clinical data regarding the efficacy of IMRT in the management of head and neck cancer is just emerging. Preliminary single-institution experience with IMRT suggests favorable outcomes (Table 2). These results must be interpreted with caution, given the small overall numbers and careful patient selection, but they suggest that head and neck IMRT appears to be safe and effective in appropriately selected patients.

Chao et al. *(19)* have reported on 126 patients who underwent head and neck IMRT. Forty-one percent of patients were treated definitively and the remainder postoperatively. Some

Table 2
Preliminary Single-Institution Experience With Intensity-Modulated Radiation Therapy

Series	No. of patients	Disease site	Definitive vs postoperative	Chemotherapy (yes/no)	Locoregional control (%)
Chao et al. *(16)*	126	General head and neck	Both	Yes[a]	89 (2-yr)
Dawson et al. *(20)*	68	General head and neck	Both	Yes[a]	79 (2-yr)
Lee et al. *(21)*	67	Nasopharynx	Definitive	Yes	98 (4-yr)
Butler et al. *(20)*	20	General head and neck	Definitive	No	85

[a]These series contain some patients who did not receive chemotherapy.

patients also received chemotherapy. The 2-yr actuarial locoregional control rate was 85%. Dawson et al. *(20)* published patterns of recurrence from a group of head and neck cancer patients treated with parotid sparing IMRT techniques at the University of Michigan. Fifty-eight patients with primary head and neck cancer were treated definitively or postoperatively and followed for a median of 27 mo. Chemotherapy was administered in 28%. A 79% local rate of control was achieved, with 12 patients developing recurrence by 2 yr. Butler et al. *(21)* reported on 20 patients with primary head and neck tumors; 19 patients had a complete response to therapy and a significant reduction of dose to parotid glands. With a median follow-up of 13.5 mo, two patients who achieved a complete response developed local recurrence at 10 and 15 mo. Treatments were generally well tolerated. Lee et al. *(22)* reported on 67 patients with nasopharyngeal carcinoma who were treated with IMRT. Fifty of 58 patients were treated with concomitant and adjuvant chemotherapy. With a median follow-up of 31 mo, a local-regional progression-free rate of 98% was observed. These results have stimulated further evaluation of head and neck IMRT in an ongoing cooperative group trial for nasopharynx cancer patients through the Radiation Therapy Oncology Group (RTOG).

These studies suggest that IMRT represents a promising new therapy in head and neck cancer. However, these early results must be viewed with some caution. Aside from the nasopharynx data, these series include a variety of head and neck disease sites, some treated definitively and some postoperatively. Chemotherapy regimens and fractionation regimens vary within and across the published series. Overall follow-up for the patients remains relatively short. The specific techniques of IMRT treatment show evolution within each of these updated series. All these factors suggest that ongoing careful and systematic evaluation regarding acute and long term outcomes with head and neck IMRT should be pursued. Indeed, several recent reports identify challenges that remain in the safe and effective advancement of head and neck IMRT *(23–25)*. Data are emerging regarding key contributing factors for disease control and treatment failure for head and neck IMRT, including tumor characteristics and treatment technique. Chao et al. *(26)* found that primary tumor GTV and nodal GTV size independently predicted for therapeutic outcome. Analysis of patterns of failure in patients treated with IMRT led Eisbruch and colleagues *(27)* to recommend careful attention to retropharyngeal nodes in patients with oropharyngeal primaries. Further reports based on clinical outcome will continue to shape the practice of head and neck IMRT.

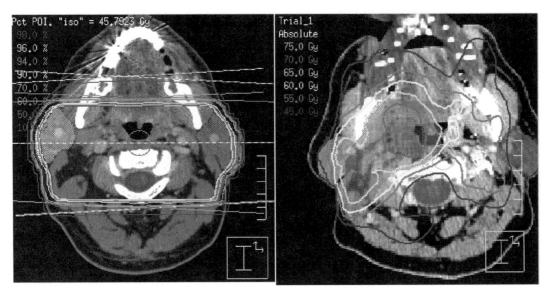

Fig. 2. Isodose distributions contrasting conventional (left) and IMRT (right) head and neck treatment plans. Dramatic reduction of dose to the left parotid gland is achieved with the IMRT plan.

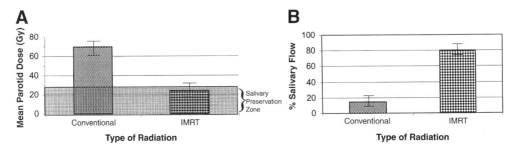

Fig. 3. **(A)** Parotid gland doses for conventional and IMRT head and neck radiation. The gray bar represents the general dose range at which preservation of salivary sparing gland function appears achievable. **(B)** Recovery pattern of salivary flow (%) following conventional vs IMRT head and neck radiation. Values represent comparison to pre-RT salivary function.

4.1. Salivary Sparing

In head and neck cancer, one of the most common rationales for IMRT is to preserve salivary gland function and thereby diminish the severity of chronic xerostomia with associated adverse impact on taste, swallowing, dentition, speech, and overall quality of life. In addition, the capacity of IMRT to limit dose to normal tissue structures may also allow dose escalation and differential dose painting, thereby accomplishing "in-field tumor boosting" *(21)*.

Xerostomia brings significant long-term consequences for the head and neck cancer patient. Lack of salivary production can lead to sore throat, decreased taste, dental decay, mandibular osteoradionecrosis, and impaired voice and swallowing functioning. IMRT techniques afford distinct opportunities for salivary gland sparing (Figs. 2 and 3). Eisbruch et al. *(17)* suggest that mean doses of 26 Gy or less to the parotid gland are necessary to spare long term parotid gland function substantially. At 26 Gy or less, excellent preservation of salivary function (unstimulated and stimulated respectively) was observed *(17)*. In addition, Eisbruch et al. *(28)* have demonstrated that salivary flow correlates with improved quality of life, suggesting that parotid sparing may be associated with improved overall clinical outcome. Chao et al. *(29)* have reported on results of a trial examining the functional outcome of salivary glands at 6 mo following radiation. Mean dose to the parotid gland was shown to correlate with ultimate salivary flow in 41 patients analyzed. More recent studies continue to suggest that salivary sparing is possible with IMRT using proper technique *(30)* and may favorably impact on overall quality of life *(31,32)*.

5. ADDITIONAL FACTORS

As with any new technology, questions remain regarding the use of IMRT. Some have voiced caution about embracing IMRT as a standard of care until the acquisition and comparative evaluation of more systematic clinical trials data *(33,34)*. Nevertheless, the general use of IMRT has increased dramatically over the last several years (Fig. 4). In a recent survey of US radiation oncologists published by Mell and colleagues in 2003 *(35)*, one-third of respondents reported that they were currently using IMRT. In addition, more than 90% of respondents who were not currently using IMRT stated that they planned to do so in the near future. Despite this increased utilization, several notable concerns regarding the use of IMRT remain, particularly in the case of head and neck cancer.

5.1. IMRT Standardization

One concern is reflected by a lack of standardization in IMRT planning and delivery. The published literature describes several different techniques, and specific aspects of IMRT planning processes remain somewhat practitioner dependent. Multiple fractionation schemes and target delineation techniques are used. Subtle technique distinctions can pose a challenge to new institutions that wish to commence use of IMRT. For these reasons, it is increasingly important to provide standardized recommendations and guidelines for head and neck IMRT planning. Indeed, guidelines are beginning to emerge with recommendations for nodal coverage targets based on tumor location and stage *(11,12)*.

5.2. IMRT Setup Precision

Radiation oncologists have been traditionally trained to use large field margins to cover unsuspected tumor infiltration and to avoid geographical miss. Since a major goal of IMRT is to limit dose to normal tissue structures that may reside very close to tumor targets, daily setup precision takes on much greater significance. A recent study by Hong et al. *(18)* suggests that the daily setup variations with conventional head and neck masking and immobilization techniques may be insufficient to ensure high quality IMRT delivery over a 6–7 wk course of treatment. Indeed, daily setup errors of several millimeters can result in underdosing of tumor or overdosing of normal tissues such as the "spared" parotid gland, underscoring the importance of rigorous quality assurance processes for IMRT.

5.3. IMRT Fractionation

Radiation therapy paradigms for head and neck cancer have undergone substantial evolution in recent years. One significant advance involves clarification regarding the importance

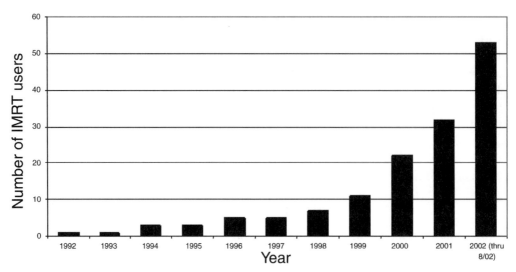

Fig. 4. Cumulative use of IMRT users by year, 1992–2002. IMRT use increased most rapidly since 1998. (Adapted from ref. *35*.)

of overall treatment time. Intensification of treatment via altered fractionation has proved valuable in improving locoregional control and disease-specific survival *(36–38)*. In order to intensify treatment with conventional radiotherapy, treatments are frequently delivered twice daily during the treatment course. In light of the increase in daily treatment time required for IMRT, and the intentional dose profile heterogeneity of IMRT, it remains unclear whether IMRT can (or should) be delivered twice daily to mimic hyperfractionation regimens. Indeed, there may be a good radiobiological rationale to maintain once-daily IMRT in light of the higher daily dose delivered to tumor (GTV) targets over elective regions.

5.4. Radiation Exposure

Another theoretical concern with IMRT involves the increased machine output (monitor units) required for IMRT delivery and the potential future risk for second malignancy. With increased modulation of the radiation beam, more monitor units are generated to deliver the prescribed dose. Consequently, there can be increased leakage from the linear accelerator, increasing the body's total exposure by two- to threefold *(39)*. In a recent publication, Hall and Wu *(39)* suggest that this increase in total body dose could potentially increase the rate of second malignancy from 1% per 10 yr to 1.75% per 10 yr, a almost doubling the second malignancy rate. Careful follow-up will be required to determine whether IMRT does in fact increase the risk of second malignancy.

5.5. Future IMRT Trials

As head and neck IMRT gradually advances into more common use, the design of clinical trials that explore the use of chemoradiation, altered fractionation, and molecular targeted therapy becomes more complex. Indeed, the cooperative oncology groups are struggling currently with systematic methodology to credential and quality-assure the process of head and neck IMRT for participating institutions. The successful accomplishment of future head and neck cancer treatment trials will need to acknowledge the steadily increasing use of IMRT despite inherent difficulties in trial design and quality assurance. This represents a significant challenge in that a broad series of promising molecular agents that may enhance radiation response are becoming available. However, the profound variation in IMRT expertise and delivery technique across institutions currently renders this an added variable that may serve to complicate the evaluation of new molecular agents with radiation.

6. CONCLUSIONS

IMRT for head and neck cancer represents a highly promising technical advance in radiation delivery providing enhanced dose conformation around tumor targets while diminishing dose to normal tissue structures. One primary objective of head and neck IMRT is to provide parotid gland sparing, which may prevent severe xerostomia and thereby improve overall quality of life. The head and neck IMRT process is labor intensive and requires an experienced team of specialists. Early clinical data suggest that head and neck IMRT may be effective in both tumor control and salivary gland sparing. However, systematic validation of early clinical results and long-term follow-up is highly desirable in controlled clinical trials.

REFERENCES

1. Greenlee RT, Hill-Harmon MB, Murray T, et al. Cancer statistics, 2001. CA Cancer J Clin 2001; 51:15–36.
2. Harari PM, Sharda NN, Brock LK, Paliwal BR. Improving dose homogeneity in routine head and neck radiotherapy with custom 3-D compensation. Radiother Oncol 1998; 49:67–71.
3. Intensity Modulated Radiation Therapy Collaborative Working Group. Intensity-modulated radiotherapy: current status and issues of interest. [Review] Int J Radiat Oncol Biol Phys 2001; 51:880–914.
4. Low DA, Chao KSC, Mutic S, et al. Quality assurance of serial tomotherapy for head and neck patient treatments. Int J Radiat Oncol Biol Phys 1998; 42:681–692.
5. Tomé WA, Meeks SL, McNutt TR, et al. Optically guided intensity modulated radiotherapy. Radiother Oncol 2001; 61:33–44.
6. Chao KS, Wippold FJ, Ozyigit G, et al. Determination and delineation of nodal target volumes for head-and-neck cancer based on patterns of failure in patients receiving definitive and postoperative IMRT. Int J Radiat Oncol Biol Phys 2002; 53:1174–1184.
7. Gregoire V, Coche E, Cosnard G. Selection and delineation of lymph node target volumes in head and neck conformal radiotherapy: Proposal for standardizing terminology and procedure based on surgical experience. Radiother Oncol 2000; 56:135–150.
8. Nowak PJ, Wijers OB, Lagerwaard FJ, et al. A three dimensional CT-based target definition for elective irradiation of the neck. Int J Radiat Oncol Biol Phys 1999; 45:33–39.
9. Wijers OB, Levendag PC, Tan T, et al. A simplified CT-based definition of the lymph node levels in the node negative neck. Radiother Oncol 1999; 52:25–42.
10. Som PM, Curtin SD, Mancuso AA. An imaging-based classification of the cervical nodes designed as an adjunct to recent clinically based nodal classifications. Arch Otolaryngol Head Neck Surg 1999; 125:388–396.
11. Levendag P, Braaksma M, Coche E, et al. Rotterdam and Brussels CT-based neck nodal delineation compared with the surgical levels as defined by the American Academy of Otolaryngology-Head and Neck Surgery. Int J Radiat Oncol Biol Phys 2004; 58:113–123.
12. Grégoire V, Levendag P, Ang KK, et al. CT-based delineation of lymph node levels and related CTVs in the node-negative neck: DAHANCA, EORTC, GORTEC, NCIC, RTOG consensus guidelines. Radiother Oncol 2003; 69:227–236.
13. Lee N, Xia P, Fischbein NJ, et al. Intensity-modulated radiation therapy for head-and-neck cancer: the UCSF experience focusing on target volume delineation. Int J Radiat Biol Phys 2003; 57:49–60.
14. Prin-Braam PM, Raaijmakers CPJ, Terhaard CHJ. Location of cervical lymph node metastases in oropharyngeal and hypopharyngeal carcinoma: implications for cranial border of elective nodal target volumes. Int J Radiat Oncol Biol Phys 2004; 58:132–138.
15. Hong TS, Tomé WA, Chappell RJ, et al. Variations in target delineation for head and neck IMRT: An international multi-institutional study.[abstract] Presented at ASTRO 2004. Int J Radiat Oncol Biol Phys 2004; 60:S157–S158.
16. Mendenhall WM, Million RR, Cassisi NJ. Squamous cell carcinoma of the head and neck treated with radiation therapy: the role of neck dissection for clinically positive neck nodes. Int J Radiat Oncol Biol Phys 1986; 12:737–740.

17. Eisbruch A, Haken RKT, Kim HM, et al. Dose, volume, and function relationships in parotid salivary glands following conformal and intensity-modulated irradiation of head-and-neck cancer. Int J Radiat Oncol Biol Phys 1999; 45:577–587.

18. Hong TS, Tomé WA, Chappell RJ, et al. The impact of daily set-up variations on head and neck IMRT. Int J Radiat Oncol Biol Phys 2005;61:779–788.

19. Chao KS, Ozyigit G, Tran BN, et al. Patterns of failure in patients receiving definitive and postoperative IMRT for head-and-neck cancer. Int J Radiat Oncol Biol Phys 2002; 55:312–3212.

20. Dawson, LA, Anzai Y, Marsh L, et al. Patterns of local-regional recurrence following parotid-sparing conformal and segmental intensity-modulated radiotherapy for head and neck cancer. Int J Radiat Oncol Biol Phys 2000; 46:1117–1126.

21. Butler EB, Teh BS, Grant WH, et al. SMART (simultaneous modulated accelerated radiation therapy) boost: a new accelerated fractionation schedule for the treatment of had and neck cancer with intensity modulated radiotherapy. Int J Radiat Oncol Biol Phys 1999; 45:21–32.

22. Lee N, Xia P, Quivey JM, Sultanem K, et al. Intensity-modulated radiotherapy in the treatment of nasopharyngeal carcinoma: an update of the UCSF experience. Int J Radiat Oncol Biol Phys 2002; 53:12–22.

23. Amosson CM, Teh BS, Van T, et al. SMART (simultaneous modulated accelerated radiation therapy) boost technique-correlation of subjective xerostmia and dosimetric parameters of the parotid glands. Int J Radiat Oncol Biol Phys 2002; 54(suppl):S18–S19.

24. Lin A, Marsh L, Dawson LA, et al. Local-regional (LR) recurrences near the base of the skull following IMRT of head and neck (HN) cancer: implications for target delineation in the high neck and for parotid sparing. Int J Radiat Oncol Biol Phys 2003; 57(suppl):S155.

25. Song S, Tome WA, Mehta MP, et al. Emphasizing conformal avoidance versus target definition for IMRT planning in head and neck cancer. Int J Radiat Oncol Biol Phys 2003; 57(suppl):S299–S300.

26. Chao KSC, Ozygit G, Blanco AI, et al. Intensity-modulated radiation therapy for oropharyngeal carcinoma: impact of tumor volume. Int J Radiat Oncol Biol Phys 2004; 59:43–50.

27. Eisbruch A, Marsh LH, Dawson LA, et al. Recurrences near base of skull after IMRT for head-and-neck cancer: implications for target delineation in high neck and for parotid gland sparing. Int J Radiat Oncol Biol Phys 2004; 59:28–42.

28. Eisbruch A, Kim HJ, Terrell JE, et al. Xerostomia and its predictors following parotid-sparing irradiation of head-and-neck cancer. Int J Radiat Oncol Biol Phys 2001; 50:695–704.

29. Chao KSC, Deasy JO, Markman J, et al. A prospective study of salivary function sparing in patients with head-and-neck cancers receiving intensity-modulated or three-dimensional radiation therapy: initial results. Int J Radiat Oncol Biol Phys 2001; 49:907–916.

30. Astreinidou E, Dehnad H, Terhaard CHJ, et al. Level II lymph nodes and radiation-induced xerostomia. Int J Radiat Oncol Biol Phys 2004; 58:124–131.

31. Reddy SP, Leman CR, Marks JE, et al. Parotid-sparing irradiation for cancer of the oral cavity-maintenance of oral nutrition and body weight by preserving parotid function. Am J Clin Oncol 2001; 24:341–346.

32. Parliament MB, Scrimger RA, Anderson SG, et al. Preservation of oral health-related quality of life and salivary flow rates after inverse-planned intensity-modulated radiotherapy (IMRT) for head-and-neck cancer. Int J Radiat Oncol Biol Phys 2004; 58:663–673.

33. Halperin HC. Overpriced technology in radiation oncology. Int J Radiat Oncol Biol Phys 2000; 48:917–918.

34. Glatstein E. The return of the snake oil salesman. Int J Radiat Oncol Biol Phys 2003; 55:561–562.

35. Mell LK, Roeske JC, Mundt AJ. A survey of intensity-modulated radiation therapy in the United States. Cancer 2003; 98:204–211.

36. Fu KK, Pajak, TF, Trotti A, et al. A Radiation Therapy Oncology Group (RTOG) phase III randomized study to compare hyperfractionation and two variants of accelerated fractionation to standard fractionation radiotherapy for head and neck squamous cell carcinomas: first report of RTOG 9003. Int J Radiat Oncol Biol Phys 2000; 48:7–16.

37. Fowler JF, Harari PM. Confirmation of improved local-regional control with altered fractionation in head and neck cancer. Int J Radiat Oncol Biol Phys 2000; 48:3–6.

38. Horiot JC, Le Fur R, N'Guyen T. Hyperfractionated versus conventional fractionation in oropharyngeal carcinoma: final analysis of a randomized trial of the EORTC cooperative group of radiotherapy. Radiother Oncol. 1992; 25:231–241.

39. Hall EJ, Wu CS. Radiation-induced second cancers: the impact of 3D-CRT and IMRT. [Review] Int J Radiat Oncol Biol Phys 2003; 56:83–88.

9

Altered Fractionation

Benefits, Pitfalls With IMRT Dosimetry, and Combined Gains With Molecular Targeting

Anesa Ahamad, MD, FRCR, David I. Rosenthal, MD, and K. Kian Ang, MD, PhD

1. INTRODUCTION

Fractionation deserves a second look in light of the explosive growth and development of radiation therapy. With the progress we have just seen in the manipulation and delivery of cytotoxic agents in conjunction with radiotherapy, there are now new avenues to explore as the classical dose and fraction size limits may no longer apply. Technological developments in physics, computing, and imaging over the past three decades culminated at the end of the 1990s in the ability to deliver elaborate 3D high-dose volumes to precisely defined targets. The traditional dose limits that are based on the tolerated dose to surrounding normal tissues may no longer be limiting since normal tissues are now avoided to a large extent. Can dose now be safely escalated using altered fractionation? Will the reduced toxicity also permit further exploration of concurrent chemotherapy with altered fractionation? Will molecular image-guided boosts to smaller subvolumes improve tolerance of "hotter" fractionation regimes? Breakthroughs in tumor biology have opened exciting new opportunities to develop specific molecularly targeted strategies to selectively enhance tumor response to radiation. With the nonoverlapping set of toxicities of these agents, can they be safely administered concurrently with more intense radiotherapy fractionation regimes?

To address these questions, a review of the results and indications of altered fraction would be useful. A survey of the key lessons may not only provide new ideas for combining these modalities to further improve the therapeutic ratio but should also underscore the key radiobiological principles that remain valid and useful in guiding everyday clinical decision making. This is especially pertinent in avoiding the potential disadvantage of the inevitable alteration of fractionation to some targets with the use of intensity-modulated radiation therapy (IMRT). Specifically, this review will summarize:

- The biological basis of altered fractionation: the reason(s) to expect an improved therapeutic ratio.
- The benefit of accelerated radiotherapy regimens.
- The benefit of hyperfractioned radiotherapy regimens.
- The combination of altered fractionation with concurrent chemotherapy.

From: *Current Clinical Oncology: Squamous Cell Head and Neck Cancer*
Edited by: D. J. Adelstein © Humana Press Inc., Totowa, NJ

- Critical fractionation issues to consider when IMRT is used:
  - Delivery of lower biologically effective dose to targets and lower probability of cure.
  - Prospect for improving the therapeutic ratio: dose escalations to targets without increased dose to normal tissues.
- Current standard of care.
- Future directions: combining the gains of molecular imaging and molecular targeting with altered fractionation.

2. THE BIOLOGICAL BASIS OF ALTERED FRACTIONATION

Until to a few years ago, the standard dose-fractionation schedule for primary treatment of head and neck cancers in the United States was 70 Gy in 35 fractions once daily, 5 d per week over 7 wk. *Accelerated radiotherapy* regimens administer the entire course in less than the standard (7-wk) overall treatment time. *Hyperfractioned radiotherapy* regimens administer a smaller dose (<2 Gy) per fraction over the same overall treatment time, usually by delivering more than one fraction per day. Both regimes improve locoregional control in head and neck squamous cell carcinoma (HNSCC). The biological mechanism of this is explained in Subheadings 2.1. and 2.2.

2.1. Accelerated Fractionation

Accelerated fractionation shortens the overall treatment time and improves outcome by counteracting the "hazard of accelerated tumor clonogen repopulation during radiotherapy" *(1)*. As tumor regresses during the course of radiation, the clonogenic surviving cells begin to proliferate more rapidly and reduce the overall net cytotoxicity of a fractionated course of radiation. This is well described in an analysis by Withers et al. *(1)*, who correlated tumor control with overall treatment time in head and neck cancer. As duration of radiotherapy is prolonged beyond 3–4 wk, the probability of local control decreases. Beyond this time the effect of each additional day is equivalent to a loss of dose effectiveness of approx 0.6 Gy. This was confirmed by a later analysis *(2)*, which showed that the lag before accelerated tumor clonogen may be less than 3 wk and that an extra 0.48 Gy/d is needed to compensate for this effect. Conversely, if the treatment duration can be reduced from the classical 7 wk, an improvement in outcome can be expected. However, to deliver treatment in less than 7 wk, it is not possible to simply give the dose in larger daily fractions because of the adverse effect of large fraction-size normal tissue late effects. Such effects on surrounding normal tissue are dose limiting in radiation therapy. To keep the level of late effects acceptable, either the total cumulative dose needs to be decreased, or a smaller dose per fraction may be given, as in the concomitant boost schema. The improvement in the therapeutic ratio by accelerated fractionation regimes is owing to the administration of the course of treatment in a time period short enough to avoid the effect of accelerated clonogenic proliferation. The probability of tumor control increases for a given total dose delivered in shorter treatment time. This leads to a therapeutic gain since overall treatment time has little influence on the probability of late normal tissue injury (when the fraction size is not increased and the interval between dose fractions is adequate for repair of sublethal DNA injury) *(3)*. However, when the overall duration of treatment is markedly reduced, acute reactions become intolerable, and it is necessary to reduce total dose or fraction size. Under these circumstances, a therapeutic gain is realized only if the dose equivalent of regeneration of tumor cells exceeds the actual reduction in dose required to keep acute reactions at a tolerable level *(4)*.

2.2. Hyperfractionation

Hyperfractionation increases the therapeutic gain by either permitting a higher total dose to be delivered or reducing the late effects by a sparing effect of small fraction size on normal tissues manifesting late complications. This is the exploitation of the subtle difference in the modes of cell kill by radiation that is a linear quadratic function of dose. The ratio of the linear and the quadratic components of cell killing, α/β, is a quantitative measure of a tissue's sensitivity to dose per fraction. Most late-responding normal tissues (for example, when fibrosis, necrosis, and demyelination are present) have a small α/β value of around 1–4 and are highly sensitive to fraction size. The administration of smaller doses per fraction allows repair of sublethal injury in normal tissue during the interfraction interval (which generally takes ≥ 6 h to approach completion in late-responding tissues). Whereas late-responding normal tissue tends to have small α/β values and be sensitive to the sparing effect of small fraction size, most human tumors *(5,6)* and acute-responding tissue, such as skin, mucosa, and hemopoetic tissue, have large α/β ratios of around 8–14 and are less capable of repair in the interfraction interval. They are less sensitive to the sparing effect of small fraction size. Therefore, hyperfractionation spares normal tissue but not tumor. Since late normal tissue complications are generally dose limiting for conventional daily fractionated radiation therapy *(7)*, reducing the dose per fraction permits a higher total dose to be given with a greater probability of tumor control for the same level of late effect. Hyperfractionation may also increase tumor radiosensitivity by redistribution of cells into more radiosensitive phases of mitosis. As the number of fractions increases, the probability of cells being hit as they progress through sensitive phases increases. Hyperfractionation may also permit improved oxygenation of tumor, which increases radiosensitivity.

By the end of the 1980s the strategy was summed up as: give as high a dose as you can without causing severe late effects, using smaller doses per fraction of around 1.8–2 Gy to keep the late effects moderate compared with tumor kill, and give this dose in as short an overall time as you can *(1)*.

Clinical experience by the end of that decade also showed that three fractions × 2 Gy per day cannot be given without causing severe late effects. The maximum dose that can be given, whatever the fractionation, appeared to be no more than 4.8–5 Gy per day. No more than 55 Gy can be given within 2 wk, or acute effects become too severe *(8)*. Based on these facts, a number of randomized trials were started. Those results are now available and are summarized in the next two sections.

3. THE BENEFIT OF ACCELERATED RADIOTHERAPY REGIMENS

Table 1 summarizes the data of four prospective trials testing pure accelerated fractionation against the conventional regimen. The key findings of accelerated fractionation regimens are summarized at the end of this section.

The regimes tested in the first two trials were found to induce unacceptable acute toxicity and have been abandoned, but the two other trials yielded positive outcomes. The Vancouver Cancer Center regimen (66 Gy as ten 2-Gy fractions per week in an overall 22–25 d instead of the conventional 45–48 d *[9]*) was terminated prematurely because the proportion of grade 4 late reactions was significantly increased in the accelerated arm. The investigators of M. Sklodowska-Curie Institute, Poland (66–72 Gy daily fractions 7 d per week at 1.8–2.0-Gy fractions) reduced the overall treatment time by 2 full weeks *(10)*. However, the incidence of

Table 1
Phase III Trials Addressing Pure Accelerated Fractionations in Patients With Head and Neck Cancer

Ref.	Tumor site and stage	No. of patients	d (Gy)	Ti (h)	n and D (Gy)	T (wk)	Tumor response	Complications
Jackson et al. (9)	Various sites, stage III–IV	82	2.0 2.0	2 (≥6) 1	66.0 66.0	3.4 6.8	CR: 35 vs 29% ($p = 0.18$). No difference in 3-yr relapse-free survival.	Grade 3–4 reactions: 27 vs 8 ($p = 0.00005$). Grade 4 late toxicity: 8 vs 2 ($p = 0.10$).
Skladowski et al. (10)	Various sites, T2–4 N0–1	100	1.8–2.0 1.8–2.0	1 1	~70.0 ~70.0	5 7	3-yr LC: 82 vs 37% ($p < 0.0001$) and 3-yr OS: 78 vs 32% ($p < 0.0001$)	Severe mucositis: 62 vs 26%. Late complications: 10 vs 0%.
Overgaard et al., Bentzen et al. (11,12)	Various sites, all stages	1485	2.0 2.0	1 1	~66.0 ~66.0	6 7	5-y LRC: 66 vs 57% . ($p = 0.01$) 5-yr DFS: 72 vs 65% ($p = 0.04$). No difference in OS	More acute mucositis with AF. No difference in late complication rate.
Hliniak et al. (13)	Larynx carcinomas, T1–3N0	395	2.0 2.0	2 (≥6) 1	66.0 66.0	5.5 6.5	No difference in LRC ($p = 0.37$)	More acute reactions with AF. No difference in late complications, except for telangiectasia.

Abbreviations: d, dose per fraction; n, number of fractions per day; Ti, time interval between fractions; D, total dose; T, overall treatment time; CR, complete response; LC, local control; LRC, locoregional control; DFS, disease-free survival; OS, overall survival; AF, accelerated fractionation.

severe confluent mucositis in the accelerated arm was more than double that of the conventional arm (62 vs 26%), and the incidence of severe late complications was 10 and 0%, respectively. The severe late complications occurred in patients who received 2 Gy per fraction in the accelerated arm (5/23 patients, or 22%). Consequently, the fraction size was decreased to 1.8 Gy per fraction in the later years of the study, and no additional late toxicity was found. The 2-wk acceleration resulted in a significant improvement in 3-yr local control (82 vs 37%, $p < 0.0001$) and overall survival (78 vs 32%, $p < 0.0001$). However, the results in the control arm might be considered rather poor, as the study did not enroll patients with N2–N3 disease, unlike most other large trials.

The experimental regimens addressed by the Danish Cooperative Group *(11,12)* and a Polish Cooperative Group *(13)* are alike and consisted of delivery of six instead of five daily fractions per week to a total dose of 66 Gy, which reduced the overall treatment time by 1 wk without reducing the radiation dose. There were more severe acute reactions, but no increase in late toxicity (e.g., edema, fibrosis), with the exception of telangiectasia ($p < 0.001$), observed in the Polish study. The larger Danish study (the Danish enrolling most patients with laryngeal cancer) demonstrated that accelerated fractionation led to a significant increase in the locoregional control rate, which so far has not had a significant impact on survival, probably because of the possibility of salvaging local relapses and a high rate of comorbidity.

The Polish Cooperative Group compared locoregional control, disease-free survival, and overall survival induced by an accelerated regimen: 66 Gy given in 33 fractions over 38 d (two fractions every Thursday) with a conventional regimen: 66 Gy given in 33 fractions over 45 d. Three hundred and ninety-five patients with T1–T3, N0, M0, glottic and supraglottic laryngeal cancer were randomized. There was no difference in terms of locoregional control ($p = 0.37$) *(13)*.

The Danish trial is one of the largest trials of altered fractionation *(11,12)*. It accrued 1485 patients with larynx, oropharynx, and oral cavity carcinomas of all stages. The sixth fraction of the week was administered either on Saturdays or as a second daily fraction during one of the weekdays. Overall 5-yr locoregional control rates improved (70 vs 60%, $p = 0.0005$). The whole benefit of shortening treatment time was seen for primary tumor control (76 vs 64%, $p = 0.0001$) but was nonsignificant for neck-node control. Treatment duration of 6 vs 7 wk improved preservation of the voice among patients with laryngeal cancer (80 vs 68%, $p = 0.007$) and improved disease-specific survival (73 vs 66%, $p = 0.01$) but not overall survival. Acute morbidity was significantly more frequent with six than with five fractions but was transient. The six fractions a week regimen has become the standard treatment in Denmark.

Multivariate analysis showed that accelerated fractionation was particularly beneficial in moderately and well-differentiated laryngeal cancer with no apparent benefit for poorly differentiated tumors (analysis of 754 larynx cancers with known differentiation). This beneficial effect of shortened treatment time for better differentiated cancers and better effect at the primary site vs nodal disease led the authors to hypothesize that the mechanism of repopulation in HNSCC is similar to the response in the normal mucosa where the tumor has originated and that, to secure such a response, the tumor needs to have a functional mechanism capable of regeneration. This capacity to respond to the trauma of irradiation is more likely to exist in well-differentiated tumors, and the process may be facilitated by signaling from the surrounding normal mucosa. Accelerated proliferation may therefore be a response of the primary tumor and not the nodal metastases *(12)*.

4. HYBRID ACCELERATED FRACTIONATION

Three forms of hybrid accelerated fractionation have been tested in randomized trials. Type A consists of an intensive short course of treatment in which the overall duration of treatment is *markedly reduced,* with a corresponding substantial decrease in the total dose. Continuous, hyperfractionated, accelerated radiotherapy (CHART) is a prototype. Types B and C represent techniques with which the duration of treatment is more *modestly reduced*, but the total dose is kept in the same range as for a conventional treatment. This is accomplished by using either a split-course twice-a-day fractionation regimen (type B) or a concomitant boost technique (type C).

Table 2 summarizes five randomized trials comparing these hybrid accelerated fractionations. Three trials addressed the type A regimen: CHART *(14)*, the Trans-Tasman Radiation Oncology Group *(15)*, and a French Cooperative Group (GORTEC) *(16)* trial. The CHART schedule *(16)* has the most drastic acceleration (54 Gy in three fractions per day in 2 wk, a reduction by 4.5 wk). The total dose was reduced by 18%. CHART did not improve tumor control or survival in head and neck cancer, but subgroup analysis revealed greater response to CHART in advanced laryngeal primaries, younger patients, and well-differentiated tumors. Poorly differentiated tumors fared better with conventional radiotherapy. The Tran-Tasman Radiation Oncology Group *(15)* (59.4 Gy in 3.5 wk) shortened the course by 3.5 wk with a 15% lower total dose. There was no gain in tumor control end points, there was more severe acute mucositis, and there was a significant reduction in some grade 2 or higher late soft tissue morbidity. The GORTEC regimen (63 Gy in 3.5 wk) also shortened the duration of treatment by a 3.5-wk acceleration but reduced the dose by only 10%, predominantly in patients with T4 oropharyngeal carcinomas *(16)*. This produced a significant improvement in the 2-yr actuarial locoregional control rate (58 vs 34%, $p < 0.01$) but no significant difference in overall survival. Acute mucositis was also more pronounced in the accelerated fractionation arm, requiring tube feeding in 90% of patients. The median follow-up was 28 mo, and late toxicity was reportedly similar between the two arms.

Two trials addressed the type B (split-course accelerated) regimen. The European Organization for Treatment of Cancer Radiotherapy Group *(17)*, and the Radiation Therapy Oncology Group (RTOG) *(18)*. The European Organization for Treatment of Cancer Radiotherapy Group tested a thrice-a-day regimen with a 1.5–2-wk treatment acceleration and a 3% total dose increment and showed a 13% improvement in the 5-yr locoregional control rate (95% CI: 3–23%). However, this regimen doubled the rate of grade 3–4 acute morbidities (including iatrogenic mortality), significantly increased the incidence of grade 3 fibrosis ($p < 0.001$), and was associated with severe neurological complications: seven cases of permanent peripheral neuropathy and two cases of radiation myelopathy. In contrast, the RTOG *(18)* tested the spit-course regimen with a 1-wk acceleration but a 4% total dose reduction. This was one of the three experimental arms compared with conventional fractionation. It failed to improve the locoregional control, and it increased acute mucositis but not late toxicity. Consequently, the two cooperative groups abandoned these two split-course regimens because of unacceptable toxicity and lack of efficacy, respectively.

One trial addressed the type C regime (concomitant boost regimen). The RTOG *(18)* trial tested 72 Gy in 42 fractions in 6.5 wk as another one of the three experimental arms compared with conventional fractionation (a 1-wk acceleration and a 3% total dose increment). This regime showed a significant improvement in 2-yr locoregional control and a trend toward improved disease-free survival, but no difference in overall survival or late toxicity.

Table 2
Phase III Trials Addressing Hybrid Accelerated Fractionations in Patients With Head and Neck Cancer

Ref.	Tumor site and stage	No. of patients	d (Gy)	n and Ti (h)		D (Gy)	T (wk)	Tumor response	Complications
				n	Ti (h)				
Accelerated fractionation with total dose reduction (type A)									
Dische et al. (14)	Various sites, mainly stage II–IV	918	1.5 2.0	3 1	(6h)	54.0 66.0	2.0 6.5	No difference in LRC, disease-free interval, and OS	More acute mucositis but less epidermis, telangiectasia, mucosal ulceration, and edema with AF
Bulsen et al. (15)	Various sites, stage III–IV	350	1.8 2	2 1	(≥6)	59.4 70	3.5 7	5-yr LRC: 52 vs 47% ($p = 0.30$). 5-yr DFS: 41 vs 35% ($p = 0.32$). 5-yr DSS: 46 vs 40% ($p = 0.40$).	More severe acute mucositis ($p = 0.00008$) but reduced incidence of grade (two late soft-tissue effects ($p < 0.05$) with AF (except for mucosal late effect).
Bourhis et al. (16)	All sites. Oropharynx- 75%; T4-70%	268	2.0 2.8	2 1		~63 70	3.3 7	2-yr LRC: 58 vs 34% ($p < 0.01$) No difference in OS.	Grade 3–4 mucositis: 83 vs 28% ($p < 0.01$) Similar late toxicity
Accelerated fractionation with split-course (type B) or concomitant boost (type C)									
Horiot et al. (17)	Various sites, T2-4 N0-1	500	1.6 2.0	3 1		72.0 70.0	5 7	5-yr LRC: 59 vs 46% ($p = 0.02$). Trend for higher 5-yr DFS ($p = 0.08$) but no difference in OS ($p = 0.96$)	More severe acute mucositis and higher incidence of severe late morbidity ($p < 0.001$) with AF
Fu et al. (18)	Various sites, stage III–IV, stage II of tongue base, hypopharynx	1073	1.8[a] 1.20 1.60 2.0	1-2 2 2 1		72.0 81.6 67.2 70.0	6 7 6 7	LRC: higher with HF and CB 54.4% ($p = 0.045$) and 54.5% ($p = 0.05$) vs 46.0% with SF.DFS: trend in favor of HF and CB ($p = 0.067$ and 0.054) but no difference in OS	More acute mucositis with all altered fractionations No difference in late complication rate

Abbreviations: d, dose per fraction; n, number of fractions per day; Ti, time interval between fractions; D, total dose; T, overall treatment time; LRC, locoregional control; DFS, disease-free survival; DSS, disease-specific survival; OS, overall survival; AF, accelerated fractionation; CB, concomitant boost; HF, hyperfractionation; SF, standard fractionation.
[a]Boost dose given in 1.5-Gy fractions.

4.1. Key Findings of Accelerated Regimens

The key findings of accelerated fractionation regimens include the following:

- Modest acceleration by 1 wk by delivering six fractions of 2 Gy per week or a concomitant boost regimen with neither dose reduction nor introduction of a treatment break yields superior locoregional control of head and neck carcinomas without appreciable increase in late toxicity but without clear impact on survival. The lack of survival advantage is perhaps because of the patient mix: a large proportion of the patients were treated for laryngeal carcinoma, for which salvage surgery is quite effective.
- Acceleration by more than 3 wk with a 10% total dose reduction (<6 to 7 Gy) also improves locoregional control without demonstrable increase in late complications. However, a further 5–8% total dose reduction abrogates the gain in tumor control but appears to reduce the severity of some late normal tissue complications, such as fibrosis and edema.
- Mucositis *per se* or its consequential late toxicity prevents delivery of more than 12 Gy per week when given in two fractions of 2 Gy per day, 5 d a week or daily fractions throughout weekends to a total dose of 66–70 Gy (pure acceleration).
- Acceleration achieves significant improved local control for well-differentiated tumors and advanced primary mucosal site tumors but may be of little benefit to advanced nodal disease and poorly differentiated tumors. This supports the existence of the accelerated proliferation phenomenon in mucosa-derived tumor cells.

5. THE BENEFIT OF HYPERFRACTIONED RADIOTHERAPY REGIMENS

Table 3 summarizes the results of four randomized trials of hyperfractionation compared with conventional regimens in intermediate to locally advanced head and neck carcinoma. The key findings of hyperfractioned fractionation regimens are summarized at the end of this section.

In all four trials *(18–21)*, hyperfractionation allowed a higher total dose to be delivered, which produced significantly improved locoregional tumor response or improved locoregional control by 8–20% associated with more severe acute mucositis but no increase in late morbidity. In two of these trials, hyperfractionation improved overall survival by 10–19%.

The Brazilian Group *(19)* tested hyperfractionated 70.4 Gy at 1.1 Gy twice daily in 6.5 d vs the 66-Gy standard. This regime improved local response by 20% and found a 3.5-yr overall survival from 8 to 27%. The European Organization for Treatment of Cancer Radiotherapy Group *(20)* tested 80.5 Gy hyperfractionated at 1.15 Gy per fraction, twice per day in 7 wk vs 70 Gy at 2 Gy per fraction. The 10.5-Gy increase in dose improved locoregional control from 40 to 59%. The Princess Margaret Hospital *(21)* tested 58.0 Gy at 1.45 Gy twice per day over 4 wk vs 51.0 Gy at 2.55 Gy per fraction once daily (a standard fractionation at that institute). The 7-Gy increase in dose improved locoregional control from 37 to 45% and improved 5-yr overall survival from 30 to 40%.

The RTOG 9003 trial *(18)* tested 81.6 Gy at 1.2 Gy per fraction twice per day over 6 wk vs 70 Gy at 2 Gy per fraction and two accelerated regimens, as shown in Table 3. The hyperfractionated regime improved locoregional control from 46 to 54.4% (similar to the improvement by accelerated fractionation with the concomitant boost arm of the trial).

This trial, which tested both alterations, provided strong evidence that total dose and treatment duration are important to outcome. Locoregional control was significantly improved by an increase of the total dose without changing overall time using hyperfractionation, or by accelerated overall treatment time without changing total dose using concomitant boost fractionation.

Table 3

Phase III Trials Addressing Hyperfractionation in Patients With Head and Neck Cancer

Ref.	Tumor site and stage	No. of patients	d (Gy)	n and Ti (h)		D (Gy)	T (wk)	Tumor response	Complications
				n	Ti (h)				
Pinto et al. (19)	Oropharynx, stage III–IV	98	1.1 2.0	2 1		70.4 66.0	6.5 6.5	Tumor response: 84 vs 64% ($p = 0.02$). 3.5-yr OS: 27 vs 8% ($p = 0.03$)	Earlier onset of acute reactions with HF. Late complications: no details
Horiot et al. (20)	Oropharynx, T2–3 N0–1	356	1.15 2.0	2 1		80.5 70.0	7 7	5-yr LRC: 59 vs 40% ($p = 0.02$). Improved local control of T3 tumors	More acute mucositis with HF. No difference in late complication rate
Cummings et al. (21)	Various sites, T3–4N0 or Any TN+	331	1.45 2.55	2 1		58.0 51.0	4 4	5-yr LRC: 45 vs 37% ($p = 0.01$). 5-yr OS: 40 vs 30% ($p = 0.01$)	More acute mucositis with HF. 5-yr grade 3–4 late toxicity: 8 vs 14% ($p = 0.31$).
Fu et al. (18)	Various sites, stage III–IV, stage II of tongue base, hypopharynx	1073	1.2 1.8[a] 1.6 2.0	2 1–2 2 1		81.6 72.0 67.2 70.0	6 7 6 7	LRC: higher with HF and CB . 54.4% ($p = 0.045$) and 54.5% ($p = 0.05$) vs 46.0% with SF and 47.5% with AFS. DFS: trend in favor of HF and CB ($p = 0.067$ and 0.054) but no difference in OS	More acute mucositis with all altered fractionations. No difference in late complication rate

Abbreviations: d, dose per fraction; n, number of fractions per day; Ti, time interval between fractions; D, total dose; T, overall treatment time; LRC, locoregional control; DFS, disease-free survival; OS, overall survival; CB, concomitant boost; HF, hyperfractionation; SF, standard fractionation; AFS, accelerated with split course.
[a]Boost dose given in 1.5-Gy fractions.

133

5.1. Key Findings of Hyperfractionated Regimens

Key findings of hyperfractioned radiotherapy regimens include the following:

- Hyperfractionation is better than standard fractionation in locoregional control of intermediate to locally advanced head and neck carcinoma. This was associated with an improvement in survival in two trials.
- Reducing the fraction size from 2 Gy to 1.1–1.2 Gy permits a 7 to 17% total radiation dose escalation without an increase in late complications. This supports the existence of a differential fractionation sensitivity (variable α/β ratios) between human late-responding normal tissues and head and neck carcinomas.

6. COMBINED ALTERED FRACTIONATION WITH CONCURRENT CHEMOTHERAPY

In light of the data in strong support of the superiority of altered fractionation to standard radiotherapy alone, it is logical to ask whether chemotherapy would further improve the gains obtained by altered fractionation. The findings of improved local control and survival with the addition of concurrent chemotherapy to radiotherapy in several randomized studies *(22–25)* and two recent metaanalyses *(26,27)* inspired investigators to combine altered fractionation schedules with chemotherapy. These trials predominantly evaluated results with the addition of chemotherapy, not results with different fractionation regimes.

Table 4 summarizes the results of six randomized studies investigating the efficacy of concurrent chemotherapy regimens with altered fractionation. The choice of fractionation regime was empirical. Radiation regimens tested so far were accelerated fractionation in three trials, hyperfractionation in one study, and split-course altered fractionation in the remaining two trials.

6.1. Accelerated Fractionalization Combined With Concurrent Chemotherapy

At least five trials using adequate doses of radiotherapy are summarized. An Austrian three-arm trial tested the addition of mitomycin C (MMC) on d 5 of treatment to accelerated fractionation: 70 Gy conventional fractionation alone vs Vienna variation of continuous hyperfractionated accelerated radiation therapy (V-CHART) alone, 55.3 Gy in 17 d vs V-CHART combined with concurrent MMC on d 5 (V-CHART + MMC) *(28)*. Locoregional tumor control was 31% after conventional fractionation, 32% after V-CHART, and 48% after V-CHART + MMC, respectively ($p < 0.05$). Overall crude survival was 24% after conventional fractionation, 31% after V-CHART, and 41% after V-CHART + MMC ($p < 0.05$). Reducing the overall treatment time from 7 wk to 17 consecutive days and radiation dose from 70 to 55.3 Gy produced equivalent results; the addition of MMC on d 5 to the accelerated fractionated treatment produced a significant improvement in local tumor control and survival. One-third of the patients treated with conventional fractionation and nearly all patients treated with accelerated fractionation developed grade 3 mucositis, which usually started at the end of or after the completion of accelerated therapy thus not causing interruption of the radiation treatment.

A German Cooperative Group compared a concomitant boost radiation regimen with or without carboplatin and 5-fluorouracil *(29)*. The addition of chemotherapy produced a trend for better locoregional control and survival rates, but it induced a significantly higher incidence of chronic dysphagia, resulting in feeding-tube dependency (51 vs 25%). A secondary randomization to receive or not receive granulocyte colony-stimulating factor to reduce mucosi-

Table 4
Phase III Trials Addressing Concurrent Chemotherapy and Altered Fractionation in Patients With Head and Neck Cancer

Ref.	Tumor site and stage	No. of patients	Therapy regimens	Tumor response	Complications
Accelerated fractionation plus chemotherapy					
Dobrowsky et al. (28)	Various sites, T1–4 N0–3	188	V-CHART 55.3 Gy/17 d (2.5 Gy on d 1, then 1.65 Gy, bid, on d 2–17) vs V-CHART + MMC vs CF: 70 Gy/7 wk	V-CHART + MMC yielded higher LRC ($p < 0.05$) and survival ($p < 0.03$) than V-CHART and CF	V-CHART induced more mucositis than CF but not intensified by MMC. Late toxicity not reported
Staar et al. (29)	Various sites, stage III–IV	240	69.9 Gy/5.5 w + carboplatin (70 mg/m^2/d) and 5-FU (600 mg/m^2/d) for 5 d × 2 69.9 Gy/ 5.5 wk (1.8 Gy qd for 3.5 wk, then bid, 1.8 Gy + 1.5 Gy, for 2 wk)	2-yr OS: 48 vs 39% ($p = 0.11$) 2-yr LC 51 vs 45% ($p = 0.14$). Patients receiving G-CSF had worse LRC ($p = 0.007$)	Grade 3–4 mucositis: 68 vs 52% ($p = 0.01$) Grade 3–4 vomiting: 8.2 vs 1.6% ($p = 0.02$) Late swallowing problems and feeding tube dependency: 51 vs 25% ($p = 0.02$)
Bourhis et al. (30)	Various sites, advanced-inoperable	109	62–64 Gy/5 wk + cisplatin (100 mg/m^2 on d 1, 16, 32) and 5-FU (1 g/m^2/d on d 1–5, 31–35) 62–64 Gy/3 wk	Not reported yet	Early cessation owing to higher treatment-related deaths in the combined arm

(continued)

Table 4 (continued)

Ref.	Tumor site and stage	No. of patients	Therapy regimens	Tumor response	Complications
Split-course accelerated fractionation plus chemotherapy					
Brizel et al. (31)	Various sites, T2–4 N0–3	122	RT: 70 Gy/47 d in 1.25 Gy bid (7–10-d break after 40 Gy) + cisplatin and 5-FU wk 1 and 6 RT alone: 75 Gy/42 d in 1.25 Gy, bid	3-yr LRC: 70 vs 44% (p = 0.01) 3-yr RFS: 61 vs 41% (p = 0.07) 3-yr OS: 55 vs 34% (p = 0.07)	Similar mucositis Increased internal feeding and sepsis Similar late complications
Wendt et al. (23)	Various sites, stage III–IV	270	70.2 Gy/51 d plus cisplatin, 5-FU, and leucovorin 70.2 Gy/51 d (23.4 Gy in 1.8-Gy fractions, bid, × 3 cycles with 10-d break)	3-yr LRC: 36 vs 17% (p < 0.004) 3-yr OS: 48 vs 24% (p < 0.0003)	Grade 3–4 acute mucositis: 38 vs 16% (p < 0.001) Serious late side effects: 10 vs 6.4% (NS)
Hyperfractionation plus chemotherapy					
Jeremic et al. (32)	Various sites, stage III–IV	130	77 Gy/7 wk + cisplatin (6 mg/m² /d) 77 Gy/7 wk (1.1 Gy, bid)	5-yr LRPFS: 50 vs 36% (p = 0.04) 5-yr PFS: 46 vs 25% (p = 0.007) 5-yr DMFS: 86 vs 57% (p = 0.001) 5-yr OS: 46 vs 25% (p = 0.008)	No significant difference in acute morbidity (except for leucopenia, p = 0.006) or late toxicity

Abbreviations: CF, conventional fractionation; V-CHART, Vienna variation of continuous hyperfractionated accelerated radiation therapy; MMC, mitomycin-C; qd, once-a-day irradiation; bid, twice-a-day irradiation; LC, local control; LRC, locoregional control; RFS, relapse-free survival; LRPFS, locoregional progression-free survival; PFS, progression-free survival; DMFS, distant metastasis-free survival; OS, overall survival; NS, not significant; G-CSF, granulocyte colony-stimulating factor.

tis produced the unexpected finding that *the administration of granulocyte colony-stimulating factor significantly reduced the probability of locoregional control in both treatment arms.*

The French Cooperative Group GORTEC tested the combination of 62–64 Gy given in 5 wk with cisplatin and fluorouracil and terminated the trial prematurely owing to unacceptable toxicity *(30)*.

Split-course altered fractionation with or without concurrent chemotherapy was tested in two trials. Both added cisplatin and fluorouracil to split-course type accelerated fractionation schedules (70 Gy in 42–51 d) *(23,31)*. Both showed that a chemotherapy regime improved locoregional control vs altered fractionation alone. The locoregional control improved, with an 18 to 26% increase in late effects. The larger trial showed improved overall survival.

6.2. Hyperfractionation and Concurrent Chemotherapy

A randomized trial by Jeremic et al. *(32)* tested the addition of low-dose daily cisplatin to 77 Gy at 1.1 Gy per fraction twice daily over 7 wk. Daily cisplatin improved the locoregional progression-free survival (50 vs 36%, $p = 0.04$), 5-yr progression-free survival (46 vs 25%, $p = 0.007$), 5-yr distant metastases free survival (86 vs 57%, $p = 0.001$), and 5-yr overall survival (46 vs 25%, $p = 0.008$). This was a true therapeutic gain because there was no difference in late side effects.

6.3. Ongoing RTOG Trial of Concurrent Chemotherapy to Select Fractionation Schedules

The optimal fractionation with concomitant chemotherapy remains unclear and must be defined by future prospective randomized trials. The RTOG is currently conducting a randomized trial to test whether altered fractionation improves the outcome of concurrent cisplatin chemotherapy, i.e., whether the benefit of altered fractionation remains true in the setting of concurrent chemotherapy *(33)*. The fractionation is based on the findings of RTOG 90-03, as given in Table 3 as presented earlier *(18)*. Patients with squamous cell carcinoma of the oral cavity, oropharynx, hypopharynx, or larynx stage III–IV disease (T2N2–3M0, T3–4 any N M0 but not T1–2N1 or T1N2–3) are randomized to either: *conventional standard radiation* (70 Gy in 35 fractions once daily over 7 wk) with three cycles of concurrent cisplatin (100 mg/ m^2 given every 3 wk during radiotherapy) or *concomitant boost* (72 Gy in 42 fractions in 6.5 wk) with two cycles of the same chemotherapy.

7. CRITICAL FRACTIONATION ISSUES TO CONSIDER WHEN USING IMRT

Advances in the accuracy of tumor delineation by diagnostic imaging and progress in dosimetry have made it possible to deliver high radiation doses that conform to the 3D shape of tumor volumes using IMRT. The new era of high-precision radiation therapy brings two major advantages: improved coverage of tumor volumes by the prescribed dose without the use of multiple matched fields, and increased sparing of normal tissues, such as parotid gland, spinal cord, brainstem, brain, optic nerve, and chiasm. However there are two important fractionation issues to be considered:

• Specification of the dose and fractionation to the primary target may result in treating secondary targets to a lower dose per fraction. This has to be corrected by alteration of the total dose to the secondary target to avoid the potentially serious disadvantage of delivering a lower biologically effective dose.

- IMRT may allow radiation dose escalation if the dose-limiting toxicity can be spared by organ avoidance. Incremental dose may be delivered as additional fractions with prolongation of the duration of treatment or by giving more than one fraction per day. Alternatively, the dose per fraction may be increased and the total escalated dose delivered in the same or shortened treatment time.

7.1. Potential Delivery of Lower Biologically Effective Dose to Targets and Lower Probability of Cure

Classic non-IMRT radiotherapy techniques for head and neck cancer deliver doses at a fixed dose per fraction to all targets. A large initial field encompasses the entire volume, then the field is reduced to cover additional regions to a higher dose. For example, a classic head and neck plan such as the one represented in Fig. 1A uses opposed lateral photon fields and abutting electron fields to deliver 50 Gy at 2 Gy per fraction to gross disease at the primary site and nodes, as well as to elective nodal regions and structures around the tumor that may contain microscopic tumor cells. A smaller pair of fields is then used to deliver an additional 16–20 Gy in 8–10 fractions to the gross tumor and nodal disease to 66–70 Gy, depending on the size of the gross tumor. A posterior electron field may be added to bring the dose adjacent to the gross nodal tumor to 56–60 Gy. This type of fractionation is used especially with concurrent chemotherapy.

In contrast with IMRT, all targets are treated in a fixed number of fractions, and difference in the total dose is achieved by varying the dose per fraction. For example, 70 Gy in 35 fractions prescribed to the gross tumor will deliver 2 Gy per fraction to this volume. The 56 and 50 Gy prescribed to secondary target volumes will also be delivered in 35 fractions in 7 wk at a smaller dose per fraction. The biologically effective dose of 56 Gy and 50 Gy in 35 fractions in 7 wk is lower using IMRT because of the effect of the smaller dose per fraction and longer treatment time, as shown in Table 5. A method to estimate the equivalent dose owing to lower dose per fraction is the linear quadratic formula:

$$BED_2 = D\{[d + (\alpha/\beta)]/[2 + (\alpha/\beta)]\}$$

Where BED_2 is the biologically isoeffective dose at 2 Gy/fraction, D is the total dose (Gy), d is the dose per fraction (Gy), and n is the number of fractions and an α/β value of 10.5 for head and neck tumor was used *(34)*. The $BED_{2,T}$ is the biologically effective dose with smaller dose per fraction in overall prolonged treatment time, assuming that D_{prolif}, the dose recovered by tumor owing to proliferation of tumor cells by prolongation, is at a rate of 0.7 Gy per day in head and neck tumors *(34)*. The $BED_{2,T}$ was calculated by the equation:

$$BED_{2,T} = D\{[d + (\alpha/\beta)]/[2 + (\alpha/\beta)]\} - (T - t) \times D_{prolif}$$

T is the prolonged time (days) and t is the original treatment time if given at 2 Gy per day. If IMRT is used, the dose to the 56- and 50-Gy targets would therefore need to be increased to approx 62.3 and 59.8, respectively, to correct for this decreased biological effect. This corrected dose (D_{corr}) is the total dose that could be given when IMRT is used. Table 5 also gives the estimated total corrected dose fraction size rounded off to 1 decimal place. If the primary target is given as 70 Gy in 35 fractions, the 56- and 50-Gy (in 2 Gy fractions) targets should be given to 63 and 59.5 Gy at 1.8 and 1.7 Gy per fraction, respectively.

For example with the multi-institutional RTOG nasopharynx protocol, RTOG H0225, which is testing the feasibility of delivering IMRT for nasopharyngeal carcinoma both the gross tumor and lymph node metastasis with a 5-mm margin will receive 70 Gy in 33 fractions

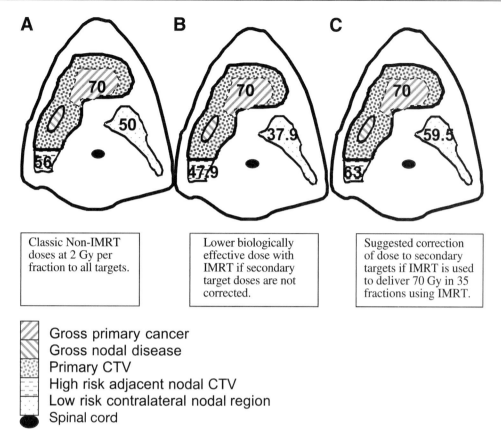

Fig. 1. Suggested adjustment of the total dose to secondary targets when intensity-modulated radiation therapy (IMRT) is used. **(A,B)** The difference between the biologically isoeffective dose (BED) at 2 Gy/fraction of plans using classic non-IMRT techniques for head and neck cancer, vs IMRT if the dose to secondary targets is not adjusted. This loss of effect is caused by smaller dose per fraction and prolonged overall treatment times. The variables used to calculate these are given in Table 6. In this example of a T3N2 base of tongue cancer, **(A)** shows doses administered using a non-IMRT technique with successive field reductions to deliver 70 Gy at 2 Gy per fraction to gross disease, 56 Gy to the high-risk region posterior to nodal disease and 2Gy per fraction and 50 Gy to an elective contralateral nodal region at 2 Gy per fraction. In **(B)**, biologically isoeffective dose at 2 Gy/fraction to these regions is shown if IMRT is used without adjustment of doses. The BED of the two secondary targets is much less than in **(A)** because the doses to secondary target volumes, 50 and 56 Gy, are delivered in 35 fractions in 7 wk using IMRT at a smaller dose per fraction. The BED is calculated from the linear quadratic formula as shown in the text. **(C)** The adjusted dose to be given to secondary targets if IMRT is used to deliver 70 Gy in 35 fractions to the primary CTV.

at 2.12 Gy per fraction. The primary subclinical first-echelon nodes or dissected neck area containing lymph node metastases will receive 59.4 Gy in 33 fractions of 1.8 Gy/fraction *(33)*.

7.2. Prospect for Improving the Therapeutic Ratio by Dose Escalations to Targets Without Increased Dose to Normal Tissues

The experience and conclusions of altered fractionation studies are based entirely on the results of traditional radiotherapy techniques and conventional conformal techniques. These techniques deliver the boost dose to a much larger volume of normal tissues. *However, IMRT*

Table 5
The Biologically Isoeffective Dose (BED) for Tumor Control to Secondary
Targets With Intensity-Modulated Radiation Therapy (IMRT)[a]

	Non-IMRT	IMRT	Non-IMRT	IMRT
Dose to secondary target (Gy)	56	56	50	50
Dose per fraction (Gy),	2	1.6	2	1.43
No. of fractions	28	35	25	35
Overall time in wk (d)	5.5 (38)	7 (47)	5 (33)	7 (47)
BED$_2$: BED for tumor control at 2 Gy/fraction without time factor ($\alpha/\beta=10.5$)	56	54.2	50	47.7
Dose recovered by tumor owing to prolongation at a rate of 0.7 Gy per day		6.3		9.8
BED in prolonged time		47.9		37.9
Total dose to be given if IMRT is used and dose to secondary target is not given at standard fractionation		62.3		59.8
Dose per fraction rounded to one decimal place		1.8		1.7
Total dose to be given with IMRT with dose per fraction rounded to one decimal place		63		59.5

[a]When the goal dose is 70 Gy in 35 fractions to primary target if the secondary targets are prescribed to 56 and 50 Gy as for non-IMRT shrinking field techniques. This takes into consideration the effect of reduced dose per fraction and the effect of prolonged overall treatment time (illustrated in Fig. 1).

The equations used to derive the BEDs for tumor control$_2$ and tumor control$_{2,T}$ are given in the text.

techniques deliver lower doses to normal structures and consequently induces for less toxicity. For example, parotid-sparing head and neck IMRT has been shown to reduce the incidence and severity of xerostomia (35–37).

Reduced dose to the brain and optic and otic apparatus may translate into fewer central nervous system complications and improved quality of life. However, a further advantage of IMRT may be its potential for dose escalation. If the toxicity that traditionally limits the total prescribed dose can be reduced, then IMRT may actually invalidate accepted limits of fractionation and dose intensity and open up a new set of boundaries. IMRT is being studied by the RTOG in two current studies:

- RTOG-H0022 is studying early oropharyngeal cancer treatment using IMRT. The prescribed dose to the primary planning target volume is 66 Gy in 30 fractions at 2.2 Gy per fraction in 6 wk. As shown in Table 6, this translates into a biologically effective dose of 69.1 Gy because the treatment is accelerated to 6 wk (33).
- RTOG-H0225 is studying nasopharyngeal cancer treatment using IMRT with concomitant chemotherapy. The prescribed dose to the primary clinical target volume is 70 Gy in 33 fractions at 2.12 Gy per fraction in 6.5 wk. As shown in Table 6, this is biologically equivalent to 73.4 Gy (33).

Table 6
Biologically Isoeffective Dose (BED) in Shortened Time,
and Higher Dose per Fraction Used in Two RTOG Studies[a]

	Non-IMRT	IMRT (RTOG H0022)	Non-IMRT	IMRT (RTOG H0225)
Dose (Gy)	66	66	70	70
Dose per fraction (Gy)	2	2.20	2	2.12
No. of fractions	33	30	35	33
Overall treatment time, in wk (d)	6.5 (45)	6 (42)	7 (49)	6.5 (45)
BED for tumor control at 2 Gy/ fraction (BED$_2$) without time factor ($\alpha/\beta = 10.5$)	66.0	67	70	70.6
Dose equivalent increase owing to shortened treatment time at a rate of 0.7 Gy per day		2.1		2.8
BED in shortened time,T (BED$_{2,T}$)		69.1		73.4

Abbreviations: RTOG, Radiation Therapy Oncology Group; IMRT, Intensity-modulated radiation therapy.

[a]1, RTOG-H0022 study of early oropharyngeal cancer treatment using IMRT to prescribe 66 Gy in 30 fractions at 2.2 Gy per fraction in 6 wk to primary target; 2, RTOG-H0225 study of nasopharyngeal cancer treatment using IMRT to prescribe 70 Gy in 33 fractions at 2.12 Gy per fraction in 6.5 wk to the primary target.

The equations used to derive BEDs for tumor control$_2$ and tumor control$_{2,T}$ are given in the text.

Both regimes will improve convenience of treatment for patients by reducing the total duration of treatment, improving the efficacy of treatment by overall acceleration, and reducing late effects by the conformality of the IMRT technique. Preclinical comparative dosimetry studies have suggested that dose escalation may be feasible using simultaneous boosts to tumor subvolumes (38). Further work is ongoing to explore whether the boost volume may be localized using metabolic or hypoxic imaging (39).

8. CURRENT STANDARD OF CARE

An analysis by the Meta-analysis of Chemotherapy on Head and Neck Cancer Collaborative Group (27) revealed a small, but statistically significant, overall benefit in survival with chemotherapy. (The absolute benefit at 2 and 5 yr was 4%.) However, concurrent chemotherapy with radiation, mainly given in conventional fractionation, yielded a significant absolute benefit at 2 and 5 yr of 8%. This benefit is seen predominantly in more locally advanced (i.e., stage IV) head and neck cancer. This is, in general, a larger survival benefit than that achieved with altered fractionation regimens. Although this is accompanied by increased acute and late toxicity in normal tissue, many head and neck oncologists recommend concurrent chemoradiation, mainly for patients with large T3 or T4 tumors or with N2–N3 nodes.

Since accelerated regimens seem to preferentially benefit local control at the primary site and not nodal control, it is reasonable to choose altered fractionation for patients with T2 or exophytic T3 or N0–1 disease and those with more advanced locoregional tumor who are unfit to receive chemotherapy (40).

The critical question of whether altered fractionation is more effective than standard fractionation when combined with concurrent chemotherapy is still being addressed based on encouraging results of phase II trials.

9. FUTURE DIRECTIONS:
COMBINING THE GAINS OF MOLECULAR IMAGING AND MOLECULAR
TARGETING WITH ALTERED FRACTIONATION

Advances in the understanding of tumor biology have opened exciting new opportunities to develop specific molecularly targeted strategies to selectively enhance tumor response to radiation. Advances in molecular imaging will also permit better delineation of selective targets.

For example, epidermal growth factor receptor (EGFR) overexpression was shown to be a strong independent prognostic indicator for overall survival and disease-free survival and a robust predictor for locoregional relapse but not for distant metastasis in a correlative study using specimens of patients with advanced HNSCCs enrolled in the RTOG 9003 trial *(18)*. When validated, EGFR immunohistochemistry could be considered for selecting patients for more aggressive combined therapies or enrollment into trials targeting EGFR or its downstream signaling pathways *(41)*.

In addition, promising preclinical and earlier phase clinical results support the use of EGFR blockade in combination with radiation for advanced HNSCC *(42–44)*.

These results were corroborated by the recently reported phase III international trial that demonstrated radiosensitization following molecular inhibition of EGFR signaling. The agent cetuximab, when added to high-dose radiation in patients with locoregionally advanced HNSCC, produced a statistically significant prolongation in overall survival and increase in locoregional control.

In this study, 424 patients were randomized to receive either radiation alone for 6–7 wk, or radiation plus weekly cetuximab. The inhibition of EGFR yielded an improved median survival of 28–54 mo, a 2-yr survival of 55 to 62%, and a 3-yr survival of 44 to 57% ($p = 0.02$) *(45)*.

Further studies are needed to explore the mechanisms behind repopulation, which will hopefully identify predictive factors to help select appropriate fractionation regimens, improve treatment strategies, and define targets. The combination of molecular imaging, image-guided radiotherapy, and molecular targeted therapy will improve the efficacy of radiotherapy.

ACKNOWLEDGMENTS

Supported in part by grant CA06294, awarded by the National Cancer Institute supplemented by the Gilbert H. Fletcher Chair. The assistance of Cynthia Holt in manuscript preparation is appreciated.

REFERENCES

1. Withers HR, Taylor JMG, Maciejewski B. The hazard of accelerated tumor clonogen repopulation during radiotherapy. Acta Oncol 1988; 27:131–46.
2. Bentzen SM, Thames HD. Clinical evidence for tumor clonogen regeneration: interpretations of the data. Radiother Oncol 1991; 22:161–166.
3. Bentzen SM, Overgaard J. Clinical normal-tissue radiobiology. In: Tobias JS, Thomas PR, eds. Current Radiation Oncology, vol 2. London: Arnold.
4. Peters LJ, Ang KK, Thames HD. Accelerated fractionation in the radiation treatment of head and neck cancer: a critical comparison of different strategies. Acta Oncol 1988; 27:185–194.
5. Thames HD, Bentzen SM, Turesson I, et al. Time-dose factors in radiotherapy: a review of the human data. Radiother Oncol 1990; 19:219–235.
6. Brenner DJ, Martinez AA, Edmundson GK, et al. Direct evidence that prostate tumours show high sensitivity to fractionation (low α/β ratio), similar to late-responding normal tissue. Int J Radiat Oncol Biol Physics 2002; 52:6–13.
7. Thames HD, Withers HR, Peters LJ, Fletcher GH. Changes in early and late radiation responses with altered dose fractionation: implications for dose-survival relationships. Int J Radiat Oncol Bio Physics 1982; 8:219–226.

8. Fowler JF. The linear-quadratic formula and progress in fractionated radiotherapy. Br J Radiol 1989; 62:679–694.

9. Jackson SM, Weir LM, Hay JH, et al. A randomized trial of accelerated versus conventional radiotherapy in head and neck cancer. Radiother Oncol 1997; 43:39–46.

10. Skladowski K, Maciejewski J, Golen M, et al. Randomized clinical trial on 7-day continuous accelerated irradiation (CAIR) of head and neck cancer: report on 3-year tumor control and normal tissue toxicity. Radiother Oncol 2000; 55:93–102.

11. Overgaard J, Hansen HS, Grau C, et al. The DAHANCA 6 & 7 trial: a randomized multicenter study of 5 versus 6 fractions per week of conventional radiotherapy of squamous cell carcinoma (scc) of the head and neck. Radiother Oncol 2000; 56(suppl):S4.

12. Bentzen J, Bastholt L, Hansen O, et al. On behalf of the Danish Head and Neck Cancer Study Group. Five compared with six fractions per week of conventional radiotherapy of squamous-cell carcinoma of head and neck: DAHANCA 6&7 randomized controlled trial. Lancet 2003; 363:933–940.

13. Hliniak A, Gwiazdowska B, Szutkowski Z, et al. A multicentre randomized/controlled trial of a conventional versus modestly accelerated radiotherapy in the laryngeal cancer: influence of a 1 week shortening overall time. Radiother Oncol 2002; 62(1):110.

14. Dische S, Saunders M, Barrett A, et al. A randomized multicentre trial of CHART versus conventional radiotherapy in head and neck cancer. Radiother Oncol 1997; 44:123–136.

15. Poulsen MG, Denham JW, Peters LJ, et al. A randomized trial of accelerated and conventional radiotherapy for stage III and IV squamous carcinoma of the head and neck: a Trans-Tasman Radiation Oncology Group Study. Radiother Oncol 2001; 60:113–122.

16. Bourhis J, Lapeyre M, Tortochaux J, et al. Very accelerated versus conventional radiotherapy in HNSCC: results of the GORTEC 94-02 randomized trial. Int J Radiat Oncol Biol Phys 2000; 48(suppl):S111.

17. Horiot JC, Bontemps P, van den Bogaert V, et al. Accelerated fractionation (AF) compared to conventional fractionation (CF) improved head and neck cancers: results of the EORTC 22851 randomized trial. Radiother Oncol 1997; 44: 111-21.

18. Fu KK, Pajak TF, Trotti A, et al. A Radiation Therapy Oncology Group (RTOG) phase III randomized study to compare hyperfractionation and two variants of accelerated fractionation to standard fractionation radiotherapy for head and neck squamous cell carcinomas: first report of RTOG 9003. Int J Radiat Oncol Biol Physics 2000; 48:7–16.

19. Pinto L, Canary P, Araujo C, et al. Prospective randomized trial comparing hyperfractionated versus conventional radiotherapy in stages II and IV oropharyngeal carcinoma. Int J Radiat Oncol Biol Phys 1991; 21:557–562.

20. Horiot JC, LeFur RN, Guyen T, et al. Hyperfractionation versus conventional fractionation in oropharyngeal carcinoma: final analysis of a randomized trial of the EORTC cooperative group of radiotherapy. Radiother Oncol 1992; 25:231–241.

21. Cummings B, O'Sullivan B, Keane T, et al. 5-year results of a 4 week/twice daily radiation schedule. Radiother Oncol 2000; 56(suppl):S8.

22. Merlano M, Benasso M, Corvo R, et al. Five-year update of a randomized trial of alternating radiotherapy and chemotherapy compared with radiotherapy alone in treatment of unresectable squamous cell carcinoma of the head and neck. J Natl Cancer Inst 1996; 88:583–589.

23. Wendt TG, Grabenbauer GG, Rodel CM, et al. Simultaneous radiochemotherapy versus radiotherapy alone in advanced head and neck cancer: a randomized multicenter study. J Clin Oncol 1998;16:1318–1324.

24. Calais G, Alfonsi M, Bardet E, et al. Randomized trial of radiation therapy versus concomitant chemotherapy and radiation therapy for advanced-stage oropharynx carcinoma. J Natl Cancer Inst 1999; 91:2081–2086.

25. Adelstein DJ, Adams GL, Li Y, et al. A phase III comparison of standard radiation therapy (RT) versus RT plus concurrent cisplatin (DDP) versus split-course RT plus concurrent DDP and 5-fluorouracil (5FU) in patients with unresectable squamous cell head and neck cancer (SCHNC): an intergroup study. Proc ASCO 2000; 19:411a (abstr).

26. El-Sayed S, Nelson N. Adjuvant and adjunctive chemotherapy in the management of squamous cell carcinoma of the head and neck region. a meta-analysis of prospective and randomized trials. J Clin Oncol 1996; 14:838–847.

27. Pignon JP, Bourhis J, Domenge C, Designe L. Chemotherapy added to locoregional treatment for head and neck squamous-cell carcinoma: three meta analyses of updated individual data. Lancet 2000; 355:949–955.

28. Dobrowsky W, Naude J. Continuous hyperfractionated accelerated radiotherapy with/without mitomycin C in head and neck cancers. Radiother Oncol 2000; 57:119–124.

29. Staar S, Rudat V, Stuetzer H, et al. Intensified hyperfractionated accelerated radiotherapy limits the additional benefit of simultaneous chemotherapy—results of a multicentric randomized German trial in advanced head and neck cancer. Int J Radiat Oncol Biol Phys 2001; 50:1161–1171.

30. Bourhis J, Lapeyre M, Tortochaux J, et al. Preliminary results of the GORTEC 96-01 randomized trial, comparing very accelerated radiotherapy versus concomitant radio-chemotherapy for locally inoperable HNSCC. Int J Radiat Oncol Biol Phys 2001; 51(suppl 1):39.

31. Brizel DM, Albers ME, Fisher SR, et al. Hyperfractionated irradiation with or without concurrent chemotherapy for locally advanced head and neck cancer. N Engl J Med 1998; 338:1798–1804.

32. Jeremic B, Shibamoto Y, Milicic B, et al. Hyperfractionated radiation therapy with or without concurrent low-dose daily cisplatin in locally advanced squamous cell carcinoma of the head and neck: a prospective randomized trial. J Clin Oncol 2000; 18: 458-64.

33. http://www.rtog.org/members/active.html#headneck

34. Bentzen S, Baumann M. Values for D_{prolif} from clinical studies. In: Basic Clinical Radiobiology, 3rd ed, 2002:138.

35. Paliament MB, Scrimger Ra, Anderson SG, et al. Preservation of oral health-related quality of life and salivary flow rates after inverse-planned intensity-modulated radiotherapy (IMRT) for head-and-neck cancer. Int J Radiat Oncol Biol Phys 2004; 58(3):663–673.

36. Munter MW, Thilmann C, Hof H, et al. Sterotactic intensity modulated radiation therapy and inverse treatment planning for tumors of the head and neck region: clinical implementation of the step and shoot approach and first clinical results. Radiother Oncol 2003; 66:313–321.

37. Lin A, Kim HM, Terrell JE, Dawson LA, Ship JA, Eisbruch A. Quality of life after parotid-sparing IMRT for head-and-neck cancer: a prospective longitudinal study. Int J Radiat Oncol Biol Phys 2003; 57:61–70.

38. Mohan R, Qiuwen W, Manning M, Schmidt-Ullrich R. Radiobiological Consideration in the design of fractionation strategies for intensity-modulated radiation therapy of head and neck cancers. Int J Radiat Oncol Biol Phys 2000; 46:619–630.

39. Chao KS, Bosch WR, Mutic S, et al. A novel approach to overcome hypoxic tumor resistance: Cu-ATSM-guided intensity-modulated radiation therapy. Int J of Radiat Oncol Biol Phys 2001; 49:1171–1182.

40. Nguyen LN, Ang KK. Radiotherapy for cancer of the head and neck: altered fractionation regimens. Lancet 2002; 3:693–701.

41. Ang KK, Berkey BA, Tu X, et al. Impact of epidermal growth factor receptor expression on survival and pattern of relapse in patients with advanced head and neck carcinoma. Cancer Res 2002; 62:7350–7356.

42. Milas L, Mason K, Hunter N, Petersen S, Yamakawa M, Ang KK, Mendelsohn J, Fan Z. In vivo enhancement of tumor radio response by C225 antiepidermal growth factor receptor antibody. Clin Cancer Res 2000; 6:701–708.

43. Nasu S, Ang KK, Fan Z, Milas L. C225 antiepidermal growth factor receptor antibody enhances tumor radiocurability. Int J Radiat Oncol Biol Phys 2001; 51:474–477.

44. Shin DM, Donato NJ, Perez-Soler R, et al. Epidermal growth factor receptor targeted therapy with C225 and cisplatin in patients with head and neck cancer. Clin Cancer Res 7:1204–1213.

45. Bonner JA, Harari PM, Giralt J, et al. Cetuximab prolongs survival in patients with locoregionally advanced squamous cell carcinoma of head and neck: a phase III study of high dose radiation therapy with or without cetuximab (abstract no. 5507) ASCO Proc 2004.

10

The Role of Tumor Hypoxia
in Head and Neck Cancer Radiotherapy

Quynh-Thu Le, MD, Amato J. Giaccia, PhD,
and J. Martin Brown, PhD

1. INTRODUCTION

Tumor hypoxia, or the condition of low tumor oxygenation, has been a focus of considerable debate in radiation therapy for almost 50 yr since the pioneering work of Gray and colleagues *(1)* demonstrating an oxygen dependency in the radiosensitivity of cells and tissues. During this period, interest among researchers has waxed and waned as promising new directions emerged from the laboratory, only to fail in clinical trials. However, with the emergence of new concepts and the development of new tools, the prospect of targeting tumor hypoxia and identifying patients who would most benefit from this approach appears more tangible clinically. This chapter discusses the significance of tumor hypoxia in head and neck squamous cell carcinomas (HNSCC) as well as past, present, and future strategies for targeting this microenvironmental factor.

2. TUMOR HYPOXIA AND MALIGNANT PROGRESSION

Poorly oxygenated regions develop within solid tumors because of aberrant blood vessel formation, changes in blood flow from intermittent closure of existing blood vessels, and increasing tumor oxygen demands for growth *(2)* (Fig. 1). The existence of hypoxia in human tumors was suggested in 1955 by Thomlinson and Gray *(3)*, who showed with histological sections that there was a constant distance (100–150 μm) across tumor tissues between blood vessels and necrosis and that this distance was the oxygen diffusion distance based on capillary oxygen partial pressure and cellular oxygen consumption. They postulated that hypoxic cells existed adjacent to necrotic areas, just beyond the oxygen diffusion distance. This is now known as chronic hypoxia. A second form of hypoxia, known as acute hypoxia, also exists owing to fluctuating flow in tumor blood vessels. This was first postulated by Brown *(4)* and subsequently demonstrated in transplanted mouse tumors using injections of two different diffusible dyes minutes apart showing that temporary reduction in flow or closure of blood vessels can be observed in solid tumors, resulting in areas of acutely hypoxic cells *(5)*. It is likely that acute and chronic hypoxia are the extremes of a continuum caused by the dynamic nature of tumor blood flow and that both can give rise to tumor cells that are prone to metastasis and resistant to conventional therapy.

From: *Current Clinical Oncology: Squamous Cell Head and Neck Cancer*
Edited by: D. J. Adelstein © Humana Press Inc., Totowa, NJ

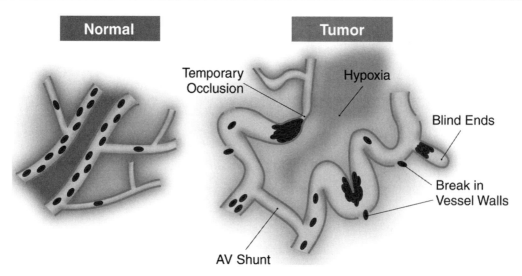

Fig. 1. Schematic representations of tumor hypoxia and necrosis that resulted from differences in the vasculature between tumor and normal tissues. (Reprinted from ref. 2, with permission from the American Association for Cancer Research.)

Laboratory studies have indicated that tumor hypoxia can play an important role in regulating cell viability and promoting cell metastatic potential. Graeber et al. *(6)* have shown that hypoxia induced apoptosis in minimally transformed mouse embryo fibroblasts with normal p53 function, but not in cells with mutant p53 proteins in both cell culture and transplantable tumors. These data suggest that hypoxia may exert a physiologic pressure for selection by clonal expansion of mutant p53 tumor cells, which, in HNSCC, have been shown to behave more aggressively than their wild-type counterparts *(7)*. Young et al. *(8)* observed that cells treated with hypoxia were more likely to invade the lungs of recipient mice than untreated cells. Likewise, acute hypoxia has been shown to enhance the formation of spontaneous nodal metastases in an orthotopic murine model or cervical carcinomas *(9)*. Clinical studies have supported the link between hypoxia and tumor metastasis: studies of soft tissue sarcomas and carcinomas of the cervix have shown that hypoxia is an independent and significant prognostic factor that correlates with metastatic spread *(10–12)*.

At the molecular level, multiple stress-response pathways are turned on when cells are exposed to hypoxia. Changes in the expression of genes and proteins are important for hypoxia-induced cellular adaptation to an anaerobic environment. One of the most well-described oxygen-response pathways is mediated by the hypoxia-inducible factor (HIF-1), which has been shown to play an important role in tumor development *(13,14)*. HIF-1 regulates genes that are involved in metabolism, angiogenesis, invasion, metastasis, and apoptosis, all of which can influence tumor growth and metastasis (Fig. 2). One of the most important HIF-1 targets is vascular endothelial growth factor (VEGF), which is a proangiogenic protein that has been implicated in poor prognosis in head and neck cancer *(15,16)*. Rapidly advancing knowledge of hypoxia-regulated genes and proteins via proteomic and genomic approaches will provide a better understanding of the molecular basis of hypoxia and give rise to novel concepts for exploiting this microenviromental factor.

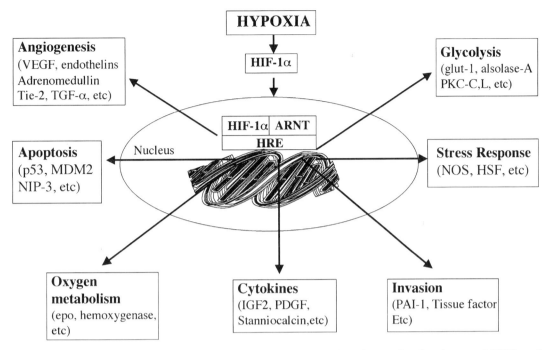

Fig. 2. Schematic representation of hypoxia-inducible factor (HIF)-1α regulated pathways. ARNT, aryl hydrocarbon receptor nuclear translocator; HRE, hypoxia responsive element; HSF, heat shock factor; IGF2, insulin-like growth factor 2; MDM2, murine double minute-2; NIP-2, Bcl-2/adenovirus E1B 19 kDa interacting protein; NOS, nitric oxide synthase; PDGF, platelet-derived growth factor; PKC, protein kinase C; PAI-1, plasminogen activator inhibitor-1; TGF-α, transforming growth factor-α; Tie-2, angioprotein receptor tie-2; Epo, erythropoetin; VEGF, vascular endothelial growth factor.

3. THE RELATIONSHIP BETWEEN TUMOR HYPOXIA AND RADIOTHERAPY OR CHEMOTHERAPY

Tumor hypoxia has been shown to confer universal resistance to radiation damage in a wide range of cells and tissues using various end points *(1)*. The oxygen enhancement ratio, which is defined as the ratio of the radiation doses required to produce the same level of cell kill under hypoxic to aerobic conditions and which reflects the difference in radiosensitivity between aerobic and hypoxic cells, is normally in the range of 2.5–3 for mammalian cells *(17)*. A typical radiation-killing curve for mammalian cells under aerobic and hypoxic conditions is shown in Fig. 3A. The reason for the universality of this effect is that oxygen reacts chemically with the unpaired electron on the free radicals produced by ionizing radiation in the DNA, thereby stabilizing, or fixing, the damage. In the absence of oxygen, the radical damage can be repaired by hydrogen donation from sulfhydryl compounds in the cell (Fig. 3B). Thus, lack of oxygen can severely compromise the efficacy of ionizing radiation.

Tumor hypoxia can also indirectly decrease the efficacy of several chemotherapy agents. Hypoxia causes cells to slow down or arrest in their progression through the cell cycle *(18)*, thereby reducing their response to anticancer drugs, which are generally more effective in proliferating cells. In addition, drug distribution is limited by perfusion distance from the blood vessels and by intermittent acute closures of existing blood vessels, thereby decreasing drug concentrations in hypoxic areas. Finally, tumor hypoxia and associated hypoglycemia

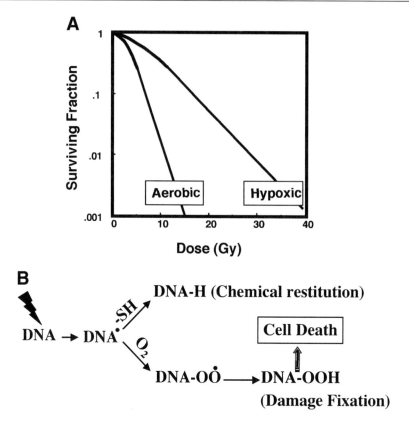

Fig. 3. (**A**) Typical survival curves for ionizing radiation for mammalian cells under aerobic and hypoxic conditions. The oxygen enhancement ratio (ratio of doses to produce the same cell kill under hypoxic to aerobic conditions) is typically 2.5–3.0 and is 2.8 in this figure. (**B**) The mechanism for decreased radiosensitivity in hypoxic cells compared with aerobic cells. Ionizing radiation produces a radical in DNA, which can be converted into permanent damage and cell death in the presence of oxygen or repaired by donation of a hydrogen from cellular nonprotein sulfhydryls (-SH) in the absence of oxygen. (Reprinted from ref. *76*, with permission from the American Association for Cancer Research.)

can activate genes that contribute to drug resistance for several chemotherapeutic agents including adriamycin *(19)*, etoposide *(20)*, and cisplatin *(21)*.

4. TECHNIQUES TO MEASURE TUMOR HYPOXIA AND THEIR CLINICAL SIGNIFICANCE IN HEAD AND NECK CANCERS

Techniques for measuring tumor oxygen can be direct and indirect. Direct approaches can be applied to tissue (needle electrodes) or blood (direct measurements or imaging of oxyhemoglobin saturation and oxygen diffusion). Indirect approaches use injectable or endogenous molecular reporters of oxygen as the end points. Injectable reporters include 2-nitroimidazole compounds such as misonidazole, pimonidazole (1-[2-nitro-1-imidazolyl]-3-*N*-piperidino-2-propanolol) *(22)*, and EF5 (2-[2-nitro-1H-imidazol-1-y1]-*N*-[2,2,3,3,3-pentafluoropropyl] acetamide) *(23)*. These compounds form stable adducts with intracellular macromolecules, and this binding is proportionally inhibited as a function of increasing oxygen concentration *(24)*. Detection of these adducts with antibodies can provide information on the relative oxygenation of tissue at a cellular resolution. Intrinsic hypoxia reporters are those genes that are induced by hypoxia including HIF-1, VEGF, CA IX (carbonic anhydrase IX), lactate, and osteopontin. Measurements of the protein expression of these markers in either tumor tissues or blood can provide indirect evidence of hypoxia in solid cancers.

4.1. Polarographic Needle Electrodes

Polarographic needles provided the first convincing evidence that hypoxia existed in human solid tumors (25,26). Since these earlier studies that used nonstandardized electrodes, the major use of the needle electrode for pO_2 measurements came with the introduction of a commercially available system (Eppendorf pO_2 histograph, Eppendorf, Hamburg, Germany). In this system, the sensing electrode, mounted on the tip of a needle (Fig. 4A), is advanced automatically through the tissue via a step motor, taking readings rapidly (within 1.4 s) to avoid changes in oxygen tension resulting from pressure artifacts or tissue damage caused by the needle. With this system, a histogram of oxygen tension can be obtained from multiple points along different tracks through the tissue. An example of measurements made in an HNSCC-involved neck node and adjacent normal subcutaneous tissue is shown in Fig. 4B. The normal tissues show a typical gaussian distribution of oxygen tensions with a median between 40 and 60 mmHg, whereas tumors invariably show a lower oxygen tension distribution (Fig. 4C).

The first information suggesting that hypoxia, as measured by the polarographic needle electrode, can be used to predict treatment outcomes was published in 1993 by Hockel et al. (27), who showed that cervical cancer patients with most hypoxic tumors (median pO_2 <10 mmHg) had a significantly lower overall and recurrence-free survival compared with patients with less hypoxic tumors. Since then, several HNSCC studies have confirmed the prognostic significance of electrode-detected tumor hypoxia. Table 1 summarizes these results. With one exception, all studies have shown that low partial oxygen tension in the tumor, defined either by median tumor pO_2 or the hypoxic fraction of the pO_2 measurements, correlate with treatment outcomes defined as locoregional control and survival in HNSCC patients treated with radiotherapy or chemoradiotherapy. Figure 5 shows representative survival curves by median tumor pO_2 for HNSCC patients from a study by Brizel et al. (28). Importantly, they also found that tumor oxygenation may help to predict for pathologically persistent neck nodes in patients undergoing a neck dissection for clinical N2–3 necks after chemoradiation treatment, strongly supporting the concept that it is the direct radiation resistance of the hypoxic cells that affects local control (28). Persistent cancer was noted in 19 of 31 patients with hypoxic tumors (median pO_2 <10 mmHg), whereas it was found in only 4 of 18 patients with well-oxygenated tumors (median pO_2 >10 mmHg).

Although the microelectrode technique can directly measure tumor pO_2 and predict treatment outcomes in HNSCC, it suffers from several drawbacks that make it difficult for general use. These include high cost, invasiveness, tumor inaccessibility, pressure dependence, interobserver variability, failure to distinguish necrosis from hypoxia, and the lack of spatial information on hypoxia. Despite these limitations, it is the most accepted method for assessing hypoxia at the present time.

4.2. Injectable and Endogenous Molecular Markers for Hypoxia

The use of 2-nitroimidazoles as hypoxia markers was first suggested in the 1970s when these agents were discovered to bind selectively to hypoxic cells (29). Two agents that are currently being tested in patients are pimonidazole and EF5. These two agents are injected intravenously up to 48 h preceding tumor biopsy or resection and have similar mechanisms

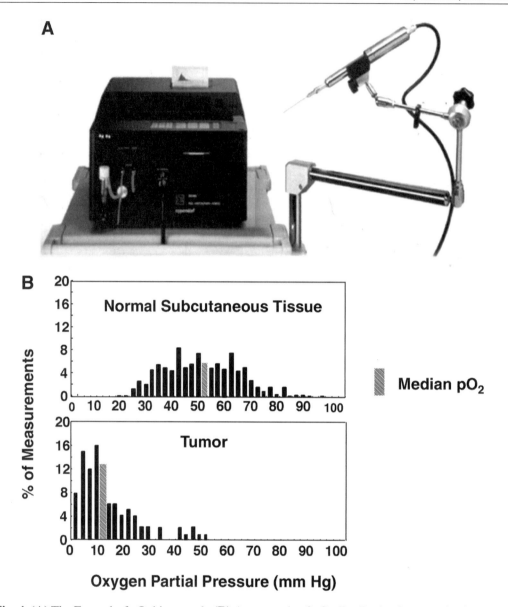

Fig. 4. (A) The Eppendorf pO$_2$ histograph. **(B)** An example of pO$_2$ distribution in normal subcutaneous tissues and a lymph node metastasis in a patient with a HNSCC. (Reprinted from ref. *76*, with permission from the American Association for Cancer Research.).

of activation but different in vivo stability, biodistribution, and pharmacokinetics. For a comprehensive review of these two agents, see Evans and Koch *(30)*. In general, 2-nitroimidazole markers stain for areas of chronic hypoxia *(31)* and are more sensitive at severe hypoxic conditions than the microelectrode *(30,32)*. At this time, there are minimal clinical data regarding the prognostic significance of these agents in HNSCC. In a small study evaluating pimonidazole, microvessel density count, and CA IX binding in 42 HNSCC tumors, pimonidazole staining was more pronounced at distances of greater than 100 μm from blood vessels than CA IX, suggesting that it is more specific for chronic hypoxia *(33)*. In addition, high pretreatment pimonidazole staining correlated with a higher risk of locoregional relapse

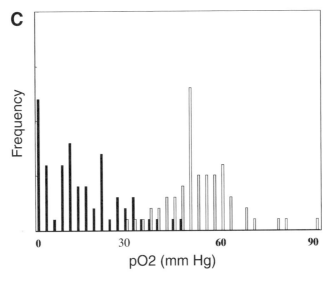

Fig. 4. (C) Distribution of median pO$_2$ values in tumor (black filled bars) and normal subcutaneous tissues (open bars) in 65 patients with HNSCC. (Reprinted from ref. *77*, with permission from Elsevier.)

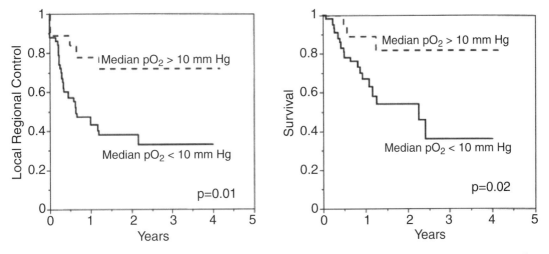

Fig. 5. Locoregional control and survival by median tumor pO$_2$ in HNSCC patients treated with radio-therapy or chemoradiotherapy. (Reprinted from ref. *78*, with permission from Elsevier.)

in patients treated with radiotherapy alone, but, importantly, not in patients treated with radiotherapy plus carbogen and nicotinamide, which are used to modulate tumor hypoxia and which improved locoregional control.

Endogenous molecular markers for tumor hypoxia are proteins whose expression is induced by hypoxic exposure. Presently, the most widely investigated proteins are HIF-1 and CA IX in tissues and VEGF and osteopontin in the blood. The advantage of this approach is that levels of these proteins can be assessed on archival materials, thereby allowing rapid correlation to treatment outcomes. In addition assessment requires neither the injection of foreign material nor any additional invasive procedure beyond that of taking blood or tumor biopsy at diagnosis. A significant drawback to these approaches is that these proteins can be regulated by

Table 1
Significance of Electrode-Based Tumor Oxygenation for Treatment Outcomes

Author	PO₂ Parameter	No. of patients	Treatment	LRC	DFS or OS	Other parameters
Nordsmark et al., 1996 (80)	HF2.5	35	RT ± ND	Yes	No	
Brizel et al., 1997 (81)	Med pO$_2$ (10 mmHg)	28	RT ± S	Yes	Yes	
Brizel et al., 1999 (78)	Med pO$_2$ (10 mmHg)	68	RT or CRT ± S	Yes	Yes	RT dose
Brizel et al., 2004 (28)	Med pO$_2$ (10 mmHg)	59	CRT ± ND			
Stadler et al., 1999 (82)	HF2.5, HF5	59	RT, CRT		Yes	Hypoxic subvol, Hb
Rudat et al., 2000 (83)	HF2.5	41	RT, CRT		Yes	
Rudat et al., 2001 (84)	HF2.5	194	RT, CRT		Yes	Age, treatment
Terris, 2000 (85)	Med pO$_2$ (10 mmHg)	63	S ± RT, CRT	No	No	

Abbreviations: HF, hypoxic fraction or % measurements < 2.5 mmHg (HF2.5) or 5 mmHg (HF5); Med pO$_2$, median pO$_2$; RT, radiotherapy; CRT, chemoradiotherapy; S, surgery; LRC, locoregional control; DFS, disease-free survival; OS, overall survival; Hb, hemoglobin; ND, neck dissection; subvol., subvolume.

factors other than hypoxia. For example, HIF-1 expression can be influenced by several nonhypoxic stimuli including nitric oxide (NO), cytokines (interleukin-1β and tumor necrosis factor-α), trophic stimuli (serum, insulin, insulin-like-growth factors), and oncogenes (p53, Vsrc, PTEN, and others) *(34–37)*. Also because HIF-1 is rapidly induced under hypoxic conditions, it is important to fix the tumor specimen very quickly after resection. In comparison studies between endogenous and injectable markers, the staining patterns of endogenous molecular markers were generally more diffuse and closer to the blood vessels than the injectable markers *(33,38)*, suggesting other modes of induction and activation at a wider range of oxygen concentration. The prognostic roles for the endogenous markers have been investigated in HNSCC, and the results have been mixed, depending on the type of therapy (Table 2). In general, overexpression of these markers portends poorer outcomes in patients treated with nonsurgical therapies but not in those treated with primary surgery. This would support the importance of a direct effect of tumor hypoxia on treatment sensitivity rather than on producing a more malignant phenotype in HNSCC.

Our laboratory focus has been on identifying secreted markers of hypoxia that can be easily measured in the blood, as these markers have the potential of being translated into universally available inexpensive laboratory tests. Two markers that have been tested in the clinic with mixed results are VEGF and osteopontin. Although circulating VEGF levels have been shown to be elevated in cancer patients *(39,40)* and in patients with acute hypoxia such as obstructive apnea *(41)*, the relationship between tumor hypoxia and systemic VEGF levels is unclear. Dunst et al. *(42)* found that serum VEGF levels significantly and independently correlated with hypoxic tumor subvolume in 56 HNSCC patients. However, it also correlated with total tumor volume, hemoglobin level, and platelet counts. They did not report on the clinical significance of serum VEGF levels in terms of treatment outcomes in this study. In contrast, we did not find a direct relationship between plasma VEGF and tumor pO_2 in 48 HNSCC patients in our study (unpublished data). We did, however, find a small but significant relationship between osteopontin level and tumor pO_2 in our patient cohort *(43)*. In addition, plasma osteopontin was an independent and significant predictor for treatment outcomes in these patients, regardless of nodal status (Fig. 6). These results were confirmed by the Danish Association of Head and Neck Cancer (DAHANCA) in a larger cohort of HNSCC patients treated with radiation therapy ± nimorazole, a hypoxic cell sensititizer *(44)*. Further validation of this promising marker is ongoing in HNSCC patients at our institution.

4.3. Imaging Hypoxia

Imaging hypoxia is important for radiation therapy in HNSCC as it theoretically provides potential targets for dose escalation. In addition, serial imaging studies can provide information on changes in tumor hypoxia during the course of therapy to help with fine-tuning of treatment delivery. Positron emission tomography (PET) and single-photon emission computed tomography (SPECT) are probably the two most extensively evaluated approaches for imaging tumor hypoxia at the moment. Most radiopharmaceuticals under development for hypoxia detection use 2-nitroimidazole compounds coupled to a radioisotope such as ^{18}F, ^{64}Cu, [60]Cu, and [123]I. The most widely used imaging agent to date is flouromisonidazole (^{18}F-miso), and data for ^{18}F-miso PET in HNSCC have demonstrated the feasibility of this technique. In a small study that combined tirapazamine (TPZ), a hypoxic cell cytotoxin, with cisplatin and radiotherapy in patients with locally advanced HNSCC, ^{18}F-miso PET scans detected hypoxia in 14 of 15 patients at baseline, with only one patient having detectable hypoxia at the end of treatment *(45)*. One disadvantage of the ^{18}F-miso PET is the high

Table 2
Significance of Endogenous Markers for Hypoxia in Head and Neck Cancers

Author	Marker	No. of patients	Tumor site	Treatment	Respond	LRC	Survival	Associated parameters
Aebersold et al., 2001 (86)	HIF-1α	98	Oropharynx	RT or CRT	Yes	Yes	Yes	Grade (inverse)
Koukourakis et al., 2002 (87)	HIF-1α, HIF-2α	75	H&N	CRT	Yes	Yes	Yes	T-stage, MVD, VEGF
Beasley et al., 2002 (88)	HIF-1α	79	H&N	Surgery			No[a]	Necrosis
Hui et al., (89)	HIF-1α, CA IX	90	Nasopharynx	RT or CRT			Yes[b]	CA IX, VEGF
Beasley et al., 2001 (90)	CA IX	79	H&N	Surgery				MVD, necrosis
Koukourakis et al., 2001 (91)	CA IX	75	H&N	CRT	Yes	Yes	Yes	MVD, necrosis
Kaanders et al., 2002 (33)	CA IX	43	H&N	RT ± ARCON	No	No	No	Pimonidazole staining

Abbreviations: H&N, head and neck; RT, radiotherapy; CRT, chemoradiotherapy; ARCON, carbogen and nicotidamide; LRC, locoregional control; MVD, microvessel density count; HIF-1α, hyoxia-inducible factor-1α; CA IX, carbonic anhydrase IX; VEGF, vascular endothelial growth factor.

[a]Improved disease-free and overall survival with HIF-1α overexpression

[b]The combination of HIF-1α and CA IX positivity (hypoxic profile) was associated with worse progression-free survival. Positivity for individual marker staining did not correlated with survival.

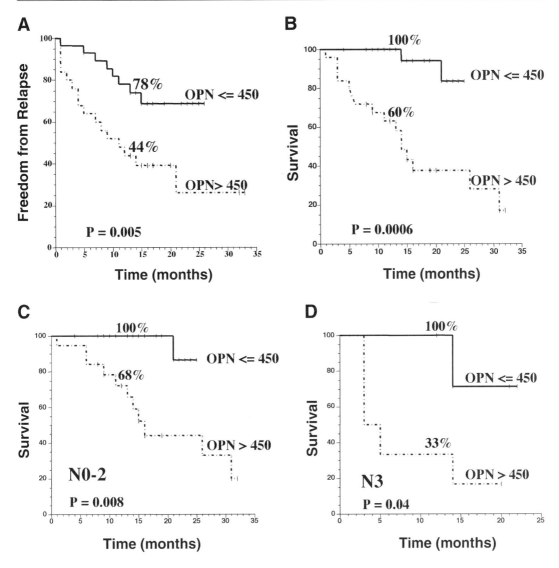

Fig. 6. Kaplan-Meier estimates. **(A)** Freedom from relapse by osteopontin (OPN) plasma levels. **(B)** Overall survival by OPN plasma levels. **(C)** Overall survival by OPN plasma levels in patients with N0–2 neck nodes. **(D)** Overall survival by OPN plasma levels in patients with N3 neck nodes. (Reprinted from ref. *43*, with permission from the American Association for Cancer Research.)

background from nonmetabolized drug. New agents such as [18]FAZA and ^{18}F-EF5 may provide better resolution with less background. Another promising PET agent is [60]Cu-ATSM, which is a nonnitro-containing bioreductive compound. It has been shown to have a correlation with oxygen electrode measurements in animal tumors and can image tumor hypoxia in HNSCC patients *(46)*. It also enjoys the advantage of having a very short half-life (23 min), which makes it feasible to perform serial imaging studies on patients. Larger studies and long-term follow-up are needed to clarify the clinical utility of imaging hypoxia and their application in radiation delivery.

5. TARGETING TUMOR HYPOXIA

Since the 1950s, enormous efforts have been devoted to develop strategies to overcome the perceived clinical problem of tumor hypoxia. These include hyperbaric oxygen treatment to increase oxygen partial pressure *(47)*, the use of specific drugs to reduce oxygen binding to hemoglobin (e.g., RSR13 *[48]*), the use of vasodilator and carbogen (ARCON) to enhance oxygen tissue delivery *(49)*, the use of electron affinity drugs as hypoxic cell radiosensitizers *(50)*, and treatment with high linear-energy transfer (LET) radiation, which is less oxygen dependent for cytotoxicity *(51)*. Although most of these strategies have not achieved general acceptance, a meta-analysis of trials using hypoxic cell sensitizers or hyperbaric oxygen showed a small but statistically significant benefit in terms of locoregional control and survival *(47)*. In this part of the chapter, we will cover some of these prior strategies (specifically hypoxic cell sensitizers), explore in detail two promising current strategies, including the concept of *exploiting* hypoxia using drugs that selectively kill hypoxic cells, such as TPZ, and touch on some future approaches for exploiting hypoxia.

5.1. Past Strategies

The most straightforward strategy for overcoming intratumoral hypoxia is the administration of oxygen at pressure higher than room air (usually three atmospheres), i.e., hyperbaric oxygen treatment. Although one study showed promising results in HNSCC patients, the results were mixed in other solid tumors *(52,53)*. In retrospect, this strategy only affects chronically hypoxic cells and is not expected to change acute hypoxia. Although a meta-analysis suggests that the use of hyperbaric oxygen breathing during radiation therapy can improve local control by 10% *(47)*, it has not gained general acceptance for clinical use owing to inconsistent response, safety issues, and the high cost and complexity of its implementation.

One of the best studied strategies for overcoming the radiation resistance of hypoxic cells is to use electron-affinic drugs (nitroimidazoles) to sensitize tumors to radiation. Xenograft studies with single large radiation doses showed significant radiosensitization with nitroimidazole compounds in tumors without enhancing normal tissue toxicity *(54,55)*. During the past two decades, nitroimidazole compounds have been extensively evaluated by the Radiation Therapy Oncology Group (RTOG) and the DAHANCA group in HNSCC as an adjunct to radiotherapy with mixed results *(50,56–59)*. Most of these trials reported disappointing local control and survival outcomes except for one large study *(50)*. In this large phase III study (DAHANCA 5-85), the addition of nimorazole to radiotherapy resulted in improved locoregional control rates (49 vs 33%, $p = 0.002$) and cancer-related survival (52 vs 41%) compared with the placebo-control arm in patients with supraglottic larynx and pharynx cancers. The main drawback to using these compounds is the neurotoxicity associated with multiple doses seen with misonidazole and to lesser extent etanidazole and nimorazole *(60,61)*. This toxicity limits the dose of drugs that can be administered to achieve maximal efficacy.

5.2. Present Strategies

5.2.1. HYPOXIC CELL CYTOTOXINS

These compounds differ from radiosensitizers in that they can directly kill hypoxic cells independent of radiation therapy. Direct killing of hypoxic cells theoretically has greater therapeutic potential than oxygenating or sensitizing these cells to conventional radiotherapy or chemotherapy for two reasons: (1) hypoxic cytotoxins kill cells that are resistant to radiation

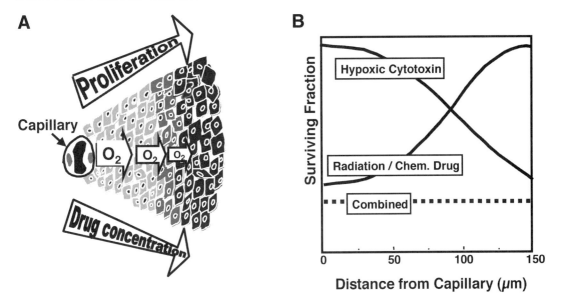

Fig. 7. (**A**) Diagramatic representation of a tumor cord surrounding a capillary showing decreasing O$_2$ concentration, proliferation, and drug concentration as a function of distance from the capillary. (**B**) The considerations in the left lead to the prediction that cell killing by radiation and conventional chemotherapy will be reduced as a function of distance from the capillary. In contrast, a hypoxic cell toxin should show the opposite profile. The combination of standard treatment with hypoxic cell toxins should be expected to produce uniform cell killing as a function of distance from capillary (combined). Such a profile has been demonstrated experimentally in xenograft models by Durand et al. *(79)*. (Reprinted from ref. *76*, with permission from the American Association for Cancer Research.)

and chemotherapy, thereby producing complementary cytotoxicity, as shown in Fig. 7; and (2) these drugs can target both acutely and chronically hypoxic cells and therefore cover a broader spectrum of hypoxic cells than hypoxic cell sensitizers. Although not developed as a specific toxin for hypoxic cells, the chemotherapy drug mitomycin C has some selective toxicity to hypoxic cells, at least in vitro *(62)*. Pooled data from two randomized trials in HNSCC suggested that the addition of mitomycin-C to radiotherapy resulted in statistically significant improvement in locoregional control and cause-specific survival at 5 yr *(63)*. Another study comparing conventional fractionated radiation alone with the Vienna continuous hyperfractionated accelerated radiation regimen (V-CHART) alone or with V-CHART plus mitomycin-C showed the best overall survival and locoregional control for the group receiving V-CHART and mitomycin-C *(64,65)*. Although promising, mitomycin-C toxicity limits the frequency of drug delivery, making it unlikely to be the ideal drug for exploiting tumor hypoxia.

A more promising strategy to exploit tumor hypoxia is through agents that have a high selectivity for killing hypoxic cells, the prototype of which is TPZ (or SR4233). TPZ is a benzotriazine with selective cytotoxicity for hypoxic cells at a relatively low drug concentration. The hypoxic cytotoxicity ratio (HCR) or the concentration of the drug that is required to produce equal cytotoxicity under normoxia relative to hypoxia is in the 50–300 range for various cell lines *(66,67)*. This is to be compared with an HCR of 1–5 for mitomycin-C *(62)*. Mechanistically, it has been demonstrated that TPZ undergoes a one-electron reduction to form a cytotoxic free radical that causes DNA breaks, chromosomal aberrations, and cell death

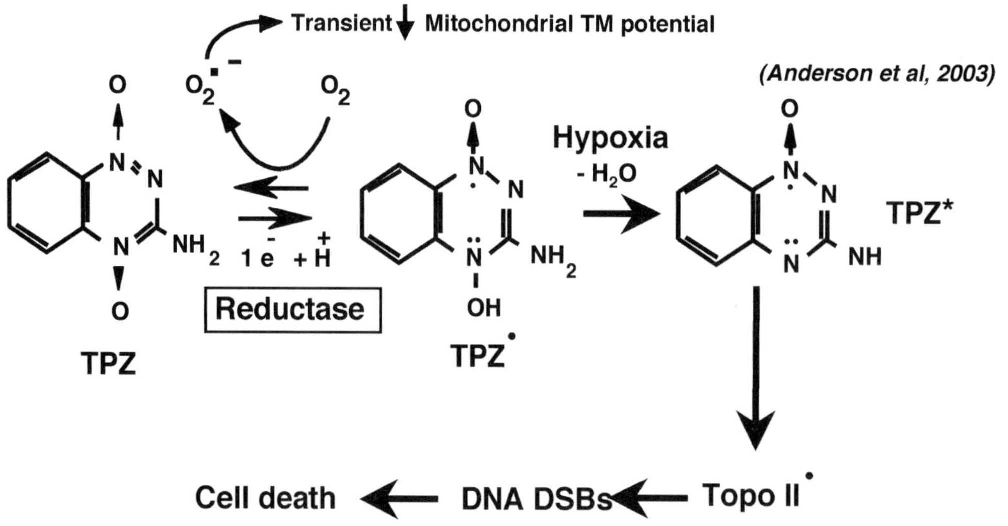

Fig. 8. Mechanism of selective hypoxic cytotoxicity of tirapazamine (TPZ).

(67) (Fig.8). In the presence of oxygen, the TPZ radical is backoxidized to the nontoxic parent compound. More recently, it has been shown to act as a topoisomerase II poison in hypoxic cells, inducing double-strand breaks in a similar fashion as etopside *(68)*. Although TPZ was first proposed to be used with radiotherapy, recent emphasis has been on TPZ's ability to potentiate the cytotoxicity of cisplatin. The maximum tolerated dose (MTD) of TPZ as a single agent or in combination with chemotherapy is 390 mg/m^2. When given concurrently with radiotherapy for head and neck cancers, toxicities were acceptable up to doses of 160 mg/m^2, administered three times a week for 12 doses *(69)*. There is a known steep dose-response relationship for TPZ-related toxicities, with vomiting, diarrhea, muscle cramps, and acute reversible hearing loss observed at a dose of 390 mg/m^2. Conversely, these side effects are uncommon with TPZ doses of 260 mg/m^2 or less *(70)*.

Early clinical results from a phase II clinical trial of TPZ plus radiotherapy in HNSCC patients are encouraging, with a reported 2-yr local control rate of 60% for patients with stage III-IV tumors *(71)*. However, the most impressive results have come from the combination of TPZ, cisplatin, and radiotherapy *(45)*. Rischin et al. *(72)* treated 16 patients with locally advanced unresectable HNSCC in a phase I study. TPZ 290 mg/m^2 was given 1 h prior to cisplatin 75 mg/m^2 followed by conventionally fractionated radiotherapy in the first, fourth, and seventh weeks of radiation. In addition TPZ 160 mg/m^2 was administered three times a week initially during wk 2, 3, 5, and 6, but for the last 10 patients it was given during wk 2 and 3 only owing to dose-limiting toxicity, which was neutropenia. The overall complete response rate was 81%; the 3-yr local progression-free rate was 88%, and overall survival was 67% at a median follow-up of 3 yr.

As a follow-up to this trial, a randomized phase II study was initiated under the auspices of the Trans-Tasman Radiation Oncology Group (TROG), in which the same regimen of TPZ, cisplatin, and radiation was compared against chemoradiotherapy using concurrent cisplatin, and 5-flourouraci (5-FU) as a chemo-boost approach during the last 2 wk of radiotherapy *(72)*. Results from this study showed a trend for improved 3-yr local-regional control. Failure-free rates (84 vs 66%, $p = 0.069$) and failure-free survival (55 vs 44%, $p = 0.16$) favoring of TPZ arm. Based on these data, a large multiinstitutional phase III trial is under way to study the efficacy of TPZ in combination with radiotherapy and cisplatin in HNSCC (Elwyn Loh, M.D., Sanofi Synthelabo, personal communication).

In contrast, a small phase II randomized study from our institution using an aggressive chemoradiotherapy regimen consisting of two cycles of induction cisplatin 100 mg/m^2, continuous infusion 5-FU (CI 5-FU) 1000 mg/m^2/d × 5 d and TPZ 300–330 mg/m^2 on d 1 and 22, followed by simultaneous chemoradiotherapy, which consisted of cisplatin 20 mg/m^2, 3×/wk (M, W, F), CI 5-FU 600 mg/m^2/d × 4 d, and TPZ 160 mg/m^2 to 260 mg/m^2 during wk 1 and 5 of conventionally fractionated radiotherapy to 66–74 Gy. This regimen was compared with the same regimen without TPZ in a total of 60 resectable HNSCC patients in the study (30 patients per arm). To date, there is no difference in treatment outcomes including locoregional control and overall survival at a median follow up of 2 yr *(73)*.

The difference between our results and those from the TROG trial may be explained by the type and schedule of chemotherapy use (i.e., induction and concomitant chemotherapy in our trial compared with concomitant chemotherapy alone in the TROG trial), the fact that we only gave TPZ for a total of six doses during the radiotherapy treatment, and the type of patients enrolled (resectable for our group vs mostly unresectable for the TROG study). The large consortium phase III randomized study will shed new light on the role of TPZ in the management of HNSCC.

5.2.2. ARCON THERAPY

Another promising approach to overcoming tumor hypoxia in HNSCC is the combined use of the nicotinamide vasodilator and carbogen breathing (ARCON) to increase the oxygen partial pressure of tumors. ARCON (accelerated radiotherapy with carbogen and nicotinamide) has produced a 3-yr local control rate in excess of 80% for advanced stage T3–4 laryngeal and oropharyngeal cancers *(49)*. Presently, a phase III clinical trial testing the efficacy of ARCON in laryngeal cancers is ongoing in Europe, with a projected accrual of 344 patients *(49)*. The results of this study will elucidate the role of ARCON in the management of some head and neck cancers.

5.3. Future Strategies

One of the future strategies for hypoxia targeting is to develop more diffusible forms of TPZ that have better tissue penetration, in order to reach most if not all the hypoxic cells. Another strategy to is exploit tumor hypoxia for drug delivery. For example, the obligate anaerobic *Clostridium* species, which have been engineered to carry prodrug-activating enzymes, can be used to target and selectively deliver cytotoxic agents to areas of hypoxia and necrosis *(74)*. Although this approach appears promising in experimental systems, it has not been tested clinically. As more is known about the molecular basis of hypoxia, another tangible future strategy will focus on targeting specific hypoxia-induced proteins such as HIF-1 *(75)* or related transcription factors.

6. CONCLUSIONS

After half a decade of efforts, tumor hypoxia continues to represent a therapeutic challenge for the head and neck oncologist. Nonetheless, the prospect of reducing its impact is looking brighter. First, an improved ability to detect and quantify tumor hypoxia allows for better selection of patients who would benefit from hypoxia-targeted therapy. The era of genomics and proteomics together with the unraveling of the human genome have significantly improved the understanding of tumor hypoxia and resulted in rapid identification of new molecular targets for therapeutic exploitation. Testing of new leads from the laboratory requires well-conducted clinical trials with innovative designs that incorporate serial novel noninvasive surrogate end points for hypoxia such as molecular makers or imaging methods. Our responsibility as oncologists is to support these trials, to improve tumor control and curability in our patients.

REFERENCES

1. Gray LH, Conger AD, Ebert M, Hornsey S, Scott OC. Concentration of oxygen dissolved in tissues at the time of irradiation as a factor in radiotherapy. Br J Radiol 1953; 26:638–648.
2. Brown JM, Giaccia AJ. The unique physiology of solid tumors: opportunities (and problems) for cancer therapy. Cancer Res 1998; 58:1408–1416.
3. Thomlinson RH, Gray LH. The histological structure of some human lung cancers and the possible implications for radiotherapy. Br J Cancer 1955; 9:539–549.
4. Brown JM. Evidence for acutely hypoxic cells in mouse tumours, and a possible mechanism of reoxygenation. Br J Radiol 1979; 52:650–656.
5. Trotter MJ, Chaplin DJ, Durand RE, Olive PL. The use of fluorescent probes to identify regions of transient perfusion in murine tumors. Int J Radiat Oncol Biol Phys 1989; 16:931–934.
6. Graeber TG, Osmanian C, Jacks T, et al. Hypoxia-mediated selection of cells with diminished apoptotic potential in solid tumours. Nature 1996; 379:88–91.
7. Koch WM, Brennan JA, Zahurak M, et al. p53 mutation and locoregional treatment failure in head and neck squamous cell carcinoma. J Natl Cancer Inst 1996; 88:1580–1586.
8. Young SD, Marshall RS, Hill RP. Hypoxia induces DNA overreplication and enhances metastatic potential of murine tumor cells. Proc Natl Acad Sci USA 1988; 85:9533–9537.
9. Cairns RA, Hill RP. Acute hypoxia enhances spontaneous lymph node metastasis in an orthotopic murine model of human cervical carcinoma. Cancer Res 2004; 64:2054–2061.
10. Brizel DM, Scully SP, Harrelson JM, et al. Tumor oxygenation predicts for the likelihood of distant metastases in human soft tissue sarcoma. Cancer Res 1996; 56:941–943.
11. Nordsmark M, Alsner J, Keller J, et al. Hypoxia in human soft tissue sarcomas: adverse impact on survival and no association with p53 mutations. Br J Cancer 2001; 84:1070–1075.
12. Fyles A, Milosevic M, Hedley D, et al. Tumor hypoxia has independent predictor impact only in patients with node-negative cervix cancer. J Clin Oncol 2002; 20:680–687.
13. Semenza GL. Targeting HIF-1 for cancer therapy. Nat Rev Cancer 2003; 3:721–732.
14. Harris AL. Hypoxia—a key regulatory factor in tumour growth. Nat Rev Cancer 2002; 2:38–47.
15. P Oc, Rhys-Evans P, Eccles SA. Expression of vascular endothelial growth factor family members in head and neck squamous cell carcinoma correlates with lymph node metastasis. Cancer 2001; 92:556–568.
16. Smith BD, Smith GL, Carter D, et al. Molecular marker expression in oral and oropharyngeal squamous cell carcinoma. Arch Otolaryngol Head Neck Surg 2001; 127:780–785.
17. Hall EA. Radiobiology for the Radiobiologist. Philadelphia: Lippincott Williams & Wilkins, 2000:91–111.
18. Pallavicini MG, Laland ME, Miller RG, Hill RP. Cell-cycle distribution of chronically hypoxic cells and determination of the clonogenic potential of cells accumulated in G2-M phases after irradiation of a solid tumor. Cancer Res. 1979; 39:1891–1897.
19. Shen J, Hughes C, Chao C, et al. Coinduction of glucose-regulated proteins and doxorubicin resistance in Chinese hamster cells. Proc Natl Acad Sci USA 1987; 84:3278–3282.
20. Hughes CS, Shen JW, Subjeck JR. Resistance to etoposide induced by three glucose-regulated stresses in Chinese hamster ovary cells. Cancer Res 1989; 49:4452–4454.
21. Murphy BJ, Laderoute KR, Chin RJ, Sutherland RM. Metallothionein IIA is upregulated by hypoxia in human A431 squamous carcinoma cells. Cancer Res 1994; 54:5808–5810.
22. Raleigh JA, Calkins-Adams DP, Rinker LH, et al. Hypoxia and vascular endothelial growth factor expression in human squamous cell carcinomas using pimonidazole as a hypoxia marker. Cancer Res 1998; 58:3765–3768.
23. Evans SM, Hahn S, Pook DR, et al. Detection of hypoxia in human squamous cell carcinoma by EF5 binding. Cancer Res 2000; 60:2018–2024.
24. Varghese AJ, Gulyas S, Mohindra JK. Hypoxia-dependent reduction of 1-(2-nitro-1-imidazolyl)-3-methoxy-2-propanol by Chinese hamster ovary cells and KHT tumor cells in vitro and in vivo. Cancer Res 1976; 36:3761–3765.

25. Gatenby RA, Kessler HB, Rosenblum JS, et al. Oxygen distribution in squamous cell carcinoma metastases and its relationship to outcome of radiation therapy. Int J Radiat Oncol Biol Phys 1988; 14:831–838.

26. Wendling P, Manz R, Thews G, Vaupel P. Heterogeneous oxygenation of rectal carcinomas in humans: a critical parameter for preoperative irradiation? Adv Exp Med Biol 1984; 180:293–300.

27. Hockel M, Knoop C, Schlenger K, et al. Intratumoral pO_2 predicts survival in advanced cancer of the uterine cervix. Radiother Oncol 1993; 26:45–50.

28. Brizel DM, Prosnitz RG, Hunter S, et al. Necessity for adjuvant neck dissection in setting of concurrent chemoradiation for advanced head-and-neck cancer. Int J Radiat Oncol Biol Phys 2004; 58:1418–1423.

29. Chapman JD. Hypoxic sensitizers—implications for radiation therapy. N Engl J Med 1979; 301:1429–1432.

30. Evans SM, Koch CJ. Prognostic significance of tumor oxygenation in humans. Cancer Lett 2003; 195:1–16.

31. Gross MW, Karbach U, Groebe K, Franko AJ, Mueller-Klieser W. Calibration of misonidazole labeling by simultaneous measurement of oxygen tension and labeling density in multicellular spheroids. Int J Cancer 1995; 61:567–573.

32. Raleigh JA, Chou SC, Arteel GE, Horsman MR. Comparisons among pimonidazole binding, oxygen electrode measurements, and radiation response in C3H mouse tumors. Radiat Res 1999; 151:580–589.

33. Kaanders JH, Wijffels KI, Marres HA, et al. Pimonidazole binding and tumor vascularity predict for treatment outcome in head and neck cancer. Cancer Res 2002; 62:7066–7074.

34. Stroka DM, Burkhardt T, Desbaillets I, et al. HIF-1 is expressed in normoxic tissue and displays an organ-specific regulation under systemic hypoxia. FASEB J 2001; 15:2445–2453.

35. Zundel W, Schindler C, Haas-Kogan D, et al. Loss of PTEN facilitates HIF-1-mediated gene expression. Genes Dev 2000; 14:391–396.

36. Zelzer E, Levy Y, Kahana C, Shilo BZ, Rubinstein M, Cohen B. Insulin induces transcription of target genes through the hypoxia-inducible factor HIF-1alpha/ARNT. EMBO J 1998; 17:5085–5094.

37. Zhong H, Chiles K, Feldser D, et al. Modulation of hypoxia-inducible factor 1alpha expression by the epidermal growth factor/phosphatidylinositol 3-kinase/PTEN/AKT/FRAP pathway in human prostate cancer cells: implications for tumor angiogenesis and therapeutics. Cancer Res 2000; 60:1541–1545.

38. Janssen HL, Haustermans KM, Sprong D, et al. HIF-1A, pimonidazole, and iododeoxyuridine to estimate hypoxia and perfusion in human head-and-neck tumors. Int J Radiat Oncol Biol Phys 2002; 54:1537–1549.

39. Riedel F, Gotte K, Schwalb J, Wirtz H, Bergler W, Hormann K. Serum levels of vascular endothelial growth factor in patients with head and neck cancer. Eur Arch Otorhinolaryngol 2000; 257:332–336.

40. Salven P, Manpaa H, Orpana A, Alitalo K, Joensuu H. Serum vascular endothelial growth factor is often elevated in disseminated cancer. Clin Cancer Res 1997; 3:647–651.

41. Imagawa S, Yamaguchi Y, Higuchi M, et al. Levels of vascular endothelial growth factor are elevated in patients with obstructive sleep apnea—hypopnea syndrome. Blood 2001; 98:1255–1257.

42. Dunst J, Stadler P, Becker A, et al. Tumor hypoxia and systemic levels of vascular endothelial growth factor (VEGF) in head and neck cancers. Strahlenther Onkol 2001; 177:469–473.

43. Le QT, Sutphin PD, Raychaudhuri S, et al. Identification of osteopontin as a prognostic plasma marker for head and neck squamous cell carcinomas. Clin Cancer Res 2003; 9:59–67.

44. Overgaard J, Nordsmark M, Alsner J, et al. Plasma osteopontin (OPN) predicts hypoxia and response to the hypoxic sensitizer Nimorazole in radiotherapy of head and neck cancer. Results from the randomized DAHANCA 5 trial (poster # 474), European Society of Therapeutic Radiology and Oncology, 2003.

45. Rischin D, Peters L, Hicks R, et al. Phase I trial of concurrent tirapazamine, cisplatin, and radiotherapy in patients with advanced head and neck cancer. J Clin Oncol 2001; 19:535–542.

46. Chao KS, Bosch WR, Mutic S, et al. A novel approach to overcome hypoxic tumor resistance: Cu-ATSM-guided intensity-modulated radiation therapy. Int J Radiat Oncol Biol Phys 2001; 49:1171–1182.

47. Overgaard J, Horsman MR. Modification of hypoxia-induced radioresistance in tumors by the use of oxygen and sensitizers. Semin Radiat Oncol 1996; 6:10–21.

48. Shaw E, Scott C, Suh J, et al. RSR13 plus cranial radiation therapy in patients with brain metastases: comparison with the Radiation Therapy Oncology Group Recursive Partitioning Analysis Brain Metastases Database. J Clin Oncol 2003; 21:2364–2371.

49. Kaanders JH, Pop LA, Marres HA, et al. ARCON: experience in 215 patients with advanced head-and-neck cancer. Int J Radiat Oncol Biol Phys 2002; 52:769–778.

50. Overgaard J, Hansen HS, Overgaard M, et al. A randomized double-blind phase III study of nimorazole as a hypoxic radiosensitizer of primary radiotherapy in supraglottic larynx and pharynx carcinoma. Results of the Danish Head and Neck Cancer Study (DAHANCA) Protocol 5-85. Radiother Oncol 1998; 46:135–146.

51. Britten RA, Peters LJ, Murray D. Biological factors influencing the RBE of neutrons: implications for their past, present and future use in radiotherapy. Radiat Res 2001; 156:125–135.

52. Watson ER, Halnan KE, Dische S, et al. Hyperbaric oxygen and radiotherapy: a Medical Research Council trial in carcinoma of the cervix. Br J Radiol 1978; 51:879–887.

53. Dische S, Anderson PJ, Sealy R, Watson ER. Carcinoma of the cervix—anaemia, radiotherapy and hyperbaric oxygen. Br J Radiol 1983; 56:251–255.

54. Sheldon PW, Foster JL, Fowler JF. Radiosensitization of C3H mouse mammary tumours by a 2-nitroimidazole drug. Br J Cancer 1974; 30:560–565.

55. Brown JM. Selective radiosensitization of the hypoxic cells of mouse tumors with the nitroimidazoles metronidazole and Ro 7-0582. Radiat Res 1975; 64:633–647.

56. Lee DJ, Pajak TF, Stetz J, Order SE, Weissberg JB, Fischer JJ. A phase I/II study of the hypoxic cell sensitizer misonidazole as an adjunct to high fractional dose radiotherapy in patients with unresectable squamous cell carcinoma of the head and neck: a RTOG randomized study (#79-04). Int J Radiat Oncol Biol Phys 1989; 16:465–470.

57. Lee DJ, Cosmatos D, Marcial VA, et al. Results of an RTOG phase III trial (RTOG 85-27) comparing radiotherapy plus etanidazole with radiotherapy alone for locally advanced head and neck carcinomas. Int J Radiat Oncol Biol Phys 1995; 32:567–576.

58. Overgaard J, Hansen HS, Anderson AP, et al. Misonidazole combined with split course radiotherapy in the treatment of invasive carcinoma of larynx and pharynx: report from the DAHANCA study. Int J Radiat Oncol Biol Phys 1989; 16:1065–1068.

59. Wasserman TH, Lee DJ, Cosmatos D, et al. Clinical trials with etanidazole (SR-2508) by the Radiation Therapy Oncology Group (RTOG). Radiother Oncol 1991; 20(Suppl 1):129–135.

60. Dische S, Saunders MI, Lee ME, Adams GE, Flockhart IR. Clinical testing of the radiosensitizer Ro 07-0582: experience with multiple doses. Br J Cancer 1977; 35:567–579.

61. Coleman CN, Wasserman TH, Urtasun RC, et al. Phase I trial of the hypoxic cell radiosensitizer SR-2508: the results of the five to six week drug schedule. Int J Radiat Oncol Biol Phys 1986; 12:1105–1108.

62. Rockwell S, Kennedy KA, Sartorelli AC. Mitomycin-C as a prototype bioreductive alkylating agent: in vitro studies of metabolism and cytotoxicity. Int J Radiat Oncol Biol Phys 1982; 8:753–735.

63. Haffty BG, Son YH, Papac R, et al. Chemotherapy as an adjunct to radiation in the treatment of squamous cell carcinoma of the head and neck: results of the Yale Mitomycin Randomized Trials. J Clin Oncol 1997; 15:268–276.

64. Dobrowsky W, Naude J, Widder J, et al. Continuous hyperfractionated accelerated radiotherapy with/without mitomycin C in head and neck cancer. Int J Radiat Oncol Biol Phys 1998; 42:803–806.

65. Dobrowsky W, Naude J. Continuous hyperfractionated accelerated radiotherapy with/without mitomycin C in head and neck cancers. Radiother Oncol 2000; 57:119–124.

66. Zeman EM, Brown JM, Lemmon MJ, Hirst VK, Lee WW. SR 4233: a new bioreductive agent with high selective toxicity for hypoxic mammalian cells. Int J Radiat Oncol Biol Phys 1986; 12:1239–1242.

67. Brown JM. SR 4233 (tirapazamine): a new anticancer drug exploiting hypoxia in solid tumors. Brit J Cancer 1993; 67:1163–1170.

68. Peters KB, Brown JM. Tirapazamine: a hypoxia-activated topoisomerase II poison. Cancer Res 2002; 62:5248–5253.

69. Shulman LN, Buswell L, Riese N, et al. Phase I trial of the hypoxic cell cytotoxin tirapazamine with concurrent radiation therapy in the treatment of refractory solid tumors. Int J Radiat Oncol Biol Phys 1999; 44:349–353.

70. Senan S, Rampling R, Graham MA, et al. Phase I and pharmacokinetic study of tirapazamine (SR 4233) administered every three weeks. Clin Cancer Res 1997; 3:31–38.

71. Lee DJ, Trotti A, Spencer S, et al. Concurrent tirapazamine and radiotherapy for advanced head and neck carcinomas: a phase II study. Int J Radiat Oncol Biol Phys 1998; 42:811–815.

72. Rischin D, Peters L, Fishter R, et al. Tirapazamine, cisplatin, and radiation versus Fluorouracil, Cisplantin, and radiation in patients with locally advanced head and neck cancer: A randomized phase II trial of the Trans-Tasman Radiation Oncology Group. J Clin Oncol 2005;23:79–87.

73. Pinto HA, Le QT, Terris DJ, Bloch D, Goffinet DR, Brown JM. Randomized trial of tirapazamine/cisplatin/fluorouracil versus cisplatin/fluorouracil for organ preservation in advanced resectable head and neck cancer (abstract # 904). In: Amercican Society of Clincical Oncology 38th Annual Meeting, Orlando, FL, 2002, vol. 21. Philadelphia, Lippincott Williams & Wilkins.

74. Liu SC, Minton NP, Giaccia AJ, Brown JM. Anticancer efficacy of systemically delivered anaerobic bacteria as gene therapy vectors targeting tumor hypoxia/necrosis. Gene Ther 2002; 9:291–296.

75. Giaccia A, Siim BG, Johnson RS. HIF-1 as a target for drug development. Nat Rev Drug Discov 2003; 2:803–811.

76. Brown JM. The hypoxic cell: a target for selective cancer therapy—eighteenth Bruce F. Cain Memorial Award lecture. Cancer Res 1999; 59:5863–5870.

77. Le QT, Kovacs MS, Dorie MJ, et al. Comparison of the comet assay and the oxygen microelectrode for measuring tumor oxygenation in head-and-neck cancer patients. Int J Radiat Oncol Biol Phys 2003; 56:375–383.

78. Brizel DM, Dodge RK, Clough RW, Dewhirst MW. Oxygenation of head and neck cancer: changes during radiotherapy and impact on treatment outcome. Radiother Oncol 1999; 53:113–117.

79. Durand RE. The influence of microenvironmental factors during cancer therapy. In Vivo 1994; 8:691–702.
80. Nordsmark M, Overgaard M, Overgaard J. Pretreatment oxygenation predicts radiation response in advanced squamous cell carcinoma of the head and neck. Radiother Oncol 1996; 41:31–39.
81. Brizel DM, Sibley GS, Prosnitz LR, Scher RL, Dewhirst MW. Tumor hypoxia adversely affects the prognosis of carcinoma of the head and neck. Int J Radiat Oncol Biol Phys 1997; 38:285–289.
82. Stadler P, Becker A, Feldmann HJ, et al. Influence of the hypoxic subvolume on the survival of patients with head and neck cancer. Int J Radiat Oncol Biol Phys 1999; 44:749–754.
83. Rudat V, Vanselow B, Wollensack P, et al. Repeatability and prognostic impact of the pretreatment pO(2) histography in patients with advanced head and neck cancer. Radiother Oncol 2000; 57:31–37.
84. Rudat V, Stadler P, Becker A, et al. Predictive value of the tumor oxygenation by means of pO_2 histography in patients with advanced head and neck cancer. Strahlenther Onkol 2001; 177:462–468.
85. Terris D. Head and neck cancer: the importance of oxygen. Laryngoscope 2000; 110:697–707.
86. Aebersold DM, Burri P, Beer KT, et al. Expression of hypoxia-inducible factor-1alpha: a novel predictive and prognostic parameter in the radiotherapy of oropharyngeal cancer. Cancer Res 2001; 61:2911–2916.
87. Koukourakis MI, Giatromanolaki A, Sivridis E, et al. Hypoxia-inducible factor (HIF1A and HIF2A), angiogenesis, and chemoradiotherapy outcome of squamous cell head-and-neck cancer. Int J Radiat Oncol Biol Phys 2002; 53:1192–1202.
88. Beasley NJ, Leek R, Alam M, et al. Hypoxia-inducible factors HIF-1alpha and HIF-2alpha in head and neck cancer: relationship to tumor biology and treatment outcome in surgically resected patients. Cancer Res 2002; 62:2493–2497.
89. Hui EP, Chan AT, Pezzella F, et al. Coexpression of hypoxia-inducible factors 1alpha and 2alpha, carbonic anhydrase IX, and vascular endothelial growth factor in nasopharyngeal carcinoma and relationship to survival. Clin Cancer Res 2002; 8:2595–2604.
90. Beasley NJ, Wykoff CC, Watson PH, et al. Carbonic anhydrase IX, an endogenous hypoxia marker, expression in head and neck squamous cell carcinoma and its relationship to hypoxia, necrosis, and microvessel density. Cancer Res 2001; 61:5262–5267.
91. Koukourakis MI, Giatromanolaki A, Sivridis E, et al. Hypoxia-regulated carbonic anhydrase-9 (CA9) relates to poor vascularization and resistance of squamous cell head and neck cancer to chemoradiotherapy. Clin Cancer Res 2001; 7:3399–3403.

11

Induction Chemotherapy in Head and Neck Cancer

A Critical Review of 25 Years of Clinical Trials

Danny Rischin, MD

1. INTRODUCTION

It has been known for more than 20 yr that cisplatin-based combination chemotherapy can achieve overall response rates of 70 to 90%, with complete response rates of 20 to 50% in patients with previously untreated locally advanced head and neck cancer *(1,2)*. The use of chemotherapy prior to radiation or surgery is commonly referred to as induction or neoadjuvant chemotherapy. Investigators hypothesized that the addition of an active induction regimen prior to definitive radiotherapy or surgery would have a significant beneficial impact on the outcome of treatment for patients with locally advanced squamous cell carcinoma of the head and neck. As well as the potential to decrease distant metastases, it was hoped that significant tumor shrinkage could contribute to improved local-regional control, and facilitate organ preservation *(3)*. Early single-arm trials confirmed the activity of platinum-based induction regimens and established that sequential induction chemotherapy and radiation was feasible, without any apparent increase in radiation toxicity *(4)*.

2. RESULTS OF PHASE III TRIALS AND META-ANALYSES

Based on promising phase II results, numerous phase III trials of induction chemotherapy have been conducted. In general, these trials have failed to demonstrate any improvement in local control or survival, although the incidence of distant metastases was frequently reduced *(3)*. Several metaanalyses, including a detailed analysis based on individual patient data, have failed to show any significant benefit with induction chemotherapy *(5–7)*. There was a risk reduction of 5% that corresponded to an absolute benefit of 2% with induction chemotherapy that was not statistically significant. None of the 31 induction trials included in the meta-analysis was significant for overall survival. However, a subgroup analysis did show that induction chemotherapy with cisplatin and 5-fluorouracil (5-FU) was different from other regimens, with a hazard ratio of 0.88 (95% CI: 0.79–0.97).

Proponents of induction chemotherapy frequently highlight two studies that they contend support the case for induction chemotherapy as a worthwhile strategy in head and neck cancer. One is the study by Domenge et al. *(8)* who reported on the Group d'Etude des Tumeurs de

From: *Current Clinical Oncology: Squamous Cell Head and Neck Cancer*
Edited by: D. J. Adelstein © Humana Press Inc., Totowa, NJ

la Tete et du Cou (GETTEC) trial that tested the addition of cisplatin and 5-FU prior to radiotherapy or surgery and radiotherapy. The GETTEC trials were included as two studies in the meta-analysis, neither of which was significant, but the two groups were pooled for publication. In the published analysis there was a significant difference in overall survival, but not in event-free survival, local-regional control, or distant metastases. These results are intriguing as it is generally much harder to show a difference in overall survival than in event-free survival in head and neck cancer trials owing to the competing causes of death in this population.

The other trial that is frequently discussed is the trial of Paccagnella et al. *(9)*, which tested the addition of induction chemotherapy prior to surgery for operable patients and prior to radiation for inoperable patients. There were no significant differences between the group that received induction chemotherapy and the group that did not. However, a subgroup analysis of the 171 inoperable patients showed an improvement in overall survival (3-yr survival 10 vs 24%, $p = 0.04$) and disease-free survival (DFS) (3 yr DFS 26 vs 34%, $p = 0.06$). There was an imbalance in the number of patients with T4 disease between the arms, and on multivariate analysis the effect of chemotherapy on overall survival became of borderline significance ($p = 0.06$). Even though 37% of patients had stage 3 disease, only 27% were deemed to be operable. Radiotherapy could be stopped for 2 wk after 40 Gy or if Grade 3 or 4 mucositis occurred, a strategy that is likely to have an adverse effect on outcome, particularly in patients being treated with radiation alone. No details about the actual duration of radiotherapy and dose delivered are included in the manuscript. The overall results in the control arm are very poor, which raises the question about whether the induction chemotherapy partly compensated for suboptimal radiation therapy.

3. DISCORDANCE BETWEEN AVAILABLE EVIDENCE AND USE OF INDUCTION CHEMOTHERAPY

Despite the largely negative results from randomized trials, induction chemotherapy has been widely used outside of clinical trials, particularly in the United States. Harari and colleagues *(10,11)* have reported on the results of community cancer specialists in the United States, who surveyed the management of patients with locoregionally advanced, nonmetastatic head and neck cancer. The specialists were equally divided among otolaryngologists, radiation oncologists, and medical oncologists. By 1996, most of the randomized trials of induction chemotherapy as well as the metaanalyses had been published. In addition, many editorials and reviews had concluded that there was no role for induction chemotherapy, apart from possibly selecting patients for larynx preservation, and that it should not be used outside of a clinical trial *(5,12,13)*. Even so, the 1996 survey revealed that 61% of respondents identified induction chemotherapy as their most common approach for the management of patients with locoregionally advanced head and neck cancer. Between 1996 and 2000, there were few new data on sequential chemoradiation, but increasing evidence of benefit for concurrent chemoradiation was found in randomized trials *(14–16)*. Metaanalyses of individual patient data published in early 2000 confirmed a benefit for concurrent but not sequential chemoradiation *(7)*. Concurrent chemoradiation was preferred by 39%; surprisingly, 31% still favored induction chemotherapy. Induction chemotherapy continues to be widely used even though its use as part of standard care has not been supported by the available evidence at any time over the last 20 yr, with the possible exception of larynx preservation.

4. WHY HAS INDUCTION CHEMOTHERAPY
HAD SUCH A LIMITED IMPACT IN HEAD AND NECK CANCER?

A number of explanations have been proposed to account for the limited impact of induction chemotherapy. Differentiated tumors such as squamous cell carcinomas of the head and neck may maintain the ability to regenerate and repopulate. During an extended period of treatment, accelerated repopulation of surviving clonogenic cells may counter any benefit from the independent cytotoxicity of chemotherapy *(17)*. Chemotherapy may be targeting a population of tumor cells that is already sensitive to radiation, and hence the addition of chemotherapy would be subadditive for local-regional control. Drug resistance may limit the impact of chemotherapy, as suggested by the fact that in the absence of definitive local therapy, chemotherapy responses are generally brief. Another explanation is that chemotherapy may have a limited impact on tumor stem cells. Chemotherapy may not be able to overcome factors that contribute to treatment failure following radiation, e.g., hypoxia. Lastly, induction chemotherapy delays the introduction of the most effective modalities for the treatment of head and neck cancer (radiation and surgery) and this may also offset any benefit from the chemotherapy.

5. LARYNX PRESERVATION TRIALS

One area in which induction chemotherapy could have been considered a reasonable approach in the past was as part of a larynx preservation strategy. This was based on the results of the Veterans Affairs (VA) randomized study demonstrating that a policy of induction chemotherapy followed by radiation for responders and surgery for nonresponders permitted larynx preservation, without any significant difference in survival compared with initial surgery *(18)*. Similar results were reported by the European Organization for Research and Treatment of Cancer (EORTC) in pyriform sinus tumors *(19)*. However, as these trials did not include a radiation-alone arm and there was no improvement in survival, the conclusions were that larynx preservation was feasible but the contribution of induction chemotherapy remained uncertain. It was postulated that the role of induction chemotherapy was to predict patients likely to do well with radiation and hence identify candidates for a larynx preservation approach. This was based on the known correlation between response to chemotherapy and favorable outcome with radiation *(20)*. Nevertheless, it had not been demonstrated that selecting patients for radiation based on response to chemotherapy gave better results than treating all patients with radiation and reserving surgery for salvage.

The other concern was that the meta-analysis showed a nonsignificant trend in favor of the control group, corresponding to an absolute negative effect in the chemotherapy arm that reduced survival at 5 yr by 6% *(7)*. Analysis by tumor site showed that this negative effect may be limited to laryngeal (VA trial) and not hypopharyngeal tumors (EORTC trial). It is important to note that patients in the VA trial proceeded to radiation after a partial or complete response, whereas in the EORTC trial only patients who achieved a complete response proceeded to radiation. These findings raise the possibility that the delay in primary treatment (surgery or radiation) in patients who achieve less than a complete response to induction chemotherapy may adversely affect outcome. Only a complete response may be adequate to counter the adverse consequences of accelerated repopulation and delayed introduction of radiation or surgery, albeit without any apparent survival benefit. An alternative explanation for the negative effect being limited to laryngeal tumors is that laryngeal tumors tend to be better differentiated than hypopharyngeal tumors and hence may have a greater capacity for accelerated repopulation following chemotherapy.

The results of the pivotal Radiation Therapy Oncology Group (RTOG) phase III larynx preservation trial (RTOG 91-11) have demonstrated that there no longer seems to be a role for induction chemotherapy as part of a larynx preservation strategy *(21)*. This trial was well designed to address some of the uncertainties that remained following the previous larynx preservation trials and also to determine the role of concurrent chemotherapy. The induction chemotherapy arm, as in the VA trial, was the control arm, with responders proceeding to radiation alone and nonresponders proceeding to laryngectomy. This approach was compared with radiation alone and with concomitant chemoradiation. Although there were no significant differences in overall survival, patients on the concurrent chemoradiation arm had improved local-regional control and a lower rate of laryngectomy. Induction chemotherapy followed by radiation did not improve local-regional control or larynx preservation rates compared with radiation alone. Although this particular trial did not show improved overall survival, the results are quite consistent with other randomized trials in locally advanced head and neck cancer, demonstrating a significant benefit with concurrent chemoradiation and little or no benefit with sequential chemoradiation.

6. REEVALUATION OF THE ROLE OF INDUCTION CHEMOTHERAPY WITH THE EMERGENCE OF CONCURRENT CHEMORADIATION AS THE STANDARD OF CARE

Concurrent chemoradiation has recently been established as the standard of care for locally advanced head and neck cancer that is treated with a primary radiation approach. The meta-analysis clearly shows that concurrent chemoradiation is far more effective than an induction approach, and this has been reinforced by an updated meta-analysis including more recent randomized trials of concurrent chemoradiation *(22)*. Hence, even if induction chemotherapy is thought to have a role in standard treatment based on a positive interpretation of the induction chemotherapy literature, e.g., emphasizing the cisplatin/5-FU subgroup analysis from the meta-analysis, its role still needs to be reevaluated in the setting of a more efficacious standard treatment than was available previously.

With improvements in local-regional control using concurrent chemoradiation and altered fractionation regimens, it has been argued that distant metastases are becoming a more common site of first relapse *(23)*. Investigators have speculated that treatments that may decrease distant metastases, such as the addition of induction chemotherapy to concurrent chemoradiation, may have an impact on survival if the rates of local-regional failure are low. Several phase II trials have reported good results with this approach *(23,24)*. However, in trials that have compared concurrent with sequential chemoradiation, the incidence of distant metastases has been similar *(21,25)*. In the larynx preservation trial, both concurrent and sequential chemoradiation decreased distant metastases compared with radiation alone *(21)*. Hence, concurrent regimens that use schedules and doses of cisplatin or cisplatin and 5-FU that have significant cytotoxic activity may be just as effective as induction chemotherapy in eradicating micrometastases. The addition of induction chemotherapy could only further decrease distant metastases if more than three cycles is more effective than three cycles, if the addition of other drugs is beneficial, e.g., taxanes, or if the concurrent chemotherapy used has minimal cytotoxic effect on distant metastases.

7. NEW INDUCTION CHEMOTHERAPY REGIMENS

There have been several reports of high response rates with taxane-containing induction regimens *(26)*. Recently, a phase III EORTC trial comparing docetaxel, cisplatin, and 5-FU with cisplatin and 5-FU as induction chemotherapy followed by radiation alone has been reported in preliminary form *(27)*. The docetaxel-containing regimen was associated with improved local-regional control, decreased distant metastases, and improved overall survival. These results suggest that more efficacious chemotherapy regimens may indeed make induction chemotherapy a more effective strategy.

Several phase III trials are planned or under way evaluating the benefit of adding taxane-containing induction chemotherapy to concurrent chemoradiation. It is important that in these trials concurrent chemoradiation regimens with proven benefit in randomized trials be used, e.g., cisplatin 100 mg/m^2 in wk 1, 4, and 7. Trials that use less intensive concurrent chemotherapy that has not been demonstrated to be of benefit may be harder to interpret. The key question to address is whether induction chemotherapy imparts additional benefit when combined with concurrent chemoradiation compared with a standard concurrent chemoradiation regimen. It is not clear whether an intensive induction regimen such as that used in the EORTC trial can be combined with an intensive concurrent regimen. The concern would be that delivery of the concurrent component may be compromised in a multicenter trial. Cumulative cisplatin toxicities such as neuropathy may also become problematic if high-dose cisplatin is included in both the induction and concurrent regimens.

8. CONCLUSIONS

The strategy of induction chemotherapy in locally advanced head and neck cancer has been evaluated in clinical trials for 25 yr, and overall the results have been disappointing. Although some data suggest that induction chemotherapy prior to radiation alone can have a positive impact (e.g., the cisplatin/5-FU subgroup analysis of the meta-analysis and the EORTC trial) the available evidence does not support its use outside of a clinical trial.

REFERENCES

1. Randolph VL, Vallejo A, Spiro RH, et al. Combination therapy of advanced head and neck cancer: induction of remissions with diamminedichloroplatinum (II), bleomycin and radiation therapy. Cancer 1978; 41:460–467.
2. Kish J, Drelichman A, Jacobs J, et al. Clinical trial of cisplatin and 5-FU infusion as initial treatment for advanced squamous cell carcinoma of the head and neck. Cancer Treat Rep 1982; 66:471–474.
3. Adelstein DJ. Induction chemotherapy in head and neck cancer. Hematol Oncol Clin North Am 1999; 13:689–698, v–vi.
4. Choksi AJ, Dimery IW, Hong WK. Adjuvant chemotherapy of head and neck cancer: the past, the present, and the future. Semin Oncol 1988; 15(suppl 3):45–59.
5. Browman GP. Evidence-based recommendations against neoadjuvant chemotherapy for routine management of patients with squamous cell head and neck cancer. Cancer Invest 1994; 12:662–670.
6. Munro AJ. An overview of randomised controlled trials of adjuvant chemotherapy in head and neck cancer. Br J Cancer 1995; 71:83–91.
7. Pignon JP, Bourhis J, Domenge C, Designe L. Chemotherapy added to locoregional treatment for head and neck squamous-cell carcinoma: three meta-analyses of updated individual data. MACH-NC Collaborative Group. Meta-Analysis of Chemotherapy on Head and Neck Cancer. Lancet 2000; 355:949–955.
8. Domenge C, Hill C, Lefebvre JL, et al. Randomized trial of neoadjuvant chemotherapy in oropharyngeal carcinoma. French Groupe d'Etude des Tumeurs de la Tete et du Cou (GETTEC). Br J Cancer 2000; 83:1594–1598.
9. Paccagnella A, Orlando A, Marchiori C, et al. Phase III trial of initial chemotherapy in stage III or IV head and neck cancers: a study by the Gruppo di Studio sui Tumori della Testa e del Collo. J Natl Cancer Inst 1994; 86:265–272.

10. Harari PM. Why has induction chemotherapy for advanced head and neck cancer become a United States community standard of practice? J Clin Oncol 1997; 15:2050–2055.
11. Harari PM CJ, Hartig GK. Evolving patterns of practice regarding the use of chemoradiation for advanced head and neck cancer patients. Proc Am Soc Clin Oncol 2001; 20.
12. Rosenthal DI, Pistenmaa DA, Glatstein E. A review of neoadjuvant chemotherapy for head and neck cancer: partially shrunken tumors may be both leaner and meaner. Int J Radiat Oncol Biol Phys 1994; 28:315–320.
13. Taylor SG. Why has so much chemotherapy done so little in head and neck cancer? J Clin Oncol 1987; 5:1–3.
14. Brizel DM, Albers ME, Fisher SR, et al. Hyperfractionated irradiation with or without concurrent chemotherapy for locally advanced head and neck cancer. N Engl J Med 1998; 338:1798–1804.
15. Calais G, Alfonsi M, Bardet E, et al. Randomized trial of radiation therapy versus concomitant chemotherapy and radiation therapy for advanced-stage oropharynx carcinoma. J Natl Cancer Inst 1999; 91:2081–2086.
16. Wendt TG, Grabenbauer GG, Rodel CM, et al. Simultaneous radiochemotherapy versus radiotherapy alone in advanced head and neck cancer: a randomized multicenter study. J Clin Oncol 1998; 16:1318–1324.
17. Peters LJ, Withers HR. Applying radiobiological principles to combined modality treatment of head and neck cancer—the time factor. Int J Radiat Oncol Biol Phys 1997; 39:831–836.
18. Induction chemotherapy plus radiation compared with surgery plus radiation in patients with advanced laryngeal cancer. The Department of Veterans Affairs Laryngeal Cancer Study Group. N Engl J Med 1991; 324:1685–1690.
19. Lefebvre JL, Chevalier D, Luboinski B, et al. Larynx preservation in pyriform sinus cancer: preliminary results of a European Organization for Research and Treatment of Cancer phase III trial. EORTC Head and Neck Cancer Cooperative Group. J Natl Cancer Inst 1996; 88:890–899.
20. Ensley JF, Jacobs JR, Weaver A, et al. Correlation between response to cisplatinum-combination chemotherapy and subsequent radiotherapy in previously untreated patients with advanced squamous cell cancers of the head and neck. Cancer 1984; 54:811–814.
21. Forastiere AA, Goepfert H, Maor M, et al. Concurrent chemotherapy and radiotherapy for organ preservation in advanced laryngeal cancer. N Engl J Med 2003; 349:2091–2098.
22. Bourhis JAC, Pignon J-P. Update of MACH-NC (Meta-Analysis of Chemotherapy in Head & Neck Cancer) database focused on concomitant chemoradiotherapy. J Clin Oncol 2004; 22:489s.
23. Vokes EE, Weichselbaum RR, Mick R, McEvilly JM, Haraf DJ, Panje WR. Favorable long-term survival following induction chemotherapy with cisplatin, fluorouracil, and leucovorin and concomitant chemoradiotherapy for locally advanced head and neck cancer. J Natl Cancer Inst 1992; 84:877–882.
24. Machtay M, Rosenthal DI, Hershock D, et al. Organ preservation therapy using induction plus concurrent chemoradiation for advanced resectable oropharyngeal carcinoma: a University of Pennsylvania Phase II Trial. J Clin Oncol 2002; 20:3964–3971.
25. Taylor SGt, Murthy AK, Vannetzel JM, et al. Randomized comparison of neoadjuvant cisplatin and fluorouracil infusion followed by radiation versus concomitant treatment in advanced head and neck cancer. J Clin Oncol 1994; 12:385–395.
26. Posner MR, Lefebvre JL. Docetaxel induction therapy in locally advanced squamous cell carcinoma of the head and neck. Br J Cancer 2003; 88:11–17.
27. Vermoken JBRE, van Herpen C, Germa Lluch J, et al. Standard cisplatin/infusional 5-fluorouracil vs docetaxel plus PF as neoadjuvant chemotherapy for nonresectable locally advanced squamous cell carcinoma of the head and neck: a phase III trial of the EORTC Head and Neck Group (EORTC #24971). J Clin Oncol 2004; 22:490.

12

The Evolution of Induction Chemotherapy in Locally Advanced Squamous Cell Cancer of the Head and Neck

The New Paradigm of Sequential Therapy

Marshall R. Posner, MD, Lori Wirth, MD, Roy B. Tishler, MD, Charles M. Norris, MD, and Robert I. Haddad, MD

1. INTRODUCTION

Squamous cell carcinoma of the head and neck (HNSCC) represents 5% of newly diagnosed cancers in adult patients seen in the United States. Although HNSCC is a highly curable malignancy when diagnosed at an early stage, many patients present with advanced local-regional disease. Locally advanced disease can be separated into either intermediate (stage III; T3N0M0 or T1–3N1M0) or advanced (stage IV; T4N0–1M0 or T1–4N2–3M0) *(1)*. Stage III patients are generally resectable, and although their prognosis is better a stage IV patients, the prognosis for all these patients, particularly those who are unresectable has remained poor *(1– 8)*. The potential for surgical resection, whether surgery is advised or not, defines a better prognosis than the presence of unresectable disease. Thus resectability, site, stage, and performance status are the major prognostic factors for patients with HNSCC. Standard therapy with surgery and/or radiotherapy can be associated with significant morbidity and functional disability, particularly when the tumor arises in the larynx, piriform sinus, or oropharynx *(9)*. In addition, despite aggressive local therapy with surgery or radiotherapy, between 50 and 60% will develop locoregional recurrences, and 20 to 30% will develop distant metastases within 2 yr. Only 20 to 45% will remain disease free and alive at 3 yr.

Over the last three decades, medical, surgical, and radiation oncologists have tried to develop a strategy to include chemotherapy in the treatment of locally advanced HNSCC to improve survival and reduce morbidity. Platinum-based chemotherapy is very active in recurrent HNSCC. Response rates to platinum-based combination chemotherapy are relatively high and, in previously untreated patients, can reach 50 to 70%, with 20 to 30% complete

From: *Current Clinical Oncology: Squamous Cell Head and Neck Cancer*
Edited by: D. J. Adelstein © Humana Press Inc., Totowa, NJ

responses *(10,11)*. These outstanding results have led to a considerable effort to develop curative and function-preserving platinum-based therapy for patients with this disease.

As a result of this long and shared endeavor, the incorporation of chemotherapy into a combined modality approach to locally advanced HNSCC has resulted in four general advantageous outcomes: (1) chemotherapy can substitute for primary site surgery, allowing primary functional organ preservation *(2,12,13)*; (2) chemotherapy can improve local regional control *(6,14,15)*; (3) chemotherapy can reduce the rate of distant failure *(13)*; and (4) chemotherapy can improve survival in patients with advanced disease *(4,6,16–19)*. Despite compelling evidence for these outcomes, optimal content and scheduling of combined modality therapy has remained extremely controversial *(20)*. Three major approaches have been investigated for the treatment of primary, locally advanced disease: (1) induction chemotherapy (IC), in which chemotherapy is given before definitive surgery and/or radiotherapy; (2) concomitant treatment with chemotherapy and radiotherapy (CRT), in which chemotherapy and radiotherapy are delivered over the same time frame; and (3) sequential chemotherapy (SCT), a combination of induction chemotherapy and CRT, followed by surgery to sites of bulky nodal or persistent primary site disease *(21,22)*.

2. INDUCTION CHEMOTHERAPY

2.1. Background

Induction chemotherapy for HNSCC has been studied for more than 25 yr. The intense interest in induction chemotherapy has been based on consistent reports of substantial response rates in patients with advanced and recurrent HNSCC. The evidence that cisplatin-based chemotherapy can rapidly shrink large tumors in patients with markedly advanced HNSCC and result in a significant fraction of pathologically negative resections supports the notion that induction chemotherapy can enhance cure rates and/or eliminate the need for surgical resection. The seminal investigations by the team of medical oncologists at Wayne State University systematically explored treatment with cisplatinum and 5-fluorouracil (5-FU) and, through a series of trials, developed the PF induction chemotherapy regimen *(10,11,23–26)*. Although a number of different schedules were tested, the combination of bolus cisplatin and a 5-d continuous infusion of 5-FU was found to be most effective, balanced with acceptable toxicity. Other schedules of these drugs or reduced doses led to lesser response rates.

The Wayne State two-drug regimen combines 100 mg/m^2 cisplatin on d 1 with 1000 mg/m^2/d continuous infusion 5-FU starting on d 1 and continuing for 5 d *(10,23)*. The toxicity of this regimen has been considerable, including nephrotoxicity, mucositis, and diarrhea. Substituting carboplatin for cisplatin to reduce toxicity has been associated with poorer survival and responses in both curable and recurrent disease *(27,28)*. Multiple phase III randomized trials in recurrent disease have combined additional drugs to improve on this regimen, without success (Table 1) *(28–34)*. The PF regimen was the most effective regimen and has remained the gold standard in advanced HNSCC until recently. In first-line therapy of patients with recurrent disease, PF is reported to produce response rates of 25–45%, with complete responses approaching 20%. Responses are short lived, with median progression free survival of 5–9 mo *(28–34)*. Although tumors shrink rapidly, acquired resistance leads to rapid regrowth. This is a reflection of the genetic plasticity and short potential doubling time of the malignant cells and explains why, in curable, untreated patients, a single modality of therapy cannot be delivered over an extended period *(35,36)*.

Table 1
Selected Randomized Phase III Trials in Recurrent Disease
Comparing PF With Other PF-Based Regimens

Study	PF dose	Comparison	PF CR + PR (%)
Paredes et al., 1988 (32)	P: 120 F: 5000	PF with DDTC protectant	41
LHNOG, 1990 (30)	P: 100 F: 4000	Cisplatin MTX Cisplatin + MTX	31
Forastiere et al., 1992 (28)	P: 100 F: 4000	Carboplatin/5-FU MTX	32
Jacobs et al., 1992 (34)	P: 100 F: 4000	Cisplatin 5-FU	40
Clavel et al., 1994 (29)	P: 100 F: 4000	CABO Cisplatin	34
Schrijvers et al., 1998 (33)	P: 100 F: 4000	PF + interferon-α2b	47
Murphy et al., 2001 (31)	P: 100 F: 4000	Cisplatin/Tp	22

Abbreviations: DDTC, diethyidithiocarbamate; MTX, methotrexate; Tp, paclitaxel; CABO, cisplatin, methotrexate, bleomycin, and vincristine; PF, cisplatinum and 5-fluorouracil; CR, complete response; PR, partial response.

The Wayne State and Stanford groups were the first clinical research teams to suggest that PF could replace surgery in curable, resectable patients (25,26). The concept of *organ preservation* gave medical oncologists a more engaged role in the curative treatment of HNSCC and drove the development of induction chemotherapy during the modern era of clinical investigation in to HNSCC. Others suggested that induction chemotherapy made biologic sense because drug delivery is better in untreated, well-vascularized tumors and, as in other tumor systems, micrometastatic disease could be eradicated by high-dose therapy. In addition, it is clearly evident that in HNSCC, the treatment-naïve patient is far more tolerant of the side effects of chemotherapy than the irradiated or postoperative patient.

The clinical benefits of PF induction chemotherapy in curable patients have been demonstrated in meta-analysis (7,19). The most recent indicated that PF regimens, including those substituting carboplatin for cisplatin, had a significant 5-yr survival advantage over standard therapy (Table 2). Close analysis reveals that only six, relatively recent, randomized trials comparing PF with standard therapy have sufficient patients (≥100/arm) and scientific rigor to allow valid conclusions to be drawn (Table 3) (4,12,13,17,18). These trials demonstrated either organ preservation, reduced distant metastases or significant improvements in survival in PF induction chemotherapy-treated patients compared with the control populations. Reported response rates have averaged 60–80%, with complete responses in 20–30% of the patients. The trials can be divided into those in which organ preservation was the major end point or survival was the major end point.

2.2. Organ Preservation in Patients With Resectable HNSCC

The phase III Veterans Affairs (VA) Larynx Preservation Trial is a two-arm study in which induction chemotherapy with PF followed by radiation was compared with initial laryngec-

Table 2
Five-Year Survival for Randomized Trials of Chemotherapy
vs Standard Therapy in HNSCC: The Results of a Meta-Analysis

Trial type	No. of trials	No. of patients	Difference (%)	p value
All trials	65	10,850	+4	<0.0001
Adjuvant	8	1854	+1	0.74
Induction	31	5269	+2	0.10
PF	15	2487	+5	0.01
Non-PF	16	2782	0	0.91
CRT	26	3727	+8	<0.0001

Abbreviations: HNSCC, head and neck squamous cell carcinoma; PF, cisplatinum and 5-fluorouracil; CRT, chemoradiotherapy.
Modified from ref. 7.

Table 3
Adequately Powered, Well-Designed Randomized Trials of Induction Platinum-Flurouracil (PF)
Chemotherapy Compared With Standard Therapy for Curable HNSCC

Preservation	Treatment regimen	No. entered	Results
Organ			
VA larynx study, 1991 (2)	PF × 3 Surgery	332	Organ preservation with PF
EORTC hypoparynx, 1994 (3)	PF × 3 Surgery	202	Organ Preservation with PF
Intergroup larynx, 2003 (6)	PF × 3 Cisplatin + SFX SFX	547	Laryngectomy free survival with CRT vs XRT No significant difference with PF
Survival			
Depondt et al., 1993 (17)	Carboplatin/5-FU Surgery and/or XRT	324	No survival advantage, total population Significant improvement in advanced disease
Paccagnella et al., 1994 (4)	PF × 4 Surgery and/or XRT	237	No survival advantage, total population Significant survival improvement in advanced disease
Domenge et al., 2000 (18)	PF × 4 Surgery and/or XRT	318	Significant survival improvement, total population

Abbreviations: SFX, standard single-fraction radiotherapy; CRT, chemoradiotherapy; XRT, X-ray therapy.

tomy followed by radiation therapy in patients with resectable, intermediate-stage larynx cancer (2). The results demonstrated that patients who received induction chemotherapy had an equivalent survival to patients treated with total laryngectomy, but organ preservation was achieved in two-thirds of the patients given induction chemotherapy. Additionally, the rate of distant metastasis was decreased in the induction chemotherapy patients. A similar study of pyriform sinus cancer performed by the European Organization for Research and Treatment of Cancer (EORTC) demonstrated an equivalent survival between the chemotherapy and surgical arms, with organ preservation achieved in one-third of the patients *(12)*. This study also included primarily patients with intermediate-stage disease. Updates of both studies confirm that the early results have held up over more than 10 yr *(37)*. These are landmark studies, which clearly established that intermediate-stage patients treated for larynx preservation with a nonsurgical approach were not penalized in terms of survival.

Prior to the most recent Intergroup 91-11 trial, attempts to replicate these data were unsuccessful for a number of reasons *(13)*. A Group d'Etude des Tumeurs de la Tete et du Cou (GETTEC) trial that studied laryngeal cancer exemplifies the flaws in design and conduct that plagued early attempts to perform clinical research in HNSCC *(38)*. This trial included very few patients, 69 in total, and had significant early morbidity, which suggested poor patient selection and treatment monitoring. This study highlights problems encountered with many trials in HNSCC, most notably, the inclusion of patients who are inappropriate for aggressive treatments by virtue of underlying morbidities or psychosocial disability. Patients being treated with an intensive therapeutic regime that includes chemotherapy and radiotherapy must be able to tolerate the treatment. In addition, when organ preservation is an outcome of importance, they must be capable of rehabilitating from the therapy. Combined-modality therapy can lead to devastating short-term toxicity and long-term morbidity, which must be addressed. Hence it is of great importance that the care in or out of clinical trials be managed by an experienced and coordinated-combined modality team skilled in the specifics of treatment for HNSCC. Importantly, late function, toxicity, and mortality are not well appreciated in many clinical trials.

More recently, induction chemotherapy for organ preservation has been compared with CRT and with standard daily fractionated radiotherapy in the Intergroup 91-11 trial *(13)*. This study reported that for the intermediate-stage patients, CRT with bolus cisplatin led to greater laryngectomy-free survival than radiotherapy alone. Induction chemotherapy was intermediate and not significantly better compared with radiotherapy or was worse than CRT. Both chemotherapy arms had diminished distant metastases compared with radiotherapy alone. This is somewhat puzzling, as CRT is not associated with a reduction in distant metastases in postoperative or advanced disease settings. Hence, this result is may be specific to the larynx as a primary site or to intermediate-stage disease. Swallowing function was significantly better at 1 yr in the induction chemotherapy group compared with radiotherapy or CRT. Surprisingly, differences in laryngectomy-free survival diminished over time. Thus, in this intermediate-stage population, CRT appears to be a more efficient and potentially effective therapy than radiotherapy alone, although with longer follow-up the difference may disappear.

Two additional studies evaluated PF in patients with both resectable and unresectable disease *(4,18)*. Patients were stratified prior to therapy into these two categories, with surgery planned to occur in the resectable patients between induction chemotherapy and radiotherapy. In the earlier Studio Trial, induction chemotherapy did not improve survival in the resectable patients, although unresectable patients did have a significant survival improvement. There are several potential reasons for these results. First, tumor mapping prior to surgery may not have been adequate. Thus, the complete original volume may not have been encompassed by the postchemotherapy surgery. Second, there was a delay to allow postsurgery healing prior to regional postoperative radiotherapy. This delay permitted the residual population of potentially resistant tumor cells to expand and repopulate their remaining tissues. Unresectable patients receiving chemotherapy on this trial did not have intervening surgery and had a significant improvement in survival. Hence, one could argue that surgery reduced survival in the resectable patients. The second trial, a GETTEC study with an identical design published 6 yr later, demonstrated a significant improvement in resectable patients who received induction chemotherapy followed by surgery and radiotherapy compared with those who did not receive PF induction chemotherapy. The improvement in survival in resectable patients receiving PF in this later trial could be the result of better pretherapy tumor mapping and more rapid movement to radiotherapy after surgery.

The biology of HNSCC must be considered when one is evaluating data from these trials. First, when comparing therapy trials for patients who have resectable disease with trials for patients who have unresectable disease, there is a critical difference in the possible end points of studies specific to larynx preservation compared with studies in patients who have unresectable disease or oropharyngeal carcinoma. In organ preservation studies, equivalent survival is an accepted end point if laryngeal or tongue function is maintained, whereas survival is the appropriate end point in unresectable disease. In addition, in larynx and pyriform sinus cancer, salvage surgery is effective in up to 30% of patients. Hence primary site surgery remains a viable therapeutic option in larynx preservation trials, whereas this is generally not the case in oropharynx or unresectable disease. In addition, the volume of disease tends to be less in resectable tumors of the larynx and pyriform sinus; hence the possibility of cure is higher. These are subtle distinctions that have implications for determining equivalence or improvement in survival in studies that include different sites or stages of HNSCC; this is an example of the complexity of therapeutic and scientific decision making in this disease. Finally, in studies with surgery or organ preservation as a planned intervention for resectable disease or after response assessment, the timing of the surgery has not been optimal. Performing primary site surgery, nodal surgery, or primary site "salvage" surgery after induction chemotherapy but before radiotherapy might negatively impact on survival by delaying the initiation of radiotherapy.

2.3. Patients With Unresectable HNSCC

The role of induction chemotherapy is well established in more advanced or unresectable HNSCC *(4,18)*. The Studio Trial and the GETTEC randomized trials have unequivocally shown that induction chemotherapy can improve survival and local disease control and can prevent the occurrence of metastasis in patients with locally advanced unresectable disease. Survival was significantly improved in the prestratified, unresectable Studio Trial patients who received induction chemotherapy over standard radiotherapy. Two-year survival was 30% in the induction arm compared with 19% in the radiotherapy arm. Updated 12-yr results of the Studio Trial were reported and the significant improvement in survival in the PF-treated patients has been maintained *(39)*.

As mentioned above, the proper sequencing of induction chemotherapy with other modalities has not been well explored. In the Studio Trial unresectable patients went directly from induction chemotherapy to radiotherapy and showed a significant improvement in survival compared with radiotherapy alone. Importantly, and radically unlike any preceding trials, patients in the unresectable group underwent a postradiation primary site biopsy. If that biopsy was negative, they went on to neck dissections if indicated prior to chemotherapy and/or radiotherapy. The notion of postradiotherapy surgery is biologically plausible, when you consider the risk of delay, potential tumor doubling times, and the nature of radiotherapy, which is regional therapy, as opposed to surgery, which is focused and structurally limited in extent. This is in marked contrast to performing surgery between induction chemotherapy and radiotherapy, which potentially allows tumor cell repopulation to occur prior to the start of radiotherapy. In addition, more restricted surgery may be viable after induction chemotherapy and aggressive radiotherapy, although this was not tested in the Studio Trial. Finally, patients are better able to tolerate more aggressive radiotherapy (or chemoradiotherapy) prior to surgery.

Primary site biopsies after induction chemotherapy for prognostic determination are underutilized. In the first study of its kind, the Wayne State group found that patients who had a complete clinical response combined with a complete *pathologic* response at the time of surgery had superior survival compared with those who still had residual disease (25). In the VA Laryngeal Cancer Study, a positive primary site biopsy after induction chemotherapy was associated with reduced locoregional control (40). Notably, one-half of partial responders had a negative postchemotherapy biopsy and a good outcome, suggesting that pathologic response was superior in predictive value to clinical assessment. Therefore, pathologic response at the primary site may be used for assessment of therapeutic efficacy and prediction for for primary site control. The predictive value may vary by site and by regimen. In newer ongoing studies, response and biopsy have been used to predict who might be a candidate for organ preservation. Primary site biopsy and response to induction chemotherapy might also be useful in setting the intensity of subsequent therapy. Newer functional imaging techniques have the potential to impact profoundly on therapeutic decision making in this setting and may serve as surrogates for primary site biopsy or may predict the need for neck dissection.

2.4. Improving PF Induction Chemotherapy

Although PF has been the standard for induction therapy, numerous phase II and phase III trials have sought to develop alternative regimens to PF to improve response or moderate toxicity. Several trials have been reported in which carboplatin was substituted for cisplatin in the PF regimen because of its simpler toxicity profile and ease of administration. In a large randomized trial reported by Depondt et al. (17), Carboplatin-based PF induction therapy led to a borderline improvement in survival in the complete population compared with standard therapy. Despite the use of an agent that is inferior for curative therapy, Depondt et al. (17) demonstrated a significant improvement in overall survival in the subset of advanced induction chemotherapy-treated patients. Cisplatin has been shown to be superior to carboplatinum in randomized trials of platinum/5-FU regimens both in the setting of induction chemotherapy and in recurrent disease (27,28). Thus, interpretation of borderline negative results with carboplatin-based PF should be performed with caution.

Other approaches have included adding a third drug, altering PF scheduling, or promoting radically new combinations. These regimens include PF with leucovorin and interferon-PF regimens (Table 1) (41); they have proved to be no better or were less effective than PF in randomized trials. Recently, the taxanes have been shown to be the most active single agents in recurrent disease. Taxanes have been investigated in combination as a doublet with carboplatinum or triplet with PF in the induction setting (3,31,42–47). One radically aggressive therapy, paclitaxel, cisplatin, and ifosfamide (TIC), has shown considerable activity and appreciable toxicity in a phase II study but has never been tested in phase III (48). A single randomized trial in the recurrent setting with cisplatin plus paclitaxel (PTp) vs PF is completed and a full report is pending (31). In this Eastern Cooperative Oncology Group (ECOG) study, response rate between PF and PTp was equivalent, and toxicity with PTp was less. However, PF had a better 1-yr survival then PTp. High-dose induction carboplatinum-taxol (CTp) regimens have been studied in phase II trials with mixed results. Although carboplatinum is inferior agent to cisplatin in combination with 5-FU, it is unclear whether, when combined with a taxane, it is less effective then cisplatin. Some carboplatin-paclitaxel regimens require cytokine support, and observed response rates are relatively low. It is therefore very surprising that carboplatin/taxane-based therapies have been accepted as standards for induction therapy, as there are no phase III data showing equivalence or improvement in response or survival, compared with standard PF.

Combinations of taxane plus PF (TPF) have been studied extensively in phase II and III trials. The majority of phase II studies in curable, previously untreated patients have shown excellent results (Table 4) *(3,43–47)*. More importantly, there are now two large, randomized phase III trials reported in abstract form demonstrating that a taxane triplet based on PF is superior to and less toxic than standard PF *(3,46)*. The EORTC trial demonstrated that a docetaxel-based TPF induction therapy, followed by radiotherapy, led to a significant improvement of survival in patients with unresectable HNSCC. A persistent relative survival improvement of 25% was associated with less nausea, vomiting, and mucositis and fewer deaths then the PF arm. The Madrid study evaluated a paclitaxel-based TPF regimen and also demonstrated, in a more mixed population, an improvement in survival and less toxicity with the triplet, compared with the PF regimen. These studies are highly significant and signal an important change in therapy for HNSCC, making TPF therapy an acceptable, more effective standard for induction chemotherapy.

3. SEQUENTIAL CHEMORADIOTHERAPY

There is compelling evidence from phase III trials and a meta-analysis that induction chemotherapy and CRT each improve survival in patients with locally advanced HNSCC *(7)*. An analysis of failures in aggressive TPF regimens followed by hyperfractionated radiotherapy revealed good control of distant metastases but disappointing locoregional failure rates, even in the face of hyperfractionated radiotherapy programs *(49)*. An analysis of multiple CRT studies reveals no effect on distant metastases by CRT treatments leading to a relative increase in distant metastases such that distant metastases account for more than 50% of failures *(6,14,15,50)*.

As opposed to CRT, induction chemotherapy provides high-dose systemic therapy, which treats distant disease and significantly reduces local and regional disease prior to the start of radiotherapy. The latter effect has the potential to lead to a better functional outcome as documented in the Intergroup Larynx Preservation Trial *(13)*. Induction chemotherapy toxicity is also usually transient, whereas CRT toxicity is significantly prolonged and frequently permanent. Induction chemotherapy is also associated with prolongation of treatment. In addition, it is possible to assess prognosis and adjust the intensity of subsequent therapy based on response to induction chemotherapy. Early studies by the Wayne State team demonstrated that CRT could salvage unresectable patients who were not responding to PF induction chemotherapy *(22)*. This group of patients would be expected to have an almost 100% mortality with standard radiotherapy; however 26% remained alive and disease free at 2 or more years, and more than half were controlled locally. Thus, CRT allows for increased locoregional dose intensity. CRT may be altered to salvage poor responses to induction chemotherapy. CRT alone is ineffective systemic therapy and is associated with considerable systemic and local toxicity. Finally, if CRT is the sole planned therapy, then there is no method to assess prognosis and adjust intensity or toxicity once CRT has started.

We, and others, have proposed and are studying methods of combining induction chemotherapy with CRT and surgery as *sequential therapy*. We have proposed a paradigm in which

Table 4
Phase III and Selected Phase II Trials of Taxane Plus PF Induction Chemotherapy for Curable Hand and Neck Squamous Cell Carcinoma

Phase II	Treatment regimen	No. entered	2-Yr survival
Posner et al., 2001 (44)	TPF	43	82%
Janinis et al., 2001 (43)	TPF	20	60%
Schrijvers et al., 2004 (45)	TPF	48	41%
Colevas et al., 2002 (47)	TPFL	34	68%
Phase III	Treatment comparison	No. entered	Summary result
Hitt et al., 2003 (46)	TpPF	383	Significant survival advantage to TpPF
			Less toxcity
Vermoken et al., 2004 (3)	TPF	358	Significant survival advantage to TPF
			Less toxicity

Abbreviations: TPF, toxane, cisplatinum, and 5-fluorouracil; TPFL, TPF plus leucouorin; TpPF, paclitaxel, cisplatinum, and 5-fluorouracil.

induction chemotherapy is followed by CRT; surgery typically is added after CRT to complete the eradication of residual cancer in areas of bulk disease, particularly in the neck, or for salvage of persistent primary site disease. We believe this paradigm optimizes therapy by attending to the known biology of HNSCC and the clinical observations of the last two decades of combined-modality therapy in this disease. Tumor growth rates are most rapid after tumor volume is decreased, as occurs in the immediate period after completion of induction chemotherapy (35). This is a biologically critical period for therapeutic intervention. Thus, the addition of a non-cross-resistant regional therapy with minimal delay, i.e. CRT after induction chemotherapy, rather than a focused treatment, i.e., surgery, at this critical time point should improve locoregional control. CRT at this point is superior to surgery because it treats the entire region, rather than specific structures. Surgery can be applied after CRT to remove any residual nidus within the sites of prior bulk disease.

Many sequential therapy plans have been investigated in phase II studies based on different treatment concepts. Schedules have varied in timing, intensity and choices of agents. These studies are summarized in Table 5 (22,46,51–57). Two phase III trials, the Madrid study and the TAX 324 studies are included, although they represent studies comparing PF with TPF (46) and do not answer questions regarding the value of the sequential therapy paradigm. The University of Pennsylvania sequential program studied very high-dose CTp followed by single-agent weekly CRT with Paclitaxel (51). Surgery was reserved for nonresponders to chemotherapy and for patients with large neck nodes, who have post-CRT neck dissections and adjuvant chemotherapy. The University of Chicago gave weekly CTp chemotherapy over 6 wk followed by THFX CRT (52). The Minnie Pearl Cancer Research Network Trial performed a study of high-dose CTp with continuous infusion of 5-FU followed by CTp weekly with radiotherapy (54). Vanderbilt University Medical Center completed a trial similar to the University of Pennsylvania trial (55). The Venice Study explored two CRT regimens in combination with TPF induction chemotherapy (57). They found two CRT cycles of a cisplatin/5-FU regimen to be more tolerable than three cycles of a carboplatinum/5-FU regimen and

Table 5
Sequential Chemotherapy Trials

	Induction chemotherapy	Concomitant chemoradiotherapy	Adjuvant chemotherapy
Wayne State phase II, 1990 (22)	PF q 3 wk × 3 SFX	Bolus cisplatin q 3 wk × 3	None
U. of Chicago phase II, 1998 (53)	PFL + interferon-α q 4 wk × 3	Split course, concomitant 5-FU, hydroxyurea	None
U. of Chicago phase II, 2003 (52)	Carboplatin/Tp q 3 wk × 6	Paclitaxel, 5-FU, hydroxyurea HF-XRT	None
U. of Penn. phase II, 2003 (51)	Carboplatin/Tp q 3 wk × 2	Paclitaxel weekly SFX	Carboplatin/Tp q 3 wk × 2
MPCRN phase II, 2003 (54)	Carboplatin/Tp q 3 wk × 2 5-FU CI d 1-42	Carboplatin/Tp weekly SFX	None
ECOG 2399 phase II, 2003 (55)	Carboplatin/Tp q 3 wk × 2	Paclitaxel weekly SFX	None
U. of Michigan phase II, 2003 (56)	PF x 1	Cisplatin q 3 wk SFX	PF × 2 q 3 wk
Madrid phase III, 2003 (46)	TpPF vs PF	Cisplatin q 3 wk SFX	None
Venice phase I/II, 2004 (57)	TPF q 3 wk × 3	Carboplatin/5-FU x 3 or PF × 2 SFX	None
TAX 324 phase III, unpublished	PF vs TPF q 3 wk × 3	Carboplatin weekly SFX	None

Abbreviations: PFL, isplatin, 5-fluorouracil (5-FU), and leucovorin; HF-XRT, hyperfractionated radiotherapy; MPCRN, Minnie Pearl Cancer Research Network; CI, continuous infusion; PF, cisplatin and 5-FU; TPF, taxane, cisplatinum, and 5-FU; TpPF, paclitaxel and PF; SFX, single-fraction radiotherapy.

plan a phase III trial comparing sequential therapy with CRT. Results for all these trials are relatively early but suggest a 60 to 70% 3-yr survival.

The University of Michigan has adopted a different approach, They are using induction chemotherapy to determine subsequent therapy (56). After one cycle of PF patients are assessed for response and nonresponders undergo laryngectomy; complete and partial responders receive CRT with bolus cisplatin. Two additional cycles of adjuvant PF are then given to complete responders. Survival and organ preservation rates are excellent. Survival at 3-yr was 80%. This population is primarily patients with resectable larynx cancer and is not directly comparable to the more advanced patients treated in the other sequential studies.

A multicenter, randomized, phase III trial, TAX 324, has been completed; it compared a sequential treatment plan of TPF (with docetaxel) vs PF induction therapy, followed by CRT with weekly carboplatinum. TAX 324 accrued over 530 patients (Fig. 1). Results should be available for initial analysis by the Fall of 2005. This trial is similar to the Madrid trial; however, the weekly CRT with carboplatin allows more regional dose intensity and less systemic toxicity was seen than with the bolus cisplatin regimen used in the Madrid study. In addition, surgery in the TAX 324 study was planned to be performed after CRT, based on the

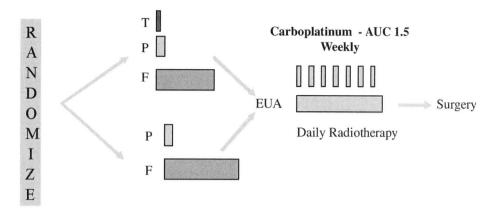

TPF: Docetaxel 75 $_{D1}$ + Cisplatin 100 $_{D1}$ + 5-FU 1000 $_{CI-D1-4}$ Q 3 weeks x3
PF: Cisplatin 100 $_{D1}$ + 5-FU 1000 $_{CI-D1-5}$ Q 3 weeks x 3

Fig. 1. Schema for the TAX 324 trial, a randomized phase III trial comparing TPF with PF in a sequential therapy paradigm. 5-FU, 5-fluorouracil; CI, continuous infusion; EUA,.

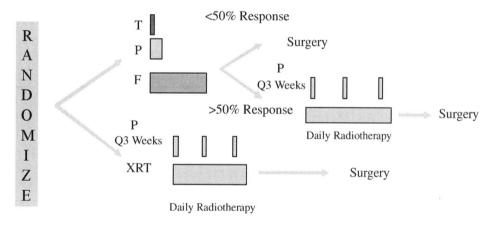

* Cisplatimum (P); Docetaxel (D); 5 -Fuorouracil (F)

Fig. 2. Schema for the SWOG trial, a randomized phase III trial comparing TPF-based sequential therapy with chemoradiotherapy. P, cisplatinum; D, docetaxel; F, 5-fluorouracil; T, taxane.

notion of enhancing regional therapy and reserving focal surgery for any residual nidus of cancer at the original sites of bulk disease.

The phase II and phase III trials of sequential therapy have reported 2- and 3-yr survival rates in advanced disease that are unprecedented. This new paradigm of treatment has not been compared with a standard CRT regimen, and phase III studies are being planned or initiated to compare the paradigms of sequential therapy and CRT. The Southwestern Oncology Group (SWOG) is a comparative trial using bolus cisplatin CRT as the standard arm and TPF induction chemotherapy followed by bolus cisplatin CRT as the experimental therapy (Fig. 2). The Dana-Farber Cancer Institute is leading an active phase III trial comparing TPF-CRT sequential therapy with cisplatin plus accelerated concomitant boost (CRT-ACB) radiotherapy (Fig. 3). The Paradigm Trial has chosen an aggressive CRT-ACB approach as the CRT control arm.

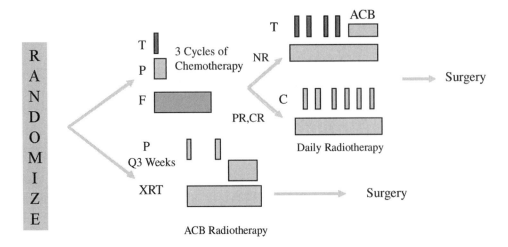

Fig. 3. Schema for the Paradigm trial, a randomized phase III trial comparing TPF-based sequential therapy with chemoradiotherapy. ACB, accelerated concomitant boose; CR, complete response; F, 5-fluorouracil; NR, no response, P, cisplatinum; PR, partial response; T, taxane; XRT, radiotherapy.

This CRT-ACB regimen is currently being compared by the Radiation Therapy Oncology Group (RTOG) with a standard arm of bolus cisplatin and once-daily radiotherapy. The Paradigm Trial takes full advantage of the prognostic value of response to induction therapy. Patients on the induction TPF arm of the Paradigm Trial with poor responses to induction therapy will be treated with a more aggressive docetaxel based CRT with ACB. Docetaxel based CRT-ACB is more locally toxic, but phase I and laboratory data indicate that taxanes are superior radiation sensitizers even when the tumor is resistant to taxane alone *(58–60)*. Unfortunately, increased normal tissue toxicity limits their utility.

4. CONCLUSIONS

Induction chemotherapy has been studied and refined over the last two decades. Induction therapy with PF leads to improved survival in patients with advanced disease. The newly studied triplets of taxane-based PF have improved the outcomes compared with PF and are a new standard of care for induction chemotherapy. The new paradigm of sequential therapy incorporates our advancing understanding of the biology of the disease and the experiences of past clinical trials and results in several potential benefits. Sequential therapy leads to improved locoregional control, organ preservation, and function by dramatically reducing tumor volume and treating systemic metastases prior to the start of CRT. By identifying patients with resistant disease before CRT, surgery or more aggressive CRT approaches can be applied. Sequential therapy and TPF induction chemotherapy will be the platforms for further investigation of the new molecularly targeted agents coming into the clinic. Sequential therapy makes sound biologic sense and represents a standard of care that is reasonable, but it remains experimental. Phase III trials will ultimately determine whether sequential therapy is truly superior to induction chemotherapy or CRT.

REFERENCES

1. Fleming ID, Cooper JS, Henson DE, et al., eds. AJCC Cancer Staging Handbook, 5th ed. Philadelphia: Lippincott Williams & Wilkins, 1998.
2. Veterans Affairs Laryngeal Cancer Study Group. Induction chemotherapy plus radiation compared with surgery plus radiation in patients with advanced laryngeal cancer. N Engl J Med 1991; 324:1685–1689.
3. Vermorken JB, Remenar E, Van Herpen C, et al. Standard cisplatin/infusional 5-fluorouracil (PF) vs docetaxel (T) plus PF (TPF) as neoadjuvant chemotherapy for nonresectable locally advanced squamous cell carcinoma of the head and neck (LA-SCCHN): a phase III trial of the EORTC Head and Neck Cancer Group (EORTC #24971). Proc ASCO 2004; 23:5508.
4. Paccagnella A, Orlando A, Marchiori C, et al. Phase III trial of initial chemotherapy in stage III or IV head and neck cancers: A study by the Gruppo di Studio sui Tumori della Testa e del collo. J Natl Cancer Inst 1994; 86:265–272.
5. Forastiere A, Koch W, Trotti A, Sidransky D. Medical progress: head and neck cancer. N Engl J Med 2001; 345:1890–1900.
6. Adelstein D, Li Y, Adams G, et al. An Intergroup Phase III comparison of standard radiation therapy and two schedules of concurrent chemoradiotherapy in patients with unresectable squamous cell head and neck cancer. J Clin Oncol 2003; 21:92–98.
7. Monnerat C, Faivre S, Temam S, Bourhis J, Raymond E. End points for new agents in induction chemotherapy for locally advanced head and neck cancers. Ann Oncol 2002; 13:995–1006, 2002.
8. Posner MR. Head and Neck Cancer. In: Goldman L, Ausiello D, eds. Cecil Textbook of Medicine, 22nd ed. Orlando, FL: WB Saunders Company, 2004: pp. 1195–2001.
9. Staar S, Rudat V, Stuetzer H, et al. Intensified hyperfractionated accelerated radiotherapy limits the additional benefit of simultaneous chemotherapy - results of a multicentric randomized German trial in advanced head and neck cancer. Int J Rad Oncol Biol Phys 2001; 50:1161–1171,
10. Kish J, Ensley J, Jacobs J, et al. A randomized trial of cisplatin (CACP) + 5-fluorouracil (5-FU) infusion and CACP + 5-FU bolus for recurrent and advanced squamous cell carcinoma of the head and neck. Cancer 1985; 56:2740–2744.
11. Kish J, Ensley J, Jacobs J, Binns P, Al-Sarraf M. Evaluation of high-dose cisplatin and 5-FU infusion as initial therapy in advanced head and neck cancer. Am J Clin Oncol 1988; 11:553–557.
12. Lefebvre J, Chevalier D, Luboinski B, et al. Larynx preservation in pyriform sinus cancer: preliminary results of a European organization for research and treatment of cancer phase III trial. J Natl Cancer Inst 1996; 88:890–898.
13. Forastiere AA, Goepfert H, Maor M, et al. Concurrent chemotherapy and radiotherapy for organ preservation in advanced larynx cancer. The N Engl J Med 2003; 349:2091–2098.
14. Calais G, Bardet E, Sire C, et al. Radiotherapy with concomitant weekly docetaxel for stages III/IV oropharynx carcinoma. Results of the 98-02 Gortec Phase II trial. Int J Rad Oncol Biol Phys 2004; 58:161–166.
15. Bernier J, Domenge C, Ozsahin M, et al. Postoperative irradiation with or without concomitant chemotherapy for locally advanced head and neck cancer. N Engl J Med 2004; 350:1945–1952.
16. Calais G, Alfonsi M, Bardet E, et al. Randomized trial of radiation therapy versus concomitant chemotherapy and radiation therapy for advanced stage oropharynx carcinoma. J Natl Cancer Inst 1999; 91:2081–2086.
17. Depondt J, Gehanno P, Martin M, et al. Neoadjuvant chemotherapy with carboplatin/5-fluorouracil in head and neck cancer. Oncology 1993; 50:23–27.
18. Domenge C, Hill C, Lefebvre J, et al. Randomized trial of neoadjuvant chemotherapy in oropharyngeal carcinoma. Br J Cancer 2000; 83:1594–1598.
19. Pignon J, Bourhis J, Domenge C, Designe L, Group M-NC. Chemotherapy added to locoregional treatment for head and neck squamous-cell cancer: three meta-analysis of updated individual data. Lancet 2000; 355:949–955.
20. Posner M, Colevas A, Tishler R. The role of induction chemotherapy in the curative treatment of squamous cell cancer of the head and neck. Sem Oncol 2000; 27(Suppl G):13–24.
21. Haddad R, Wirth L, Posner M. The integration of chemotherapy in the curative treatment of locally advanced head and neck cancer. Exp Rev Anticancer Ther 2003; 3:331–338.
22. Ensley J, Ahmed K, Kish J, Tapazoglou E, Al-Sarraf M. Salvage of patients with advanced squamous cell cancers of the head and neck (SCCHN) following induction chemotherapy failure using radiation and concurrent cisplatinum (CACP). In: Salmon S, ed. Adjuvant Therapy of Cancer VI, Philadelphia: WB Saunders, 1990: pp. 92–100:
23. Rooney M, Kish J, Jacobs J, et al. Improved complete response rate and survival in advanced head and neck cancer. Cancer 1985; 55:1123–1128.
24. Kish J, Weaver A, Jacobs J, Cummings G, Al-Sarraf M. Cisplatin and 5-fluorouracil infusion in patients with recurrent and desseminated epidermoid cancer of the head and neck. Cancer 1984; 53:1819–1824.

25. Al-Kourainy K, Kish J, Ensley J, et al. Achievement of superior survival for histologically negative versus histologically positive clinically complete responders to cisplatin combination in patients with locally advanced head and neck cancer. Cancer 1987; 59:233–238.

26. Jacobs C, Goffinet D, Goffinet L, Kohler M, Fee W. Chemotherapy as a substitute for surgery in the treatment advanced resectable head and neck cancer. A report from the Northern California Oncology Group. Cancer 1987; 60:1178–1183.

27. De Andres L, Brunet J, Lopez-Pousa A, et al. Randomized trial of neoadjuvant cisplatin and flourouracil versus carboplatin and fluorouracil in patients with stage IV-M0 head and neck cancer. J Clin Oncol 1995; 13:1493–1500.

28. Forastiere A, Metch B, Schuller D, et al. Randomized comparison of cisplatin plus fluorouracil and carboplatin plus fluorouracil versus methotrexate in advanced squamous cell carcinoma of the head and neck: a Southwest Oncology Group study. J Clin Oncol 1992; 10:1245–1251.

29. Clavel M, Vermorken J, Cognetti F, et al. Randomized comparison of cisplatin. methotrexate, bleomycin, and vincristine (CABO) versus cisplatin and 5-fluorouracil (CF) versus csiplatin (C), in recurrent or metastatic squamous cell carcinoma of the head and neck. A Phase III stduy of the EORTC head and neck cancer cooperative group. Ann Oncol 1994; 5:521–526.

30. LHNOG. A phase III randomized trial of cisplatin, methotrexate, cisplatin + methotrexate and cisplatin + 5-FU in end stage squamous carcinoma of the head and neck. Br J Cancer 1990; 61:311–315.

31. Murphy B, Li Y, Cella D, Karnad A, Hussain M, Forastiere A. Phase iii study comparing cisplatin (C) and 5-flurouracil (F) versus cisplatin and paclitaxel (T) in metstatic/recurrent head and neck cancer (MHNC). Proc Am Soc Clin Oncol 2001; 20.

32. Paredes J, Hong W, Felder T, et al. Prospective randomized trial of high-dose cisplatin and fluorouracil infusion with or without sodium diethyldithiocabramate in recurrent and/or metastatic squamous cell cancer of the head and neck. J Clin Oncol 1988; 6:955–962.

33. Schrijvers D, Johnson J, Jimenez U, et al. Phase III trial of modulation of cisplatin/fluorouracil chemotherapy by interferon alfa-2b in patients with recurrent or metastatic head and neck cancer. J Clin Oncol 1998; 16:1054–1059.

34. Jacobs C, Lyman G, Velez-Garcia E, et al. A Phase III randomized study comparing cisplatin and fluorouracil as single agents and in combination for advanced squamous cell carcinoma of the head and neck. J Clin Oncol 1992; 10:257–263.

35. Takimoto C, Rowinsky E. Dose-intense paclitaxel: deja vu all over again? J Clin Oncol 2003; 21:2810–2814.

36. Kotelnikov V, Coon J IV, Haleem A, et al. Cell kinetics of head and neck cancer. Clin Cancer Res 1995; 1:527–537.

37. Lefebvre J, Chevalier D, Luboinski B, et al. Is laryngeal preservation with induction chemotherapy safe in the treatment of hypopharyngeal SCC? Final results of the phase III EORTC 24891. Proc ASCO 2004; 23:5531.

38. Richard J, Sancho-Garnier H, Pessey J, et al. Randomized trial of induction chemotherapy in larynx cancer. Oral Oncol 1998; 34:224–228.

39. Zorat P, Loreggian L, Paccagnella A, et al. Randomized phase III trial of neoadjuvant chemotherapy (CT) in head and neck (H&N) cancer patients: an update based on 10 years' follow up. Proc ASCO 2004; 23:5532.

40. Spaulding M, Fischer S, Wolf, G. Tumor response, toxicity, and survival after neoadjuvant organ-preserving chemotherapy for advanced laryngeal carcinoma. J Clin Oncol 1994; 12:1592–1599.

41. Clark J, Busse P, Norris C, et al. Induction chemotherapy with cisplatin, fluorouracil, and high-dose leucovorin for squamous cell carcinoma of the head and neck: long-term results. J Clin Oncol 1997; 15:3100–3110.

42. Clark JI, Hofmeister C, Choudhury A, et al. Phase II evaluation of paclitaxel in combination with carboplatin in advanced head and neck carcinoma. Cancer 2001; 92:2334–2340.

43. Janinis J, Papadakou M, Panagos G, et al. Sequential chemoradiotherapy with docetaxel, cisplatin, and 5-fluorouracil in patients with locally advanced head and neck cancer. Am J Clin Oncol 2001; 24:227–231.

44. Posner M, Glisson B, Frenette G, et al. A multi-center phase I-II trial of docetaxel, cisplatinum , and 5-fluorouracil induction chemotherapy for patients with locally advanced squamous cell cancer of the head and neck. J Clin Oncol 2001; 19:1096–1104.

45. Schrijvers D, Van Herpen C, Kerger J, et al. Docetaxel, cisplatin, and 5-fluorouracil in patients with locally advanced unresectable head and neck cancer: a phase I-II feasibility study. Ann Oncol 2004; 15:638–645.

46. Hitt R, Lopez-Pousa A, Rodriguez M, et al. Phase III study comparing cisplatin (P) & 5-fluoruracil (F) versus P, F and paclitaxel (T) as induction therapy in locally advanced head and neck cancer (LAHNC). Proc ASCO 2003; 22:496.

47. Colevas AD, Norris CM, Tishler RB, et al. Phase I/II trial of outpatient docetaxel, cisplatin, 5-fluorouracil, leucovorin (opTPFL) as induction for squamous cell carcinoma of the head and neck (SCCHN). Am J Clin Oncol 2002; 25:153–159.

48. Shin DM, Glisson BS, Khuri FR, et al. Phase II study of induction chemotherapy with paclitaxel, ifosfamide, and carboplatin (TIC) for patients with locally advanced squamous cell carcinoma of the head and neck. Cancer 2002; 95:322–330.

49. Haddad R, Norris C, Sulivan C, et al. Docetaxel, cisplatin and 5-fluorouracil based induction chemotherapy in patients with locally advanced squamous cell carcinoma of the head and neck: the Dana-Farber Cancer Institute experience. Cancer 2003; 97:412–418.

50. Cooper J, Pajak TF, Forastiere A, et al. Postoperative concurrent radiotherapy and chemotherapy for high-risk squamous-cell carcinoma of the head and neck. N Engl J Med 2004; 350:1937–1944.

51. Machtay M, Rosenthal DI, Hershock D, et al. Organ preservation therapy using induction plus concurrent chemoradiation for advanced resectable oropharyngeal carcinoma: a University of Pennsylvania phase II trial. J Clin Oncol 2002; 20:3964–3971.

52. Vokes EE, Stenson K, Rosen FR, et al. Weekly carboplatin and paclitaxel followed by concomitant paclitaxel, fluorouracil, and hydroxyurea chemoradiotherapy: curative and organ-preserving therapy for advanced head and neck cancer. J Clin Oncol 2003; 21:320–326.

53. Kies MS, Haraf DJ, Athanasiadis I, et al. Induction chemotherapy followed by concurrent chemoradiation for advanced head and neck cancer: improved disease control and survival. J Clin Oncol 1998; 16:2715–2721.

54. Hainsworth JD, Meluch AA, McClurkan S, et al. Induction paclitaxel, carboplatin and infusional 5-FU followed by concurrent radiation therapy and weekly paclitaxel/carboplatin in the treatment of locally advanced head and neck cancer: a phase II trial of the Minnie Pearl Cancer Research Network. Cancer J 2002.

55. Cmelak A, Murphy BA, Burkey B, Douglas S, Netterville J. Induction chemotherapy (IC) followed by concurrent chemoradiation (CCR) for organ preservation (OP) in locally advanced squamous head and neck cancer (SHNC): results of a phase II trial. Proc ASCO 2003; 22.

56. Urba S, Wolf G, Bradford C, et al. Improved survival and decreased late salvage surgery using chemo-selection of patients for organ preservation in advanced laryngeal cancer. Proc ASCO 2003; 22:497.

57. Grazia M, Paccagnells A, D'Amanzo P, et al. Neoadjuvant docetaxel, cisplatin, 5-flurorucil before concurrent chemoradiotherapy in locally advanced squamous cell carcinoma of the head and neck versus concomitant chemoradiotherapy: a phase II feasibility study. Int J Rad Oncol Biol Phys 2004; 59:481–487.

58. Mason K, Hunter N, Milas M, Abbruzzese J, Milas L. Docetaxel enhances tumor radioresponse in vivo. Clin Cancer Res 1997; 12:2431–2438.

59. Milross C, Mason K, Hunter N, et al. Enhanced radioresponse of pacitaxel-sensitive and -resistant tumors in vivo. Eur J Cancer 1997; 8:1299–1308.

60. Tishler RB, Norris CM, Haddad R, et al. A phase I/II trial of docetaxel and concomitant boost radiation therapy for patients with squamous cell cancer of the head and neck following induction chemotherapy. Proc ASCO 2003; 22:506.

13

Concurrent Chemoradiotherapy

Impact on Survival and Organ Preservation

David J. Adelstein, MD

1. INTRODUCTION

Initial efforts to integrate systemic chemotherapy into the definitive management of squamous cell head and neck cancer focused on sequential treatment schedules. Given the impressive response rates seen with multiagent chemotherapy in previously untreated patients, considerable effort went into the study of induction or neoadjuvant treatment schedules *(1)*. Numerous randomized trials have now been completed. Although induction chemotherapy has been generally well tolerated, and appears to decrease the likelihood of distant metastatic disease, no consistent survival benefit has been demonstrated from this treatment approach alone *(2)*.

Increasingly the focus of multimodality treatment for this disease has been on the use of concurrent rather than sequential schedules. This approach, commonly referred to as chemoradiotherapy (CRT), is based on the potential for synergism between the two treatment modalities, i.e., chemotherapeutic radiosensitization *(3)*.

A number of mechanisms for radiosensitization have been suggested *(4)*. These include the potential ability of chemotherapy to decrease tumor cell repopulation following radiation fractionation. The possibility that chemotherapy might recruit cancer cells into a more radiation-sensitive phase of their cell cycle has also been suggested, as has the ability of chemotherapy to inhibit repair of sublethal radiation damage. Both laboratory and/or clinical models of radiosensitization have been demonstrated for several chemotherapeutic agents including cisplatin, 5-fluorouracil (5-FU), mitomycin, hydroxyurea, bleomycin, and the taxanes. Concurrent treatment approaches have been found to be valuable not just in head and neck cancer but also in several of the gastrointestinal tumors including esophageal cancer, rectal cancer, anal cancer, and pancreatic cancer as well as in lung, genitourinary, and gynecologic malignancies.

The theoretical advantages of concurrent treatment also include the fact that both chemotherapy and radiation therapy are independently active treatment modalities and may act on different cell populations. The use of chemotherapy in conjunction with radiation also allows for the treatment of microscopic metastatic disease not addressed by locoregional treatment. Furthermore, the concurrent rather than sequential use of these two treatment modalities provides for a shorter overall treatment duration, an issue of considerable importance in the relatively noncompliant head and neck cancer population.

From: *Current Clinical Oncology: Squamous Cell Head and Neck Cancer*
Edited by: D. J. Adelstein © Humana Press Inc., Totowa, NJ

There is, however, a significant disadvantage to concurrent treatment *(1)*. The simultaneous use of two independently toxic treatment modalities will necessarily result in greater toxicity than either treatment modality used alone. This has often resulted in a compromise of the dose intensity of the radiation, the chemotherapy, or both. These compromises have included the use of single-agent rather than combination chemotherapy, a reduction in chemotherapy dose, or an alteration in radiation scheduling, most notably the use of split radiotherapy courses. Such compromises in dose intensity also compromise overall treatment results. It is therefore important that any benefit achieved by the concurrent use of these two treatment modalities be more than just additive, in order to compensate for the increased resultant toxicity.

2. SINGLE-AGENT CHEMORADIOTHERAPY TRIALS

The initial exploration of concurrent chemoradiotherapy utilized a full course of conventional, uninterrupted radiation therapy as the definitive management along with simultaneous single-agent chemotherapy. Although it was recognized that the chemotherapy was, by itself, suboptimal, it was felt to be potentially sensitizing in conjunction with the radiation. A number of randomized phase III trials have been reported comparing radiation therapy with radiation and single-agent 5-FU *(5–7)*, bleomycin *(8–11)*, and platinum *(12–15)* (Table 1).

5-FU was the first chemotherapy drug studied in this fashion. A randomized trial begun in 1961 at the University of Wisconsin demonstrated an improvement in both local control and survival in patients treated with bolus 5-FU and concurrent radiation compared with radiation therapy alone *(5)*. The benefit appeared to be restricted to those patients with oral cavity tumors. A survival benefit was also demonstrated in a large trial reported by Sanchiz et al. *(6)* comparing 60 Gy of radiation with the same radiation dose and single-agent 5-FU. In this study, a third treatment arm using hyperfractionated radiation to a larger total dose (70.4 Gy) produced results similar to those of the CRT arm. Browman et al. *(7)* reported their trial of conventional radiation compared with radiation and two concurrent 72-h, 5-FU infusions. The concurrent group experienced greater toxicity but a statistically improved complete response rate with marginally improved progression-free and overall survival.

The experience using concurrent single-agent bleomycin has been inconsistent. Locoregional control and relapse-free survival were improved in the Northern California Oncology Group Trial *(10)*, whereas results reported by the European Organization for Research and Treatment of Cancer (EORTC) were negative, with no benefit identified from the addition of bleomycin *(11)*. This latter trial, however, was compromised by frequent protocol deviations. The Northern California Oncology Group study also used additional adjuvant chemotherapy with methotrexate and bleomycin, thus making it difficult to interpret the results fully.

Encouraging phase II trials have been reported using several schedules of single-agent cisplatin and concurrent radiation therapy. The Eastern Cooperative Oncology Group (ECOG) studied a weekly low-dose cisplatin treatment schedule *(16)*, and the Radiation Therapy Oncology Group (RTOG) utilized high-dose cisplatin given every 3 wk *(17)*. A large randomized Intergroup study was subsequently performed comparing radiation therapy alone and the ECOG regimen of cisplatin (20 mg/m^2/wk) along with radiation in patients with locally advanced but unresectable cancer *(12)*. No survival benefit resulted from the concurrent treatment despite a higher overall response rate. One explanation for this lack of benefit was the relatively small dose of cisplatin ultimately given (140 mg/m^2). Subsequent randomized trials employing radiation and daily cisplatin chemotherapy *(13,14)* or the RTOG, every 3-wk

Table 1
Randomized Trials of Radiotherapy vs Radiotherapy and Concurrent Single-Agent Chemotherapy

Author	Yr	No. of patients	Radiation (Gy)	Survival benefit
5-Fluorouracil				
Lo et al. (5)	1976	136	60-70	Yes
Sanchiz et al. (6)	1990	859	60	Yes
Browman et al. (7)	1994	175	66	Marginal
Bleomycin				
Shanta et al. (8)	1980	157	55–60	Yes
Vermund et al. (9)	1985	222	65	No
Fu et al. (10)	1987	104	70	Yes[a]
Eschwege et al. (11)	1988	199	70	No
Platinum				
Haselow et al. (12)	1990	319	68–78	No
Jeremic et al. (13)	1997	159	70	Yes
Jeremic et al. (14)	2000	130	77	Yes
Adelstein et al. (15)	2000	295	70	Yes

[a]Relapse-free survival.

regimen have demonstrated a clear survival benefit for the concurrent chemotherapy arms (15).

This last experience was studied in a second-generation Intergroup randomized trial for patients with locally advanced unresectable tumors (15). This trial compared (1) radiation therapy alone (given in a conventional fractionation schedule), (2) the same radiation therapy plus concurrent high-dose cisplatin (100 mg/m^2) given every 3 wk, and (3) an unconventional split course of radiation plus concurrent 5-FU and cisplatin combination chemotherapy. The third treatment schedule had been designed with the hope that patients initially deemed unresectable might be rendered surgical resectable after limited preoperative CRT.

This study enrolled 295 patients from the ECOG and the Southwest Oncology Group (SWOG), and clearly demonstrated an improved survival for patients treated with the concurrent high-dose cisplatin regimen compared with radiation therapy alone. The split-course radiation therapy and combination chemotherapy arm was not statistically different from either of the other two treatment arms. The lack of improvement seen from the use of a multiagent chemotherapy regimen was felt to reflect the detrimental impact of the split course of radiation therapy, which was not compensated for by the number of surgical resections ultimately performed. This Intergroup study also allowed salvage surgical procedures to be performed in patients with less than a complete response, or in those with a locoregional recurrence after definitive nonoperative management. Such salvage surgery proved possible, although the surgical procedure was most often only a neck dissection, performed after achievement of a complete response at the primary site. The clear improvement demonstrated from the addition of high-dose single-agent cisplatin to conventional radiation therapy established a new standard of care for the management of patients with unresectable disease.

3. MULTIAGENT CHEMORADIOTHERAPY TRIALS

What stands out from these single-agent trials is the reproducible survival benefit achieved by the addition of either concurrent single-agent 5-FU or single-agent platinum. Unlike the

Table 2
Randomized Trials of Radiotherapy vs Radiotherapy and Concurrent Multiagent Chemotherapy

Author	Yr	No. of patients	Chemotherapy	Radiation (Gy)	Survival benefit	Locoregional control benefit
Weissler et al. (19)	1992	32	PF	72 (bid, split)	Yes[a]	—
Adelstein et al. (20)	1997	100	PF	66–72	Yes[b]	Yes
Wendt et al. (21)	1998	270	PFL	70.2 (bid, split)	Yes	Yes
Brizel et al. (22)	1998	116	PF	70–75 (bid)	Yes	Yes
Calais et al. (23)	1999	226	CpF	70	Yes	Yes
Staar et al. (24)	2001	240	CpF	69.9 (bid CB)	Yes[c]	Yes[c]

Abbreviations: CB, concomitant boost; Cp, carboplatin: F, 5-fluorouracil; L, leucovorin; P, cisplatin.
[a]Disease-specific survival.
[b]Relapse-free survival.
[c]Oropharynx cancer subset.

experience using induction chemotherapy schedules, this represents a clear demonstration that chemotherapy has a role in the definitive management of patients with head and neck cancer. The next logical step was the use of concurrent combination chemotherapy regimens.

Multiagent CRT has been approached somewhat more tentatively, however, in view of significant and realistic concerns about toxicity (18), Many of the initial efforts employed suboptimal drug combinations, chemotherapy doses, or radiotherapy treatment schedules. Despite these compromises, reproducible success, using predominantly 5-FU and platinum combinations, has been reported, demonstrating a survival benefit compared with radiation alone (Table 2) (19–24).

Perhaps the most convincing of these studies was initially reported by Calais et al. in 1999 (23) and updated by Denis et al. in 2004 (25). This study randomized 226 patients to either radiation therapy alone (70 Gy in 35 fractions) or concurrent CRT using the same radiation therapy schedule and three cycles of concurrent carboplatin and 5-FU. All reported end points statistically favored the CRT arm, with a 5-yr overall survival of 22% compared with 16% for those patients treated with radiation therapy alone. Planned surgical salvage or neck dissection was not part of this treatment protocol and may explain the relatively poor overall survival. Nonetheless, the study serves as a proof of principle and validates the additional benefit possible with concurrent combination chemotherapy. In this study, as in all others, the acute toxicity seen with concurrent CRT was significantly greater than after radiation therapy alone.

Although planned salvage surgery is important in patient management, it has a confounding impact on the results of these kinds of studies. In 1997, Adelstein et al. (20), reported results from a phase III trial comparing radiation therapy alone with radiation and two cycles of concurrent 5-FU and cisplatin. Patients with resectable stage III and IV disease were eligible, and surgical resection was planned for all patients with less than a complete response or with locoregional disease recurrence after treatment. Although the overall survival rate was unaffected by the addition of concurrent chemotherapy, relapse-free survival, distant metastatic control, and overall survival with primary site preservation were significantly improved in those patients treated with the CRT. The lack of an overall survival benefit was felt to represent the important contribution of surgical salvage in patients treated with radiation alone.

Several randomized trials have been performed comparing concurrent CRT with sequential treatment schedules using induction chemotherapy followed by definitive management. Both

Taylor et al. *(26)* and Adelstein et al. *(27)* used a 5-FU plus cisplatin chemotherapy combination with a split course of radiation therapy, and reported a suggestive but inconclusive benefit for the concurrent treatment group. Pinnaro et al. *(28)* compared single-agent cisplatin and concurrent radiation to induction 5-FU and cisplatin followed by radiation. No differences in survival were identified.

Metaanalysis data have been confirmatory. The largest of these metaanalyses, from the Meta-Analysis of Chemotherapy on Head and Neck Cancer (MACH-NC) group based in France, reviewed 63 randomized trials, including more than 10,000 patients, using updated individual patient data *(29)*. No survival advantage was identified from either a neoadjuvant or adjuvant treatment schedule, except for the subgroup of patients treated with induction platinum and 5-FU (hazard ratio 0.88; 95% CI:0.79–0.97). Patients treated with concomitant CRT however, had an absolute 5-yr survival benefit of 8% with a $p < 0.0001$ (HR 0.81; 95% CI: 0.76–0.88). It is important to point out that this metaanalysis did not include most of the trials reported in Table 2.

A variation on this theme of concurrent CRT has been the reemergence of intraarterial chemotherapy regimens. The RADPLAT (intraarterial cisplatin and concurrent radiation therapy) regimen devised by Robbins et al. *(30)* at the University of Tennessee uses high-dose intraarterial cisplatin, systemic thiosulfate neutralization, and concurrent radiation in patients with advanced head and neck cancers. The phase II experience suggests excellent locoregional control but has raised concern for the possibility of distant metastases.

This concern about distant metastatic disease has also emerged as a direct result of the locoregional success achieved by aggressive concurrent CRT regimens. Two recent phase II studies of multiagent chemotherapy and altered fractionation radiation therapy have reported locoregional control in more than 90% of patients *(31,32)*. As a result, and in contrast to all previous experience in this disease, the most common cause of treatment failure in these two series was distant metastases. This observation has suggested to some that there is a possible role for the reintroduction of induction chemotherapy prior to definitive concurrent treatment in an effort both to increase locoregional control and to decrease distant metastases. Studies of this approach are currently under way.

Most of the concurrent CRT trials that have been reported have utilized conventional radiation fractionation. Several of the more recent studies have explored altered radiation fractionation schedules *(22,24,32)*, a radiation therapy approach of proven, albeit modest additional benefit *(33)*. Whether this intensification of radiation therapy will improve results or will only produce additional toxicity remains to be seen.

It must be stressed that these kinds of concurrent treatment schedules are associated with significant toxicity, far in excess of that seen after single-modality treatment. The success of these approaches has only been possible because of growing familiarity with the necessary intensive supportive-care measures. Close nursing and physician follow-up, active dental prophylaxis, early aggressive and appropriate antibiotic usage, and vigorous nutritional support are critical. Feeding tubes are now routinely employed in these patients in an effort to avoid the treatment breaks that would have previously been required because of mucositis and dysphagia *(34)*. The importance of maintaining dose intensity and avoiding radiation therapy treatment breaks cannot be overemphasized.

Although our ability to manage these acute toxic affects has improved, there is growing recognition of the consequential late toxic manifestations from these kinds from treatments *(35)*. In particular there is concern about persistent posttreatment dysphagia, including persistent feeding tube dependence. Although in some patients this may reflect the locally advanced nature of the tumor at presentation, and a baseline compromise in swallowing, it may also reflect the protracted period during which CRT-induced mucosal inflammation precludes oral intake. When coupled with the tumor-induced functional change, treatment-induced stricturing and scarring of the hypopharyngeal and proximal esophageal structures can result. Subsequent dysphagia may be irreversible. Aggressive diagnostic and therapeutic measures, with vigorous rehabilitation are required. The observed improvement in survival from concurrent CRT has also come at the price of an increase in radiation fibrosis of the neck, xerostomia, and laryngeal dysfunction, with an incidence that varies widely depending on the chemotherapeutic agents and radiation therapy schedules chosen. Intensive investigation of the impact of these treatments on long-term functioning is a major focus of current investigations.

4. POSTOPERATIVE ADJUVANT CONCURRENT CHEMORADIOTHERAPY

Although concurrent CRT has improved patient survival compared with radiation therapy alone, definitive surgical resection remains the most appropriate intervention for many patients with this disease. There are, however, no studies that have compared definitive surgery with concurrent CRT, and no statement can be made as to their relative efficacy. Patients who have early-stage disease and patients who have advanced tumors with significant preexisting organ dysfunction may be better served by definitive resection followed by postoperative adjuvant treatment. For patients with high-risk tumors after surgical resection, including patients with positive surgical margins, multiple lymph node involvement, extracapsular disease extension, or angiolymphatic invasion, postoperative radiation therapy is indicated. The addition of concurrent chemotherapy to this postoperative radiation has been intensively studied and is the subject of Chapter 14 in this volume.

5. CONCURRENT CHEMORADIOTHERAPY FOR ORGAN PRESERVATION

Next to survival, organ function conservation is the most important treatment goal. The loss of speech, swallowing, or nonstomal breathing is a significant price to pay. It is important, however, to distinguish between *organ* preservation and organ *function* preservation (36). Although a total laryngectomy is a terribly multilating procedure, postoperative rehabilitation will often allow successful restoration of intelligible speech. A definitive nonoperative approach, on the other hand, might obviate surgical resection but still result in significant functional disability, such as in the patient with long-term feeding tube dependence.

Chemotherapy has been increasingly legitimized as a tool that might allow for the wider application of definitive radiation and the elimination or modification of surgery, with the hope that organ function conservation might be improved. This approach has been best tested in patients with larynx and hypopharynx cancer who would require a total laryngectomy for surgical control. Both the Veterans Affairs Laryngeal Cancer Study Group (37) and the EORTC (38) have demonstrated a role for induction chemotherapy in predicting those patients most likely to benefit from definitive radiation rather than surgical resection.

It has, however, been unclear from these studies whether radiation therapy alone might be equally successful in allowing patients to avoid a laryngectomy. This question was addressed by the recently reported second-generation, three-arm laryngeal preservation Intergroup study (RTOG 91–11) (39). This trial compared definitive radiation alone, induction chemotherapy followed by radiation therapy (with surgical salvage for nonresponders), and definitive concurrent CRT, in patients with advanced larynx cancer. Induction chemotherapy consisted of 5-FU and cisplatin, and the concurrent treatment schedule used single-agent high-dose

Table 3
RTOG 91-11: Overall Survival and Surgical Salvage

	Treatment arms		
	Induction chemotherapy	Concurrent chemotherapy	Radiotherapy alone
No. of patients	173	172	173
5-yr projected survival (%)	55	54	56
Underwent salvage laryngectomy	48 (28%)	27 (16%)	54 (31%)
Failure-free after laryngectomy	25 (14%)	18 (10%)	35 (20%)

Data from refs. *39* and *40*.

cisplatin alone. Clear superiority of the radiotherapy/concurrent cisplatin arm was demonstrated in laryngeal preservation and locoregional control compared with both the induction chemotherapy and the radiation therapy alone arms. Both of the chemotherapy-containing arms suppressed the incidence of distant metastases and resulted in a better disease-free survival than radiation therapy alone. Both chemotherapy-containing arms also produced significantly more acute toxicity.

Despite this improvement in organ preservation, no survival benefit was found from the use of concurrent chemotherapy. Indeed, survival was the same for all three treatment arms. It should be pointed out, however, that salvage laryngectomy was performed in 25% of the patients entered on this study and was successful in more than 60% *(40)*. It was also required in fewer patients on the concurrent treatment arm, again pointing out the confounding influence of surgical salvage on our interpretation of these multimodality studies (Table 3).

The potential for concurrent CRT to allow for organ preservation (and organ function conservation) in nonlaryngeal head and neck cancers has not been well tested *(36)*. Many of the phase III trials reported have demonstrated an improvement in organ preservation compared with radiation therapy alone. However, survival equivalence with primary surgical approaches has not been studied, and the ultimate functional benefit derived from aggressive concurrent CRT is unknown.

6. CONCLUSIONS

There is little doubt that the concurrent use of systemic chemotherapy with radiation produces a survival benefit compared with radiation therapy alone. Further efforts must be directed toward defining those patients best suited for this kind of intervention as opposed to primary surgical resection. The optimal combination of chemotherapy and radiation that will produce both the best survival and best functional result also needs to be identified. Efforts to modify both the acute and late toxicities must be coupled with continued efforts to define the long-term functional implications of both surgical and nonsurgical approaches. The recognition that distant metastases are now a more frequent cause of treatment failure must continue to prompt the search for better systemic agents, whether these are conventional chemotherapeutic drugs or the newer targeted therapies.

REFERENCES

1. Adelstein DJ, Tan EH, Lavertu P. Treatment of head and neck cancer: the role of chemotherapy. Crit Rev Oncol Hematol 1996;24:97–116.

2. Adelstein DJ. Induction chemotherapy in head and neck cancer. Hematol Oncol Clin N Am 1999;13:689–698.

3. Kinsella TJ. An approach to the radiosensitization of human tumors. Cancer J Sci Am 1996;2:184–193.

4. Vokes EE, Weichselbaum RR. Concomitant chemoradiotherapy: Rationale and clinical experience in patients with solid tumors. J Clin Oncol 1990;8:911–934.

5. Lo TCM, Wiley AL, Ansfield FJ, et al. Combined radiation therapy and 5-fluorouracil for advanced squamous cell carcinoma of the oral cavity and oropharynx: a randomized study. Am J Roentgenol 1976;126:229–235.

6. Sanchiz F, Millá A, Torner J, et al. Single fraction per day versus two fractions per day versus radiochemotherapy in the treatment of head and neck cancer. Int J Radiat Oncol Biol Phys 1990;19:1347–1350.

7. Browman GP, Cripps C, Hodson DI, et al. Placebo-controlled randomized trial of infusional fluorouracil during standard radiotherapy in locally advanced head and neck cancer. J Clin Oncol 1994;12:2648–2653.

8. Shanta V, Krishnamurthi S. Combined bleomycin and radiotherapy in oral cancer. Clin Radiol 1980;31:617–620.

9. Vermund H, Kaalhus O, Winther F, et al. Bleomycin and radiation therapy in squamous cell carcinoma of the upper aero-digestive tract: a phase III clinical trial. Int J Radiat Oncol Biol Phys 1985;11:1877–1886.

10. Fu KK, Phillips TL, Silverberg IJ, et al. Combined radiotherapy and chemotherapy with bleomycin and methotrexate for advanced inoperable head and neck cancer: update of a Northern California Oncology Group randomized trial. J Clin Oncol 1987;5:1410–1418.

11. Eschwege F, Sancho-Garnier H, Gerard JP, et al. Ten-year results of randomized trial comparing radiotherapy and concomitant bleomycin to radiotherapy alone in epidermoid carcinomas of the oropharynx: experience of the European Organization for Research and Treatment of Cancer. NCI Monogr 1988;6:275–278.

12. Haselow RE, Warshaw MG, Oken MM, et al. Radiation alone versus radiation with weekly low dose cis-platinum in unresectable cancer of the head and neck cancer. In: Fee WE, Jr, Goepfert H, Johns ME, et al., eds. Head and Neck Cancer, vol II. Philadelphia: JB Lippincott, 1990: pp. 279–281.

13. Jeremic B, Shibamoto Y, Stanisavljevic B, et al. Radiation therapy alone or with concurrent low-dose daily either cisplatin or carboplatin in locally advanced unresectable squamous cell carcinoma of the head and neck: a prospective randomized trial. Radiother and Oncol 1997;43:29–37.

14. Jeremic B, Shibamoto Y, Milicic B, et al. Hyperfractionated radiation therapy with or without concurrent low-dose daily cisplatin in locally advanced squamous cell carcinoma of the head and neck: a prospective randomized trial. J Clin Oncol 2000;18:1458–1464.

15. Adelstein DJ, Li Y, Adams GL, et al. An Intergroup phase III comparison of standard radiation therapy and two schedules of concurrent chemoradiotherapy in patients with unresectable squamous cell head and neck cancer. J Clin Oncol 2003;21:92–98.

16. Haselow RE, Adams GS, Oken MM, et al. Cis-platinum (DDP) with radiation therapy (RT) for locally advanced unresectable head and neck cancer. Proc ASCO 1983;2:160 (Abstr).

17. Marcial VA, Pajak TF, Mohiuddin M, et al. Concomitant cisplatin chemotherapy and radiotherapy in advanced mucosal squamous cell carcinoma of the head and neck. Cancer 1990;66:1861–1868.

18. Adelstein DJ. Recent randomized trials of chemoradiation in the management of locally advanced head and neck cancer. Curr Opin Oncol 1998;10:213–218.

19. Weissler MC, Melin S, Sailer SL, et al. Simultaneous chemoradiation in the treatment of advanced head and neck cancer. Arch Otolaryngol Head Neck Surg 1992;118:806–810.

20. Adelstein DJ, Saxton JP, Lavertu P et al. A phase III randomized trial comparing concurrent chemotherapy and radiotherapy with radiotherapy alone in resectable stage III and IV squamous cell head cancer: Preliminary results. Head Neck 1997;19:567–575.

21. Wendt TG, Grabenbauer GG, Rödel CM, et al. Simultaneous radiochemotherapy versus radiotherapy alone in advanced head and neck cancer: a randomized multicenter study. J Clin Oncol 1998;16:1318–1324.

22. Brizel DM, Albers ME, Fisher SR, et al. Hyperfractionated irradiation with or without concurrent chemotherapy for locally advanced head and neck cancer. N Engl J Med 1998;338:1798–1804.

23. Calais G, Alfonsi M, Bardet E, et al. Randomized trial of radiation therapy versus concomitant chemotherapy and radiation therapy for advanced-stage oropharynx carcinoma. J Natl Cancer Inst 1999;91:2081–2086.

24. Staar S, Rudat V, Stuetzer H, et al. Intensified hyperfractionated accelerated radiotherapy limits the additional benefit of simultaneous chemotherapy—results of a multicentric randomized German trial in advanced head and neck cancer. Int J Radiat Oncol Biol Phys 2001;50:1161–1171.

25. Denis F, Garaud P, Bardet E, et al. Final results of the 94-01 French Head and Neck Oncology and Radiotherapy Group randomized trial comparing radiotherapy alone with concomitant radiochemotherapy in advanced stage oropharynx carcinoma. J Clin Oncol 2004;22:69–76.

26. Taylor SG, Murthy AK, Vannetzel J-M, et al. Randomized comparison of neoadjuvant cisplatin and fluorouracil infusion followed by radiation versus concomitant treatment in advanced head and neck cancer. J Clin Oncol 1994;12:385–395.

27. Adelstein DJ, Sharan VM, Earle AS, et al. Long-term follow-up of a prospective randomized trial comparing simultaneous and sequential chemoradiotherapy for squamous cell head and neck cancer. In: Salmon SE, ed. Adjuvant Therapy of Cancer VII. Philadelphia: JB Lippinott, 1993: pp. 82–91.

28. Pinnarò P, Cercato MC, Giannarelli D, et al. A randomized phase II study comparing sequential versus simultaneous chemo-radiotherapy in patients with unresectable locally advanced squamous cell cancer of the head and neck. Ann Oncol 1994;5:513–519.

29. Pignon JP, Bourhis J, Domenge C, et al. Chemotherapy added to locoregional treatment for head and neck squamous-cell carcinoma: three meta-analyses of updated individual data. Lancet 2000;355:949–955.

30. Robbins KT, Kumar P, Regine WF, et al. Efficacy of targeted supradose cisplatin and concomitant radiation therapy for advanced head and neck cancer: the Memphis experience. Int J Radiat Oncol Biol Phys 1997;38:263–271.

31. Vokes EE, Kies MS, Haraf DJ, et al. Concomitant chemoradiotherapy as primary therapy for locoregionally advanced head and neck cancer. J Clin Oncol 2000;18:1652–1661.

32. Adelstein DJ, Saxton JP, Lavertu P, et al. Maximizing local control and organ preservation in stage IV squamous cell head and neck cancer with hyperfractionated radiation and concurrent chemotherapy. J Clin Oncol 2002;20:1405–1410.

33. Fu KK, Pajak TF, Trotti A, et al. A Radiation Therapy Oncology Group (RTOG) phase III randomized study to compare hyperfractionation and two variants of accelerated fractionation to standard fractionation radiotherapy for head and neck squamous cell carcinomas: First report of RTOG 9003. Int J Radiat Oncol Biol Phys 2000;48:7–16.

34. Mekhail TM, Adelstein DJ, Rybicki LA, et al. Enteral nutrition during the treatment of head and neck carcinoma. Cancer 2001;91:1785–1790.

35. Trotti A, Bentzen SM. The need for adverse effects reporting standards in oncology clinical trials. J Clin Oncol 2004;22:19–22.

36. Adelstein DJ. Oropharyngeal cancer: the role of the medical oncologist in organ-function conservation. In: Perry MC, ed. American Society of Clinical Oncology Education Book. Alexandria, VA: American Society of Clinical Oncology 1999: pp. 544–550.

37. Wolf GT, Hong WK, Fisher SG, et al. Induction chemotherapy plus radiation compared with surgery plus radiation in patients with advanced laryngeal cancer. N Engl J Med 1991;324:1685–1690.

38. Lefebvre JL, Chevalier D, Luboinski B, et al. Larynx preservation in pyriform sinus cancer: preliminary results of a European Organization for Research and Treatment of Cancer phase III trial. J Natl Cancer Inst 1996;88:890–899.

39. Forastiere AA, Goepfert H, Maor M, et al. Concurrent chemotherapy and radiotherapy for organ preservation in advanced laryngeal cancer. N Engl J Med 2003;349:2091–2098.

40. Weber RS, Berkey BA, Forastiere A, et al. Outcome of salvage total laryngectomy following organ preservation therapy. The Radiation Therapy Oncology Group trial 91-11. Arch Otolaryngol Head Neck Surg 2003;129:44–49.

14

Postoperative Treatment of Locally Advanced Head and Neck Cancers

Jacques Bernier, MD, PD
and Søren M. Bentzen, PhD, DSc

1. INTRODUCTION

With about half a million cases diagnosed yearly worldwide *(1)*, head and neck squamous cell cancers (HNSCCs) represent 4 to 5% of all solid malignancies. The prognosis of locally advanced stages, which are found in at least 40% of oral cavity and pharynx carcinomas, remains dismal: in the United States the 5-yr relative survival rates for the period 1989–1995 hardly reached 50%. At the time of diagnosis, distant metastases are found in less than 10% of the cases and until the late 1980s, this disease feature led investigators to focus on local treatment.

Throughout the 1960s and 1970s, surgery and/or radiotherapy were the mainstay of locoregional treatment in patients with locally advanced HNSCC. Stage I–II lesions were treated efficiently with one of these two modalities, and about 60 to 90% of the patients with early disease were free of cancer at 5 yr. Throughout the past century, the treatment of stage III–IV tumors remained a matter of debate, and their management was sometimes highly controversial.

With the advent of megavoltage units in the 1950s, tumors considered *unresectable* were routinely treated with definitive radiation therapy. With time, both treatment machines and irradiation techniques improved, which led radiooncologists both to consolidate their knowledge of conventional treatments and to investigate novel altered fractionation regimes, either accelerated or hyperfractionated. Definitive radiotherapy used to achieve 5-yr overall survival rates of less than 30% *(2)*, but the significant number of patients in poor general conditions and with lifestyle-related comorbidity certainly accounted for this.

In the late 1970s, various cytotoxic drugs were found to produce promising overall response rates. Among them cisplatin and 5-fluorouracil (5-FU) were extensively investigated both as definitive treatment and in combination with radiotherapy. In a metaanalysis of chemotherapy in head and neck cancer *(3)*, which included more than 10,000 patients with locally advanced HNSCC, the overall survival at 5 yr was 32%.

On the other hand, surgery is the first-line treatment of choice in *resectable* tumors, and traditionally postoperative radiotherapy is delivered in case of locally advanced tumor or in the presence of close resection margins. In the 1980s, there were some indications that adding cytotoxic agents to the locoregional treatment might have an impact on treatment outcome, but, in terms of evidence-based medicine, no clear conclusions could be drawn from the scarce

From: *Current Clinical Oncology: Squamous Cell Head and Neck Cancer*
Edited by: D. J. Adelstein © Humana Press Inc., Totowa, NJ

prospective trials that had addressed this issue. It is only within the last few years that new evidence has emerged in favor of adjuvant treatments based on a multidisciplinary approach.

Recently we have improved our knowledge in several areas such as the clinical and pathologic features of importance for the prognosis after primary line surgery and the impact of various adjuvant treatments on treatment outcome.

Obviously a number of gray zones remain in the field of adjuvant treatment in patients with locally advanced tumors, especially regarding the indication for chemotherapy in intermediate-risk disease. However, recent trials have produced level I evidence for improved outcome after postoperative chemoradiotherapy (CRT) in high-risk patients. We concentrate here on patients operated on with curative intent and do not discuss the outcome in patients with gross residual disease after surgery, since these cases receive palliative treatment.

Some conclusions can now be drawn from the most recent studies, especially those that addressed prospectively the issues mentioned above. We show how a transatlantic collaboration, developed in the last decade between a European and a US cooperative group, has probably given a definitive answer to the long-lasting dilemma of the adjuvant treatment of head and neck cancers.

2. THE ROAD TO CHEMORADIOTHERAPY IN THE ADJUVANT SETTING

2.1. Postoperative Radiotherapy

In the early 1970s, Fletcher and Evers (4) pioneered the use of radiosurgical approaches, especially in patients with stage II–IV HNSCC. A prompt confirmation that postoperative radiotherapy significantly reduced the risk of failure above the clavicles was offered by other institutions, both in Europe and in the United States (5–7).

Throughout the next 20 yr, operable patients were usually managed with surgery followed by postoperative radiotherapy. Interestingly, the range of locoregional control rates reported in the literature for surgery combined with radiotherapy is astonishingly broad; from 35 to 75%, depending on tumor stage and histopathological pattern (8–10). This marked variation in outcome suggests that, in addition to heterogeneities in tumor- and patient-related factors, variations in surgeon and radiotherapist expertise may have affected the prognosis of these patients.

After primary surgery the prognosis of HNSCC is essentially determined by the clinical stage and presence of unfavorable histopathological features. Prognostic factors for survival are tumor location and stage, quality of surgical resection, and, in some studies, age and gender (8,11–15). Indeed, it has been repeatedly shown that, although most small T1–2 tumors with no evidence of neck node involvement can be adequately treated by surgery alone, the incidence of locoregional failures and distant metastases is high in patients locally advanced disease (5,6,8,10).

Careful retrospective analyses conducted by Fletcher and colleagues (4) at the M.D. Anderson Cancer Center showed that a dose of 50 Gy was required to eradicate malignant microfoci in 95% of the cases with negative surgical margins. It was also found that high doses, up to 70 Gy, had to be delivered postoperatively in patients with oropharyngeal or oral cavity squamous cell carcinomas, and in case of positive surgical margins (16).

What about preoperative radiotherapy? Few controlled trials have looked at the optimal sequencing of surgery and radiation. Tupchong et al. (17) found in a phase III study that preoperative irradiation (50 Gy) was inferior to postoperative radiation therapy (60 Gy) in patients presenting with supraglottic larynx and hypopharynx disease. Note, however, the lower total dose in the preoperative arm. This being said, preoperative radiotherapy has only been used in a few institutions in the last two decades.

Thus radiotherapy is traditionally delivered as an adjuvant therapy to surgery, and the benefit from this combination in patients with poor prognostic factors is now well documented (4–7). The parallel development of both surgical techniques "à la carte" and novel radiation techniques such as 3D CRT and intensity modulated radiotherapy (IMRT) has reinforced the role of postoperative radiotherapy, especially regarding the quality of life of patients after treatment.

The incidence of treatment sequelae, such as functional impairment of swallowing or speech or a poor cosmetic outcome is linked to the extent of the surgical procedure. However, in choosing between primary line vs salvage surgery, we should never lose sight of the fact that cure represents the overall goal of therapeutic management and that surgery with postoperative radiotherapy is a key element in the achievement of that objective.

2.2. Chemotherapy

The rationale for the inclusion of chemotherapy in the therapeutic management of locally advanced tumors springs from three main observations: (1) even if 70 to 75 % of these cases remain free of disease at 2 yr, their long-term prognosis is poor: 5-yr survival rates rarely exceed 30 to 35%; (2) although a fairly high number of deaths are linked to intercurrent diseases, the incidence of metastases can reach 15 to 20% (5); and (3) a variety of cytotoxic agents have demonstrated efficacy against epithelial cell cancers.

Systemic treatments not only increase cell killing through an additive effect to that of radiotherapy but also improve disease-free survival rates through a reduction in distant metastases. From the late 1970s on, various schemes of adjuvant chemotherapy were tested first in sequence and thereafter concomitantly with radiation therapy.

Interestingly enough, the actual role of adjuvant chemotherapy remained to be defined when investigators decided, in the 1990s, to move more consistently to modalities combining concurrent chemo- and radiotherapy (18,19): indeed the encouraging results obtained in nonrandomized studies (20–22) had not been fully consolidated in randomized trials, at least in terms of a significant gain in survival (10,23,24).

Nonrandomized studies essentially focused on the impact of 5-FU in the adjuvant setting. For instance, Johnson et al. (22), tested the sequential administration of methotrexate with leucovorin rescue, and 5-FU for 6 mo after surgery and radiotherapy. Beyond the fact that the CRT was shown to be well tolerated, the adjusted 2-yr disease-free survival was 67%, comparing favorably with the 36% disease-free survival for concurrent controls, treated with surgery and radiotherapy alone. Among the randomized studies (23–25), the effect of adjuvant chemotherapy on survival was highest for resectable tumors with unfavorable histopathological factors. For instance, Intergroup study 0034 (25) clearly showed that, whereas adjuvant chemotherapy given sequentially to radiotherapy did not affect prognosis in terms of locoregional failures and survival rates in the whole group, the high-risk group benefited more from adjuvant chemotherapy than the low-risk group, for both tumor control and survival.

Another strong message from the Intergroup study related to the pattern of failure, which had been significantly modified by the addition of chemotherapy: a reduction of recurrences in the nodes and of distant metastases was indeed observed in the chemotherapy-containing arm. This reduction in distant metastases had been shown in a previous report (26) for the treatment arm using maintenance chemotherapy. These observations provided the first convincing evidence that high-dose regimes of chemotherapy had to be used in the postoperative setting if the targets were both an effect on local control and a significant impact on microscopic cell deposits at the systemic level. This trial was undoubtedly a milestone in the developmental work on the adjuvant treatment of head and neck cancers.

In parallel, a number of institutions were attempting to overcome the dismal prognosis of locally advanced carcinomas by investigating regimes combining chemo- and radiotherapy concomitantly. They were actually aiming to gain a significant benefit from the so-called supraadditive (or synergistic or radiosensitizing) effect (27,28) that is observed when the cytotoxic effect of the combination is greater than the sum of the effects of radiotherapy and chemotherapy considered separately.

In patients treated conservatively, early metaanalyses had shown that this coadministration was able to increase both locoregional control and survival rates significantly (3,29–32); this led various institutions and cooperative groups to activate prospective trials investigating the role of cytotoxic drugs as adjuvant treatment to primary line surgery as well.

2.3. Concomitant Chemo- and Radiotherapy

A series of potential interactions between chemo- and radiotherapy in coadministration indeed justified this approach (33), among them: (1) changes in the cell survival curve; (2) cooperation to prevent the emergence of resistant clones; (3) decrease in tumor mass and reoxygenation; (4) selective toxicity for hypoxic cells; (5) selective toxicity depending on cell cycle phase; (6) cytokinetic cooperation; (7) action on DNA repair; and (8) increased apoptosis (34).

In the 1990s, both neoadjuvant and sequential chemotherapy failed to increase local control for head and neck cancer patients treated conservatively (35–38). Many investigators assumed that the higher progression-free survival rates reported for patients treated conservatively with concomitant single-agent chemotherapy and radiotherapy (referred to here as CRT) could be extrapolated to the postoperative situation.

2.3.1. CHOICE OF DRUGS

As mentioned above, platinum-derivate compounds and 5-FU combined concurrently with radiotherapy have been most studied by prospective trials (18–24). The activity of both drugs against head and neck cancer is thought to stem from the following properties: (1) inhibition of repair of lethal and sublethal damage induced by radiotherapy; (2) capacity to radiosensitize hypoxic cells; (3) reduction of tumor burden, leading to an improved blood supply; (4) synchronization and redistribution of tumor cells into the more sensitive G2-M cell cycle phase; and (5) induction of apoptosis (34).

Platinum-derived analogs, specifically cis-diamminoplatinum [II] (cisplatin) and cis-diammine-1,1-cyclobutane dicarboxyplatinum [II] (carboplatin), are the agents most often delivered concomitantly to radiation in the treatment of locally advanced HNSXC. Among these analogs, cisplatin has been the most extensively investigated by far in the postoperative setting.

Interactions of these agents with ionizing radiation are not still fully understood and, a number of recent laboratory studies focus on their administration before or after cell irradiation. Among the potential mechanisms associated with cisplatin- and carboplatin-mediated radiation sensitization under both oxic and hypoxic conditions were the enhanced formation of toxic platinum intermediates in the presence of radiation-induced free radicals (27,39–43) and a radiation-induced increase in cellular platinum uptake.

2.3.2. THE TIME FACTOR

In patients with rapidly proliferating tumors such as HNSCC, therapeutic efficacy may be improved with shorter overall treatment time. These so-called *accelerated radiotherapy* regimes are more efficient in counterbalancing cell repopulation *(33,44–46)*.

There are good reasons to believe that accelerated repopulation of any remaining tumor cells may be a particular problem in postoperative radiotherapy for HNSCC *(46)*. This is partly based on retrospective studies of the importance of the interval between surgery and radiotherapy for tumor control probability although patient selection bias is a major concern in these studies. From a biological point of view, the release of growth factors and cytokines after surgery and the possible effect of tumor debulking on a putative homeostatic control also provide indirect support for the importance of overall time in the postoperative setting. However, the most convincing evidence comes from recent randomized phase III trials showing a marked benefit from acceleration of postoperative radiotherapy *(47,48)*. One possible benefit of CRT is the intensification of therapy, which effectively causes a treatment acceleration.

2.3.3. CHEMORADIOTHERAPY SCHEMES

Platinum-derived compounds thus represent reference agents to combine with radiotherapy in HNSCC since they are both potentially strong "radiosensitizers" and active chemotherapeutic compounds in their own right. In trials of first-line postoperative CRT, the dose/delivery schedules of platinum varied dramatically, ranging from every 3 wk (100 mg/m^2) to low-dose daily (6 mg/m^2) administration *(33)*.

One of the first prospective studies on the combination of postoperative radiotherapy with cisplatin, as single-agent therapy, was completed by Bachaud and colleagues, in 1996 *(49,50)*. They randomized 83 patients with stage III or IV head and neck carcinomas with histological evidence of extracapsular spread of tumor in lymph node metastases to receive either radiotherapy using a daily dose of 1.7 Gy for the first 54 Gy and 1.8–2 Gy until the completion of the treatment (up to a total dose of 65–70 Gy to the primary site). In the combined modality arm, cisplatin 50 mg iv with forced hydration was given every week (i.e., seven to nine cycles) concurrently with radiotherapy. Fourty-four patients were treated by radiation only and 39 by radiation with chemotherapy. The radiotherapy group displayed a higher locoregional failure rate than the second group (41 vs 23%; $p = 0.08$). Survival without locoregional failure was better in the CRT group ($p = 0.05$).

Meanwhile, in the late 1980s, two groups *(51,52)* investigated the feasibility and efficacy of regimens combining radiotherapy concomitantly with cisplatin or mitomycin C at various dose levels and intensities. Table 1 lists the results of randomized studies conducted in the late 1980s and 1990s comparing postoperative radiotherapy with CRT in an attempt to achieve radiosensitization and spatial cooperation *(38,49–52)*. The cytostatic agents most frequently administered were cisplatin and mitomycin C. In the two studies that accrued the largest number of patients, disease-free survival rates were increased in the CRT arm *(50,52)*.

In the early 1990s, the encouraging results of the study conducted by Al-Sarraf et al. *(53)*, giving cisplatin in single high doses (100 mg/m^2) repeated every 3 wk (d 1, 22, and 43), led the European Organization for Research and Treatment of Cancer (EORTC) and the Radiation Therapy Oncology Group (RTOG) cooperative groups to consider this regime as the reference CRT approach for adjuvant treatment of head and neck carcinomas and to activate two randomized trials measuring treatment outcome for this regime after curative surgery in patients with locally advanced tumors.

Table 1
First Generation Trials on Adjuvant Treatments Comparing Chemoradiotherapy to Radiotherapy
Alone After Primary Line Surgery

Author	No. of patients	Site	Type of CT	LRC p value	Survival
Weissberg et al., 1989 (51)	120	Oral cavity, naso-, oro-, and hypopharynx, larynx	Mitomycin C	< 0.01	NS
Bachaud et al., 1991 (49,50)	88	Oral cavity, oro- and hypopharynx, larynx	Cisplatin	< 0.01	NS
Weissler et al., 1992 (38)	26	Oral cavity, oro- and hypopharynx, larynx	Cisplatin, 5-FU	NS	NS
Haffty et al., 1993[a] (52)	120	Oral cavity, oro- and hypopharynx, larynx	Mitomycin C	< 0.01	NS

Abbreviations: CT, chemotherapy; 5-FU, 5-fluorouracil; LRC, locoregional control.
[a]Update of Weissberg's study.

3. THE POSTOPERATIVE MANAGEMENT AT THE TURN OF THE CENTURY

3.1. Can We Predict Treatment Outcome in Patients Primarily Treated With Curative Surgery?

The "more is better" principle does not always apply to the adjuvant treatment in head and neck oncology, especially in the postoperative setting. For instance, two randomized studies conducted in the 1990s failed to demonstrate any significant benefit for either higher doses of radiotherapy or the addition of chemotherapy to radiotherapy, as adjuvant treatments. Nevertheless, these studies demonstrated the clear need to stratify the patient population according to their level of risk before any treatment (54): they strongly supported the value of data from previous retrospective analyses on the critical importance of various disease patterns such as primary tumor site and extension, surgical margin status, perineural invasion, vascular embolisms, number and location of positive lymph nodes, and presence of extracapsular extension (ECE) of nodal disease.

L.J. Peters et al. (54) showed that risk assessment by clusters of surgical-pathologic features usefully indicated the need for postoperative radiotherapy. Two main messages emerged from their analysis: first, ECE was the only significant independent variable and combinations of two or more risk factors were associated with a progressively higher risk of recurrence. Second, patients with no adverse surgical-pathologic features were shown not to need postoperative radiotherapy, because the 5-yr actuarial locoregional control and survival rates achieved with surgery alone were 90 and 83%, respectively.

3.2. Is There a Dose–Effect Relationship in Postoperative Setting?

The dose–effect relationship for postoperative radiotherapy is not well established. For instance, the study by Peters et al. (54), showed no significant dose–response relationship for total doses ranging from 57.6 to 68.4 Gy in the whole irradiated population. It can be speculated that the beneficial effect on tumor control of doses more than 57.6 Gy was partly offset by tumor cell regeneration occurring during the additional time taken to deliver the higher doses (given at 1.8 Gy/d).

Moreover, in the study mentioned above, patients with one adverse feature other than ECE who received 57.6 Gy postoperatively had a 5-yr actuarial locoregional control rate of 94%: this moderate dose, which induces a lower incidence of acute and late morbidity than did 63 Gy in their patient cohort, appears to be sufficient to cure a significant number of patients with an intermediate risk of recurrence. Finally, even after higher radiation dose (63 Gy), the prognosis of high-risk patients (i.e., those with ECE or two or more other adverse features) remains rather dismal, with a 5-yr actuarial locoregional control rates of only 65–70%.

3.3. The Concept of "Treatment Package"

The overall duration of the "treatment package," i.e., the total treatment time from the time of the surgical procedure until completion of the radiotherapy, should be considered at the time of treatment planning. Ang et al. *(47)* randomized high-risk patients to a total dose of 63 Gy delivered in 5 wk ($n = 76$) or 7 wk ($n = 75$). In the 7-wk schedule, a prolonged interval between surgery and postoperative radiotherapy was associated with significantly lower local control ($p = 0.03$) and survival ($p = 0.01$). Overall treatment time had a major influence on the 5-yr locoregional control rate: for overall time less than 11 wk, locoregional control was achieved in 76% compared with 62% for 11–13 wk, and 38% for more than 13 wk ($p = 0.002$). Ang et al.'s study *(47)*, together with those by Awwad et al. *(48)*, Sanguineti et al. *(55)*, Trotti et al. *(56)*, Shah et al. *(57)*, and Rosenthal et al. *(58)* thus supports the concept that microscopic tumor cell aggregates escaping surgical excision repopulate quickly before treatment completion.

The treatment package should be delivered in a short overall time *(55–58)*, and Ang and colleagues *(47)* recommend completion of the combined treatment in less than 11 wk. One way to achieve this is by acceleration of the radiotherapy schedule. As an alternative, acceleration based on the concomitant delivery of cytotoxic drugs and ionizing radiation could reach equivalent or better results at both the local and systemic levels.

3.4. A Dilemma: Dose Intensities and Densities in Chemoradiotherapy

Whereas CRT based on low doses of cytostatic agents mainly aims for only a chemo- and/or radiosensitizing effect, the goal of high-dose CRT is to achieve better control of locoregional disease as well as a prevent metastasis and treat occult metastatic deposits efficiently.

Since distant metastases are the cause of failure in one of five patients with locally advanced, stage III–IV, head and neck cancers, the delivery of high-dose chemotherapy is preferable in the adjuvant setting, since the gain from a pure radiosensitizing effect of the combined cytotoxic agent(s) is limited by the competing risk of distant failure. Still, the delivery of high doses of chemotherapy, certainly in combination with high doses of radiation, and possibly in the framework of multidrug regimes, has to be carefully evaluated by the physician before treatment is started. Compliance with aggressive adjuvant therapy may be low in this category of patients, whose general condition is often influenced by the surgery as well as comorbid conditions. This is reflected in dose intensity reductions in some 25 to 33% of patients receiving postoperative CRT (33).

Regarding the type of chemotherapy used in the adjuvant setting, there are no strong data on the efficacy level of the various chemotherapy regimes: cisplatin-based schedules are generally accepted as the first choice, and there are no convincing data showing that multidrug regimes are superior to cisplatin or carboplatin alone. The addition of 5-FU is likely to account for an undue increase in acute mucosal reactions in this fragile category of patients and might be responsible for a dose-intensity reduction *(24)*.

3.5. Toxicity of Adjuvant Treatments

Acute reactions from adjuvant treatments are known to be markedly increased with CRT *(59)*. The need for intravenous rehydration, gastric feeding tubes during treatment, and narcotics for severe pain implies an intensive supportive care that not all in- and outpatient units are able to manage. Caution is therefore needed when introducing this type of therapeutic management in community hospitals.

Unfortunately, late side effects are often poorly reported in the literature *(60)* and although most reports show only a limited increase in severe late side effects after CRT *(61,62)*, it is likely that late toxicity is underreported. This situation may improve when prolonged follow-up becomes available. Also, current attempts to develop guidelines for the side effects of cancer therapy will hopefully improve the information content of published reports on novel therapies.

A more detailed appraisal of these acute and late toxicities is given in the next section.

4. ADJUVANT TREATMENT OF LOCALLY ADVANCED HEAD AND NECK CANCERS: NEW EVIDENCE, NEW CHALLENGES

4.1. Objectives of Recent Prospective CRT Studies in the Adjuvant Setting

Two randomized controlled trials *(63,64)*, conducted by the EORTC and the RTOG, have recently been reported. Both trials were designed to evaluate the role of CRT in the postoperative setting. The EORTC study *(63)* compared the addition of concomitant high doses of cisplatin plus radiotherapy vs radiotherapy alone in high-risk head and neck cancers of the oral cavity, oropharynx, larynx, or hypopharynx. The end points were disease-free survival (primary end point) and overall survival, local control rates, and treatment toxicity as secondary end points. The study was open from 1994 to 2000, and 334 patients were randomly assigned to either radiotherapy (66 Gy in 33 fractions more than 6.5 wk) or CRT, using the same radiotherapy schedule combined with three courses of cisplatin, 100 mg/m^2, on d 1, 22, and 43.

In the experimental arm, grade 3–4 functional mucosal reactions were significantly more frequent (44 vs 21%; $p = 0.0004$), but there was no difference in objective mucosal reactions between the two arms ($p = 0.2$). Grade 3–4 chemotherapy-related acute toxicity was mainly hematological, with 11% granulocytopenia and 2% thrombocytopenia.

Regarding treatment outcome, progression-free survival was the primary end point. At a median follow up of 60 mo, there was a significant ($p = 0.044$) difference in progression-free survival in favor of the CRT group: the estimated median progression-free survival was 23 mo (95% CI: 18-30) in the radiotherapy and 55 mo (95% CI: 33–75) in the CRT group; the 5-yr Kaplan-Meier estimates were 36 and 47%, respectively. In terms of overall survival, there was a significant ($p = 0.02$) difference in overall survival in favor of the CRT group: the 5-yr estimates were 40% for the control arm and 53% in the experimental one. Finally, regarding the local outcome, the 5-yr cumulative incidence estimates of locoregional relapses were 31% for the radiotherapy and 18% for the CRT group ($p = 0.007$). Time to progression was also significantly improved ($p = 0.14$) after CRT compared with radiotherapy alone (Fig. 1). Adding chemotherapy to postoperative irradiation did not significantly affect the incidence of metastases.

Finally, the cumulative incidences of late complications were not significantly different across the two groups. Although a higher incidence of grade 3+ muscular fibrosis was found after CRT (10 vs 5%), severe xerostomia was observed less often in this group (14% vs 22%).

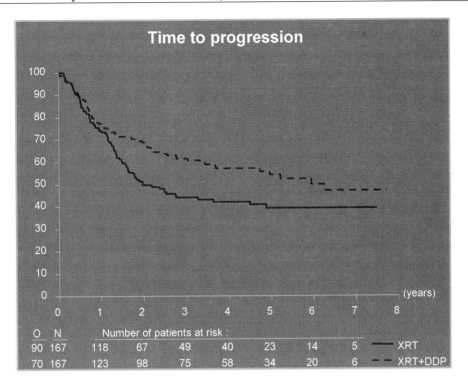

Fig. 1. Kaplan-Meier estimates for time to progression rates in EORTC trial 22931. Patients assigned to CRT (dashed curve) experienced longer times to progression compared with those randomized to radiotherapy (XRT; solid curve; $p = 0.014$, log-rank test). N, number of patients; o, number of observed events; DDP, carboplatin.

The RTOG 95-01 study *(64)* yielded a clear benefit in terms of disease-free survival, overall survival and local control, although the magnitude was less than that observed in the EORTC 22931 study (Figs. 2 and 3). A preliminary comparison of these two trials shows that notwithstanding an apparently similar design, inclusion criteria were different in the two studies; indeed, the RTOG based its selection of risk factors on the presence of tumor in two or more lymph nodes, and/or extracapsular spread of nodal disease, and/or microscopic-size tumor involvement of the surgical margins of resection as the factors most significantly associated with a high risk of locoregional relapse. In contrast, the EORTC selected the risk factors based on literature data, especially from the study conducted in the early 1990s by Peters et al. *(35)*: vascular embolisms, perineural disease, and oral cavity and oropharynx carcinomas with positive lymph nodes at level IV or V. This means that, in addition to the presence of stage III or IV disease, the common high-risk criteria in the EORTC and RTOG trials were extracapsular spread, and positive surgical margins.

There was also a marked difference in N-stage distribution between the two trials: in the RTOG trial, more than 93% of the cases presented with N2–3 stage compared with only 56% in the EORTC trial. Likewise, positive surgical margins were found in 29% of the cases treated in the EORTC study (arm 1: 32%; arm 2: 27%). In the RTOG trial the corresponding figures were lower, 19 and 17% in the control and experimental arms, respectively.

This comparison shows that patient selection and the distribution of clinical characteristics differed between the two studies, including tumor sites, neck disease stage, and risk factor

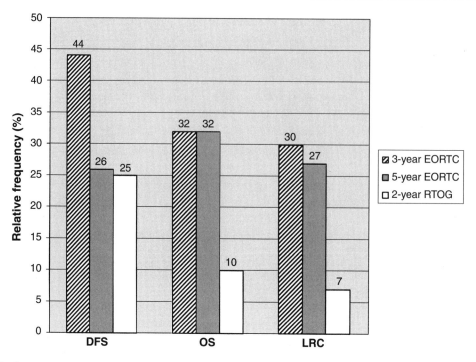

Fig. 2. Compared with radiotherapy alone, relative gain obtained by CRT in terms of disease-free survival (DFS), overall survival (OS), and locoregional control (LRC) rates in EORTC trial 22931 and RTOG trial 9501.

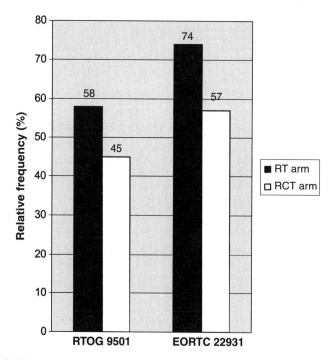

Fig. 3. Impact of CRT on cancer-related death rates in EORTC trial 22931 and RTOG trial 9501. Compared with those radomized to radiotherapy alone, patients assigned to CRT experienced an absolute reduction in cancer-related death rates of 17% at 5 yr in the EORTC trial and a 13% reduction at 2 yr in the RTOG trial.

selection. Also, the proportion of patients with positive surgical margins was higher in the EORTC trial. These differences are likely to influence the absolute gain from postoperative CRT.

5. CURRENT POLICY

In patients with locally advanced HNSCC, postoperative radiotherapy produced largely unsatisfactory survival rates until the late 1990s. As a result, various strategies have been proposed to improve treatment outcome in patients with resectable tumors at high risk of recurrence or metastasis. Most recent reports on postoperative CRT have suggested a change in the pattern of failure, with a relative increase in distant metastases as a cause of death in up to 25% of cases with locally advanced disease. This is likely to result from the application of more intensive locoregional treatments.

The recent EORTC and RTOG CRT trials with high-dose cisplatin (100 mg/m^2 on d 1, 23, and 45 of radiotherapy) and radiation doses of at least 60–66 Gy have shown that this combination is more effective than radiotherapy alone in HNSCC patients with unfavorable clinical and/or pathological factors treated with primary surgery. The addition of chemotherapy resulted in a significant increase in local control and disease-specific and overall survival rates. Even if longer follow-up is needed to assess accurately the late morbidity after CRT, this therapeutic approach can be considered the standard adjuvant treatment for this population of patients.

The outcomes observed in these two trials must obviously be interpreted in the light of various tumor and treatment factors that may potentially modulate the magnitude of the CRT effect, as demonstrated by the RTOG 95-01 trial results.

6. FUTURE OPTIONS FOR ADJUVANT TREATMENT

Despite the improvement seen with CRT, locoregional control levels reached so far remain unsatisfactory, even after high-intensity multimodality treatments. A first complementary approach is the addition of more active drugs that may further improve the efficiency of the combination, such as hypoxic cell killing agents (tirapazamine) or topoisomerase 1 inhibitors (33).

Overexpression of the epidermal growth factor receptor (EGFR) has been correlated with more aggressive behavior and poor clinical outcome (45). Blockade of EGFR—an interesting therapeutic target—by the monoclonal antibody C225 (cetuximab) was shown to increase the cell radiosensitivity in vitro (33), and this approach could also be tested in the postoperative setting.

With respect to radiotherapy side effects, there has been some interest in compounds that could possible reduce treatment toxicity: agents such as amifostine (65) and pilocarpine (66) are currently under investigation, but it is too early to draw definitive conclusions on the value of these agents in sparing the salivary gland function.

As mentioned above, distant metastases have now become the most common cause of treatment failure and death and now emerge as a real impediment to cure in patients with locally advanced tumors. As a consequence, more effective drugs such as taxanes, which demonstrate a high level of activity in head and neck carcinoma patients, should be investigated more extensively in the adjuvant setting.

After surgery, one of the main concerns is the delay in starting radiotherapy (7). Although it seems logical to begin radiation therapy as soon as possible to avoid any tumor cell repopulation, delayed wound healing can postpone the start of adjuvant treatment beyond 6–7 wk in a number of cases. It seems logical to try to address the potential problem of accelerated tumor cell repopulation after surgery. Very few studies, however, have taken this parameter into consideration (7). Delivery of perioperative chemotherapy begun no later than 10 d after surgery and protracted, on a weekly basis, until onset of CRT should be investigated prospectively.

Finally, further investigations on treatments combining altered fractionation with either cytotoxic drugs or noncytotoxic compounds could give us useful indications on what can be expected from an increase in cell killing and/or attempts to counterbalance tumor cell proliferation.

It might be that, with the increasing locoregional efficacy of combined treatments, the relative importance of local failures as causes of cancer-related death is reduced and that metastases become the main concern of oncologists when they try to optimize the adjuvant treatment of high-risk, resectable head and neck cancer.

REFERENCES

1. Parkin DM, Muir CS, Whelan SL, Gao YT, Ferlay J, Powell J. Cancer Incidence in Five Vontinents, vol. 6. Lyon: IARC, 1992.
2. Al-Sarraf M, Hussein M. Head and neck cancer:present status and future prospects of adjuvant chemotherapy. Cancer Invest 1995; 13:41–53.
3. Pignon JP, Bourhis J, Domenge C, Designe L. Chemotherapy added to locoregional treatment for head and neck squamous-cell carcinoma:three meta-analyses of updated individual data. MACH-NC Collaborative Group. Meta-Analysis of Chemotherapy on Head and Neck Cancer. Lancet 2000; 355(9208):949–955.
4. Fletcher GH, Evers W. Radiotherapeutic management of surgical recurrences and post-operative residuals in tumors of the head and neck. Radiology 1970; 95:185–188.
5. Kramer S, Gelber RD, Snow JB, et al. Combined radiation therapy and surgery in the management of head and cancer: final report of study 73-03 of the radiation therapy oncology group. Head Neck Surg 1987; 10:19–30.
6. Snow GB, Annyas AA, van Slotten EA, Bartelink H, Hart AA. Prognostic factors of neck node metastases. Clin Otolaryngol 1982; 185–192.
7. Vikram B, Strong EW, Shah JP, Spiro R. Failure at the primary site following multimodality treatment in advanced head and neck cancer. Head Neck Surg 1984; 6:720–723.
8. Johnson JT, Barnes EL, Myers EN, Schramm VL, Borochovitz D, Sigler BA. The extracapsular spread of tumors in cervical node metastasis. Arch Otolaryngol 1981; 107:725–729.
9. Barkley HT, Fletcher GH, Jesse RH, Lindberg RD. Management of cervical lymph node metastases in squamous cell carcinomas of the tonsillar fossa, base of tongue, supraglottic larynx and hypopharynx. Am J Surg 1972; 124:462–467.
10. Bitter K. Post-operative chemotherapy versus post-operative cobalt-60 radiation therapy in patients with advanced oral carcinoma. Head Neck Surg 1981; 3:260 (abstract).
11. Shah JT, Cendon AA, Farr HW, Strong EW. Carcinoma of the oral cavity: factors affecting treatment failure at the primary site and neck. Am J Surg 1976; 132:1401–1410.
12. Bartelink H, Breur K, Hart G. Radiotherapy of lymph node metastases in squamous cell carcinomas of the tonsillar fossa, base of tongue, supraglottic larynx and hypopharynx. Int J Radiat Oncol Biol Phys 1982; 8:983–990.
13. Bataini JP, Asselain B, Jaulerry C, et al. A multivariate primary tumor control analysis in 465 patients treated by radical radiotherapy for carcinoma of the tonsillar region: clinical and treatment parameters as prognostic factors. Radiother Oncol 1989; 14:265–277.
14. Bernier J, Bataini JP. Regional outcome in oropharyngeal and pharyngolaryngeal cancers treated with high dose per fraction radiotherapy. Analysis of neck disease response in 1646 cases. Radiother Oncol 1986; 6:87–103.
15. Griffin TW, Pajak TF, Gillespie BW, et al. Predicting the response of head and neck cancers to radiation therapy with a multivariate modelling system: an analysis of the RTOG head and neck cancer registry. Int J Radiat Oncol Biol Phys 1984; 10:481–487.
16. Marcus RB, Million RR, Cassisi NJ. Post-operative irradiation for squamous cell carcinoma of head and neck: analysis of time-dose factors related to control above the clavicles. Int J Radiat Oncol Biol Phys 1979; 5:1943–1949.
17. Tupchong L, Scott CB, Blitzer PH, et al. Randomized study of preoperative versus post-operative radiation therapy in advanced head and neck carcinoma:long-term follow-up of RTOG study 73-03. Int J Radiat Oncol Biol Phys 1991; 20:21–28.
18. Fu KK, Phillips TL, Silverberg IY, et al. Combined radiotherapy and chemotherapy with bleomycin and methotrexate for advanced inoperable head and neck cancers. Update of a Northern California oncology group randomized trial. J Clin Oncol 1987; 5:1410–1418.

19. Tannock IF. Combined modality treatment with radiotherapy and chemotherapy. Radiother Oncol 1989; 16:83–101.
20. Huanq AT, Cole TB, Fishburn R, et al. Adjuvant chemotherapy after surgery and radiation far stage III and IV H&N cancer. Ann Surg 1984; 100:195–199.
21. Jacobs JR, Pajak TF, Al Sarraf M, et al. Chemotherapy following surgery in head and neck cancer. Am J Clin Oncol, 1989; 12:185–189.
22. Johnson JT, Myers EN, Schramm VL, et al. Adjuvant chemotherapy for high risk squamous cell carcinomas of the head and neck. J Clin Oncol 1987; 5:456–458.
23. Rossi A, Molinari R, Boracchi P, et al. Adjuvant chemotherapy with vincristine, cyclophosphamide, and doxorubicin after radiotherapy in loco-regional nasopharyngeal cancer:results of a four-year multicenter randomized study. J Clin Oncol 1988; 6:1401–1410.
24. Szpirglas H, Chastang CL, Bertrand JC. Adjuvant treatment of tongue and floor of mouth cancer. Cancer Res 1978; 68:309–317.
25. Laramore GE, Scott CB, Al Sarraf M, et al. Adjuvant chemotherapy for resectable squamous cell carcinomas of the head and neck: report on intergroup study 0034. Int J Radiat Oncol Biol Phys 1991; 21(Suppl 1):190.
26. Jacobs C, Makuch R. Efficacy of adjuvant chemotherapy for patients with resectable H&N cancer. A subset analysis of head and neck contract programs. J Clin Oncol 1990; 8:838–843.
27. Dewitt L. Combined treatment of radiation and cis-diamminedichloroplatinum (II): a review of experimental and clinical data. Int J Radiat Oncol Biol Phys 1987; 13:403–426.
28. Vokes EE, Awan AM, Weichselbaum RR. Radiotherapy with concomitant chemotherapy for head and neck cancer. Oncol Clin North AM 1991; 5:5753–767.
29. Stell PM, Rawson NS. Adjuvant chemotherapy in head and neck cancer. Br J Cancer 1990; 61:779–787.
30. Munro AJ. An overview of randomised controlled trials of adjuvant chemotherapy in head and neck cancer. Br J Cancer 1995; 71:83–91.
31. El Sayed S, Nelson N. Adjuvant and adjunctive chemotherapy in the management of squamous cell carcinoma of the head and neck region. A meta-analysis of prospective and randomized trials. J Clin Oncol 1996; 14:838–847.
32. Browman GP, Hodson DI, Mackenzie RJ, Bestic N, Zuraw L. Choosing a concomitant chemotherapy and radiotherapy regimen for squamous cell head and neck cancer: a systematic review of the published literature with subgroup analysis. Head Neck 2001; 23:579–589.
33. Bernier J, Bentzen SM. Head and Neck Cancer Management: Which Post-operative Treatment Best Serves Your Patient? ASCO 2003: 306–312.
34. Blank K, Rudoltz M, Kao G, Muschel R, McKenna G. The molecular regulation of apoptosis and implications for radiation therapy. Int J Radiat Biol 1997; 71:455–466.
35. Bourhis J, Mornex F. The biological basis for chemoradiation. In: Mornex F, Mazeron JJ, Droz JP, Marty M, eds. Concomitant Chemoradiation: Current Status and Future. Paris: Editions Scientifiques et Médicales Elsevier SAS, 1999:16–25.
36. Haselow RE, Marshaw MG, Okin MM, et al. Radiation alone versus radiation plus weekly low-dose cis-platinum in unresectable cancer of the head and neck. In: Fee WE, Goepfert H, Johns ME, Strong EW, Ward PH, eds. Head and Neck Cancer. 1st ed. Toronto: Marcel Dekker, 1990:279–281.
37. Wendt TG. The radiochemotherapy of advanced head and neck tumors. What is certain? Strahlenther Onkol 1996; 172:409–416.
38. Weissler M, Melin S, Sailer S, et al. Simultaneous Chemo-radiation in the treatment of advanced head and neck cancer. Arch Otolaryngol Head Neck Surg 1992; 118:806–810.
39. Brizel DM, Albers ME, Fisher SR, et al. Hyperfractionated irradiation with or without concurrent chemotherapy for locally advanced head and neck cancer. N Engl J Med 1998; 338:1798–1804.
40. Begg AC. Cisplatin and radiation: interaction probabilities and therapeutic possibilities. Int J Radiat Oncol Biol Phys 1990; 19:1183–1189.
41. Creagan ET, Fountain KS, Frytak S, DeSanto LW, Earle JD. Concomitant radiation therapy and cis-diamminedichloroplatinum (II) in patients with advanced head and neck cancer. Med Pediatr Oncol 1981; 9:119,120.
42. Denham JW, Abbott RL. Concurrent cisplatin, infusional 5-fluorouracil, and conventionally fractionated radiation therapy in head and neck cancer: dose limiting mucosal toxicity. J Clin Oncol 1991; 9:458–463.
43. Leipzig B. Cisplatin sensitization to radiotherapy of squamous cell carcinomas of the head and neck. Am J Surg 1983; 146:462–465.
44. Marcial VA, Pajak TF, Mohiuddin M, et al. Concomitant cisplatin chemotherapy and radiotherapy in advanced mucosal squamous cell carcinoma of the head and neck: long-term results of the RTOG study 81-17. Cancer 1990; 66:1861–1868.

45. Horiot JC, Bontemps P, Van den Bogaert W, et al. Accelerated fractionation (AF) compared with conventional fractionation (CF) improves loco-regional control in the radiotherapy of advanced head and neck cancers: results of the EORTC 22851 randomized trial. Radiother Oncol 1997; 44:111–121.

46. Bentzen SM. Repopulation in radiation oncology: perspectives of clinical research. Int J Radiat Biol 2003; 79:581–585.

47. Ang KK, Trotti A. Brown BW, et al. Randomized trial addressing risk features and time factors of surgery plus radiotherapy in advanced head-and-neck cancer. Int J Radiat Oncol Biol Phys 2001; 51:571–578.

48. Awwad HK, Lotayef M, Shouman T, et al. Accelerated hyperfractionation (AHF) compared to conventional fractionation (CF) in the post-operative radiotherapy of locally advanced head and neck cancer:influence of proliferation. Br J Cancer 2002; 86:517–523.

49. Bachaud JM, David JM, Boussin G, Daly N. Combined post-operative radiotherapy and weekly cisplatin infusion for locally advanced squamous cell carcinoma of the head and neck:preliminary report of a randomized trial. Int J Radiat Oncol Biol Phys 1991; 20:243–246.

50. Bachaud JM, Cohen-Jonathan E, Alzieu C, et al. Combined postoperative radiotherapy and weekly cisplatin infusion for locally advanced head and neck carcinoma: final report of a randomized trial. Int J Radiat Oncol Biol Phys 1996; 36:999–1004.

51. Weissberg J, Son Y, Papac R. Randomized clinical trial of mitomycin C as an adjunct to radiotherapy in head and neck cancer. Int J Radiat Oncol Biol Phys 1989; 17:3–9.

52. Haffty B, Son Y, Sasaki C, Fisher R. Mitomycin C as an adjunct to post-operative radiation therapy in squamous cell carcinoma of the head and neck: results from two randomized clinical trials. Int J Radiat Oncol Biol Phys 1993; 27:241–250.

53. Al-Sarraf M, Pajak TF, Byhardt RW, et al. Post-operative radiotherapy with concurrent cisplatin appears to improve locoregional control of advanced, resectable head and neck cancers: RTOG 88-24. Int J Radiat Oncol Biol Phys 1997; 37:777–782.

54 . Peters LJ, Goepfert H, Ang KK, et al. Evaluation of the dose for post-operative radiation therapy of head and neck cancer: first report of a prospective randomized trial. Int J Radiat Oncol Biol Phys 1993; 26:3–11.

55. Sanguineti G, Corvo' R, Vitale V, et al. Post-operative radiotherapy for head and neck squamous cell carcinomas: feasibility of a biphasic accelerated treatment schedule. Int J Radiat Oncol Biol Phys 1996; 36:1147–1153.

56. Trotti A, Klotch D, Endicott J, et al . Post-operative accelerated radiotherapy in high-risk squamous cell carcinoma of the head and neck: long-term results of a prospective trial. Head Neck 1998; 20:119–123.

57. Shah N, Saunders MI, Dische S. A pilot study of post-operative CHART and CHARTWEL in head and neck cancer. Clin Oncol 2000; 12:392–396.

58. Rosenthal DI, Liu L, Lee JH, et al. Importance of the treatment package time in surgery and post-operative radiation therapy for squamous carcinoma of the head and neck. Head Neck 2002; 24:115–126.

59. Bieri S, Bentzen SM, Huguenin P, et al. Early morbidity after radiotherapy with or without chemotherapy in advanced head and neck cancer: experience from four nonrandomized studies. Strahl Onkol 2003; 179:390–395.

60. Trotti A, Bentzen SM. The need for adverse effects reporting standards in oncology clinical trials. (Editorial) J Clin Oncol 2004; 22:19–22.

61. Peters LJ, Withers HR. Applying radiobiological principles to combined modality treatment of head and neck cancer. The time factor. Int J Radiat Oncol Biol Phys 1997; 39:831–836.

62. Laramore GE, Scoot CB, Al-Sarraf M, et al. Adjuvant chemotherapy for respectable squamous cell carcinoma of the head and neck: report on intergroup study 0034. Int J Radiat Oncol Biol Phys 1992; 23:705–713.

63. Bernier J, Domenge C, Eschwege F et al. Chemo-radiotherapy, as compared to radiotherapy alone, significantly increases disease-free and overall survival in head and neck cancer patients after surgery:results of EORTC phase III trial 22931. (Abstract). Int J Rad Oncol Biol Phys 2001; 51(Suppl 1):1.

64. Cooper JS, Pajak TF, Forastiere AA, et al. Postoperative concurrent radiochemotherapy in high-risk SCCA of the head and neck:initial report of RTOG 9501/intergroup phase III trial. (Abstract). Journal of Clinical Oncology 2002; 21:226a.

65. Chao KS, Ozygit G, Thorsdad WL. Toxicity profile of intensity-modulated radiation therapy for head and neck carcinoma and potential role of amifostine. Sem Oncol 2003; 30:101–108.

66. Bardet E, Martin L, Calais G, et al. Preliminary data of the GORTEC 2000-02 phase III trial comparing intravenous and subcutaneous administration of amifostine for head and neck tumors treated by external radiotherapy. Semin Oncol 2002; 29:57–60.

15

Multimodality Management of Nasopharyngeal Carcinoma

Eng-Huat Tan, MRCP, *Swan-Swan Leong,* MRCP, *Terence Tan,* FRCR, *Kam-Weng Fong,* FRCR, *and Joseph Wee,* FRCR

1. INTRODUCTION

Nasopharyngeal carcinoma (NPC) of the endemic type (World Health Organization [WHO] type II and III) is considered separately from head and neck squamous cell cancer (HNSCC) because of certain distinctive features that confer a different biological behavior in terms of treatment responses and disease outcome. The most important feature that probably accounts for this difference is its strong association with the Epstein-Barr virus (EBV) *(1–3)*. This virus is probably the key etiological agent in the pathogenesis of this cancer, with genetic predisposition and other environmental factors as important cofactors *(4–13)*. This is in line with the peculiar geographic distribution and racial predilection of this disease.

Owing to the location of the primary site, it is not surprising that the vast majority of such patients would be diagnosed with advanced-stage disease at presentation. An estimated 50 to 65% of these patients would present with locally advanced disease, and about 5 to 8% would have disseminated disease at the outset *(14,15)*. The more aggressive systemic nature of NPC compared with HNSCC is another distinctive feature that has been well described *(16,17)*. Cvitkovic et al. *(16)*, in their series of 255 consecutive patients with newly diagnosed advanced NPC who underwent uniform staging procedures inclusive of a unilateral posterior iliac crest bone marrow aspiration and biopsy, found that 44% of these patients had disseminated disease. Bone wass the most common site for metastatic involvement, accounting for 65% of all patients with disseminated disease, which is similar to our series (74%) *(16,17)*. Bone marrow involvement was found in about 25% of these patients *(16)*. More than 50% of the patients with disseminated disease had more than one site of metastasis *(17)*.

The high rate of responsiveness to chemotherapy and/or radiotherapy is the third distinctive feature of NPC. This has been shown reproducibly in various phase II studies of metastatic/recurrent disease in which response rates of 50 to 80% to platinum-based regimens were demonstrated with complete responses of up to about 20% *(18–21)*. However, despite the initial high response rates, the duration of response is generally short, not exceeding 8 mo in most studies. The use of three or more first-generation cytotoxics in combination has resulted in unacceptably significant toxicities, including treatment-related deaths, but also a median survival that exceeded 12 mo *(18,19,22–24)*. A feature of note is the sustained

From: *Current Clinical Oncology: Squamous Cell Head and Neck Cancer*
Edited by: D. J. Adelstein © Humana Press Inc., Totowa, NJ

Table 1
Activity of New Cytotoxic Agents

Agent	Ref.	Response rate (%)
Paclitaxel	26	21.7
Gemcitabine	27	28
Capecitabine	28	23.5
Irinotecan	29	17

chemoresponsiveness of NPC in the second-line and even third-line setting (25). Since the early 1990s, a series of studies have added new active agents to the armamentarium (26–29). Paclitaxel, capecitabine, gemcitabine, and irinotecan are the agents found to be active in the first- and/or second-line setting in patients with disseminated disease (Table 1). Combination of these second-generation agents with a platinum resulted in comparable response rates and duration of response, compared with the first-generation combination regimens, at acceptable toxicities (30–33). Preliminary results of a phase II study using a triplet combination of paclitaxel, gemcitabine, and carboplatin showed an overall response rate of 78%, with one complete responder (34). Although the time to progression of 8 mo is not improved compared to historical data, the median survival of 18.5 mo with this triplet combination is rather encouraging. A phase III randomized study to assess these novel combinations is clearly required. Bringing these new agents forward in the primary treatment of patients with locoregionally confined disease is also warranted. The use of cetuximab (C225), an epidermal growth factor receptor (EGFR)-targeted form of treatment, has also been studied, but its role in NPC is still ill defined (35).

2. RADIOTHERAPY IN NPC

The primary treatment for locoregionally confined NPC is radiotherapy, mainly because of its high radiosensitivity and the technical difficulty with surgery. Radiosensitivity of NPC is dependent on histological type. The WHO type I or keratinizing squamous cell type is less sensitive and holds a poorer prognosis (36,37). Endemic NPC in East Asia and the Mediterranean is primarily type II or III (or the undifferentiated type) and carries a better prognosis, with a 5-yr survival rate of about 60% (38–40).

The radiotherapy technique adopted in Singapore and Hong Kong is generally quite similar and more aggressive than what radiation oncologists from nonendemic areas would prescribe (41,42). In Singapore, patients are treated with external beam radiotherapy using 6-MV linear accelerators. The primary tumor is treated with two lateral opposed facial fields to 20 Gy, followed by a three-field technique (anterior facial and lateral opposed facial fields) to a total dose of 66 Gy for T1 and T2 lesions and 70 Gy for T3 and T4 lesions. The neck is treated to a dose of 60 Gy, and lymph nodes are boosted with electrons for another 10 Gy. Treatment is at a rate of 2 Gy per fraction 5 d a week, and all fields are treated daily. Patients with high cervical lymph nodes or inferior extension of their tumor toward the oropharynx are treated with a shrinking field technique, using long faciocervical fields for the first 40 Gy, followed by a three-field plan for the rest of the tratment. Patients with bulky parapharyngeal disease are boosted with a "parapharyngeal boost technique," as described by Tsao (15,43). The addition of intracavitary brachytherapy for early primary tumors (T1–2) is also commonly prescribed in a bid to improve control (44,45).

The results of radiotherapy in early-stage disease are good, with 5-yr survival rate of greater than 80 and 70% for stages I and II, respectively *(14,15)*. As expected, this 5-yr survival rate drops markedly to less than 30% for those with locally advanced stage IV disease. This is largely because of the higher risk of distant relapse in those with locally advanced disease—30 to 60% at 5 yr, with most relapses occurring within the first 2 yr of diagnosis *(46)*. Locoregional relapse is also common, with a local relapse rate of about 50% in those with more advanced primary tumors.

Several strategies were explored in a bid to improve locoregional control, especially in those with locally advanced disease. The addition of parapharyngeal boost or stereotactic radiosurgery in selected groups as consolidation after external beam radiotherapy was reported to result in improved locoregional control *(47,48)*. The use of radiobiological principles to improve tumor control has also been studied. Wang *(49)*, from the Massachusetts General Hospital in Boston, first reported improved local control using an accelerated fractionation scheme. However, when a group from Hong Kong attempted to repeat this regimen, the study was stopped prematurely because of increased neurological toxicity (probably from the larger radiation portals commonly used in East Asia) *(50)*. However another attempt at accelerating the radiotherapy by treating patients 6 d a week resulted in a promising rate of local control with acceptable toxicity and is currently the subject of a phase III randomized study involving centers in Hong Kong, China, Singapore, Canada, and the United Kingdom *(51)*. The use of intensity-modulated radiotherapy (IMRT) and inverse treatment planning has also reported excellent tumor control with the added advantage of sparing normal tissues like the parotid glands. Series using chemo-IMRT from the University of California (San Francisco), Washington University, and Memorial Sloan Kettering Cancer Center reported excellent local control rates for locally advanced tumors *(52–54)*.

3. CHEMOTHERAPY IN COMBINED MODALITY MANAGEMENT

Because of the systemic nature of NPC, especially in those with locoregionally advanced disease, it is unlikely that radiotherapy as a single modality will be able to address the therapeutic hurdles sufficiently *(16)*. In view of the high chemoresponsiveness of NPC, the addition of cytotoxics to radiation has been a subject of intense study in this subset of patients over the past few decades. Despite the initial hurdles and controversies, significant strides have been made in this area. The various ways of sequencing chemotherapy with radiation have been investigated in phase III randomized studies, and the picture that has emerged is that definitive treatment with radiation of the locoregional disease should be instituted earlier rather than later (with exceptions, as will be explained later) and that sensitization of this important modality with chemotherapy is probably crucial.

4. NEOADJUVANT CHEMOTHERAPY

There are sound reasons for considering neoadjuvant chemotherapy in patients who present with locally advanced disease. Neoadjuvant chemotherapy aims to (1) eradicate distant micrometastases that are likely to be present in this subset of patients, (2) reduce primary and regional tumor bulk and hence improve oxygenation with resultant higher sensitivity and response to definitive radiation, and (3) reduce the extent of radiation, especially at critical structures at the brainstem and hence reduce the morbidity of the radiation. The high response rates observed with platinum-based chemotherapy in the metastatic/recurrent setting and the even higher responses seen in the locoregionally advanced setting gave strong support for such an approach.

Table 2
Randomized Studies of Neoadjuvant Chemotherapy

Study	Yr	Treatment	No. of patients	Response to NACT (%)	OS rate (%)		
					2-yr	3-yr	5-yr
Chan et al.	1995	2 PF > RT > 4 PF	37	81	80	NR	NR
(61)		RT alone	40	—	80.5 (p = NS)	NR	NR
Hareyama	2001	2 PF > RT	40	NR	NR	NR	60
et al. (62)		RT alone	40	—	NR	NR	48 (p = NS)
Cvitkovic,	1996	3 BEP > RT	171	91	NR	NR	NR
(63)[a]		RT alone	168	—	NR	NR	NR
Chua et al.	1998	2/3 PE > RT	134	84	NR	78	NR
(64)		RT alone	152	—	NR	71 (p = 0.57)	NR
Ma et al.	2001	2/3 PBF > RT	224	82.6	NR	NR	63
(65)		RT alone	225	—	NR	NR	56 (p = 0.11)

Abbreviations: >, Followed by; NACT, neoadjuvant chemotherapy; OS, overall survival; PF, cisplatin, 5-fluorouracil; BEP, bleomycin, epirubicin, cisplatin; PE, cisplatin, epirubicin; PBF, cisplatin, bleomycin, 5-fluorouracil; RT, radiotherapy; NR, not reported; NS, not significant.

[a]Overall survival not statistically significant, but the number of events to determine its final significance had not yet been reached at the time of report.

Single-arm phase II studies have reproducibly shown very high responses to neoadjuvant platinum-based combination regimens of 75–98%, with some reporting promising survival outcome (55–60). However, these initial impressions were not borne out by the results of prospective randomized studies (Table 2). Two small studies done in Hong Kong and Japan, respectively, used two cycles of an induction regimen comprising cisplatin and 5-fluorouracil (5-FU) before radical radiotherapy in the experimental arm. A further four cycles of the same chemotherapy was given as consolidation after radiotherapy in the Hong Kong study. No significant difference in outcome was observed in both studies. However, a major flaw with both studies is the small sample size, which may lack the statistical power to show a difference (61,62).

Three large randomized studies have been reported to date that probably helped to answer this question more definitively (63–65). The first large international study, led by the French, randomized 339 patients to three cycles of induction chemotherapy (cisplatin, bleomycin, and epirubicin) before radiotherapy or to radiotherapy alone (63). An excess of treatment-related deaths was noted in the chemotherapy arm (8 vs 1%), implying the importance of experience and caution with the use of this chemotherapy combination. Although there was a significant difference in disease-free survival (favoring the chemotherapy arm), no difference in overall survival was observed at a median follow-up of 49 mo (range 23–70 mo). There has been no follow-up on this report to date.

The second large international study, led by investigators from Hong Kong, randomized 334 patients to two to three cycles of induction chemotherapy comprising cisplatin and epirubicin followed by radiotherapy or to radiotherapy alone (64). At a median follow-up of 41 mo (range 5–77 mo) at the time of the report, the median overall survival time had not yet been reached. However, the investigators observed a trend toward an improved relapse-free survival at 3 yr favoring the chemotherapy arm (58 vs 46%, p = 0.053). A longer follow-up period would be required to determine any impact on overall survival, if any.

The largest trial to date was a single-institution study conducted at the Sun Yat-Sen University of Medical Sciences, Guangzhou, People's Republic of China, where the world's highest incidence of NPC is found *(65)*. A total of 456 patients, accrued over a 1-yr period, were randomized to receive either induction chemotherapy (cisplatin, bleomycin, and 5-FU) before radiotherapy or radiotherapy alone. The median follow-up period for patients alive was 66 mo (range 35–75 mo). There was good compliance with the treatment, with about 98% of patients in each arm completing the planned radiation, and all the patients in the chemotherapy arm had at least two cycles of the induction chemotherapy. There was a trend towards improved overall survival (63 vs 58%; $p = 0.11$) and relapse-free survival (59 vs 49%; $p = 0.05$) at 5 yr in the chemotherapy arm.

The main impression of the studies reported to date is that the use of induction chemotherapy followed by radiotherapy is probably not an optimal way to sequence these treatment modalities. Although there appears to be a trend toward a positive biological effect with two to three cycles of induction chemotherapy that is platinum based, this effect is probably at best mild to modest. It is possible that there is an overestimation of this effect, resulting in sample sizes in these studies that lack the statistical power to show its true effect.

We have not excluded the usefulness of using chemotherapy as induction before definitive treatment in the locally advanced setting despite the negative results of the studies just described. As mentioned, this sequencing may allow the avoidance of undue toxicity to nervous tissue from high-dose radiation in patients with intracranial extension. It is possible that the use of induction chemotherapy to effect downsizing of the tumor followed by concurrent chemoradiotherapy (CRT) as definitive treatment may achieve the dual results of improved outcome with minimal long-term injury to critical nervous tissues. This method of scheduling has not been well studied, and hence it is uncertain whether radiotherapy, which is the more important treatment modality, would be compromised with this approach. A well-designed randomized study should be able to answer this important question.

5. ADJUVANT CHEMOTHERAPY

The main aim of adjuvant chemotherapy is to eradicate distant micrometastatic disease in patients who are at risk. Two studies looking specifically at this issue have been reported, which unfortunately did not help in the clarification of this important matter *(66,67)*.

Rossi et al. *(66)* randomized 229 patients to receive radiotherapy alone or radiotherapy followed by adjuvant chemotherapy comprising vincristine, cyclophosphamide, and doxorubicin. This study failed to show any survival benefit with the addition of adjuvant chemotherapy. However, the main criticism of this study is the use of a nonplatinum chemotherapy combination.

The investigators from Taiwan studied the effect of adjuvant cisplatin, 5-FU, and leucovorin given on a weekly schedule *(67)*. Although they planned to randomize 240 patients in this study, they decided on the early termination after 157 patients were randomized over a 4-yr period owing to the slow accrual rate and the low compliance with chemotherapy in the experimental arm. At a median follow-up of 49.5 mo, there was no difference in overall survival or relapse-free survival at 5 yr between the combined and standard arm (54.5 vs 60.5% and 54.4 vs 49.5%, respectively). The poor progress and the small sample size of this study make it difficult to arrive at any meaningful conclusion regarding the role of adjuvant treatment.

6. CONCURRENT CHEMORADIOTHERAPY

The use of concurrent cisplatin with radiotherapy has been well established in HNSCC as an effective way to preserve organs and as a superior treatment method compared with radiotherapy alone *(68–70)*. However, significant toxicity is associated with this form of sequencing, and proper patient selection is of paramount importance to reduce the potential fatal complication rate with the use of concurrent CRT.

Because of the wide radiation portal and the more aggressive radiation technique alluded to above in Subheading 2. that is used in the treatment of NPC, the use of cisplatin as a single agent or in combination with 5-FU concurrently can result in significant toxicities. The use of cisplatin and 5-FU at 20 mg/m^2/d and 1 g/m^2/d, respectively, on d 1–4 administered during the first and fifth weeks of radiotherapy was deemed too toxic from our pilot study, with a 14% toxic death rate *(71)*.

Al-Sarraf et al. *(72)* reported acceptable toxicities with no compromise of radiation delivered in a series of 27 patients treated at Wayne State University; cisplatin was administered at 100 mg/m^2 every 3 wk for three cycles during radiation. The survival outcome appeared to be improved compared with historical data *(72)*. A phase III Intergroup study (0099) followed (reported in 1998) in which standard radiotherapy was compared with the same radiotherapy and concurrent cisplatin as above, followed by three further cycles of cisplatin and 5-FU postradiation *(73)*. The study closed early when the first interim analysis of 147 randomized patients showed a significant survival benefit in favor of CRT. At a minimum follow-up of 5 yr, the overall survival rate was 67 vs 37% in favor of the CRT arm (74). Sixty-three and 55% of the patients were able to receive the three cycles of the cisplatin during the concurrent phase and three cycles of the adjuvant cisplatin/5-FU, respectively. However, what is unclear from this study is the relative benefit of concurrent and adjuvant chemotherapy.

Despite the significant survival benefit with chemoradiotherapy demonstrated in the Intergroup 0099 study, this treatment strategy did not find wide acceptance among the oncologists from the Asian region for the following reasons. The most important reason is the less aggressive form of radiotherapy technique used in the 0099 study that could have led to an inferior result in the radiotherapy arm. Compared with the historical results of the more aggressive radiotherapy technique used in Singapore and Hong Kong, the survival outcome of patients treated with radiation only in these endemic areas appears similar to the CRT arm in the 0099 study. The second reason is the histological subtypes in the 0099 study: less than half of the patients have the endemic WHO type III undifferentiated carcinoma. Although this could explain the inferior results in the radiotherapy-alone arm, it was felt that the results of the Intergroup 0099 study should not be adopted as a new standard in the Asian context without further investigations.

Nevertheless, it was clear that despite the use of a more aggressive radiation technique, a significant proportion of patients with locoregionally advanced endemic NPC would fail locoregionally and/or systemically. It was therefore important to address the role that chemotherapy should play in the primary treatment. We performed a pilot study using a slightly modified form of the chemotherapy regimen used in the Intergroup 0099 study *(75)*. The aim of this study was to determine the feasibility of administering chemotherapy without altering the aggressive radiation technique in our patients. Cisplatin was used at the same dose but fractionated at 25 mg/m^2/d on d 1–4 every 3 wk during radiotherapy and at 20 mg/m^2/d on d 1–4 every 4 wk together with 5-FU 1000 mg/m^2/d during the adjuvant phase. We found that this treatment schedule was feasible, with acceptable toxicities. Seventy-five percent and 63% of the 57 patients treated were able to complete all three cycles of the cisplatin during radiation and all three cycles of the adjuvant chemotherapy, respectively.

We proceeded to conduct a phase III randomized study (SQNP01 study) to determine the applicability of the Intergroup 0099 results in Singapore *(76)*. A total of 221 patients with stage III/IV disease (according to the American Joint Commission for Cancer /Union International Contre Cancer 1997 stage groupings) were randomized between September 1997 and May 2003. Only two patients in the radiotherapy arm (R) were noncompliant with treatment. However, 40% of those in the chemotherapy arm (C) had either dose reduction or reduced cycles of chemotherapy during the concurrent phase. Thirty-one percent of these patients did not receive any adjuvant chemotherapy, and another 27% had dose reduction, or reduced or delayed cycles of chemotherapy. Six patients in C required a reduction of the radiotherapy dose. At the time of interim analysis in October 2003, 59 patients (37 in R, 22 in C) had died. The cause of death was disease-related for 51 of them. The median survival time for those in R was 49.9 mo, but this has not been reached for those in C. The 2-yr disease-free survival rates for the two regimens were 62% for R and 76% for C. The hazard ratio (HR) was 0.67 (95% CI: 0.42–1.08, $p = 0.10$). The 2-yr cumulative incidence rate for distant metastasis was 28% (95% CI: 18–37%) for R and 14% (95% CI: 7–21%) for C. The difference in incidence of distant metastasis between the two groups was statistically significant ($p = 0.034$). The 2-yr overall survival rates were 77% for R and 85% for C, respectively (Fig. 1). Patients who were randomized to receive C had a longer survival time than those on R. The HR estimate was 0.54 (95% CI: 0.32–0.89, $p = 0.02$). It is hence clear that the CRT treatment schedule as used in the Intergroup 0099 study confers survival benefit in patients with locally advanced NPC in the endemic region as well and should be adopted as the standard of care with the caveat that only patients with good performance status be selected and that good supportive measures be readily available to treat potential complications. However, the relative importance of concurrent vs adjuvant chemotherapy remains unclear.

Kwong et al. *(77)*, from Queen Mary Hospital, Hong Kong, attempted to address the relative importance of concurrent and adjuvant chemotherapy in a four-arm randomized study. The three study arms were: (1) concurrent CRT using uracil-tegafur (UFT) at 200 mg q8h throughout radiation, (2) radiotherapy followed by adjuvant chemotherapy consisting of a cisplatin/ 5-FU combination alternating with a vincristine, bleomycin, and methotrexate combination for six cycles, and (3) concurrent CRT followed by adjuvant chemotherapy as detailed in (1) and (2). This study was terminated early after 222 out of the targeted 350 patients were randomized owing to a slow accrual rate and the significant toxicities encountered with the adjuvant chemotherapy. Sixty-five percent of the patients experienced grade 3/4 toxicities during adjuvant treatment that were mainly of the hematological or gastrointestinal type. When the two arms that received concurrent UFT and radiation were compared with the other two arms that did not, the investigators found that concurrent CRT reduced the distant metastasis rate at 3 yr significantly compared with radiotherapy alone (29.4 vs 14.8%; $p = 0.026$). However, there was only a borderline impact on the 3-yr overall survival rate (86.5 vs 76.8%; $p = 0.06$). The addition of adjuvant chemotherapy has no significant impact on the outcome in this study. However, the negative impact of the smaller than expected sample size on a definite conclusion in this study implies that the jury is still out regarding the relative role of concurrent and adjuvant chemotherapy.

Two recent reports from Hong Kong and Taiwan looked specifically at concurrent CRT in a phase III randomized fashion *(78–80)*. Chan et al. *(78)* used weekly cisplatin at 40 mg/m^2 during the radiation in their study; 350 patients were randomized between April 1997 and

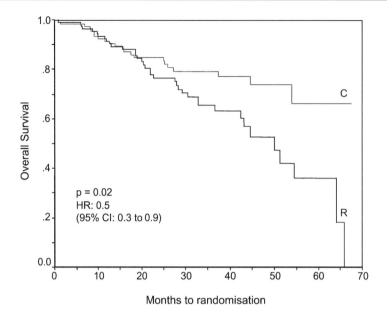

Fig. 1. Overall survival comparison between chemoradiotherapy (C) and radiotherapy (R) in the SQNP01 study.

No. at risk (Death)

C	111 (0)	93 (8)	70 (7)	54 (4)	32 (1)	15 (1)	6 (1)	0
(0)								
R	109 (0)	93 (7)	67 (8)	46 (10)	24 (4)	9 (4)	2 (2)	0
(2)								

Treatment	No. of patients (n)	Observed no. of deaths (O)	Expected no. of deaths (E)	O/E	HR	95% C. I.
C	111	22	31.04	0.71	0.54	0.32 to 0.89
R	109	37	27.96	1.32	-	-
Total	220	58				

November 1999, with progression-free survival (PFS) as the end point. As expected, toxicities were higher in the CRT arm, and 78% of the patients were able to receive at least four weekly doses of cisplatin. Only 44% of the patients were able to complete at least six weekly doses of cisplatin. At the time of data analysis, the median follow-up was 2.71 yr (range 0.52–6.36 yr). The number of events for overall survival analysis was not yet reached and hence was not reported. However, there was no significant difference in the 2-yr progression-free survival between the CRT arm (76%) and the radiotherapy-alone arm (69%), with an estimated HR of 1.367 (95% CI: 0.93–2.00, $p = 0.1$). There was no difference in time to local failure between the two arms as well. The progression-free survival for patients who received less than six weekly doses of cisplatin was also not statistically different from those who received at least six doses (HR 1.348; $p = 0.299$). However, subgroup analysis revealed a clear benefit in favor of those with T3–T4 stages with improvement of the 2-yr progression-free survival from 46 to 68% (HR 2.328); this was attributable to a reduction in distant metastases in this group of patients. An update on the overall survival outcome was presented at the 40th American Society of Clinical Oncology Annual Meeting in June 2004 *(79)*. At a median follow-up of 5.5 yr, the 5-yr overall survival was 72% for those on the CRT arm, in contrast to 59% for those treated with radiotherapy alone (HR 1.41; 95% CI: 1.00–2.00, $p = 0.0479$). However, the 5-yr progression-free survival was of borderline significance in favor of CRT (62 vs 52%; $p = 0.0764$).

Lin et al. *(80)* used a combination of cisplatin at 20 mg/m^2/d and 5-FU at 400 mg/m^2/d over a 96-h infusion in their study. Those randomized to CRT would receive two cycles of the chemotherapy regimen during wk 1 and 5 of the radiation. Two hundred and eighty-four patients were randomized during a 5-yr period from December 1993 to April 1999. Despite the expected higher acute toxicities with concurrent chemotherapy, the compliance with radiotherapy was not reduced and the number of patients requiring delay in radiotherapy was not increased compared with radiotherapy-alone arm (11 vs 16 patients). The compliance with chemotherapy was also very good, with 93.6% of the patients completing the planned two cycles with a delay of 1 wk or more of the second cycle in only nine patients. At a median follow-up of 65 mo (range 36–100 mo), there was significant improvement in the 5-yr overall survival rate and progression-free survival (72.3 vs 54.2% and 71.6 vs 53%, respectively). This was mainly attributable to the significant improvement in local control rates at 5 yr (89.3 vs 72.6%, $p = 0.0009$), although there was also a nonsignificant trend toward improved distant control (78.7 vs 69.9%, $p = 0.0577$).

It is difficult to make firm statements regarding the merits of these two trials, given the different trial designs and the levels of maturity of the data. However, taking the results of our study *(76)* into consideration as well (which showed a highly significant improvement in overall survival in favor of CRT attributable to significant improvement in the distant control rate despite the short follow-up period), it is perhaps justifiable to make some preliminary observations.

First, it is likely that concurrent CRT is the major contributor to the improved outcome, as observed in the Intergroup 0099, the Singapore, and the Taiwan studies (Table 3). This is also in line with experience in the treatment of locally advanced HNSCC *(68,69)*. However, is cisplatin as a single agent used during radiation sufficient without the addition of the adjuvant cisplatin, and 5-FU combination? This question is difficult to answer without a randomized study. However, based on experience with treatment of metastatic disease, the high risk of systemic disease in high-risk groups at diagnosis, and the fact that systemic relapse is a major contributor to mortality, using multiagent combination to address systemic control is a more tenable position.

Second, early, rapid, and effective locoregional treatment is probably crucial to improve the outcome of those with advanced locoregional disease. Radiation treatment is still the more important modality in primary treatment and should be instituted earlier rather than later; this concept is supported by the lack of benefit shown in the large randomized neoadjuvant chemotherapy studies reported *(63–65)*. Augmentation of radiation effect by administering chemotherapy concurrently has been shown conclusively by four well-conducted randomized studies to impact positively on overall survival *(73,76,78–80)*. Whether an accelerated fractionation schedule of radiotherapy would help improve survival is a question that is best left to the outcome of the ongoing multicenter study led by the investigators from Hong Kong alluded to above in Subheading 2. *(51)*.

Table 3
Randomized Studies of Concurrent Chemoradiotherapy

Study	Yr	Treatment	No. of patients	OS rate (%)		
				2-yr	3-yr	5-yr
Al-Sarraf	1998	P/RT > 3 PF	78	NR	78	67
et al.		RT	68	NR	47 (p = 0.005)	37 (p = 0.001)
(73,74)						
Wee et al.	2004	P/RT > 3 PF	111	85	NA	NA
(76)		RT	109	77 (p = 0.02)	NA	NA
Kwong et al.	2003	UFT/RT	53	NR	83.5	NR
(77)		UFT/RT > PF/VBM	57	NR	89	NR
		RT > PF/VBM	55	NR	82.7 (p = NS)	NR
Chan et al.	2003	P/RT	174	NR	NR	72
(78,79)		RT	176	NR	NR	59 (p = 0.0479)
Lin et al.	2003	PF/RT	141	NR	NR	72.3
(80)		RT	143	NR	NR	54.2 (p = 0.002)

Abbreviations: >, followed by; P/RT, cisplatin and concurrent radiation; PF, cisplatin, 5-fluorouracil; UFT/RT, uracil-tegafur and concurrent radiation; PF/VBM, cisplatin, 5-fluorouracil alternate with vincristine, bleomycin, methotrexate; PF/RT, cisplatin, 5-fluorouracil and concurrent radiation; NR, not reported; NS, not significant; OS, overall survival.

7. CONCURRENT CHEMORADIOTHERAPY FOR LOCOREGIONALLY RECURRENT DISEASE

Local relapse is a significant problem, ranging from about 10 to 50% at 5 yr depending on the T stage at presentation (46). Teo et al. (81), in his series of 903 patients, found that skull base invasion and cranial nerve involvement at diagnosis independently predicted for local recurrence after a standard course of radiotherapy. Of note, in our series (82), patients who developed locoregional relapse as the sole site of recurrence after primary treatment tend to be bothered mainly by the problem of locoregional control on follow-up, with only 14% developing disseminated disease at a median interval of 12 mo from the time of first recurrence. Locoregional disease with the resultant complications is the major contributor to mortality in this group of patients.

Management of patients with locoregional relapse is fraught with difficulties. The decision regarding the management plan depends on several factors. The first factor is the disease-free interval after the radical radiotherapy received at diagnosis. A disease-free interval of less than 1 yr generally precludes the use of a second course of radiation. The second factor is the extent of the locoregional recurrence. An extensive area of recurrence requiring a large radiation portal can result in significant morbidity and is generally unacceptable. Third, patients who have undergone more than one prior radical course of radiotherapy to the same subsite(s) are not suitable for further radiation. Finally, good performance status is an important requisite for any radical form of salvage therapy.

Treatment options are limited. Surgery is usually limited to neck dissection for patients with cervical nodal recurrence only. Nasopharyngectomy is usually performed in patients who have failed a repeat course of radiation and who have very limited persistent or recurrent local disease. Very few patients are suitable for this latter option. A repeat course of radiotherapy is a well-established option and is often prescribed for those with first local or locoregional relapse, with successful salvage in a small proportion of appropriately selected patients. Lee et al. *(83)*, from Hong Kong, reported an 11% 5-yr local control rate in the largest series of patients with recurrent NPC treated with reirradiation. They found that the extent of local recurrence was the most significant factor affecting local salvage. The 5-yr freedom from local failure rate for those with early recurrent primary tumor was 28 to 35%. The Taiwan group of Chang et al. *(84)*, in their experience with 186 patients found that advanced stage of recurrence, short disease-free interval of less than 2 yr before retreatment, and inability to deliver at least 50 Gy of radiation during retreatment predicted for a significantly poorer outcome. The overall 5-yr survival rate for all the patients was 12.4%. The survival outcome declined markedly to 3.7% at 3 yr for those with evidence of intracranial extension or cranial nerve palsy at the time of reirradiation.

The use of concurrent CRT as salvage therapy has been reported to be capable of salvaging a small proportion of patients who had undergone prior radical treatments for HNSCC *(85,86)*. We recently reported a small series of 35 patients with locoregionally recurrent nasopharyngeal carcinoma who were retreated with reirradiation and concurrent cisplatin (80 mg/m^2) with/without subsequent consolidation chemotherapy using the standard cisplatin and 5-FU combination *(87)*. Most of these patients had extensive locally recurrent rT3–T4 disease (66%) and hence the resultant multiple cranial nerve palsies (51%). Most of the patients (77%) were able to receive at least two cycles of cisplatin during the reirradiation, and 69% of the patients were able to proceed to the consolidation cisplatin/5-FU. Almost all patients (97%) received at least 50 Gy of reirradiation to the site(s) of disease recurrence using various techniques. At a median follow-up of 46 mo, the 5-yr overall survival rate and progression-free survival rate were 29 and 16%, respectively, for those with rT3–T4 lesions. As expected, late toxicities were not uncommon. These included cranial neuropathies (31%), temporal lobe necrosis (14%), and endocrine abnormalities (14%). Of those with temporal lobe necrosis, only one patient had grade 4 toxicity, which occurred 82 mo after retreatment. The other four patients were diagnosed as having incidental radiologic findings without significant clinical consequences. Of the five patients with endocrine abnormalities, four had grade 3 hypopituitarism, and one had grade 4 diabetes insipidus. Hence the calculated actuarial incidences of any grade 3–4 late toxicity were 12 and 23% at 2 and 5 yr after retreatment, respectively.

The treatment of locoregionally recurrent NPC remains a therapeutic challenge owing to the prior high dose of radiotherapy. The presence of significant morbidities from the extensive locoregional recurrence compounds the problem further. The use of reirradiation alone yields results that are far from ideal, even in those with early local recurrences. The concurrent use of chemotherapy and an adequate dose of reirradiation is a promising treatment schedule in this context, although late neurological and endocrine toxicities can be problematic. The use of IMRT in this context may be able to obviate these long-term problems and improve the therapeutic ratio of concurrent CRT.

8. CONCLUSIONS

The treatment of NPC has made significant strides over the past decade. Concurrent CRT has been shown to improve the survival outcome of patients with locally advanced disease. There are still hurdles to overcome, which should be possible with recent changes and advances. Advances in technology have made possible a more targeted delivery of high-dose radiotherapy, avoiding critical structures; this may improve locoregional control with lower acute and, more importantly, long-term toxicities. Newer active cytotoxics with proven activity in NPC have been added to the armamentarium, and studies are under way to determine whether they can effect improved systemic control as primary treatment and in the metastatic setting. With the improvement in the infrastructure for the conduct of clinical trials in the Asian region and greater collaboration between different centers, we can await more exciting results ahead.

REFERENCES

1. Henle G, Henle W. Epstein-Barr virus-specific IgA serum antibodies as an outstanding feature of nasopharyngeal carcinoma. Int J Cancer 1976; 17:1–7.
2. Zeng Y, Zhang LG, Wu YC, et al. Prospective studies on nasopharyngeal carcinoma in Epstein-Barr virus IgA/VCA antibody-positive persons in Wuzhou City, China. Int J Cancer 1985; 36:545–547.
3. Young LS, Murray PG. Epstein-Barr virus and oncogenesis: from latent genes to tumours. Oncogene 2003; 22:5108–5121.
4. Simons MJ, Wee GB, Da NE, Morris PJ, Shanmugaratnam K, De-The GB. Immunogenetic aspects of nasopharyngeal carcinoma:I. Differences in HL-A antigen profiles between patients and control groups. In J Cancer 1974; 13:122–134.
5. Simons MJ, Wee GB, Chan SH, Shanmugaratnam K. Probable identification of an HL-A second-locus antigen associated with a high risk of nasopharyngeal carcinoma. Lancet 1975; 1:142–143.
6. Simons MJ, Wee GB, Goh EH, et al. Immunogenetic aspects of nasopharyngeal carcinoma: IV. Increased risk in Chinese of nasopharyngeal carcinoma associated with a Chinese-related HLA profile (A2, Singapore 2). J Natl Cancer Inst 1976; 57:977–980.
7. Hildesheim A, Apple RJ, Chen CJ, et al. Association of HLA class I and II alleles and extended haplotypes with nasopharyngeal carcinoma in Taiwan. J Natl Cancer Inst 2002; 94:1780–1789.
8. Feng BJ, Huang W, Shugart YY, et al. Genome-wide scan for familial nasopharyngeal carcinoma reveals evidence of linkage to chromosome 4. Nat Genet 2002; 31:395–399.
9. Armstrong RW, Imrey PB, Lye MS, Armstrong MJ, Yu MC, Sani S. Nasopharyngeal carcinoma in Malaysian Chinese: salted fish and other dietary exposures. Int J Cancer 1998; 77:228–235.
10. Farrow DC, Vaughan TL, Berwick M, Lynch CF, Swanson GM, Lyon JL. Diet and nasopharyngeal cancer in low-risk population. Int J Cancer 1998; 78:675–679.
11. Yuan JM, Wang XL, Xiang YB, Gao YT, Ross RK, Yu MC. Preserved foods in relation to risk of nasopharyngeal carcinoma in Shanghai, China. Int J Cancer 2000; 85:358–363.
12. Ward MH, Pan WH, Cheng YJ, et al. Dietary exposure to nitrite and nitrosamines and risk of nasopharyngeal carcinoma in Taiwan. Int J Cancer 2000; 86:603–609.
13. Zou XN, Lu SH, Liu B. Volatile N-nitrosamines and their precursors in Chinese salted fish—a possible etiological factor for NPC in China. Int J Cancer 1994; 59:155–158.
14. Sham JST, Choy D. Prognostic factors of nasopharyngeal carcinoma: a review of 759 patients. Br J Radiol 1990; 63:51–58.
15. Heng DMK, Wee J, Fong KW, et al. Prognostic factors in 677 patients in Singapore with non-disseminated nasopharyngeal carcinoma. Cancer 1999; 86:1912–1920.
16. Cvitkovic E, Bachouchi M, Bousson H, et al. Leukemoid reaction, bone marrow invasion, fever of unknown origin, and metastatic pattern in the natural history of advanced undifferentiated carcinoma of the nasopharyngeal type: a review of 255 consecutive cases. J Clin Oncol 1993; 12:2434–2442.
17. Ong YK, Heng DM, Chung B, et al. Design of a prognostic index score for metastatic nasopharyngeal carcinoma. Eur J Cancer 2003; 39:1535–1541.
18. Boussen H, Cvitkovic E, Wendling JL, et al. Chemotherapy of metastatic and/or recurrent undifferentiated nasopharyngeal carcinoma with cisplatin, bleomycin and fluorouracil. J Clin Oncol 1991; 9:1675–1681.
19. Mahjoubi R, Azli N, Bachouchi M, et al. Metastatic undifferentiated carcinoma of the nasopharyngeal type treated with bleomycin, epirubicin and cisplatin. Final report (abstract). Proc Am Soc Clin Oncol 1992; 11:240.
20. Au E, Ang PT. A phase II trial of 5-fluorouracil and cisplatin in recurrent or metastatic nasopharyngeal carcinoma. Ann Oncol 1994; 5:87–89.
21. Yeo W, Leung TW, Leung SF, et al. Phase II study of the combination of carboplatin and 5-fluorouracil in metastatic nasopharyngeal carcinoma. Cancer Chemother Pharmacol. 1996; 38:466–470.
22. Wang CH, Wang HM, Chen JS, Chang WJ, Lai GM. Intensive chemotherapy plus recombinant human granulocyte colony stimulating factor support for distant metastatic nasopharyngeal carcinoma. A preliminary report. Oncology 1997; 54:34–37.

23. Siu LL, Czaykowki PM, Tannock IF. Phase I/II study of CAPABLE regimen for patients with poorly differentiated carcinoma of the nasopharynx. J Clin Oncol 1998; 16:2514–2521.

24. Hasbini A, Mahjoubi R, Fandi A, et al. Phase II trial of combining mitomycin with 5-fluorouracil, epirubicin, and cisplatin in recurrent and metastatic undifferentiated carcinoma of the nasopharyngeal type. Ann Oncol 1999; 10:421–425.

25. Tay MH, Ong YK, Foo KF, et al. The role of salvage chemotherapy in metastatic nasopharyngeal carcinoma (abstract). Proc Am Soc Clin Oncol 2001; 20:199b.

26. Au E, Tan EH, Ang PT. Activity of paclitaxel by three-hour infusion in Asian patients with metastatic undifferentiated nasopharyngeal cancer. Ann Oncol 1998; 9:327–329.

27. Foo KF, Tan EH, Leong SS, et al. Gemcitabine in metastatic nasopharyngeal carcinoma of the undifferentiated type. Ann Oncol 2002; 13:150–156.

28. Chua DT, Sham JS, Au GK. A phase II study of capecitabine in patients with recurrent and metastatic nasopharyngeal carcinoma pretreated with platinum-based chemotherapy. Oral Oncol 2003; 39:361–366.

29. Poon D, Chowbay B, Leong SS, et al. Phase II study of irinotecan (CPT-11) as salvage therapy for advanced nasopharyngeal carcinoma (NPC). Proc Am Soc Clin Oncol 2004; 23:505

30. Tan EH, Khoo KS, Wee J, et al. Phase II trial of a paclitaxel and carboplatin combination in Asian patients with metastatic nasopharyngeal carcinoma. Ann Oncol 1999; 10:235–237.

31. Yeo W, Leung TWT, Chan ATC, et al. A Phase II study of combination paclitaxel and carboplatin in advanced nasopharyngeal carcinoma. Eur J Cancer 1998; 34:2027–2031.

32. Ngan RK, Yiu HH, Lau WH, et al. Combination gemcitabine and cisplatin chemotherapy for metastatic or recurrent nasopharyngeal carcinoma:report of a phase II study. Ann Oncol 2002; 13:1252–1258.

33. Ma BBY, Tannock IF, Pond GR, Edmonds MR, Siu LL. Chemotherapy with gemcitabine-containing regimens for locally recurrent or metastatic nasopharyngeal carcinoma. Cancer 2002; 95:2516–2523.

34. Leong SS, Foo KF, Wee J, et al. Phase II study of gemcitabine, paclitaxel and carboplatin in patients with metastatic nasopharyngeal carcinoma—updated results (abstract). Proc Am Soc Clin Oncol 2003; 22:497.

35. Chan ATC, Hsu MM, Goh BC, et al. A phase II study of cetuximab (C225) in combination with carboplatin in patients with recurrent or metastatic nasopharyngeal carcinoma who failed to a platinum-based chemotherapy. Proc Am Soc Clin Oncol 2003; 22:497.

36. Hoppe RT, Williams J, Warnke R, Goffinet DR, Bagshaw MA. Carcinoma of the nasopharynx—the significance of histology. Int J Radiat Oncol Biol Phys 1978; 4:199–205.

37. Shanmugaratnam K, Chan SH, de-The G, et al. Histopathology of nasopharyngeal carcinoma: correlations with epidemiology, survival rates and other biological characteristics. Cancer 1979; 44:1029–1044.

38. Ozyar E, Yildiz F, Akyol FH, Atahan IL. Comparison of AJCC 1988 and 1997 classifications for nasopharyngeal carcinoma. Int J Radiat Oncol Biol Phys 1999; 44:1079–1087.

39. Lee AW, Poon YF, Foo W, et al. Retrospective analysis of 5037 patients with nasopharyngeal carcinoma treated during 1976-1985: overall survival and patterns of failure. Int J Radiat Oncol Biol Phys 1992; 23:261–270.

40. Wee J, Heng D, Tan T, et al. Review of the 1997 AJCC/UICC Staging System for NPC—the Singapore experience. J HK Coll Radiol Suppl 2003; 6:40.

41. Chan ATC, Teo PML, Leung TWT, Johnson PJ. The role of chemotherapy in the management of nasopharyngeal carcinoma. Cancer 1998; 82:1003–1012.

42. Al-Sarraf M, McLaughlin PW. Nasopharynx carcinoma: choice of treatment. Int J Radiat Oncol Biol Phys 1995; 33:761–763.

43. Tsao SY. Technical details for radiotherapy delivery. In: Hasselt CA, Gibb AG, edis. Nasopharyngeal Carcinoma. Hong Kong: The Chinese University Press,1991:207–208.

44. Teo PM, Leung SF, Fowler J. Improved local control for early T-stage nasopharyngeal carcinoma—a tale of two hospitals. Radiother Oncol 2000; 57:155–166.

45. Wee J, Yeo R, Tan T et al. A review of intracavitary brachytherapy for nasopharyngeal cancer (abstract). Proc Am Soc Clin Oncol 2001; 20:235a.

46. Fong KW, Chua EJ, Chua ET, et al. Patient profile and survival in 270 computer-tomography-staged patients with nasopharyngeal cancer treated at the Singapore General Hospital. Ann Acad Med Singapore 1996; 25:341–346.

47. Teo P, Tsao SY, Shiu W. A clinical study of 407 cases of nasopharyngeal carcinoma in Hong Kong. Int J Radiat Oncol Biol Phys 1989; 17:515–530.

48. Chang SD, Tate DJ, Goffinet DR. Treatment of nasopharyngeal carcinoma: stereotactic radiosurgical boost following fractionated radiotherapy. Stereotact Funct Neurosurg 1999; 73:64–67.

49. Wang CC. Accelerated hyperfractionation radiation therapy for carcinoma of the nasopharynx. Techniques and results. Cancer 1989; 63:2461–2467.

50. Teo PM, Leung SF, Chan AT, et al. Final report of a randomized trial on altered-fractionated radiotherapy in nasopharyngeal carcinoma prematurely terminated by significant increase in neurologic complications. Int J Radiat Oncol Biol Phys 2000; 48:1311–1322.

51. Lee AW, Sze WM, Yau TK. Retrospective analysis on treating nasopharyngeal carcinoma with accelerated fractionation (6 fractions per week) in comparison with conventional fractionation (5 fractions per week):report on 3-year tumor control and normal tissue toxicity. Radiother Oncol 2001; 58:121–130.

52. Lee N, Xia P, Quivey JM, et al. Intensity-modulated radiotherapy in the treatment of nasopharyngeal carcinoma:an update of the UCSF experience. Int J Radiat Oncol Biol Phys 2002; 53:12–22.

53. Cengiz M, Chao C, Perez CA. Intensity-modulated radiotherapy (IMRT) with concurrent cisplatin chemotherapy (CT) yields superior therapeutic outcome than conventional techniques with or without chemotherapy in locally advanced nasopharyngeal carcinoma (abstract). Int J Radiat Oncol Biol Phys 2000; 48:3.

54. Wolden S, Pfister D, Zelefsky M, et al. Intensity modulated radiation therapy improves locoregional control for nasopharyngeal carcinoma (abstract). Proc Am Soc Clin Oncol 2002; 21:240a.

55. Clark JR, Norris CM, Dreyfuss AI, et al. Nasopharyngeal carcinoma: the Dana-Farber Cancer Institute experience with 24 patients treated with induction chemotherapy and radiotherapy. Ann Otol Rhinol Laryngol 1987; 96:608–614.

56. Bachouchi M, Cvitkovic E, Azli N, et al. High complete response in advanced nasopharyngeal carcinoma with bleomycin, epirubicin and cisplatin before radiotherapy. J Natl Cancer Inst 1990; 82:616–620.

57. Dimery IW, Peters LJ, Goepfert H, et al. Effectiveness of combined induction chemotherapy and radiotherapy in advanced nasopharyngeal carcinoma. J Clin Oncol 1993; 11:1919–1928.

58. Garden AS, Lippman SM, Morrison WH, et al. Does induction chemotherapy have a role in the management of nasopharyngeal carcinoma? Results of treatment in the era of computerized tomography. Int J Radiat Oncol Biol Phys 1996; 36:1005–1012.

59. Geara FB, Glisson BS, Sanguineti G, et al. Induction chemotherapy followed by radiotherapy versus radiotherapy alone in patients with advanced nasopharyngeal carcinoma. Results of a matched cohort study. Cancer 1997; 79:1279–1286.

60. Hong RL, Ting LL, Ko JY, et al. Induction chemotherapy with mitomycin, epirubicin, cisplatin, fluorouracil and leucovorin followed by radiotherapy in the treatment of locoregional advanced nasopharyngeal carcinoma. J Clin Oncol 2001; 19:4305–4313.

61. Chan ATC, Teo PML, Leung TWT, et al. A prospective randomized study of chemotherapy adjunctive to definitive radiotherapy in advanced nasopharyngeal carcinoma. Int J Radiat Oncol Biol Phys 1995; 33:569–577.

62. Hareyama M, Sakata K, Shirato H, et al. A prospective randomized trial comparing neoadjuvant chemotherapy with radiotherapy alone in patients with advanced nasopharyngeal carcinoma. Cancer 2002; 94:2217–2223.

63. International Nasopharynx Cancer Study Group: VUMCA I Trial. Preliminary results of a randomized trial comparing neoadjuvant chemotherapy (cisplatin, epirubicin, bleomycin) plus radiotherapy vs. radiotherapy alone in stage IV ($\geq$ N2, M0) undifferentiated nasopharyngeal carcinoma: a positive effect on progression-free survival. Int J Radiat Oncol Biol Phys 1996; 35:463–469.

64. Chua DTT, Sham JST, Choy D, et al. Preliminary report of the Asian-Oceanian Clinical Oncology Association randomized trial comparing ciplatin and epirubicin followed by radiotherapy versus radiotherapy alone in the treatment of patients with locoregionally advanced nasopharyngeal carcinoma. Cancer 1998; 83:2270–2283.

65. Jun Ma, Mai HQ, Hong MH, et al. Results of a prospective randomized trial comparing neoadjuvant chemotherapy plus radiotherapy with radiotherapy alone in patients with locoregionally advanced nasopharyngeal carcinoma. J Clin Oncol 2001; 19:1350–1357.

66. Rossi A, Molinari R, Boracchi P, et al. Adjuvant chemotherapy with vincristine, cyclophosphamide, and doxorubicin after radiotherapy in local-regional nasopharyngeal cancer:results of a 4-year multicenter randomized study. J Clin Oncol 1988; 6:1401–1410.

67. Chi KH, Chang YC, Guo WY, et al. A phase III study of adjuvant chemotherapy in advanced nasopharyngeal carcinoma patients. Int J Radiat Oncol Biol Phys 2002; 52:1238–1244.

68. Forastiere A, Koch W, Trotti A, Sidransky D. Head and neck cancer. N Eng J Med 2001; 26:1890–900.

69. Adelstein DJ, Li Y, Adams GL, et al. An intergroup phase III comparison of standard radiation therapy and two schedules of concurrent chemoradiotherapy in patients with unresectable squamous cell head and neck cancer. J Clin Oncol 2003; 21:92–98.

70. Forastiere AA, Goepfert H, Maor M, et al. Concurrent chemotherapy and radiotherapy for organ preservation in advanced laryngeal cancer. N Engl J Med 2003; 349:2091–2098.

71. Ong YK, Tan EH, Wee J, et al. Concurrent chemoradiotherapy in patients with locally advanced nasopharyngeal carcinoma of the undifferentiated type. Ann Acad Med Singapore 1999; 28:525–528.

72. Al-Sarraf M, Pajak TF, Cooper JS, Mohiuddin M, Herskovic A, Ager PJ. Chemo-radiotherapy in patients with locally advanced nasopharyngeal carcinoma:a radiation therapy oncology group study. J Clin Oncol 1990; 8:1342–1351.

73. Al-Sarraf M, LeBlanc M, Giri PG, et al. Chemoradiotherapy versus radiotherapy in patients with advanced nasopharyngeal cancer: phase III randomized Intergroup study 0099. J Clin Oncol 1998; 16:1310–1317.
74. Al-Sarraf M, LeBlanc M, Giri PGS, et al. Superiority of five year survival with chemo-radiotherapy (CT-RT) vs radiotherapy in patients (Pts) with locally advanced nasopharyngeal cancer (NPC). Intergroup (0099) (SWOG 8892, RTOG 8817, ECOG 2388) phase III study: final report. Proc Am Soc Clin Oncol 2001; 20:227a.
75. Tan EH, Chua ET, Wee J, et al. Concurrent chemoradiotherapy followed by adjuvant chemotherapy in Asian patients with nasopharyngeal carcinoma:toxicities and preliminary results. Int J Radiat Oncol Biol Phys 1999; 45:597–601.
76. Wee J, Tan EH, Tai BC, et al. Phase III randomized trial of radiotherapy versus concurrent chemo-radiotherapy followed by adjuvant chemotherapy in patients with AJCC/UICC (1997) Stage 3 and 4 nasopharyngeal cancer of the endemic variety. Proc Am Soc Clin Oncol 2004; 23:487.
77. Kwong DLW, Sham JST, Au GKH. Concurrent and adjuvant chemotherapy for nasopharyngeal carcinoma:a factorial study. Proc Am Soc Clin Oncol 2003; 22:495.
78. Chan AT, Teo PM, Ngan RK, et al. Concurrent chemotherapy-radiotherapy compared with radiotherapy alone in locoregionally advanced nasopharyngeal carcinoma: progression-free survival analysis of a phase III randomized trial. J Clin Oncol 2002; 20:2038–2044.
79. Chan AT, Ngan R, Teo P, et al. Final results of a phase III randomized study of concurrent weekly cisplatin-RT versus RT alone in locoreginoally advanced nasopharyngeal carcinoma (NPC). Proc Am Soc Clin Oncol 2004; 23:492.
80. Lin JC, Jan JS, Hsu CY, Liang WM, Jiang RS, Wang WY. Phase III study of concurrent chemoradiotherapy versus radiotherapy alone for advanced nasopharyngeal carcinoma: positive effect on overall and progression-free survival. J Clin Oncol 2003; 21:631–637.
81. Teo PML, Kwan WH, Yu P, Lee WY, Leung SF, Choi P. A retrospective study of the role of intracavitary brachytherapy and prognostic factors determining local tumour control after primary radical radiotherapy in 903 non-disseminated nasopharyngeal carcinoma patients. Clin Oncol 1996; 8:160–166.
82. Wong ZW, Tan EH, Yap SP, et al. Chemotherapy with or without radiotherapy in patients with locoregionally recurrent nasopharyngeal carcinoma. Head Neck 2002; 24:549–554.
83. Lee AWM, Foo W, Law SCD, et al. Reirradiation for recurrent nasopharyngeal carcinoma:factors affecting the therapeutic ratio and ways for improvement. Int J Radiat Oncol Biol Phys 1997; 38:43–52.
84. Chang JTC, See LC, Liao CT, et al. Locally recurrent nasopharyngeal carcinoma. Radiother Oncol 2000; 54:135–142.
85. Haraf DJ, Weichselbaum RR, Vokes EE. Re-irradiation with concomitant chemotherapy of unresectable recurrent head and neck cancer: a potentially curable disease. Ann Oncol 1996; 7:913–918.
86. Tan EH, Adelstein DJ, Saxton JP, et al. Concurrent chemoradiotherapy for salvage in relapsed squamous cell head and neck cancer. Cancer Invest 1997; 15:422–428.
87. Poon D, Yap SP, Wong ZW, et al. Concurrent chemoradiotherapy in locoregionally recurrent nasopharyngeal carcinoma. Int J Radiat Oncol Biol Phys 2004;59:1312–1318.

16

Strategies for Protecting Normal Tissue in the Treatment of Head and Neck Cancer

David M. Brizel, MD

1. INTRODUCTION

Normal tissue tolerance limits the delivery of both ionizing radiation and cytotoxic chemotherapy for virtually all types of cancer including squamous cell carcinoma of the head and neck (HNSCC). The concept of the therapeutic ratio (TR) is fundamental to the understanding of this issue. The TR can be qualitatively defined as the TCP/NTCP where TCP is the tumor control probability and NTCP is the normal tissue complication probability. Both of these parameters have sigmoid dose-response curves (Fig. 1). The horizontal separation between these two curves for any given treatment will often determine the efficacy of that treatment. As the curves separate from one another, the likelihood increases that treatment will be effective and not cause an unacceptable level of morbidity. Conversely, the closer together these two curves are, the less the likelihood is that treatment will be effective without causing an unacceptable level of morbidity.

Radiotherapy plus concurrent chemotherapy has been demonstrated to be superior to either sequential combined-modality therapy or single-modality therapy in multiple disease categories in well-designed randomized trials. Disease sites include uterine cervix *(1–4)*, esophagus *(5)*, and lung *(6)*. Perhaps the greatest volume of data supporting the value of concurrent chemoradiotherapy (CRT) exists for the curative intent treatment of HNSCC. A metaanalysis published by Pignon et al. *(7)* evaluated more than 10,000 patients treated in randomized trials that were completed and reported through 1993. An 8% absolute survival benefit over radiotherapy alone was observed in patients who received concurrent therapy. A smaller, but significant, benefit was also seen in patients treated with sequential neoadjuvant chemotherapy. The metaanalysis also suggested that concurrent treatment was superior to sequential therapy *(7)*.

A recent three-arm randomized trial conducted by the Radiation Therapy Oncology Group (RTOG) in advanced larynx cancer demonstrated the superiority of concurrent therapy over both single-modality radiation and sequential CRT in head-to-head comparisons *(8)*. Several randomized trials that cumulatively enrolled more than 1500 patients have been published since the 1993 metaanalysis cutoff date. These trials all used both state of the art radiotherapy (many with modified fractionation and chemotherapy, all with either platinum and/or 5-

From: *Current Clinical Oncology: Squamous Cell Head and Neck Cancer*
Edited by: D. J. Adelstein © Humana Press Inc., Totowa, NJ

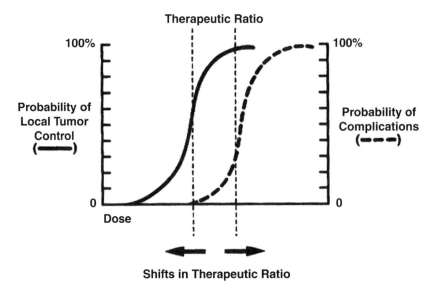

Fig. 1. A graphic representation of the therapeutic index (TI). The tumor control probability (TCP) is to the left of the normal tissue complication probability (NTCP) and both are displayed as sigmoid dose-response curves. Larger separations are indicative of higher TIs. Ideally, normal tissue protection strategies would move the NTCP curve to the right without compromising TCP (moving the TCP curve to the right). Ideal therapeutic intensification strategies would move the TCP curve to the left without worsening NTCP (moving the NTCP curve to the left).

fluorouracil [5-FU]). They all show statistically significant improvement in local regional control, failure-free survival, and overall survival in the range of 10 to 20% (8–15).

Radiotherapy with concurrent chemotherapy is rapidly evolving into a significant component in the adjuvant therapy of patients who undergo primary surgical resection. Pathologic characteristics including positive surgical margins and extracapsular nodal spread determine high risk for locoregional recurrence. Randomized trials conducted by the European Organization for the Research and Treatment of Cancer (EORTC) and RTOG have demonstrated that the addition of concurrent chemotherapy to postoperative irradiation improves locoregional control, failure-free survival, and overall survival. These improvements again come at the cost of increased acute and chronic toxicity (16,17).

The availability of hematologic growth factor support has made it possible to combine more intensive/optimal radiotherapy and chemotherapy regimens in the concurrent scheduling format. Nonetheless, treatment intensification still clearly increases toxicity in the context of concurrent CRT. Two of the most significant toxicities that arise during the treatment of head and neck cancer are mucositis and xerostomia, both of which develop acutely during the course of treatment.

A trial conducted at Duke University randomized patients with advanced head and neck cancer to either accelerated hyperfractionation alone or accelerated hyperfractionation with concurrent cis-diaminedichloroplatinum (CDDP)/5-FU chemotherapy. The incidence of confluent grade 3 mucositis was the same in both treatment arms (74 vs 77%, respectively) but the mean time to resolution of mucositis was 50% longer in the patients receiving combined-modality therapy (6 vs 4 wk). The University of Munich conducted a randomized trial comparing split-course accelerated fractionation vs split-course accelerated fractionation with concurrent CDDP, 5-FU, and leucovorin in patients with unresectable head and neck cancer. The incidence of confluent mucositis more than doubled in the patients receiving combined-modality therapy (38 vs 16%, $p < 0.001$) *(14)*. A French randomized trial in advanced oropharynx cancer (GORTEC 94-01) compared once-daily radiotherapy against once-daily radiotherapy with concurrent carboplatin and 5-FU. Confluent mucositis increased from 39 to 71% ($p = 0.005$) with the addition of chemotherapy *(18)*. The University of Vienna compared standard fractionation radiotherapy vs accelerated fractionation with concurrent mitomycin C and 5-FU *(11)*. Although there was a survival benefit in the combined modality arm, confluent mucositis also increased from 33 to 90%.

The GORTEC 94-01 trial demonstrated that chronic morbidity is also more severe with concurrent therapy *(18)*. Grade 3/4 cervical fibrosis increased from 12 to 27% ($p = 0.04$). Grade 3/4 xerostomia was comparable between the standard and experimental arms (35 vs 41%), but severe dental complications were significantly higher in patients receiving combined-modality therapy (37 vs 18%, $p = 0.01$). Overall, 32% of the patients receiving radiotherapy alone had grade 3/4 late effects vs 49% for those patients treated with combined-modality therapy ($p = 0.02$).

The data clearly demonstrate that disease control and survival are improved with radiation and concurrent chemotherapy over radiation alone or sequential chemotherapy followed by radiation. The added morbidity of this treatment reveals, however, that there is a pressing need for the development of strategies to ameliorate treatment-induced toxicity. Some investigators have coined the term "toxic cure" to describe the effects of concurrent therapy *(19)*. These toxicities arise primarily from radiotherapy and are exacerbated with the addition of chemotherapy.

Normal tissue-protective strategies have been employed in radiation oncology almost since the inception of this discipline. These strategies can be classified on the basis of the physical manipulation of the beam, alteration of the fractionation schedule, and pharmacologic manipulation of the radiation response. Physical radiation protection schemes are based on the simple principle that exclusion of normal tissue from the target volume is the most effective form of radioprotection. Standard techniques for achieving this goal include the placement of lead alloy blocks into the path of the radiation beam in order to prevent radiation from passing through tissues that lie underneath the block. The use of multiple treatment fields is another standard technique for protecting normal tissues. The intent is to include the entire tumor within the volume of tissue that is irradiated by all the beams while exposing critical normal tissues to radiation from less than the full complement of beams. Multiple shaped treatment fields may not provide adequate normal tissue protection in a setting in which the tumor volume and normal tissues are immediately adjacent to one another or even wrapped around one another. In these circumstances, techniques such as conformal radiotherapy or intensity-modulated radiotherapy (IMRT) may be more effective means of minimizing normal tissue dose.

Standard fractionation radiotherapy for head and neck cancer consists of the delivery of one fraction per day in the range of 180–200 cGy. Acute morbidity from radiotherapy is a function of the total dose delivered in a given period and is relatively independent of the fractionation scheme utilized. Late or chronic morbidity is dependent on the total dose delivered too, but it also is highly dependent on the size of the dose per fraction. For a given cumulative dose of irradiation, a larger number of small doses per fraction will create less chronic toxicity than a smaller number of larger doses per fraction. Hyperfractionation is the term employed to describe the use of a significantly greater number of smaller multiple daily doses of radiation. The rationale for the use of hyperfractionation is that such a scheme will improve the TR by allowing the delivery of a larger cumulative dose to improve treatment efficacy over standard fractionation while maintaining a constant risk of late toxicity. EORTC Trial 22791 confirmed the validity of this concept in patients with oropharyngeal cancer who were randomized to receive either standard fractionation 2 Gy per day to 70 Gy in 7 wk or 80.5 Gy in 7 wk at 1.15 Gy bid. Local regional control was increased from 40 to 59% ($p = 0.02$) with the utilization of hyperfractionation. The incidence of confluent mucositis was also higher with hyperfractionation, but there was no difference in late morbidity between the two treatment arms (20).

The other approach to normal tissue protection in the treatment of head and neck cancer is pharmacologic in nature. Controversy exists as to whether modification of treatment delivery, e.g., IMRT or altered fractionation, or pharmacologic manipulation of radiation response is the optimal strategy for normal tissue protection. Prior to exploring the data relating to physical manipulation of the radiation beam, a review of the Food and Drug Administration (FDA) guidelines for approval and marketing of devices is in order. The hardware and software necessary for the delivery of radiotherapy, including IMRT, is regulated by the FDA through the 510k mechanism. The FDA requirement for the approval of a new device for marketing and sale is that the ". . . device is substantially equivalent (for the indications for use stated in the enclosure) to legally marketed predicate devices marketed in interstate commerce . . .." In other words, if the new treatment planning software or beam shaping collimation devices produce radiation dose distributions in a target volume equivalent to those that can be produced by devices already on the market, then the new devices in question will be approved for marketing and sale. No type of clinical trial, randomized or otherwise, is required. Demonstration of efficacy or clinical benefit is not required.

A search of the National Library of Medicine PubMed database indicates that several hundred articles relating to the topic of IMRT (cancers of all sites) have been published since 1997. Virtually none of these is a prospective clinical trial, and not one is a randomized trial. Nonetheless, IMRT has proved to be a useful tool in improving our understanding of dose-volume-function relationships for normal tissues in the radiotherapy of head and neck cancer. Specifically, traditional "wisdom" stated that the tolerance of the parotid glands to radiotherapy was 50 Gy. Eisbruch et al. (21) have elegantly demonstrated, however, that that when the mean dose to the parotids exceeds 26 Gy, there is usually little if any recovery of function. These data should prove quite useful in the design of future trials directed toward preservation of salivary gland function.

Similarly, Garden et al. (22) demonstrated that the use of IMRT with once-daily standard fractionation in the treatment of 54 patients with early-stage (T1 and T2) oropharyngeal carcinoma resulted in less irradiation to the parotid glands than would have arisen from conventional radiotherapy. Acute mucosal toxicity was not improved, however, and may actually have been worse, as 42% of the patients required placement of feeding gastrostomies (22). These data force one to keep in mind that a physical improvement in the radiation dose distribution in and around the target volume and critical normal tissues may or may not lead to an improvement in clinical outcome.

IMRT-mediated reductions in dose to tissues such as the parotid are accomplished at the expense of irradiating much larger volumes of normal tissue, not necessarily in the vicinity of the target, to doses as high as 10 to 30% of the prescribed target dose. This "dose dumping" effect may deliver 700–2000 cGy to anatomic regions that would not receive any dose at all with conventional or even conformal treatment techniques. These doses are potentially carcinogenic, and the carcinogenicity of radiation cannot be ignored, especially in the head and neck population, in which the risk of developing a second malignant neoplasm approaches 20 to 30%.

The FDA requirements for the approval and marketing of a new drug are considerably more rigorous than those for the approval of a new device or technology. A series of phase I, II, and III trials must be performed to demonstrate both the safety and efficacy of the drug with respect to a prespecified prospective end point. In some circumstances, a second confirmatory phase III trial may be required. The safety of a conventional cytotoxic drug relates to the side effects that are directly attributable to its administration. There is an additional dimension to the safety profile of a potential radioprotective drug: specifically, is the activity of the drug selective enough to prevent the damaging effects of ionizing irradiation on normal tissues but not on the tumor? Consequently, a clinical trial designed to test the effectiveness of a pharmacologic radioprotective agent must also demonstrate that the agent does not impair the efficacy of the radiotherapy itself. This consideration injects an aspect of treatment equivalence into the study design and typically leads to the requirement of a larger study population than would otherwise be necessary (23).

Pharmacologic radioprotective strategies can be loosely classified into three categories: protection, mitigation, and treatment. A review of randomized trials of prototypical agents in each group will illustrate the different strategies. The bellwether pharmacologic radioprotector is amifostine (WR-2721; Ethyol®, Medimmune, Inc., Gaithersburg, MD). Amifostine is a thiol-containing compound long recognized to have radioprotective potential (24). It functions as a classical radiation protector via free radical scavenging. It preferentially accumulates in the saliva glands. A pivotal open-label phase III trial conducted from 1995 to 1997 randomized patients to receive curative intent or postoperative irradiation with or without iv amifostine (200 mg/m^2) given 15–30 min prior to each radiotherapy fraction daily. The primary end points of this trial were reduction in the incidence of grade 2 or higher acute and late xerostomia and grade 3 or higher acute mucositis. Preservation of antitumor efficacy of the radiotherapy was also assessed along with the acute toxicity of the drug itself.

This trial enrolled 303 patients, and the minimum follow-up for all surviving patients is 2 yr. Administration of amifostine did not reduce the incidence of grade 3 mucositis (25). It did, however, result in diminished xerostomia. There was no compromise of locoregional disease control, failure-free survival, survival (Table 1). The FDA approved amifostine in 1999 for use in conjunction with postoperative irradiation in settings in which a substantial portion of the saliva glands would be in the radiation field.

Severe toxicity (>CTC grade 3) attributable to amifostine occurred in less than 10% of patients on this trial and consisted of nausea and vomiting and transient hypotension. Nearly two-thirds of the patients had less severe grades of these side effects, and drug-related toxicity did cause approx 20% of patients to discontinue amifostine prior to completing radiotherapy. Subcutaneous administration of the drug may cause fewer side effects than intravenous dosing (26).

Critics of this trial contend that its size made it underpowered to detect a very small compromise in survival and that it was neither placebo controlled nor blinded (27). The first argument is technically correct but overlooks the reality that absolute refutation of a small compromise of antitumor efficacy attributable to amifostine would have required an equivalence trial. Demonstration that amifostine reduced survival from a hypothetical 45 to 40% (α = 0.05, 80% power) would have necessitated 1246 patients per study arm (28). Such a large study cannot be performed in head and neck cancer. Patient resources are too scarce. The largest randomized head and neck trial ever conducted, RTOG 90-03, required 8 yr to enroll 1113 patients into four treatment arms (29).

Table 1
Phase III Trial Results for Amifostine

Parameter	Amifostine (n = 153) vs control (n = 150)			
	12 mo (%)	18 mo (%)	24 mo (%)	Overall p value
Locoregional tumor control	72 vs 71	61 vs 64	54 vs 58	0.863
Progression-free survival	75 vs 70	63 vs 63	56 vs 59	0.911
Overall survival	89 vs 82	81 vs 73	72 vs 67	0.145
RTOG grade ≥2 xerostomia	32 vs 56	29 vs 51	20 vs 36	0.002
Unstimulated saliva (>0.1 g)	70 vs 49	69 vs 60	76 vs 56	0.011

The second contention regarding the absence of blinding and placebo control is valid. Xerostomia is a physician-assessed, semiquantitative parameter, and the scoring of an individual patient can vary between different assessors. The absence of a blinded placebo control arm created the potential for physician bias in the assessment of this end point. Fortunately, prospective secondary end points in the trial included both serial patient self-assessment of symptoms associated with dry mouth and quantitation of salivary production, the latter of these being an objective, quantitative measure not subject to variation among different assessors. Those patients who had the least severe xerostomia as scored by the investigators were also the ones who had the greatest production of unstimulated saliva. Similarly, the patients who assessed themselves as having the least severe xerostomia-related symptoms had the greatest salivary production. All three of these end points were highly correlated with one another, which helps to validate the results in the absence of a placebo control arm.

Small phase II and III studies suggest that amifostine may reduce CRT-induced salivary, pulmonary, mucosal, and hematologic toxicity (30–32). A metaanalysis of all these trials may help to clarify the tumor protection concerns associated with the use of this drug.

Another approach to the management of radiation-induced toxicity is the utilization of substances that mitigate damage caused by prior radiation exposure. This strategy contrasts to the classical free radical scavenging radioprotective mechanism of drugs such as amifostine. The leading drug under development in this category is palifermin. Palifermin is a recombinant human keratinocyte growth factor that belongs to the fibroblast growth factor family of cytokines (FGF-7). It stimulates cellular proliferation and differentiation in a variety of epithelial tissues including mucosa throughout the alimentary tract, salivary glands, and type II pneumocytes. Palifermin also regulates intrinsic glutathione-mediated cytoprotective mechanisms. Administration of palifermin in preclinical rodent models leads to a significant thickening of oral tongue mucosa (Fig. 2) (33). Preclinical studies of fractionated radiotherapy have revealed that the administration of palifermin leads to increases in the dose of radiotherapy necessary to induce ulcerative mucositis and also to reduce the duration of this ulceration when it does occur (34,35). Parotid gland production of saliva is also preserved when palifermin is administered in the setting of radiotherapy in preclinical systems.

The ability of palifermin to reduce mucositis in a clinical setting has been tested in a pivotal phase III double-blind placebo-controlled trial of patients with non-Hodgkin's lymphoma undergoing bone marrow transplantation. The bone marrow ablative regimen consisted of 1200 cGy of total body irradiation (TBI) given at 150 cGy bid. Thereafter, VP-16 and cyclophosphamide were administered. Palifermin was delivered prior to the initiation of TBI and again after the completion of chemotherapy, which also corresponded to 5 d after the completion of TBI. The dose schedule of palifermin was 60 µg/kg/d three times for both

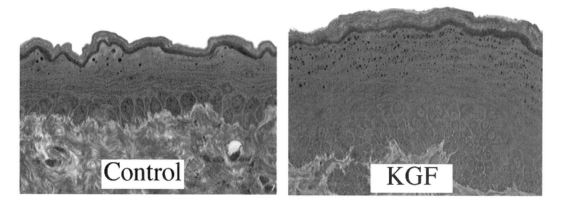

Fig. 2. Enhanced mucosal proliferation in rodent tongue after 3 d of administration of recombinant human kertinocyte growth factor (KGF; 5 mg/kg/d) *(33)*. The mucosal thickness has doubled secondary to the cytokine exposure.

administrations. This trial enrolled 212 patients who were equally divided between the placebo and palifermin arms. The WHO scoring system was used. The incidence of grade 3/4 mucositis approached 90% in the placebo arm as opposed to approx 60% in the palifermin arm. For those patients who developed this level of toxicity, the duration was significantly reduced from 10.4 d in the placebo arm to 3.7 d in the palifermin arm ($p > 0.001$). Grade IV mucositis developed in 62% of the placebo arm patients and only 20% of the palifermin arm patients ($p > 0.001$). Mean duration of grade IV mucositis was reduced from 6.2 d to 3.3 d with the use of this drug ($p > 0.001$).

The clinical experience with palifermin in head and neck cancer is limited to one phase I and one phase II trial. Both of these trials integrated palifermin into regimens of radiation and concurrent CDDP/5-FU chemotherapy for patients with American Joint Commission for Cancers (AJCC) stages III/IV nonmetastatic squamous carcinoma of the head and neck. Both trials utilized a dose of palifermin prior to the initiation of chemoradiation and then delivered an additional dose at the end of each week of radiotherapy. The primary end point of the phase I trial was safety and tolerability of the drug. The dose of palifermin was escalated from 20 to 80 μg/kg. The most common toxicity of the drug was an erythema of the face, which occurred in 9/60 patients (50%) and was a non-dose-limiting toxicity. Hypersalivation occurred as a dose-limiting toxicity in one patient. Transient, asymptomatic elevations of amylase and lipase were observed. The maximum tolerated dose was not determined in the dose schedule tested in this trial. There was a 3:1 randomization to palifermin and placebo in this trial and no evidence of compromise of treatment outcome in patients receiving palifermin.

A phase II trial was subsequently performed in which the same type of patient population received concurrent chemoradiation. Patients were randomized 2:1 between palifermin and placebo. Institutions had the discretion to deliver radiotherapy via conventional once-daily 2-Gy fractions or with an accelerated hyperfractionated regimen of 1.25 Gy bid. One hundred patients were enrolled on this trial, of whom 34 received accelerated hyperfractionation and the remainder received standard fractionation. Palifermin was delivered at a dose of 60 μg/kg. Again, the first dose was delivered prior to the initiation of CRT and then every Friday afternoon after the last fraction of radiation. Two additional doses of palifermin were given 1 and 2 wk after the completion of radiotherapy for a total of 10 doses of the drug. Palifermin did not reduce the incidence or duration of mucosal or salivary gland toxicity. The subset of patients receiving hyperfractionated radiation, however, showed significant improvements in the duration and severity of mucositis. They also had improved swallowing function and less salivary gland toxicity relative to patients who received placebo.

The relative lack of success of palifermin in the head and neck setting in the transplant context would appear to be multifactorial. To begin with, the dose intensity of palifermin was significantly greater in the transplant trial than in the head and neck studies. Cumulative doses of 180 μg/kg were sandwiched around a dose of 1200 cGy of radiotherapy. This contrasts with doses of 60–80 μg/kg that were sandwiched around 1000–1200 cGy in the head and neck studies. The effect of this lesser dose intensity of palifermin would then have been amplified by the significantly larger doses of mucosal irradiation that are delivered for head and neck cancer as opposed to bone marrow transplant conditioning. Lastly, the head and neck trials used the RTOG/CTCT version 2.0 scale for mucositis assessment. This scale mandates a cutoff of assessment 90 d after the initiation of therapy. Mucositis after concurrent CRT for head and neck cancer will commonly persist for more than 6 wk beyond the completion of treatment, the implications of which are that mucositis is still present at the end of the 90-day cutoff date. Thus, the scoring system used in these trials was insensitive in terms of distinguishing a difference between a patient whose mucositis resolved 91 d after the initiation of therapy vs 120 d after the completion of therapy. Further investigation of palifermin is indicated in head and neck cancer. Future strategies will probably include more intensive administration of the drug and utilization of the more up-to-date CTC version 3.0 toxicity scoring scheme.

Radioprotectors and radiation mitigators are both designed with the intent of minimizing the risk of clonogenic death of normal cells and subsequent disruption of the protective mucosal barrier. Head and neck radiotherapy also initiates a local cytokine cascade, which includes interleukin-1, and -6, and tumor necrosis factor (TNF)-α. An inflammatory response results, which contributes to the ultimate anatomic disruption of the mucosa. Secondary bacterial and fungal overgrowth are thought to exacerbate the local pathophysiology.

Sucralfate, a basic aluminum salt of sucrose, has long been used in the treatment of peptic ulcer disease. It provides a protective coating to ulcerated tissue by means of binding to exposed proteins in damaged cells (36). It also stimulates mucus production, mitosis, and surface migration of cells. Sucralfate has been tested in several double-blind placebo-controlled randomized trials. Despite the attractive conceptual nature of using it to ameliorate mucositis, the clinical data do not show any benefit from sucralfate (37–40).

Benzydamine HCl is a nonsteroidal antiinflammatory drug that also posses antimicrobial activity (41). It is a potent inhibitor of TNF-α (42). This particular proinflammatory cytokine is upregulated in mucosal tissue of the head and neck regions, with peak levels typically peak at approx 2000 cGy (conventionally fractionated) just prior to the first signs of mucosal ulceration. The ability of benzydamine to reduce mucositis during head and neck radiotherapy was tested in a randomized double-blind placebo-controlled trial (43). The primary end point of this trial was the area under the curve for the mean mucositis score over a cumulative radiotherapy dose up to a total dose of 5000 cGy. Secondary end points included use of concomitant pain medication, oral pain at rest and with eating, body weight, and the use of enteral nutritional support.

Benzydamine therapy resulted in a 30% reduction in mucosal erythema and ulceration. Most of this benefit was observed once doses greater than 2500 cGy had been delivered. One-third of the benzydamine patients did not develop any mucosal ulceration at all, compared with only 18% of the placebo-treated patients ($p = 0.04$). There was a nonsignificant trend toward reduction in mouth pain at rest for the patients who received benzydamine. Importantly, benzydamine was no more effective than placebo with respect to the reduction of pain during meals. Cumulative weight loss during radiotherapy was equivalent in the two treatment groups. There was no difference in the proportion of patients who required enteral nutritional support between the two treatment arms.

The data from the benzydamine trials suggest that this agent is active against mucositis but are clearly inconclusive with respect to whether or not it has any clinical role in the treatment of this condition. There was no significant benefit regarding the functional sequelae of mucositis. Most patients received radiotherapy doses of 6400–7400 cGy. Mucosal assessment was not performed beyond 5000 cGy. This aspect of the study design may explain the discordance between the improvement in the anatomic assessment of mucosal integrity associated with benzydamine and the lack of any functional benefit, as the latter parameters were assessed throughout a patient's entire course of radiotherapy. The most severe mucositis during a course of head and neck radiotherapy occurs beyond the 5000-cGy level. Fewer than 10% of the patients enrolled in this trial received concurrent chemotherapy, even though most of them had stage III/IV disease. Concurrent CRT has become the standard of care for most patients with this extent of disease. Thus, the clinical value of benzydamine has not been proved for patients receiving high-dose radiotherapy with or without concurrent chemotherapy.

Endogenous oral flora may exacerbate the mucosal inflammatory process once the mucosal integrity is disrupted. This secondary infection may prolong the course of mucositis. Protegrins are naturally occurring peptides that have broad-spectrum antimicrobial activity *(44)*. Iseganan is a synthetic analog of this class of compounds. A placebo-controlled trial in patients receiving chemotherapy suggested that iseganan reduced the incidence of ulcerative stomatitis and decreased both mouth pain and swallowing difficulty. Consequently, a phase III double-blind, placebo-controlled trial was launched in patients receiving head and neck radiotherapy *(45)*.

This trial allowed different fractionation schemes but mandated that a minimum dose of 6000 cGy be delivered. Forty percent of the patients enrolled received concurrent chemotherapy. The study contained three treatment arms: iseganan plus standard oral care, placebo plus standard oral care, and supportive oral care only.

Iseganan and placebo were completely equivalent to one another with respect to all end points in the trial. Interestingly enough, iseganan and placebo were both superior to standard oral care. Two-thirds of the patients in both arms had confluent mucositis compared with 79% in the supportive oral care arm ($p = 0.02$). Only 2% of the SOC patients had no mucosal ulceration vs 9% in both the iseganan and placebo arms ($p = 0.04$). Peak mouth pain and difficulty swallowing were also significantly worse for the patients assigned to supportive oral care. Radiotherapy dose reductions were also significantly more common in the supportive oral care patients.

The iseganan trial did not show any benefit associated with the administration of the study drug, but it did, however, demonstrate the importance of adherence to a strict regimen of oral hygiene during head and neck radiotherapy. Patients on both the drug and placebo arms were instructed to swish and gargle prior to each administration of study drug. They also maintained study diaries to help ensure adequate compliance with administration of the study drug. These interventions were not performed in the patients assigned to supportive oral care. Despite the absence of benefit associated with iseganan therapy, this trial has made a very important contribution toward the development of new therapies for mucositis through its demonstration of the value of organized and systematic attention to the maintenance of good oral hygiene throughout a course of head and neck CRT.

REFERENCES

1. Thomas GM. Improved treatment for cervical cancer—concurrent chemotherapy and radiotherapy. N Engl J Med 1999; 340:1198–1200.
2. Rose PG, Bundy BN, Watkins EB, et al. Concurrent cisplatin-based radiotherapy and chemotherapy for locally advanced cervical cancer. N Engl J Med 1999; 340:1144–1153.
3. Morris M, Eifel PJ, Lu J, et al. Pelvic radiation with concurrent chemotherapy compared with pelvic and para-aortic radiation for high-risk cervical cancer. N Engl J Med 1999; 340:1137–1143.
4. Keys HM, Bundy BN, Stehman FB, et al. Cisplatin, radiation, and adjuvant hysterectomy compared with radiation and adjuvant hysterectomy for bulky stage IB cervical carcinoma. N Engl J Med 1999; 340:1154–1161.
5. Cooper JS, Guo MD, Herskovic A, et al. Chemoradiotherapy of locally advanced esophageal cancer: long-term follow-up of a prospective randomized trial (RTOG 85-01). Radiation Therapy Oncology Group. JAMA 1999; 281:1623–1627.
6. Murray N, Coy P, Pater JL, et al. Importance of timing for thoracic irradiation in the combined modality treatment of limited-stage small-cell lung cancer. The National Cancer Institute of Canada Clinical Trials Group. J Clin Oncol 1993; 11:336–344.
7. Pignon JP, Bourhis J, Domenge C, et al. Chemotherapy added to locoregional treatment for head and neck squamous-cell carcinoma: three meta-analyses of updated individual data. MACH-NC Collaborative Group. Meta-Analysis of Chemotherapy on Head and Neck Cancer. Lancet 2000; 355:949–955.
8. Forastiere AA, Goepfert H, Maor M, et al. Concurrent chemotherapy and radiotherapy for organ preservation in advanced laryngeal cancer. N Engl J Med 2003; 349:2091–2098.
9. Al-Sarraf M, LeBlanc M, Giri PG, et al. Chemoradiotherapy versus radiotherapy in patients with advanced nasopharyngeal cancer: phase III randomized Intergroup study 0099. J Clin Oncol 1998; 16:1310–1317.
10. Brizel DM, Albers ME, Fisher SR, et al. Hyperfractionated irradiation with or without concurrent chemotherapy for locally advanced head and neck cancer. N Engl J Med 1998; 338:1798–1804.
11. Dobrowsky W, Naude J. Continuous hyperfractionated accelerated radiotherapy with/without mitomycin C in head and neck cancers. Radiother Oncol 2000; 57:119–124.
12. Jeremic B, Shibamoto Y, Milicic B, et al. Hyperfractionated radiation therapy with or without concurrent low-dose daily cisplatin in locally advanced squamous cell carcinoma of the head and neck: a prospective randomized trial. J Clin Oncol 2000; 18:1458–1464.
13. Budach VG DS, Haake K, Stuschke M, et al. Accelerated chemoradiation to 70.6 Gy is more effective than accelerated radiaiton to 77.6 Gy alone- two year results of a German multicenter randomized trial. Int J Radiat Oncol Biol Phys 2000; 48(Supp):150.
14. Wendt TG, Grabenbauer GG, Rodel CM, et al. Simultaneous radiochemotherapy versus radiotherapy alone in advanced head and neck cancer: a randomized multicenter study. J Clin Oncol 1998; 16:1318–1324.
15. Denis F, Garaud P, Bardet E, et al. Final results of the 94-01 French Head and Neck Oncology and Radiotherapy Group randomized trial comparing radiotherapy alone with concomitant radiochemotherapy in advanced-stage oropharynx carcinoma. J Clin Oncol 2004; 22:69–76.
16. Bernier J, Domenge C, Ozsahin M, et al. Postoperative irradiation with or without concomitant chemotherapy for locally advanced head and neck cancer. N Engl J Med 2004; 350:1945–1952.
17. Cooper JS, Pajak TF, Forastiere AA, et al. Postoperative concurrent radiotherapy and chemotherapy for high-risk squamous-cell carcinoma of the head and neck. N Engl J Med 2004; 350:1937–1944.
18. Denis F, Garaud P, Bardet E, et al. Late toxicity results of the GORTEC 94-01 randomized trial comparing radiotherapy with concomitant radiochemotherapy for advanced-stage oropharynx carcinoma: comparison of LENT/SOMA, RTOG/EORTC, and NCI-CTC scoring systems. Int J Radiat Oncol Biol Phys 2003, 55:93–98.
19. Maguire PD, Meyerson MB, Neal CR, et al. Toxic cure: hyperfractionated radiotherapy with concurrent cisplatin and fluorouracil for stage III and IVA head-and-neck cancer in the community. Int J Radiat Oncol Biol Phys 2004; 58:698–704.
20. Horiot JC, Le Fur R, N'Guyen T, et al. Hyperfractionation versus conventional fractionation in oropharyngeal carcinoma: final analysis of a randomized trial of the EORTC cooperative group of radiotherapy. Radiother Oncol 1992; 25:231–241.
21. Eisbruch A, Ten Haken RK, Kim HM, et al. Dose, volume, and function relationships in parotid salivary glands following conformal and intensity-modulated irradiation of head and neck cancer. Int J Radiat Oncol Biol Phys 1999; 45:577–587.

22. Garden AS, Morrison WH, Wong P, et al. Preliminary results of intensity modulated radiation therapy for small primary oropharyngeal carcinoma. Int J Radiat Oncol Biol Phys 2003; 57:S407.

23. Millar JA, Burke V. Relationship between sample size and the definition of equivalence in non-inferiority drug studies. J Clin Pharm Ther 2002; 27:329–333.

24. Yuhas JM, Spellman JM, Culo F. The role of WR-2721 in radiotherapy and/or chemotherapy. Cancer Clin Trials 1980; 3:211–216.

25. Brizel DM, Wasserman TH, Henke M, et al. Phase III randomized trial of amifostine as a radioprotector in head and neck cancer. J Clin Oncol 2000; 18:3339–3345.

26. Anne PR, Curran WJ, Jr. A phase II trial of subcutaneous amifostine and radiation therapy in patients with head and neck cancer. Semin Radiat Oncol 2002; 12:18,19.

27. Lindegaard JC, Grau C. Has the outlook improved for amifostine as a clinical radioprotector? Radiother Oncol 2000; 57:113–118.

28. Simon RM. Clinical trials in cancer. In: DeVita H, Rosenberg, eds. Cancer Priniciples and Practice of Oncology. Philadelphia: Lippincott-Raven, 1997:520–521.

29. Fu KK, Pajak TF, Trotti A, et al. A Radiation Therapy Oncology Group (RTOG) phase III randomized study to compare hyperfractionation and two variants of accelerated fractionation to standard fractionation radiotherapy for head and neck squamous cell carcinomas: first report of RTOG 9003. Int J Radiat Oncol Biol Phys 2000; 48:7–16.

30. Koukourakis MI, Kyrias G, Kakolyris S, et al. Subcutaneous administration of amifostine during fractionated radiotherapy: a randomized phase II study. J Clin Oncol 2000; 18:2226–2233.

31. Antonadou D, Pepelassi M, Synodinou M, et al. Prophylactic use of amifostine to prevent radiochemotherapy-induced mucositis and xerostomia in head-and-neck cancer. Int J Radiat Oncol Biol Phys 2002; 52:739–747, 2002

32. Buntzel J, Glatzel M, Kuttner K, et al. Amifostine in simultaneous radiochemotherapy of advanced head and neck cancer. Semin Radiat Oncol 2002; 12:4–13.

33. Potten CS, O'Shea JA, Farrell CL, et al. The effects of repeated doses of keratinocyte growth factor on cell proliferation in the cellular hierarchy of the crypts of the murine small intestine. Cell Growth Differ 2001; 12:265–275, 2001

34. Dorr W, Spekl K, Farrell CL. Amelioration of acute oral mucositis by keratinocyte growth factor: fractionated irradiation. Int J Radiat Oncol Biol Phys 2002; 54:245–251.

35. Dorr W, Spekl K, Farrell CL. The effect of keratinocyte growth factor on healing of manifest radiation ulcers in mouse tongue epithelium. Cell Prolif 2002; 35(Suppl 1):86–92.

36. Martin F, Farley A, Gagnon M, et al. Comparison of the healing capacities of sucralfate and cimetidine in the short-term treatment of duodenal ulcer: a double-blind randomized trial. Gastroenterology 1982; 82:401–405.

37. Carter DL, Hebert ME, Smink K, et al. Double blind randomized trial of sucralfate vs placebo during radical radiotherapy for head and neck cancers. Head Neck 1999; 21:760–766.

38. Pfeiffer P, Madsen EL, Hansen O, et al. Effect of prophylactic sucralfate suspension on stomatitis induced by cancer chemotherapy. A randomized, double-blind cross-over study. Acta Oncol 1990; 29:171–173.

39. Meredith R, Salter M, Kim R, et al. Sucralfate for radiation mucositis: results of a double-blind randomized trial. Int J Radiat Oncol Biol Phys 1997; 37:275–279.

40. Makkonen TA, Bostrom P, Vilja P, et al. Sucralfate mouth washing in the prevention of radiation-induced mucositis: a placebo-controlled double-blind randomized study. Int J Radiat Oncol Biol Phys 1994; 30:177–182.

41. Segre G, Hammarstrom S. Aspects of the mechanisms of action of benzydamine. Int J Tissue React 1985; 7:187–193.

42. Sironi M, Pozzi P, Polentarutti N, et al. Inhibition of inflammatory cytokine production and protection against endotoxin toxicity by benzydamine. Cytokine 1996; 8:710–716.

43. Epstein JB, Silverman S, Jr., Paggiarino DA, et al. Benzydamine HCl for prophylaxis of radiation-induced oral mucositis: results from a multicenter, randomized, double-blind, placebo-controlled clinical trial. Cancer 2001; 92:875–885.

44. Bellm L, Lehrer RI, Ganz T. Protegrins: new antibiotics of mammalian origin. Expert Opin Investig Drugs 2000; 9:1731–1742.

45. Trotti A, Garden A, Warde P, et al. A multinational, randomized phase III trial of iseganan HCl oral solution for reducing the severity of oral mucositis in patients receiving radiotherapy for head-and-neck malignancy. Int J Radiat Oncol Biol Phys 2004; 58:674–681.

17

Targeted Therapies
in Head and Neck Cancer

Tanguy Y. Seiwert, MD and Ezra E. W. Cohen, MD

1. INTRODUCTION

Squamous cell carcinoma of the head and neck (HNSCC) can be treated with various modalities including radiotherapy, chemotherapy, and surgery. These are often employed in combination, with each playing a substantial and complementary role. Using a multidisciplinary approach, investigators have recently been able to achieve improved survival outcomes for patients with locally advanced, nonmetastatic disease—including both increased long-term survival rates (now approaching 70% in recent reports) *(1–3)* and organ preservation *(4,5)*. Nevertheless, in approx 50% of high-risk patients tumors will recur *(1–3,6)*, often with distant metastasis, making the cancer incurable and shifting the treatment goal toward palliation. In addition, short- and long-term toxicities of combination therapy are significant, with xerostomia, esophageal strictures, dysphagia, and increased aspiration risk commonly encountered.

The last decade has witnessed startling advances in so-called targeted therapies in oncology. The approval of agents such as imatinib, rituximab, trastuzumab, erlotonib, bevacizumab, and cetuximab has started to change management significantly in several solid and liquid tumors. In fact, we are still in the process of establishing the best way to integrate these novel options with existing therapies. Unlike cytotoxic chemotherapy, which interrupts normal mitotic activity in all dividing cells, targeted therapies are rationally designed to interfere with cancer-specific markers or signaling pathways. Given their higher specificity, they are expected to be better tolerated, have a higher therapeutic index, be effective at doses lower than the maximum tolerated dose, and differ from cytotoxics in their side effect profile.

Given the current treatment limitations in HNSCC, the hope is that the introduction of targeted therapies will further improve clinical outcomes and at the same time reduce toxicities. This chapter gives an overview of novel compounds that are being investigated in HNSCC, some of which are in late-stage clinical trials and may be considered for regulatory approval in the near future. Integrating these targeted therapies with radiotherapy or chemoradiotherapy (CRT) will be vital for the advancement of HNSCC treatment.

2. MOLECULAR BIOLOGY OF HNSCC

It has been estimated that in order for HNSCC to develop, cells require the accumulation of 6–10 genetic alterations *(7)*. In HNSCC, as in all cancers, these fall into two categories—

From: *Current Clinical Oncology: Squamous Cell Head and Neck Cancer*
Edited by: D. J. Adelstein © Humana Press Inc., Totowa, NJ

Table 1
Selected Oncogenes Involved in HNSCC

Oncogene	Description	Timing in carcinogenesis	Chromosomal location	Prevalence in HNSCC	Comments
CyclinD1	Cell cycle regulator—G1/S transition leads to tumor progression	Late	11q13	30% of tumors have gene amplification	Rb and p16 are negative regulators of cyclin D1
				Lack of inhibition (p16, Rb) in majority of tumors	Rb and p16 are frequently inactivated
EGFR	Receptor tyrosine kinase—heterodimerizes with other members of erb family activates multiple oncogenic signaling pathways (e.g., MAPK, Akt, Stat-3)	Early to mid	7p12	10–20% mutated or amplified	Target for multiple agents (e.g., gefitinib, cetuximab)
				80–90% overexpressed	Mutations found in lung cancer, but none seen in HNSCC in early tests
				Early studies suggest over-expression does not correlate with responsiveness	Overexpression increases progressively from precancerous lesions to invasive tumor
Met	Receptor tyrosine kinase—with role in progression, invasion, metastasis, angiogenesis	Unclear	7q31	>50% overexpress met receptor	Potent activity in vitro, small-molecule inhibitors in development
				~11% harbor mutations	
Cyclooxygenase 2 (COX-2)	Prostagladin synthesis	Early	1q25	Overexpressed in most tumors	COX-2 inhibitors (e.g., celecoxib) being investigated regarding chemoprevention
p63	Involved in epithelial renewal oncogenic possibly via β catenin pathway	Early	3q	~30%	Together with 9p altered early in carcinogenesis

Abbreviations: EGFR, epidermal growth factor receptor; HNSCC, head and neck squamous cell carcinoma; MAPK, mitogen-activated protein kinase.

Table 2
Selected Tumor Suppressor Genes Altered in HNSCC

Tumor suppressor gene	Description	Timing	location	Chromosomal HNSCC	Prevalence in Comments
p16^{ink4a}	Negative regulator of cyclin D1; physiologically leads to senescence; if abrogated, cell cycle progression	Early	9p21	~80% inactivation through deletion, point mutations, methylation	Most common genetic change in HNSCC. Commonly found in premalignant lesions
p53	Central role in cell cycle regulation and cell survival	Early to mid	17p13	Mutations in >50% of HNSCC	p53 mutations occur between preinvasive and invasive stage; implicated in tumor progression. Mutations predict chemotherapy treatment failures
3p (chromosome location)	Location of multiple tumor suppressor genes (e.g., FHIT, RASSF1A)	Early	3p21	Altered in most HNSCC	Together with alterations in 9p21 early and common event in HNSCCs carcinogenesis
PTEN	Phosphatase that negatively regulates signaling/migration via PI3K signaling to AKT and PKB	Unclear	10q23	10–29%	Inactivated through multiple mechanisms—methylation, monoallelic loss, mutations
Rb	Regulates cell cycle at stage of G1/S transition (via p16)	Unclear	13q	13q loss in ~60% of tumors; Rb altered only in subgroup	Second TSG may exist adjacently
TGF-β	Receptor serine/threonine kinase negative growth regulator leading to G1/S arrest via downstream regulators	Unclear	9q22	Mutations found in one series in 6 of 28	Alteration in chromosomes 3p and 9p occur early in carcinogenesis
RAR-β	Involved in cell differentiation via induction of multiple gene products	Early	3p	Downregulated, e.g., via promoter hyper-methylation	Investigated regarding role in chemoprevention. Involved in genesis of leukoplakia lesions

Abbreviations: HNSCC, hean and neck squamous cell carcinoma; PI3K, phosphatidylinositol 3 kinase; RAR, retinoic acid receptor; TGF, transforming growth factor.

241

activation of protooncogenes and inactivation of tumor suppressor genes. Tables 1 and 2 give an overview of genetic changes that are frequently reported and felt to be important in HNSCC carcinogenesis.

Although most HNSCC tumors are smoking and alcohol related, tumors of the palatine tonsils and the base of the tongue frequently contain oncogenic human papilloma virus (HPV) DNA and form a distinct subgroup found frequently in nonsmokers (8). These are less likely to harbor p53 mutations and are correlated with an improved stage- and disease-specific survival. In contrast, tumors of the larynx, hypopharynx, and floor of mouth are nearly always substance use related (9,10).

The hypothesized progression from normal mucosa to hyperplasia, dysplasia, carcinoma in situ, and invasive carcinoma has been studied extensively. Early carcinogenic molecular events include 9p (p16) inactivation and 3p loss—both of which involve tumor suppressor genes central to HNSCC genesis (11,12). This is apparently followed by alterations on chromosome 17p, which is seen in the progression of preinvasive to invasive lesions (13,14). Other events follow, as outlined in Tables 1 and 2. The exact sequence of events varies and may be different for different molecular subgroups.

Early insults are felt to induce field cancerization—the expansion of a common clonal progenitor to a large area—and may explain the frequent occurrence of metachronous or synchronous tumors (15–18). Field cancerization therefore forms the rationale for the use of primary prophylaxis with chemopreventative agents. Retinoic acid derivates have been most extensively studied in this regard; however, they have thus far either been ineffective at low doses or associated with unacceptable mucocutaneous toxicity at high doses.

Chemoprevention may be best aimed at premalignant lesions showing 3p and 9p alterations; persistence of these changes has been shown to correlate with progressive lesions and poor outcome (19). More recently it has also been suggested that DNA content and aneuploidy can be powerful predictors of progression to invasive cancer as well as treatment failure and mortality (20,21). How this will be integrated with previous molecular progression models needs to be further elucidated.

Many of these alterations are currently being investigated as targets for novel, targeted therapies. Thus far relatively few drugs have been approved, but it is expected that many more will follow. This chapter provides an overview of the current status of these agents and the various stages of clinical development.

3. EPIDERMAL GROWTH FACTOR RECEPTOR

The epidermal growth factor receptor (EGFR; synonymous with erbB1 or Her1) is a membrane-bound receptor tyrosine kinase. It is part of a family of four receptors (erbB1–B4) that are activated after binding of their respective ligands by dimerization (homo- or heterodimerization) and phosphorylation of intracellular tyrosine residues (Fig. 1). erbB2 (her2/neu) does not have a known ligand in vivo and is activated by heterodimerization with other family members (e.g., EGFR). Upon activation, intracellular signaling cascades mediate a multitude of functions including cell proliferation, survival, invasion, metastasis, and angiogenesis (Fig. 1). Invoked signaling cascades include the Ras/Raf/mitogen-activated protein kinase (MAPK), phosphatidylinositol 3 kinase (PI3K)/AKT/mammalian target of rapamycin (mTOR), and Janus kinase (Jak)/signal activator and transducer of infection (Stat)/protein kinase C (PKC) pathways (22). EGFR and other erbB receptors are deregulated in multiple solid tumors including lung, breast, colorectal, and also HNSCC. In fact, 80 to 90% of HNSCC

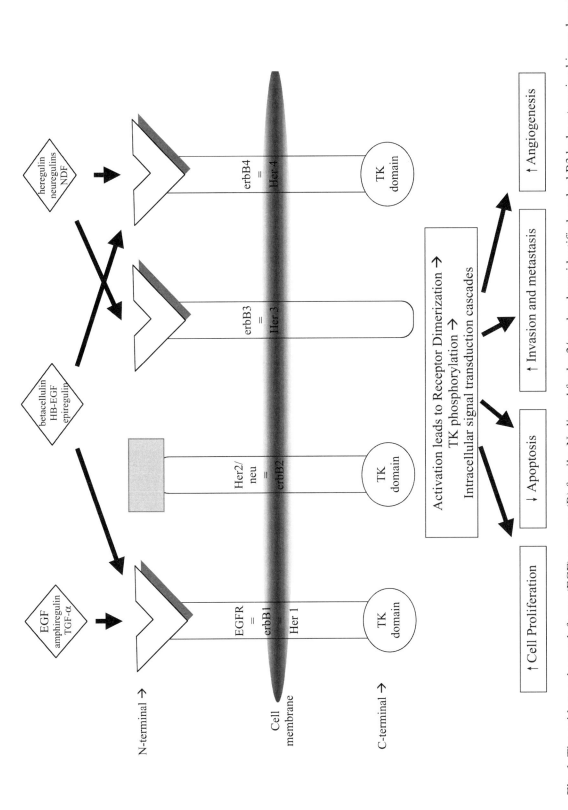

Fig. 1. The epidermaol growth factor (EGF) receptor (R) family. No ligand for her2/neu has been identified, and erbB3 lacks a tyrosine kinase domain. TK, tyrosine kinase; TGF-α, transforming growth factor-α.

overexpress EGFR, and overexpression increases progressively from early precancerous lesions to invasive tumors *(23,24)*. Overexpression of its ligands is also frequently present, suggesting an autocrine signaling loop. EGFR expression has been suggested to confer an adverse prognosis, as it correlates with increased tumor size, presentation with more advanced stage, decreased survival, increased risk of recurrence, and decreased radiation sensitivity *(25–29)*. In general, four mechanisms of increased activity have been described: receptor overexpression, receptor mutations, overproduction of ligand (auto- and paracrine), and activation through other receptor systems (e.g., uPA receptor [UPAR]).

Given the role EGFR plays in the progression of tumors and its importance in early precancerous lesions, EGFR quickly became an interesting target for the development of novel therapies. Multiple strategies have been pursued with the aim of inhibiting EGFR signaling. Only two strategies have so far come to clinical fruition: monoclonal antibodies to the extracellular domain of EGFR and small-molecule inhibitors of the intracellular tyrosine kinase domain. An overview of the agents undergoing clinical trials is shown in Table 3. Alternative approaches using inhibition of receptor trafficking and EGFR synthesis have so far not been used outside of preclinical model systems. In the future it may be possible to improve the efficacy of antibodies by attaching bacterial toxins or radionuclides allowing specific delivery to tumor cells. The EGFR ligand, transforming growth factor (TGF)-α has been linked to the *Pseudomonas* endotoxin TP-38 and is currently in phase I/II clinical trials (TGF-α-PE38 immunotoxin [TP-38]) employing intratumoral administration.

Both EGFR small-molecule inhibitors and anti-EGFR monoclonal antibodies lead to inhibition of the signal transduction, but only antibodies achieve downregulation of EGFR expression. Observed effects of these agents include cell cycle arrest in the G1 phase, decreased tumor vascularization (presumably by downregulation of vascular endothelial growth factor [VEGF]), and increased apoptosis *(30–35)*. The small-molecule inhibitors are available orally for daily dosing, whereas monoclonal antibodies are administered intravenously with half-lives that allow weekly to every 3-wk dosing. Both classes of EGFR inhibitors have a favorable side effect profile, with very few grade 3 and 4 toxicities reported. Both classes of agents cause a characteristic acneiform rash that has been correlated in clinical trials with response and survival *(36–38)*. Small-molecule EGFR inhibitors have been reported to cause gastrointestinal upset *(37–39)*, and gefitinib has been associated in rare cases with severe pulmonary pneumonitis. This has only been observed in patients with lung cancer with an approx 1% incidence rate, although one-third of cases are fatal *(40)*. This toxicity appears to be far more common in the Japanese population, for unknown reasons.

3.1. Clinical Trial Results With EGFR Inhibitors

The use of cetuximab in HNSCC was first reported in a dose-finding phase IB study in combination with cisplatin *(41)*. No dose-limiting toxicities were observed; therefore surrogates such as receptor saturation (measured by immunohistochemistry), tyrosine kinase assays, and EGF/EGFR immunoblots were used to establish the current dosing of 400 mg/m^2 loading and 250 mg/m^2 maintenance administered weekly. Even in patients with high EGFR expression, this dose achieved approx 95% receptor saturation. In 6 of 9 patients with known cisplatin-refractory metastatic disease, partial responses were observed (12 patients total in the trial). Subsequently, in larger phase II trials, response rates in refractory metastatic disease of 11–14% were reported *(42–44)*. The combination of cetuximab with cisplatin vs cisplatin alone was reported in an ECOG trial in 200 treatment-naïve patients. Despite a significantly improved

Table 3
Novel Agents Targeting the EGFR Pathway

EGFR inhibitor	Class	Administration	Common toxicities	Comments
Monoclonal antibodies				
Cetuximab (C225, Erbitux™)	Chimeric monoclonal antibody	Intravenous	Cutaneous, allergic	FDA approved for colorectal cancer In combination with radiation (vs radiation alone) shown to have improved survival in HNSCC (45)
EMD 72000	Humanized monoclonal antibody	Intravenous	Cutaneous	
h-R3	Humanized monoclonal antibody	Intravenous	Hemodynamic, systemic	
Panitumumab (ABX-EGF)	Humanized monoclonal antibody	Intravenous	Cutaneous	
Immunotoxins				
TGF-α-PE38 immunotoxin (TP-38)	TGF-α linked to toxin	Intratumoral	Phase I study ongoing	TGF-α linked to *Pseudomonas* entotoxin TP-38 protein; administered intratumorally
Small molecules				
Gefitinib (ZD1839 Iressa™)	Reversible tyrosine kinase inhibitor	Oral	Cutaneous, gastrointestinal, rare pneumonitis described mostly in Japanese patients with lung cancer	FDA approved for third line treatment in NSCLC Response rates as single agent in first and second line therapy 3–10%, with larger proportion of patients having disease stabilization
Erlotinib (OSI-774 Tarceva™)	Reversible tyrosine kinase inhibitor	Oral	Cutaneous, gastrointestinal	
PKI-166	Reversible tyrosine kinase inhibitor	Oral	Cutaneous, gastrointestinal, systemic, liver	

(continued)

Table 3 (continued)

EGFR inhibitor	Class	Administration	Common toxicities	Comments
Lapatinib (GW572016)	Reversible tyrosine kinase inhibitor	Oral	Cutaneous, gastrointestinal, systemic	Inhibits both EGFR and her-2/neu
Canertinib (CI-1033)	Irreversible tyrosine kinase inhibitor	Oral	Cutaneous, oral, systemic, gastrointestinal	Pan-erbB inhibitor

Abbreviations: EGF(R), epidermal growth factor receptor; FDA, Food and Drug Administration; NSCLC, non-small cell lung cancer; TGF-α, transforming growth factor-α.
Modified from ref. 22.

response rate and a trend in favor of the experimental arm, statistical significance in progression-free survival was not established.

Recently, the activity of cetuximab activity in HNSCC was demonstrated most clearly in a trial of cetuximab in combination with radiation vs radiation alone in locally advanced HNSCC. The results, presented in abstract form only, revealed a marked benefit with respect to local control and median overall survival of 54 vs 28 mo in the experimental and control arms, respectively (45). Although these observations will not immediately alter the standard of care, this trial suggests that EGFR inhibitory strategies enhance the beneficial effect of radiotherapy with manageable toxicity. The integration of these agents with current approaches should follow.

The second class of anti-EGFR agents, small-molecule EGFR inhibitors, block intracellular ATP binding to EGFR and prevent phosphorylation and activation of the receptor. Gefitinib (Iressa™) and erlotinib (Tarceva™) were approved for nonsmall cell lung cancer (NSCLC) in 2003 and 2004 (46). In HNSCC cell lines as well as xenograft models, gefitinib showed highly potent antitumor activity (47). In cell lines, combination with chemotherapy and radiation was synergistic (48,49).

Two phase II trials of gefitinib therapy in patients with recurrent or metastatic HNSCC showed modest response rates (38,50), with the higher dose of gefitinib appearing to be more active. In the trial using the higher 500-mg daily dose, a response rate of 11% was reported, with a clinical benefit in 53% of patients and a median overall survival of 8.1 mo. A subsequent trial administering 250 mg/d and enrolling a similar cohort of patients, however demonstrated a response rate of only 1%, with a 5.2-mo median overall survival. These findings would suggest that a dose–response relationship exists for gefitinib in HNSCC and that 500 mg is a more optimal dose than 250 mg. Nevertheless, both trials reported a correlation of the development of rash with clinical benefit. Randomized trials are currently ongoing to evaluate the role of gefitinib in recurrent or metastatic HNSCC.

Recently, early data of a phase I trial combining gefitinib with celecoxib were reported (51). The regimen was well tolerated, without dose-limiting toxicities. Three of nine patients had a response (33%), suggesting potentially enhanced activity over gefitinib alone, and phase II testing is planned. Furthermore, gefinitib has been used in combination with chemotherapy as well as chemoradiotherapy (CRT). The University of Chicago has tested gefitinib as part of a 5-fluorouracil (5-FU), hydroxyurea, twice-daily radiation (FHX) platform in treatment-naïve, curative-intent patients. Efficacy results are premature, but it appears that gefitinib is well tolerated as part of a CRT regimen.

Erlotonib is the second reversible EGFR inhibitor that has been studied in HNSCC and has shown overall results comparable to those of gefitinib. In a 29-center, phase II study comprising 114 patients with advanced HNSCC, erlotinib showed partial responses in 4% and disease stabilization in 38% of patients *(52)*. Common side effects again were acneiform rash and diarrhea *(52)*. Increased rash severity was also correlated with an increase in survival *(36,52)*. Recently investigators from the University of Chicago reported early data on a phase I trial combining erlotinib and bevacizumab *(53)*, with encouraging results (nine evaluable patients: one partial response, seven stable disease, and one progressive disease). Bevacizumab is discussed further in Subheading 4.

Other agents, including PKI-66, lapatinib (GW572016), and CI-1033 are in phase I and II clinical trials. They may be somewhat different in their activity, as they inhibit additional members of the erbB family and CI-1033 binds irreversibly.

In summary, anti-EGFR agents, including both monoclonal antibodies and small-molecule inhibitors, are in the process of finding their role in HNSCC. Single agent activity has been demonstrated and, based on ongoing and recent trials, approval of these agents is likely in the near future. Cetuximab, gefitinib, and erlotinib are most advanced in their development and clinical evaluation.

4. ANGIOGENESIS

Angiogenesis is the process of forming new blood vessels to support growth in both normal and tumor tissue. During the past decade it has been increasingly appreciated to what degree tumors rely on angiogenesis for their continued growth. In fact, it has been demonstrated that solid tumors will not grow larger than 2–3 mm in diameter in the absence of new blood vessels and furthermore rely on angiogenesis to form metastases *(54–57)*. The process of angiogenesis is mediated by a multitude of pro- and antiangiogenic factors, many of which are redundant and stand in a well-regulated balance with each other *(58)*. The proangiogenic factors that are known to play a role in HNSCC are listed in Table 4. Among the proangiogenic factors, VEGF plays a central role in neovascularization. After more than 15 yr of research the anti-VEGF antibody bevacizumab (Avastin™) was recently approved in the treatment of colon cancer *(59)* but has also shown activity in several other tumors. The importance of VEGF in HNSCC biology is also well established *(60–63)*.

VEGF signals primarily via a transmembrane tyrosine kinase receptor called VEGFR-2 (also known as KDR or Flk-1) and induces endothelial cell proliferation and survival *(55,64)*. Inhibition of the VEGF pathway markedly decreases angiogenesis and inhibits the growth of tumors (including HNSCC) in nude mice *(65,66)*. Multiple antiangiogenic strategies have been pursued including antibodies to VEGF (e.g., bevacizumab), the inhibition of the receptor (VEGFR-2) via monoclonal antibodies or small-molecule inhibitors, the administration of natural or synthetical antiangiogenic factors to counterbalance proangiogenic stimuli, inhibition of enzymes that degrade the extracellular matrix, integrin antagonists, and therapies with direct endothelial cell toxicity. In HNSCC so far only the first two strategies have been employed.

Somewhat particular to HNSCC was the concern that, because of the central role of radiation therapy, which relies on adequate oxygenation, inhibition of angiogenesis could potentially create larger hypoxic areas, leading to radiation resistance. However, recent data suggest

Table 4
Angiogenic Factors Secreted by Keratinocytes and HNSCC

Factor	Alternate name	Function
AFGF	FGF1	Universal FGFR ligand
BFGF	FGF2	Wide-spectrum mitogenic, angiogenic, and neurotrophic factor; high brain concentrations
VEGF		Vascular endothelial cell mitogen
PDGF		Wide-spectrum mitogen
PD-ECGF	Thymidine phosphorylase	Highly restricted endothelial cell mitogen
TGF-α		Principal EGFR ligand
TGF-β		Multifunctional; controls proliferation and differentiation; negative autocrine growth factor
IGF-I	Somatomedin C	Wide-spectrum mitogen, especially skeletal muscle
IGF-II	Somatomedin A	Wide-spectrum mitogen, especially muscle growth and differentiation
HGF	Scatter factor	Wide-spectrum mitogen
TNF-α		Multifunctional proinflammatory cytokine, with effects on lipid metabolism, coagulation, insulin resistance, and endothelial function
IL-1		Potent mediator of inflammation and immune response
IL-8		Mediates neutrophil activation and migration
G-CSF, GM-CSF		Stimulate proliferation and differentiation of granulocyte progenitors

Abbreviations: FGF(R), fibroblast growth facot (receptor); G(M)CSF, granulocyte (macrophage) colony-stimulating factor; HGF, hepatocyte growth factor; IGF, insulin-like growth factor; IL, interleukin; PD-ECGF, platelet-derived endothelial cell growth factor; PDGF, platelet-derived growth factor; TGF, transforming growth factor; TNF, tumor necrosis factor; VEGF, vascular endothelial growth factor.

that radioresistance is partly owing to new vessel formation by the tumor *(67–70)*. Weichselbaum and colleagues *(71–73)* confirmed that the combination of angiostatin or an anti-VEGF antibody with radiation was synergistic and decreased radioresistance of tumors. These results have also been confirmed for antiangiogenic small-molecule tyrosine kinase inhibitors *(74)*. In xenograft HNSCC models, antiangiogenic strategies have had encouraging results *(74–79)* and have led to the incorporation of novel antiangiogenic agents into clinical HNSCC trials.

SU5416 is a small-molecule inhibitor of the VEGFR2 receptor tyrosine kinase and was studied in HNSCC in a single-agent phase II trial. The abstract reported one response in 20 patients. As with other antiangiogenic drugs, this trial demonstrates that angiogenesis inhibition by itself has little activity *(80)*. Combinations with standard therapies are more promising, as has been demonstrated for bevacizumab in colon cancer *(59)*. The development of SU5416 has been discontinued owing to marked toxicities (dose reductions in 50% of patients *[81]*) and administration difficulties (intravenous, with vehicle causing hypersensitivity). Several other agents in this class, however, are promising, such as the orally available small-molecule inhibitors PTK-787 or ZD6474, which are currently in phase I and II trials. Another oral antiangiogenic agent, sorafanib (Bay 43-9006), was originally conceived as a Raf-1 kinase inhibitor but does target other kinases including VEGFR-2. Trials in renal cell carcinoma (82) and melanoma (83,84) (both highly vascular tumors) have shown activity. Sorafenib is currently in phase II study for HNSCC, and results should be available in the next 1–2 yr.

Bevacizumab, an antibody against the VEGF protein, is approved by the Food and Drug Administration (FDA) for colon cancer and is actively being studied in HNSCC. Its incorporation with CRT in locally advanced HNSCC and with an EGFR inhibitor (erlotinib) in recurrent or metastatic disease has been undertaken. In a phase I trial in poor-risk patients, bevacizumab was given concurrently with 5-FU, hydroxyurea, and split-course radiation (BFHX) (85); a response rate of 75% was reported, suggesting activity and proving the feasibility of this approach. The side effect profile included mucositis, dermatitis, and elevation of transaminases, as frequently seen with FHX. However, hypertension, thrombosis, and bleeding events were also observed, probably related to bevacizumab. A phase II trial, using bevacizumab at a dose of 10 mg/kg, again in poor-prognosis patients, and a phase II randomized trial of FHX with or without bevacizumab in intermediate-stage disease are now ongoing.

As mentioned earlier, EGFR induces angiogenesis via VEGF expression (86,87). EGFR inhibition has also demonstrated the ability to decrease VEGF production and vessel formation in vivo (88–94). Based on in vitro and in vivo evidence of synergism and reversal of EGFR resistance (76,95,96), the combination of anti-EGFR and anti-VEGF therapies is also now being studied. Preliminary data on a phase I trial combining erlotinib and bevacizumab have been reported (53). Overall the regimen was very well tolerated, but one patient experienced a grade 4 hemorrhage from a base of tongue tumor. Of nine evaluable patients, one patient had a partial response, seven patients had stable disease, and one patient had progressive disease.

5. HYPOXIA: HIF-1α

Hypoxia is a major mechanism of tumor radiation- and chemoresistance (97). Hypoxic HNSCC tumors show a propensity to metastasize, have higher local failure rates, and carry an overall worse prognosis (97–99). Multiple strategies have been pursued to target this phenomenon, including hypoxic cell sensitizers (100), as well as agents that interfere with hypoxia-inducible factor (HIF)-1α. HIF-1α is the central protein coordinating the response to hypoxia (101). HIF-1α levels rise markedly and rapidly under hypoxic conditions and induce the transcription of multiple genes including VEGF, endothelin-1 (102), and c-Met (103). HIF-1α is regulated by the von Hippel-Lindau protein, mdm-2 through p53, the PI3 kinase/AKT pathway (104), and thioredoxin (Trx)-1 (105). The activation of HIF-1α via Trx-1 is poorly understood, but inhibition decreases HIF-1α levels, VEGF levels, and angiogenesis in experimental models (106–109). HIF-1α expression has been correlated with increased failure rates, decreased survival, and resistance to therapy (110–113).

Inhibitors of HIF-1α that have been studied include the small-molecule antibiotic quinocarmycin monicitrate (KW2152) and its analog (DX-52-1). These were promising in preclinical models, but development was discontinued owing to the lack of effect or severe toxicity (114–116). Small-molecule inhibitors of Trx-1 have also been developed, one of which, PX-478, has demonstrated promising preclinical activity in vitro and in in vivo models and is currently in phase I clinical trials (109).

6. OTHER NOVEL TARGETS AND DRUGS IN DEVELOPMENT

An overview of potential novel targets is given in Table 5. The development of drugs for many of these targets is still in the early stages.

Table 5
Novel Targets (Other Than EGFR) and Respective Drugs in Development for HNSCC

General target	Specific protein/ target	Type of agent(s)	Example(s)	Phase of development in HNSCC
Growth factors	Met	Small molecule	RTK inhibitors: SU11274, PHA-665752	Preclinical
			Protein stability: 17-AAG	I
	IGFR	Monoclonal antibody	EM164	Preclinical
		Small molecule	NVP-ADW742	Preclinical
Signal transduction	Ras	FTI	SCH66336	II
	Raf	Small molecule	BAY 43-9006	II
	STAT3	Antisense		Preclinical
		Small molecule		Preclinical
	mTOR	Small molecule	CCI-779, RAD001, AP23573, rapamycin	II
	MEK	Small molecule	PD0325901	Preclinical
	PKC	Small molecule	LY317615, UCN-01, bryostatin-1	II
		Antisense	ISIS 3521	Preclinical
Cell cycle		Small molecule	Bryostatin-1, flavopiridol, UCN-01, peri-fosine, roscovitine, Ro31-7453	II
	Cyclin D1	Antisense		Preclinical
	p16	Gene therapy		Preclinical
p53		Gene therapy	ONYX-015, Ad-p53	II
Apoptosis	Bcl-X$_l$	Small molecule	gossypol	Preclinical
	Bcl-2	Antisense	Oblimersen	Preclinical
Proteasome	NF-κB	Small molecule	bortezomib	I
Prostaglandin synthesis	COX-2	Small molecule	Celecoxib, rofecoxib	II
Hypoxia		Hypoxic cell sensitizers	Mitomycin C, tirapazamine	III
	HIF-1α	Small molecule	PX-478, AW464	Preclinical
Angiogenesis	VEGF	Monoclonal antibody	Bevacizumab	II
	VEGFR2	Monoclonal antibody	IMC-1C11	Preclinical
		Small molecule	ZD6474, NVP-AEE788, SU5416, PTK-787	II
	MMP	Small molecule	Marimastat, ONO-4817, MMI-166	Preclinical
	Natural inhibitors	Small molecule	ABT-510, angiostatin, endostatin	Preclinical
	Endothelial cell	Small molecule	Combratostatin, ZD6126	Preclinical

Abbreviations: COX, cyclooxygenase; FTI, farmesyltransferase inhibitor; HIF-1α, hypoxia-inducible factor-1α; HNSCC, head and neck squamous cell carcinoma; IGFR, insulin-like growth factor receptor; MMP, matrix metalloproteinase; mTOR, mammalian target of rapamycin; NF-κB, nuclear factor-κB; RTK, receptor tyrosine kinase; STAT, signal transducer and activator of infection; VEGFR, vascular endothelial growth factor.

6.1. Growth Factors and Their Receptors: Met

Met is a potent cell surface receptor tyrosine kinase implicated in many solid tumors and leukemias (117–119). Met signaling is similar to that of other tyrosine kinase receptors with respect to activation of the Ras-Raf-MAPK, PI3-K-Akt-mTOR, and Jak-Stat-PKC pathways. Overexpression has been linked to a poor prognosis in HNSCC (120–122), and mutations of Met have been described in HNSCC (123) (mostly in the tyrosine kinase domain) and have been linked with metastasis (124), inhibition of anoikis (125), cell migration (126), and angiogenesis (127). Small-molecule inhibitors of Met (128,129) as well as antibodies to both Met and its ligand hepatocyte growth factor, are in development and will probably enter clinical trials within the next 1–2 yr. An alternative approach to targeting this pathway has been taken with 17-AAG, a geldanamycin derivative. This agent inhibits heat shock protein 90 (HSP90), a chaperone protein involved in the maintenance of functional Met. Clinical trials of 17-AAG are ongoing, with acceptable toxicities in early reports in other advanced solid tumors (130,131).

6.2. Signal Transducers: Ras, Raf, TOR, and PKC

Ras, Raf, and mTOR are part of the downstream signaling cascades of both the EGFR and the Met receptor tyrosine kinases. Novel drugs are being developed to inhibit these targets. H-Ras is dependent on posttranslational farnesylation, forming the rationale for using farnesyltransferase inhibitors (FTIs) in HNSCC, although it is likely that FTIs primarily target other proteins. FTIs have been found to be radiosensitizers in preclinical models (132) and a phase I trial using the agent L-778,123 in combination with radiation in a cohort of NSCLC and HNSCC showed good tolerability (133). Another study by Kies et al. (134) used SCH66336 starting 2 wk prior to definitive surgery in locally advanced disease. A reduction in farnesylation of two proteins (DNAJ-2 and Prelamin A) was observed; interestingly, despite the short administration design, two partial and two minor responses were reported in 28 patients. A phase II trial evaluating SCH66336 in recurrent/metastatic disease is ongoing.

Raf signals downstream from Ras, and overexpression of c-Raf has been described in HNSCC (135). Sorafenib is an orally available small-molecule inhibitor of Raf-1 and BRAF kinases (136), that is currently undergoing phase II testing in HNSCC (137). A phase I study that included three HNSCC patients showed one prolonged disease stabilization (138).

The PI3K/AKT pathway has been implicated in HNSCC growth and development (139–142). The mammalian target of rapamycin (mTOR) regulates protein translation downstream of AKT and has been of interest in cancer therapy. There are currently at least three mTOR inhibitors in early clinical trials: CCI-779, RAD001, and AP23573. CCI-779 and RAD001 have entered phase II clinical trials in several solid tumors. Specific trials in HNSCC are scheduled.

The PKC family of serine/threonine kinases mediates many key physiological processes such as growth, death, differentiation, and transformation. Recent work showed that inhibition of PKC isoforms using a global PKC inhibitor (chelerythrine chloride), leads to apoptosis of HNSCC cell lines and in vivo produces significant growth delay (143). Furthermore, PKC inhibition is additive when combined with cisplatin in HNSCC (144). Given the potential for toxicities by broadly inhibiting the PKC family, attempts are being made to target the isoforms more specifically (145).

6.3. Broad Cell Cycle Inhibitors

A number of molecules that target the cyclin-dependent kinases (CDKs) are being evaluated in HNSCC including bryostatin-1, flavopiridol, UCN-01, and perifosine. It is unclear whether the antineoplastic effects of these agents are due to inhibition of CDKs or other targets. So far none of these agents has demonstrated single-agent activity.

6.4. Tumor Suppressors: p53, p16

TP53 is a known tumor suppressor gene and, as outlined earlier, plays a vital role in HNSCC *(146,147)*. The p53 protein functions in multiple cellular processes including DNA repair, apoptosis, and induction of cell cycle arrest *(148)*. Trying to capitalize on a nonfunctional p53 protein/TP53 gene, two adenoviral constructs, ONYX-015 and Adp53, have been developed and tested in HNSCC.

ONYX-015 is thought to replicate only in p53-deficient cells *(149)* and has demonstrated activity in clinical trials *(150)*, with a 13% response rate as a single agent *(151)* and a 63% response rate (27% complete responses) in combination with cisplatin and 5-FU *(152)*. ONYX-015 has also been employed as a mouthwash for chemoprevention in patients with oral leukoplakia and dysplasia *(153)*. Histologic resolution of dysplasia was seen in 37% of patients and was very well tolerated. Unfortunately, lesions recurred after discontinuation. Adp53 restores the TP53 gene and was evaluated in two phase I/II studies in patients with recurrent HNSCC, with modest activity: 12% response rate in unresectable patients and a 27% 18-mo survival in resectable patients *(154,155)*.

As mentioned earlier aberrations of the CDK inhibitor p16 (INK4) are vital as an early event in the transformation of normal mucosa to carcinoma. Viral constructs restoring p16 expression in experimental models have been described and can reverse tumor growth and induce apoptosis *(156–158)*. These constructs have not yet been evaluated clinically.

6.5. Other Targets

6.5.1. COX-2

Prostaglandins are produced by cyclooxygenase (COX) and regulate inflammation as well as other physiological processes. Prostagladins have been implicated in carcinogenesis and tumor progression. Nonsteroidal antiinflammatory drugs inhibit COX, and because of their availability have been investigated as chemopreventative agents for multiple tumors *(159–166)*. COX-2, the inducible form of COX, is the isoform thought to be mostly involved in tumorigenesis *(167)* and is overexpressed in pathological HNSCC specimens *(168)*. COX-2 inhibition has been described to decrease or stop tumor formation, growth, survival, metastasis, angiogenesis, and immune evasion *(169–175)*. COX-2 inhibitors were able to prevent tongue carcinomas in a rat tongue carcinogenesis model *(176)* and growth of HNSCC in a mouse xenograft model *(177)*. Interestingly, COX-2 inhibitors have also demonstrated radiosensitizing properties in other tumor models *(178–180)*. Phase II human trials are under way or planned to test the efficacy of celecoxib in primary and secondary prevention of HNSCC, as well as in combination with other agents and radiation *(181)*. The safety of long-term use of higher doses remains to be determined; cardiovascular side effects may be problematic.

6.5.2. The Proteasome

Many cellular proteins are marked for degradation by a process called polyubiquitination and subsequently are broken down into smaller fragments by the proteasome. The 26S proteasome eliminates the majority of intracellular proteins *(182–185)* and inhibition results in unusually strong apoptotic effects in preclinical cancer models *(186–190)*. The proteasome inhibitor bortezomib, a synthetic peptide boronate, is selective for the 26S proteasome and has recently been approved in the United States for refractory multiple myeloma *(191)*. The mechanism of action of bortezomib is probably mediated by interference with multiple pathways, but targeting nuclear factor κb (NFκB) through inhibitor κb (IκB) has been proposed. Proteasome inhibition may also decrease angiogenesis owing to preferential toxicity in proliferating endothelial cells *(191)*.

In HNSCC models, bortezomib was able to demonstrate apoptosis induction in vitro *(188)*, tumor growth inhibition in vivo *(192)*, and radiosensitization *(193–195)*. Accordingly, a phase I trial of bortezomib in combination with radiation in patients with recurrent HNSCC was undertaken *(196)*. Thus far, no severe toxicities were observed in the initial seven patients, and proteasome inhibition was demonstrated in peripheral blood mononuclear cells.

7. CONCLUSIONS AND FUTURE DIRECTIONS

Despite the recent advances in the management of patients with head and neck cancer, much room for improvement remains. Efforts are being made to reduce recurrence rates in patients with high-risk tumors as well as lessen the debilitating consequences of current therapies. The rapid evolution in the understanding of the molecular biology of HNSCC offers hope and promise for patients. Several agents, most notably the EGFR inhibitors, have shown promising results and will undoubtedly find their role in the management of HNSCC. However, many challenges lie ahead. The sheer number (some estimates suggest up to 1000 compounds) of novel agents in development has the potential to overwhelm our research and regulatory institutions, ultimately, and paradoxically, depriving HNSCC patients of beneficial therapies. The costs associated with developing targeted agents discourage exploration in less common malignancies such as HNSCC. Moreover, integrating agents with the intensive radiotherapy regimens often used in HNSCC adds toxicity and scheduling dilemmas that must be dealt with. It is imperative that we streamline the testing processes and efficiently integrate the changes that lie ahead into clinical trials and patient care. Approaches based on proper subject selection and early determination of active agents must be adopted. A multidisciplinary approach that advances the field and allows patients to access novel therapies early in their treatment via clinical trials is mandated.

REFERENCES

1. Bernier J, Domenge C, Ozsahin M, et al. Postoperative irradiation with or without concomitant chemotherapy for locally advanced head and neck cancer. N Engl J Med 2004; 350:1945–1952.
2. Cooper JS, Pajak TF, Forastiere AA, et al. Postoperative concurrent radiotherapy and chemotherapy for high-risk squamous-cell carcinoma of the head and neck. N Engl J Med 2004; 350,:1937–1944.
3. Haraf DJ, Rosen FR, Stenson K, et al. Induction chemotherapy followed by concomitant TFHX chemoradiotherapy with reduced dose radiation in advanced head and neck cancer. Clin Cancer Res 2003; 9:5936–5943.
4. Forastiere AA, Goepfert H, Maor M, et al. Concurrent chemotherapy and radiotherapy for organ preservation in advanced laryngeal cancer. N Engl J Med 2003; 349:2091–2098.
5. Saunders MI, Rojas AM. Management of cancer of the head and neck—a cocktail with your PORT? N Engl J Med 2004; 350:1997–1999.
6. Vokes EE, Stenson KM. Therapeutic options for laryngeal cancer. N Engl J Med 2003; 349:2087–2089.
7. Renan MJ. How many mutations are required for tumorigenesis? Implications from human cancer data. Mol Carcinog 1993; 7:139–146.
8. Gillison ML, Koch WM, Capone RB, et al. Evidence for a causal association between human papillomavirus and a subset of head and neck cancers. J Natl Cancer Inst 2000; 92:709–720.
9. Brennan JA, Boyle JO, Koch WM, et al. Association between cigarette smoking and mutation of the p53 gene in squamous-cell carcinoma of the head and neck. N Engl J Med 1995; 332:712–717.

10. Koch WM, Lango M, Sewell D, Zahurak M, Sidransky D. Head and neck cancer in nonsmokers: a distinct clinical and molecular entity. Laryngoscope 1999; 109:1544–1551.

11. Mao L, Lee JS, Fan YH, et al. Frequent microsatellite alterations at chromosomes 9p21 and 3p14 in oral premalignant lesions and their value in cancer risk assessment. Nat Med 1996; 2:682–685.

12. Rosin MP, Lam WL, Poh C, et al. 3p14 and 9p21 loss is a simple tool for predicting second oral malignancy at previously treated oral cancer sites. Cancer Res 2002; 62:6447–6450.

13. Koch WM, Brennan JA, Zahurak M, et al. p53 mutation and locoregional treatment failure in head and neck squamous cell carcinoma. J Natl Cancer Inst 1996; 88:1580–1586.

14. Boyle JO, Hakim J, Koch W, et al. The incidence of p53 mutations increases with progression of head and neck cancer. Cancer Res 1993; 53:4477–4480.

15. Partridge M, Pateromichelakis S, Phillips E, Emilion G, Langdon J. Profiling clonality and progression in multiple premalignant and malignant oral lesions identifies a subgroup of cases with a distinct presentation of squamous cell carcinoma. Clin Cancer Res 2001; 7:1860–1866.

16. Tabor MP, Brakenhoff RH, Ruijter-Schippers HJ, Kummer JA, Leemans CR, Braakhuis BJ. Genetically altered fields as origin of locally recurrent head and neck cancer: a retrospective study. Clin Cancer Res 2004; 10:3607–3613.

17. Braakhuis BJ, Tabor MP, Kummer JA, Leemans CR, Brakenhoff RH. A genetic explanation of Slaughter's concept of field cancerization: evidence and clinical implications. Cancer Res 2003; 63:1727–1730.

18. Tabor MP, Brakenhoff RH, van Houten VM, et al. Persistence of genetically altered fields in head and neck cancer patients: biological and clinical implications. Clin Cancer Res 2001; 7:1523–1532.

19. Mao L, El-Naggar AK, Papadimitrakopoulou V, et al. Phenotype and genotype of advanced premalignant head and neck lesions after chemopreventive therapy. J Natl Cancer Inst 1998; 90:1545–1551.

20. Sudbo J, Lippman SM, Lee JJ, et al. The influence of resection and aneuploidy on mortality in oral leukoplakia. N Engl J Med 2004; 350:1405–1413.

21. Sudbo J, Kildal W, Risberg B, Koppang HS, Danielsen HE, Reith A. DNA content as a prognostic marker in patients with oral leukoplakia. N Engl J Med 2001; 344:1270–1278.

22. Pomerantz RG, Grandis JR. The role of epidermal growth factor receptor in head and neck squamous cell carcinoma. Curr Oncol Rep 2003; 5:140–146.

23. Shin DM, Ro JY, Hong WK, Hittelman WN. Dysregulation of epidermal growth factor receptor expression in premalignant lesions during head and neck tumorigenesis. Cancer Res 1994; 54:3153–3159.

24. Rubin Grandis J, Tweardy DJ, Melhem MF. Asynchronous modulation of transforming growth factor alpha and epidermal growth factor receptor protein expression in progression of premalignant lesions to head and neck squamous cell carcinoma. Clin Cancer Res 1998; 4:13–20.

25. Chen BK, Ohtsuki Y, Furihata M, et al. Co-overexpression of p53 protein and epidermal growth factor receptor in human papillary thyroid carcinomas correlated with lymph node metastasis, tumor size and clinicopathologic stage. Int J Oncol 1999; 15:893–898.

26. Ang KK, Berkey BA, Tu X, et al. Impact of epidermal growth factor receptor expression on survival and pattern of relapse in patients with advanced head and neck carcinoma. Cancer Res 2002; 62:7350–7356.

27. Etienne MC, Pivot X, Formento JL, et al. A multifactorial approach including tumoural epidermal growth factor receptor, p53, thymidylate synthase and dihydropyrimidine dehydrogenase to predict treatment outcome in head and neck cancer patients receiving 5-fluorouracil. Br J Cancer 1999; 79:1864–1869.

28. Rubin Grandis J, Melhem MF, Gooding WE, et al. Levels of TGF-alpha and EGFR protein in head and neck squamous cell carcinoma and patient survival. J Natl Cancer Inst 1998; 90:824–832.

29. Gupta AK, McKenna WG, Weber CN, et al. Local recurrence in head and neck cancer: relationship to radiation resistance and signal transduction. Clin Cancer Res 2002; 8:885–892.

30. Wu X, Fan Z, Masui H, Rosen N, Mendelsohn J. Apoptosis induced by an anti-epidermal growth factor receptor monoclonal antibody in a human colorectal carcinoma cell line and its delay by insulin. J Clin Invest 1995; 95:1897–1905.

31. Busse D, Doughty RS, Ramsey TT, et al. Reversible G(1) arrest induced by inhibition of the epidermal growth factor receptor tyrosine kinase requires up-regulation of p27(KIP1) independent of MAPK activity. J Biol Chem 2000; 275:6987–6995.

32. Perrotte P, Matsumoto T, Inoue K, et al. Anti-epidermal growth factor receptor antibody C225 inhibits angiogenesis in human transitional cell carcinoma growing orthotopically in nude mice. Clin Cancer Res 1999; 5:257–265.

33. Ciardiello F, Caputo R, Troiani T, et al. Antisense oligonucleotides targeting the epidermal growth factor receptor inhibit proliferation, induce apoptosis, and cooperate with cytotoxic drugs in human cancer cell lines. Int J Cancer 2001; 93:172–178.

34. Moyer JD, Barbacci EG, Iwata KK, et al. Induction of apoptosis and cell cycle arrest by CP-358,774, an inhibitor of epidermal growth factor receptor tyrosine kinase. Cancer Res 1997; 57:4838–4848.

35. Liu B, Fang M, Schmidt M, Lu Y, Mendelsohn J, Fan Z. Induction of apoptosis and activation of the caspase cascade by anti-EGF receptor monoclonal antibodies in DiFi human colon cancer cells do not involve the c-jun N-terminal kinase activity. Br J Cancer 2000; 82:1991–1999.

36. Clark G.M. P-SR, Siu L.L., et al. Rash severity is predictive of increased survival in erlotinib HCl. Proc Am Soc Clin Oncol 2003; 22:196 (Abstract 786).

37. Kane MA, et al. Phase II study of 250 mg gefitinib in advanced squamous cell carcinoma of the head and neck (SCCHN). ASCO 2004, New Orleans, LA, abstract 5586.

38. Cohen EE, Rosen F, Stadler WM, et al. Phase II trial of ZD1839 in recurrent or metastatic squamous cell carcinoma of the head and neck. J Clin Oncol 2003; 21:1980–1987.

39. Soulieres D, Senzer NN, Vokes EE, Hidalgo M, Agarwala SS, Siu LL. Multicenter phase II study of erlotinib, an oral epidermal growth factor receptor tyrosine kinase inhibitor, in patients with recurrent or metastatic squamous cell cancer of the head and neck. J Clin Oncol 2004; 22:77–85.

40. Cohen MH, Williams GA, Sridhara R, et al. United States Food and Drug Administration Drug Approval summary: gefitinib (ZD1839; Iressa) tablets. Clin Cancer Res 2004; 10:1212–1218.

41. Shin DM, Donato NJ, Perez-Soler R, et al. Epidermal growth factor receptor-targeted therapy with C225 and cisplatin in patients with head and neck cancer. Clin Cancer Res 2001; 7:1204–1213.

42. Baselga J, Pfister D, Cooper MR, et al. Phase I studies of anti-epidermal growth factor receptor chimeric antibody C225 alone and in combination with cisplatin. J Clin Oncol 2000; 18:904–914.

43. Baselga J ea. Cetuximab (C225) plus cisplatin/carboplatin is active in patients (pts) with recurrent/metastatic squamous cell carcinoma of the head and neck (SCCHN) progressing on a same dose and schedule platinum-based regimen. Proc Am Soc Clin Oncol 2002; 21:226 (abstract 900).

44. Kies MS, et al. Final report of the efficacy and safety of the anti-epidermal growth factor antibody Erbitux (IMC-C225), in combination with cisplatin in patients with recurrent squamous cell carcinoma of the head and neck (SCCHN) refractory to cisplatin containing chemotherapy. Proc Am Soc Clin Oncol 2002; 21:232 (abstract 925).

45. Bonner JA, et al. Cetuximab prolongs survival in patients with locoregionally advanced squamous cell carcinoma of head and neck: a phase III study of high dose radiation therapy with or without cetuximab. ASCO 2004 Annual Meeting, New Orleans, abstract 5507.

46. Shepherd F. A randomized placebo-controlled trial of erlotinib in patients with advanced non-small cell lung cancer (NSCLC) following failure of 1st or 2nd line chemotherapy. A National Cancer Institute of Canada Clinical Trials Group (NCIC CTG) trial. ASCO, 2004.

47. Magne N, Fischel JL, Dubreuil A, et al. Influence of epidermal growth factor receptor (EGFR), p53 and intrinsic MAP kinase pathway status of tumour cells on the antiproliferative effect of ZD1839 ("Iressa"). Br J Cancer 2002; 86:1518–1523.

48. Magne N, Fischel JL, Dubreuil A, et al. Sequence-dependent effects of ZD1839 ('Iressa') in combination with cytotoxic treatment in human head and neck cancer. Br J Cancer 2002; 86:819–827.

49. Huang SM, Li J, Armstrong EA, Harari PM. Modulation of radiation response and tumor-induced angiogenesis after epidermal growth factor receptor inhibition by ZD1839 (Iressa). Cancer Res 2002; 62:4300–4306.

50. Cohen EE, et al. A phase II study of 250-mg gefitinib (ZD1839) monotherapy in recurrent or metastatic squamous cell carcinoma of the head and neck (SCCHN). Proc Am Soc Clin Oncol 2003; 22:502.

51. Wirth LJ, et al. Phase I study of gefitinib plus celecoxib in patients with metastatic and/or locally recurrent squamous cell carcinoma of the head and neck (SCCHN). ASCO 2004 Annual Meeting New Orleans, abstract 5540.

52. Soulieres D, Senzer NN, Vokes EE, Hidalgo M, Agarwala SS, Siu LL. Multicenter phase II study of erlotinib, an oral epidermal growth factor receptor tyrosine kinase inhibitor, in patients with recurrent or metastatic squamous cell cancer of the head and neck. J Clin Oncol 2004; 22:77–85.

53. Mauer AM, Cohen E.E., et al. Phase I study of epidermal growth factor receptor (EGFR) inhibitor erlotonib, and vascular endothelial growth factor monoclonal antibody, bevacizumab, in recurrent and/or metastatic squamous cell carcinoma of the head and neck (SCCHN). ASCO 2004 Annual Meeting, New Orleans, abstract 5539.

54. Folkman J. What is the evidence that tumors are angiogenesis dependent? (editorial). J Natl Cancer Inst 1990; 82:4–6.

55. Folkman J. Angiogenesis in cancer, vascular, rheumatoid and other disease. Nat Med 1995; 1:27–31.

56. Folkman J. Clinical applications of research on angiogenesis. N Engl J Med 1995; 333:1757–1763.

57. Folkman J, Hanahan D. Switch to the angiogenic phenotype during tumorigenesis. Princess Takamatsu Symp 1991; 22:339–347.

58. Bouck N, Stellmach V, Hsu SC. How tumors become angiogenic. Adv Cancer Res 1996; 69:135–174.

59. Hurwitz H, Cartwright T, Hainsworth J, et al. Bevacizumab (a monoclonal antibody to vascular endothelial growth factor) prolongs survival in first-line colorectal cancer (CRC): results of a phase III trial of bevacizumab

in combination with bolus IFL (irinotecan, 5-fluorouracil, leucovorin) as first-line therapy in subjects with metastatic CRC. American Society of Clinical Oncology, Chicago, IL, June 2003, 2003.

60. Moriyama M, Kumagai S, Kawashiri S, Kojima K, Kakihara K, Yamamoto E. Immunohistochemical study of tumour angiogenesis in oral squamous cell carcinoma. Oral Oncol 1997; 33:369–374.

61. Denhart BC, Guidi AJ, Tognazzi K, Dvorak HF, Brown LF. Vascular permeability factor/vascular endothelial growth factor and its receptors in oral and laryngeal squamous cell carcinoma and dysplasia. Lab Invest 1997; 77:659–664.

62. Inoue K, Ozeki Y, Suganuma T, Sugiura Y, Tanaka S. Vascular endothelial growth factor expression in primary esophageal squamous cell carcinoma. Association with angiogenesis and tumor progression. Cancer 1997; 79:206–213.

63. Petruzzelli GJ, Benefield J, Taitz AD, et al. Heparin-binding growth factor(s) derived from head and neck squamous cell carcinomas induce endothelial cell proliferations. Head Neck 1997; 19:576–582.

64. Millauer B, Shawver LK, Plate KH, Risau W, Ullrich A. Glioblastoma growth inhibited in vivo by a dominant-negative Flk-1 mutant. Nature 1994; 367:576–59.

65. Riedel F, Gotte K, Li M, Hormann K, Grandis JR. Abrogation of VEGF expression in human head and neck squamous cell carcinoma decreases angiogenic activity in vitro and in vivo. Int J Oncol 2003; 23:577–583.

66. Kim KJ, Li B, Winer J, et al. Inhibition of vascular endothelial growth factor-induced angiogenesis suppresses tumour growth in vivo. Nature 1993; 362:841–84.

67. Auerbach R, Arensman R, Kubai L, Folkman J. Tumor-induced angiogenesis: lack of inhibition by irradiation. Int J Cancer 1975; 15:241–245.

68. Kerbel RS. Inhibition of tumor angiogenesis as a strategy to circumvent acquired resistance to anti-cancer therapeutic agents. Bioessays 1991; 13:31–36.

69. Kakeji Y, Teicher BA. Preclinical studies of the combination of angiogenic inhibitors with cytotoxic agents. Invest New Drugs 1997; 15:39–48.

70. Koukourakis MI, Giatromanolaki A, Sivridis E, et al. Squamous cell head and neck cancer: evidence of angiogenic regeneration during radiotherapy. Anticancer Res 2001; 21:4301–4309.

71. Mauceri HJ, Hanna NN, Beckett MA, et al. Combined effects of angiostatin and ionizing radiation in antitumour therapy. Nature 1998; 394:287–291.

72. Gorski DH, Mauceri HJ, Salloum RM, et al. Potentiation of the antitumor effect of ionizing radiation by brief concomitant exposures to angiostatin. Cancer Res 1998; 58:5686–5689.

73. Gorski DH, Beckett MA, Jaskowiak NT, et al. Blockage of the vascular endothelial growth factor stress response increases the antitumor effects of ionizing radiation. Cancer Res 1999; 59:3374–3378.

74. Ning S, Laird D, Cherrington JM, Knox SJ. The antiangiogenic agents SU5416 and SU6668 increase the antitumor effects of fractionated irradiation. Radiat Res 2002; 157:45–51.

75. Katori H, Baba Y, Imagawa Y, et al. Reduction of in vivo tumor growth by MMI-166, a selective matrix metalloproteinase inhibitor, through inhibition of tumor angiogenesis in squamous cell carcinoma cell lines of head and neck. Cancer Lett 2002; 178:151–159.

76. Orhan G, Yigitbasi MNY, Bradley A, et al. Dual inhibition of EGFR and VEGFR in squamous cell carcinoma of the head and neck: the role of the new EGFR/VEGFR inhibitor NVP-AEE788. 2003 AACR-NCI-EORTC International Conference, Molecular Targets and Cancer Therapeutics, Boston, November 17–21, 2003.

77. Kawano T, Furukawa S, Matsuda H, et al. [Antitumor effect of the angiogenesis inhibitor, TNP470, on squamous cell carcinoma cells in head and neck cancer]. Nippon Jibiinkoka Gakkai Kaiho 2000; 103:821–828.

78. Ueda N, Kamata N, Hayashi E, Yokoyama K, Hoteiya T, Nagayama M. Effects of an anti-angiogenic agent, TNP-470, on the growth of oral squamous cell carcinomas. Oral Oncol 1999; 35:554-60.

79. Zips D, Westphal J, Bruechner K, et al. Inhibition of VEGFR tyrosine kinase by ZK 222584/ ptk 787 (PTK/ZK) combined with fractionated radiotherapy (RT) in human squamous cell carcinoma (hSCC) in nude mice. 14th EORTC-NCI-AACR Symposium, Molecular Targets and Cancer Therapeutics, Frankfurt, Germany, November 19–22, 2002.

80. Zahalsky AJ, et al. Phase II trial of SU5416 in patients with advanced incurable head and neck cancer. ASCO 2002 Annual Meeting New Orleans, abstract 902.

81. Zahalsky A, Wong RJ, Lis E, et al. Phase II trial of SU5416 in patients with advanced incurable head and neck cancer. American Society of Clinical Oncology Annual Meeting 2002:21.

82. Ratain MJ, et al. Preliminary antitumor activity of BAY 43-9006 in metastatic renal cell carcinoma and other advanced refractory solid tumors in a phase II randomized discontinuation trial (RDT). ASCO 2004 Annual Meeting, New Orleans, abstract 4501.

83. Ahmad T, et al. BAY 43-9006 in patients with advanced melanoma: the Royal Marsden experience. ASCO 2004 Annual Meeting, New Orleans, abstract 7506.

84. Flaherty KT, et al. Phase I/II trial of BAY 43-9006, carboplatin (C) and paclitaxel (P) demonstrates preliminary antitumor activity in the expansion cohort of patients with metastatic melanoma. ASCO 2004 Annual Meeting, New Orleans, abstract 7507.

85. Gustin DM, Haraf D, Stenson K, Dekker A, Stadler W, Vokes E. Phase I study of bevacizumab, fluorouracil, hydroxyurea and radiotherapy (B-FHX) for patients with poor prognosis head and neck cancer. Proceedings of the AACR, Washington, DC, 2003, vol. 44.

86. Zhong H, Chiles K, Feldser D, et al. Modulation of hypoxia-inducible factor 1alpha expression by the epidermal growth factor/phosphatidylinositol 3-kinase/PTEN/AKT/FRAP pathway in human prostate cancer cells: implications for tumor angiogenesis and therapeutics. Cancer Res 2000; 60:1541–1545.

87. Jiang BH, Jiang G, Zheng JZ, Lu Z, Hunter T, Vogt PK. Phosphatidylinositol 3-kinase signaling controls levels of hypoxia-inducible factor 1. Cell Growth Differ 2001; 12:363–469.

88. Ciardiello F, Bianco R, Damiano V, et al. Antiangiogenic and antitumor activity of anti-epidermal growth factor receptor C225 monoclonal antibody in combination with vascular endothelial growth factor antisense oligonucleotide in human GEO colon cancer cells. Clin Cancer Res 2000; 6:3739–3747.

89. Huang SM, Harari PM. Modulation of radiation response after epidermal growth factor receptor blockade in squamous cell carcinomas: inhibition of damage repair, cell cycle kinetics, and tumor angiogenesis. Clin Cancer Res 2000; 6:2166–2174.

90. Bruns CJ, Harbison MT, Davis DW, et al. Epidermal growth factor receptor blockade with C225 plus gemcitabine results in regression of human pancreatic carcinoma growing orthotopically in nude mice by antiangiogenic mechanisms. Clin Cancer Res 2000; 6:1936–1948.

91. Perrotte P, Matsumoto T, Inoue K, et al. Anti-epidermal growth factor receptor antibody C225 inhibits angiogenesis in human transitional cell carcinoma growing orthotopically in nude mice. Clin Cancer Res 1999; 5:257–265.

92. Petit AM, Rak J, Hung MC, et al. Neutralizing antibodies against epidermal growth factor and ErbB-2/neu receptor tyrosine kinases down-regulate vascular endothelial growth factor production by tumor cells in vitro and in vivo: angiogenic implications for signal transduction therapy of solid tumors. Am J Pathol 1997; 151:1523–530.

93. Huang SM, Li J, Armstrong EA, Harari PM. Modulation of radiation response and tumor-induced angiogenesis after epidermal growth factor receptor inhibition by ZD1839 (Iressa). Cancer Res 2002; 62:4300–4306.

94. Ciardiello F, Caputo R, Bianco R, et al. Inhibition of growth factor production and angiogenesis in human cancer cells by ZD1839 (Iressa), a selective epidermal growth factor receptor tyrosine kinase inhibitor. Clin Cancer Res 2001; 7:1459–1465.

95. Viloria-Petit A, Crombet T, Jothy S, et al. Acquired resistance to the antitumor effect of epidermal growth factor receptor-blocking antibodies in vivo: a role for altered tumor angiogenesis. Cancer Res 2001; 61:5090–5101.

96. Ciardiello RB, Caputo R, Caputo R, et al. Antitumor activity of ZD6474, a small molecule VEGF receptor tyrosine kinase inhibitor, in human cancer cells with acquired resistance to EGF receptor-targeted drugs. Proc Am Soc Clin Oncol, Chicago, IL, 2003, vol. 22.

97. Peters LJ. Targeting hypoxia in head and neck cancer. Acta Oncol 2001; 40:937–940.

98. Brizel DM, Dodge RK, Clough RW, Dewhirst MW. Oxygenation of head and neck cancer: changes during radiotherapy and impact on treatment outcome. Radiother Oncol 1999; 53:113–117.

99. Brizel DM, Sibley GS, Prosnitz LR, Scher RL, Dewhirst MW. Tumor hypoxia adversely affects the prognosis of carcinoma of the head and neck. Int J Radiat Oncol Biol Phys 1997; 38:285–289.

100. Brown JM. Exploiting the hypoxic cancer cell: mechanisms and therapeutic strategies. Mol Med Today 2000; 6:157–162.

101. Semenza GL. Targeting HIF-1 for cancer therapy. Nat Rev Cancer 2003; 3:721–732.

102. Semenza GL. HIF-1 and tumor progression: pathophysiology and therapeutics. Trends Mol Med 2002; 8:S62–S67.

103. Pennacchietti S, Michieli P, Galluzzo M, Mazzone M, Giordano S, Comoglio PM. Hypoxia promotes invasive growth by transcriptional activation of the met protooncogene. Cancer Cell 2003; 3:347–361.

104. Mottet D, Dumont V, Deccache Y, et al. Regulation of hypoxia-inducible factor-1alpha protein level during hypoxic conditions by the phosphatidylinositol 3-kinase/Akt/glycogen synthase kinase 3beta pathway in HepG2 cells. J Biol Chem 2003; 278:31,277–31,285.

105. Ema M, Hirota K, Mimura J, et al. Molecular mechanisms of transcription activation by HLF and HIF1alpha in response to hypoxia: their stabilization and redox signal-induced interaction with CBP/p300. EMBO J 1999; 18:1905–1914.

106. Welsh SJ, Bellamy WT, Briehl MM, Powis G. The redox protein thioredoxin-1 (Trx-1) increases hypoxia-inducible factor 1alpha protein expression: Trx-1 overexpression results in increased vascular endothelial growth factor production and enhanced tumor angiogenesis. Cancer Res 2002; 62:5089–5095.

107. Welsh SJ, Williams RR, Birmingham A, Newman DJ, Kirkpatrick DL, Powis G. The thioredoxin redox inhibitors 1-methylpropyl 2-imidazolyl disulfide and pleurotin inhibit hypoxia-induced factor 1alpha and vascular endothelial growth factor formation. Mol Cancer Ther 2003; 2:235–243.

108. Mukherjee A, Westwell AD, Stevens MF, Martin SG. Characterizing the anti-tumor and anti-angiogenic activity of AW464 (NSC 706704), a novel thioredoxin inhibitor, 2003 AACR-NCI-EORTC International Conference, Molecular Targets and Cancer Therapeutics, Boston, November 17–21, 2003.

109. Welsh SJ, Berggren M, Kirkpatrick DL, Powis G. The antitumor activity of PX-478, an inhibitor of hypoxia-inducible factor-1a (HIF-1a) is associated with decreased tumor HIF-1a and plasma VEGF, Proceedings of the AACR, Washington, DC, 2003, vol. 44.

110. Koukourakis MI, Giatromanolaki A, Sivridis E, et al. Hypoxia-inducible factor (HIF1A and HIF2A), angiogenesis, and chemoradiotherapy outcome of squamous cell head-and-neck cancer. Int J Radiat Oncol Biol Phys 2002; 53:1192–1202.

111. Hui EP, Chan AT, Pezzella F, et al. Coexpression of hypoxia-inducible factors 1alpha and 2alpha, carbonic anhydrase IX, and vascular endothelial growth factor in nasopharyngeal carcinoma and relationship to survival. Clin Cancer Res 2002; 8:2595–2604.

112. Ueno T, Higashino F, Kohgo T, Shindoh M. Expression of HIF-1a in squamous cell carcinoma of the tongue: a new parameter for predicting cancer cell metastasis. Proceedings of the AACR, July 2003, vol. 44.

113. Nordsmark M, Overgaard J. The prognostic value of pO2 measurements and endogeneous hypoxia marker HIF-a in advanced head and neck cancers. Proceedings of the AACR, July 2003, vol. 44.

114. Plowman J, Dykes DJ, Narayanan VL, et al. Efficacy of the quinocarmycins KW2152 and DX-52-1 against human melanoma lines growing in culture kand in mice. Cancer Res 1995; 55:862–867.

115. Lunt SJ, Stratford IJ. The efficacy of small molecule inhibitors of HIF-1 on overall metastases presentation, hypoxic fraction, and HIF-1 mediated gene expression. 2003 AACR-NCI-EORTC International Conference, Molecular Targets and Cancer Therapeutics, Boston, November 17–21, 2003.

116. Brown LM, Cowen R, Melillo G, Sausville E, Stratford IJ. The potential therapeutic application of targeting HIF-1 using gene therapy or small molecule approaches. Proceedings of the AACR, Washington, DC, 2003, vol. 44.

117. Sattler M, Ma PC, Salgia R. Therapeutic targeting of the receptor tyrosine kinase Met. Cancer Treat Res 2004; 119:121–138.

118. Ma PC, Maulik G, Christensen J, Salgia R. c-Met: structure, functions and potential for therapeutic inhibition. Cancer Metastasis Rev 2003; 22:309–325.

119. http://www.vai.org/vari/metandcancer/index.aspx.

120. Uchida D, Kawamata H, Omotehara F, et al. Role of HGF/c-met system in invasion and metastasis of oral squamous cell carcinoma cells in vitro and its clinical significance. Int J Cancer 2001; 93:489–496.

121. Aebersold DM, Kollar A, Beer KT, Laissue J, Greiner RH, Djonov V. Involvement of the hepatocyte growth factor/scatter factor receptor c-met and of Bcl-xL in the resistance of oropharyngeal cancer to ionizing radiation. Int J Cancer 2001; 96:41–54.

122. Morello S, Olivero M, Aimetti M, et al. MET receptor is overexpressed but not mutated in oral squamous cell carcinomas. J Cell Physiol 2001; 189:285–290.

123. Aebersold DM, Landt O, Berthou S, et al. Prevalence and clinical impact of Met Y1253D-activating point mutation in radiotherapy-treated squamous cell cancer of the oropharynx. Oncogene 2003; 22:8519–8523.

124. Di Renzo MF, Olivero M, Martone T, et al. Somatic mutations of the MET oncogene are selected during metastatic spread of human HNSC carcinomas. Oncogene 2000; 19:1547–1555.

125. Zeng Q, Chen S, You Z, et al. Hepatocyte growth factor inhibits anoikis in head and neck squamous cell carcinoma cells by activation of ERK and Akt signaling independent of NFkappa B. J Biol Chem 2002; 277:25,203–25,208.

126. Fleigel J, Sedwick J, Kornberg LJ. Hepatocyte growth factor/scatter factor stimulates mitogenesis and migration of a head and neck squamous cell carcinoma cell line. Otolaryngol Head Neck Surg 2002; 127:271–278.

127. Dong G, Chen Z, Li ZY, Yeh NT, Bancroft CC, Van Waes C. Hepatocyte growth factor/scatter factor-induced activation of MEK and PI3K signal pathways contributes to expression of proangiogenic cytokines interleukin-8 and vascular endothelial growth factor in head and neck squamous cell carcinoma. Cancer Res 2001; 61:5911–5918.

128. Sattler M, Pride YB, Ma P, et al. A novel small molecule met inhibitor induces apoptosis in cells transformed by the oncogenic TPR-MET tyrosine kinase. Cancer Res 2003; 63:5462–5469.

129. Christensen JG, Schreck R, Burrows J, et al. A selective small molecule inhibitor of c-Met kinase inhibits c-Met-dependent phenotypes in vitro and exhibits cytoreductive antitumor activity in vivo. Cancer Res 2003; 63:7345–7355.

130. Ehrlichman C, et al. A phase I trial of 17-allylamino-geldanamycin (17AAG) in patients with advanced cancer. ASCO 2004 Annual Meeting, New Orleans, abstract 3030.

131. Solit D, B., et al. Phase I trial of 17-AAG (17-allylamino-17-demethoxygeldanamycin) in patients (pts) with advanced cancer. ASCO 2003 Annual Meeting, New Orleans, abstract 795.

132. Brunner TB, Gupta AK, Shi Y, et al. Farnesyltransferase inhibitors as radiation sensitizers. Int J Radiat Biol 2003; 79:569–576.

133. Hahn SM, Bernhard EJ, Regine W, et al. A Phase I trial of the farnesyltransferase inhibitor L-778,123 and radiotherapy for locally advanced lung and head and neck cancer. Clin Cancer Res 2002; 8:1065–1072.

134. Kies M, Clayman GL, El-Naggar AK, et al. Induction Therapy with SCH 66336, a Farnesyltransferase Inhibitor, in Squamous Cell Carcinoma (SCC) of the Head and Neck. American Society of Clinical Oncology Annual Meeting, San Francisco, CA, 2001, vol. 20.

135. Riva C, Lavieille JP, Reyt E, Brambilla E, Lunardi J, Brambilla C. Differential c-myc, c-jun, c-raf and p53 expression in squamous cell carcinoma of the head and neck: implication in drug and radioresistance. Eur J Cancer B Oral Oncol 1995; 31B:384–391.

136. Lyons JF, Wilhelm S, Hibner B, Bollag G. Discovery of a novel Raf kinase inhibitor. Endocr Relat Cancer 2001; 8:219–225.

137. Lee JT, McCubrey JA. BAY-43-9006 Bayer/Onyx. Curr Opin Investig Drugs 2003; 4:757–763.

138. Awada A HA, Gil T, Munoz R, et al. Final results of a clinical and pharmacokinetic (PK) phase I study of the Raf kinase inhibitor BAY 43-9006 in refractory solid cancers: a promising anti-tumor agent. 14th EORTC-NCI-AACR Symposium, Molecular Targets and Cancer Therapeutics, Frankfurt, Germany, November 19–22, 2002.

139. Redon R, Muller D, Caulee K, Wanherdrick K, Abecassis J, du Manoir S. A simple specific pattern of chromosomal aberrations at early stages of head and neck squamous cell carcinomas: PIK3CA but not p63 gene as a likely target of 3q26-qter gains. Cancer Res 2001; 61:4122–4129.

140. Singh B, Reddy PG, Goberdhan A, et al. p53 regulates cell survival by inhibiting PIK3CA in squamous cell carcinomas. Genes Dev 2002; 16:984–993.

141. Woenckhaus J, Steger K, Werner E, et al. Genomic gain of PIK3CA and increased expression of p110alpha are associated with progression of dysplasia into invasive squamous cell carcinoma. J Pathol 2002; 198:335–342.

142. Worsham MJ, Pals G, Schouten JP, et al. Delineating genetic pathways of disease progression in head and neck squamous cell carcinoma. Arch Otolaryngol Head Neck Surg 2003; 129:702–708.

143. Chmura SJ, Dolan ME, Cha A, Mauceri HJ, Kufe DW, Weichselbaum RR. In vitro and in vivo activity of protein kinase C inhibitor chelerythrine chloride induces tumor cell toxicity and growth delay in vivo. Clin Cancer Res 2000; 6:737–742.

144. Hoffmann TK, Leenen K, Hafner D, et al. Antitumor activity of protein kinase C inhibitors and cisplatin in human head and neck squamous cell carcinoma lines. Anticancer Drugs 2002; 13:93–100.

145. Cohen EEW GS, Rosner MR. The effects of protein kinase C zeta inhibition on MAPK activation and growth in squamous cell carcinoma of the head and neck (SCCHN). Annual Meeting of the American Association of Cancer Research, Washington, DC, 2003, vol. 44.

146. Boyle JO, Hakim J, Koch W, et al. The incidence of p53 mutations increases with progression of head and neck cancer. Cancer Res 1993; 53:4477–4480.

147. Koch WM, Brennan JA, Zahurak M, et al. p53 mutation and locoregional treatment failure in head and neck squamous cell carcinoma. J Natl Cancer Inst 1996; 88:1580–1586.

148. Vogelstein B, Lane D, Levine AJ. Surfing the p53 network. Nature 2000; 408:307–310.

149. Bischoff JR, Kirn DH, Williams A, et al. An adenovirus mutant that replicates selectively in p53-deficient human tumor cells. Science 1996; 274:373–376.

150. Cohen EE, Rudin CM. ONYX-015. Onyx Pharmaceuticals. Curr Opin Investig Drugs 2001; 2:1770–1775.

151. Nemunaitis J, Khuri F, Ganly I, et al. Phase II trial of intratumoral administration of ONYX-015, a replication-selective adenovirus, in patients with refractory head and neck cancer. J Clin Oncol 2001; 19:289–298.

152. Khuri FR, Nemunaitis J, Ganly I, et al. a controlled trial of intratumoral ONYX-015, a selectively-replicating adenovirus, in combination with cisplatin and 5-fluorouracil in patients with recurrent head and neck cancer. Nat Med 2000; 6:879–885.

153. Rudin CM, Cohen EE, Papadimitrakopoulou VA, et al. An attenuated adenovirus, ONYX-015, as mouthwash therapy for premalignant oral dysplasia. J Clin Oncol 2003.

154. Clayman GL, Frank DK, Bruso PA, Goepfert H. Adenovirus-mediated wild-type p53 gene transfer as a surgical adjuvant in advanced head and neck cancers. Clin Cancer Res 1999; 5:1715–1722.

155. Clayman GL, el-Naggar AK, Lippman SM, et al. Adenovirus-mediated p53 gene transfer in patients with advanced recurrent head and neck squamous cell carcinoma. J Clin Oncol 1998; 16:2221–2232.

156. Mobley SR, Liu TJ, Hudson JM, Clayman GL. In vitro growth suppression by adenoviral transduction of p21 and p16 in squamous cell carcinoma of the head and neck: a research model for combination gene therapy. Arch Otolaryngol Head Neck Surg 1998; 124:88–92.

157. Wolf JK, Kim TE, Fightmaster D, et al. Growth suppression of human ovarian cancer cell lines by the introduction of a p16 gene via a recombinant adenovirus. Gynecol Oncol 1999; 73:27–34.

158. Rocco JW, Li D, Liggett WH, Jr., et al. p16INK4A adenovirus-mediated gene therapy for human head and neck squamous cell cancer. Clin Cancer Res 1998; 4:1697–1704.

159. Schreinemachers DM, Everson RB. Aspirin use and lung, colon, and breast cancer incidence in a prospective study. Epidemiology 1994; 5:138–146.

160. Giovannucci E, Egan KM, Hunter DJ, et al. Aspirin and the risk of colorectal cancer in women. N Engl J Med 1995; 333:609–614.

161. Rao CV, Rivenson A, Simi B, et al. Chemoprevention of colon carcinogenesis by sulindac, a nonsteroidal anti-inflammatory agent. Cancer Res 1995; 55:1464–1472.

162. Giardiello FM, Hamilton SR, Krush AJ, et al. Treatment of colonic and rectal adenomas with sulindac in familial adenomatous polyposis. N Engl J Med 1993; 328:1313–1316.

163. Steinbach G, Lynch PM, Phillips RK, et al. The effect of celecoxib, a cyclooxygenase-2 inhibitor, in familial adenomatous polyposis. N Engl J Med 2000; 342:1946–1952.

164. Thun MJ, Namboodiri MM, Heath CW, Jr. Aspirin use and reduced risk of fatal colon cancer. N Engl J Med 1991; 325:1593–1596.

165. Church RD, Fleshman JW, McLeod HL. Cyclo-oxygenase 2 inhibition in colorectal cancer therapy. Br J Surg 2003; 90:1055–1067.

166. Mohan S, Epstein JB. Carcinogenesis and cyclooxygenase: the potential role of COX-2 inhibition in upper aerodigestive tract cancer. Oral Oncol 2003; 39:537–546.

167. Lin DT, Subbaramaiah K, Shah JP, Dannenberg AJ, Boyle JO. Cyclooxygenase-2: a novel molecular target for the prevention and treatment of head and neck cancer. Head Neck 2002; 24:792–799.

168. Chan G, Boyle JO, Yang EK, et al. Cyclooxygenase-2 expression is up-regulated in squamous cell carcinoma of the head and neck. Cancer Res 1999; 59:991–994.

169. Kawamori T, Rao CV, Seibert K, Reddy BS. Chemopreventive activity of celecoxib, a specific cyclooxygenase-2 inhibitor, against colon carcinogenesis. Cancer Res 1998; 58:409–412.

170. Oshima M, Murai N, Kargman S, et al. Chemoprevention of intestinal polyposis in the Apcdelta716 mouse by rofecoxib, a specific cyclooxygenase-2 inhibitor. Cancer Res 2001; 61:1733–740.

171. Harris RE, Alshafie GA, Abou-Issa H, Seibert K. Chemoprevention of breast cancer in rats by celecoxib, a cyclooxygenase 2 inhibitor. Cancer Res 2000; 60:2101–2103.

172. Sawaoka H, Kawano S, Tsuji S, et al. Cyclooxygenase-2 inhibitors suppress the growth of gastric cancer xenografts via induction of apoptosis in nude mice. Am J Physiol 1998; 274:G1061–1067.

173. Nishimura G, Yanoma S, Mizuno H, Kawakami K, Tsukuda M. A selective cyclooxygenase-2 inhibitor suppresses tumor growth in nude mouse xenografted with human head and neck squamous carcinoma cells. Jpn J Cancer Res 1999; 90:1152–1162.

174. Sheng H, Shao J, Kirkland SC, et al. Inhibition of human colon cancer cell growth by selective inhibition of cyclooxygenase-2. J Clin Invest 1997; 99:2254–2259.

175. Liu XH, Kirschenbaum A, Yao S, Lee R, Holland JF, Levine AC. Inhibition of cyclooxygenase-2 suppresses angiogenesis and the growth of prostate cancer in vivo. J Urol 2000; 164:820–825.

176. Shiotani H, Denda A, Yamamoto K, et al. Increased expression of cyclooxygenase-2 protein in 4-nitroquinoline-1-oxide-induced rat tongue carcinomas and chemopreventive efficacy of a specific inhibitor, nimesulide. Cancer Res 2001; 61:1451–1456.

177. Nishimura G, Yanoma S, Satake K, et al. An experimental model of tumor dormancy therapy for advanced head and neck carcinoma. Jpn J Cancer Res 2000; 91:1199–1203.

178. Petersen C, Petersen S, Milas L, Lang FF, Tofilon PJ. Enhancement of intrinsic tumor cell radiosensitivity induced by a selective cyclooxygenase-2 inhibitor. Clin Cancer Res 2000; 6:2513–2520.

179. Kishi K, Petersen S, Petersen C, et al. Preferential enhancement of tumor radioresponse by a cyclooxygenase-2 inhibitor. Cancer Res 2000; 60:1326–1331.

180. Pyo H, Choy H, Amorino GP, et al. A selective cyclooxygenase-2 inhibitor, NS-398, enhances the effect of radiation in vitro and in vivo preferentially on the cells that express cyclooxygenase-2. Clin Cancer Res 2001; 7:2998–3005.

181. Choy H, Milas L. Enhancing radiotherapy with cyclooxygenase-2 enzyme inhibitors: a rational advance? J Natl Cancer Inst 2003; 95:1440–1452.

182. Naujokat C, Hoffmann S. Role and function of the 26S proteasome in proliferation and apoptosis. Lab Invest 2002; 82:965–980.

183. Spataro V, Norbury C, Harris AL. The ubiquitin-proteasome pathway in cancer. Br J Cancer 1998; 77:448–455.

184. Hochstrasser M. Ubiquitin-dependent protein degradation. Annu Rev Genet 1996; 30:405–439.

185. Wilkinson KD. Ubiquitin-dependent signaling: the role of ubiquitination in the response of cells to their environment. J Nutr 1999; 129:1933–1936.

186. Masdehors P, Omura S, Merle-Beral H, et al. Increased sensitivity of CLL-derived lymphocytes to apoptotic death activation by the proteasome-specific inhibitor lactacystin. Br J Haematol 1999; 105:752–757.

187. Delic J, Masdehors P, Omura S, et al. The proteasome inhibitor lactacystin induces apoptosis and sensitizes chemo- and radioresistant human chronic lymphocytic leukaemia lymphocytes to TNF-alpha-initiated apoptosis. Br J Cancer 1998; 77:1103–1107.

188. Kudo Y, Takata T, Ogawa I, et al. p27Kip1 accumulation by inhibition of proteasome function induces apoptosis in oral squamous cell carcinoma cells. Clin Cancer Res 2000; 6:916–923.

189. Orlowski RZ, Eswara JR, Lafond-Walker A, Grever MR, Orlowski M, Dang CV. Tumor growth inhibition induced in a murine model of human Burkitt's lymphoma by a proteasome inhibitor. Cancer Res 1998; 58:4342–4348.

190. Murray RZ, Norbury C. Proteasome inhibitors as anti-cancer agents. Anticancer Drugs 2000; 11:407–417.

191. Richardson PG, Hideshima T, Anderson KC. Bortezomib (PS-341): a novel, first-in-class proteasome inhibitor for the treatment of multiple myeloma and other cancers. Cancer Control 2003; 10:361–369.

192. Sunwoo JB, Chen Z, Dong G, et al. Novel proteasome inhibitor PS-341 inhibits activation of nuclear factor-kappa B, cell survival, tumor growth, and angiogenesis in squamous cell carcinoma. Clin Cancer Res 2001; 7:1419–1428.

193. Russo SM, Tepper JE, Baldwin AS, Jr., et al. Enhancement of radiosensitivity by proteasome inhibition: implications for a role of NF-kappaB. Int J Radiat Oncol Biol Phys 2001; 50:183–193.

194. Pajonk F, Pajonk K, McBride WH. Apoptosis and radiosensitization of hodgkin cells by proteasome inhibition. Int J Radiat Oncol Biol Phys 2000; 47:1025–1032.

195. Pervan M, Pajonk F, Sun JR, Withers HR, McBride WH. Molecular pathways that modify tumor radiation response. Am J Clin Oncol 2001; 24:481–485.

196. Lebowitz PF, Conley B, Headlee D, et al. Concomitant therapy with proteasome inhibitor, bortezomib, and radiation in patients with recurrent or metastatic head and neck squamous cell carcinoma (HNSCC). American Society of Clinical Oncology Annual Meeting, Chicago, IL, 2003, vol. 22.

18

Gene Therapy for Patients
With Head and Neck Cancer

Andrew Iskander, MD and George H. Yoo, MD

1. INTRODUCTION

1.1. Genetics of Cancer

It is generally recognized that the unregulated growth of cancer cells results from sequential acquisition of mutations in genes that control growth and/or differentiation of cells or are involved in protection of the genome. Cancer develops when the accumulation of these alterations allows for a growth advantage over normal surrounding cells *(1)*. The pathogenesis of cancer can be described as follows: *Oncogenes* are altered normal genes (called protooncogenes) that mediate normal cell growth and differentiation. Gain-of-function (dominant) mutations affect these genes to induce the neoplastic phenotype. *Tumor suppressor genes* are genes that normally inhibit cellular function. Loss-of-function (recessive) mutations alter their inhibitory properties, leading to unimpeded proliferation. Gene therapy aims to change these genetic alterations so that cancer cell growth can be suppressed. After a gene is transfected into a cell, mRNA is transcribed, and then its protein product is translated.

Alterations of the tumor suppressor genes p53 and p16 have been implicated in the development of head and neck squamous cell cancer (HNSCC) *(2,3)*. The p53 gene is mutated in approx 33 to 45% of HNSCC *(2–4)*. The p53 protein acts by inhibiting the cell cycle, promoting apoptosis, and regulating transcription *(5)*. The p53 protein upregulates the cell cycle inhibitor p21, which further acts on cyclin-dependent kinases (cdks) to cause cell cycle arrest. The p53 gene also causes apoptosis in cells that have undergone severe DNA damage from radiation or chemotherapy exposure and inhibits DNA repair and synthesis. Furthermore, p53 regulates transcription by stimulating transactivator proteins *(5)*. The suppressive effects of p53 genes lead one to believe that clinical behavior can be correlated to alterations in the gene. A handful of protooncogenes have been implicated in the development of HNSCC, e.g., Her2/neu and cyclin D1. Her2/neu, a transmembrane tyrosine kinase receptor that functions to promote cellular proliferation, is overexpressed in approx 40 to 50% of HNSCC *(6,7)*. Cyclin D1 (a promoter of cdk 4/6 and the cell cycle) is overexpressed in 12 to 54% of HNSCC *(8)*, because of the amplification of chromosomal area 11q13 *(9,10)*.

1.2. Tumor Immunology

The body's immune system has a surveillance function that seeks out and destroys tumor cells. A "hierarchy of immunosuppression" exists in patients with HNSCC *(11)* that enables tumor cells to avoid detection. Immune reactivity is maximally suppressed in tumor infiltrat-

From: *Current Clinical Oncology: Squamous Cell Head and Neck Cancer*
Edited by: D. J. Adelstein © Humana Press Inc., Totowa, NJ

ing lymphocytes (TILs), followed by lymph node lymphocytes (LNLs) and peripheral blood lymphocytes (PBLs) *(11)*. Immune cells, such as cytotoxic T lymphocytes (CTLs) and natural killer (NK) cells, attack cancer cells. Cytokines, such as interleukins and interferons, activate the immune system. Tumor-specific antigens are expressed on tumor cells and help the host recognize and mount a specific immune response against these cells.

Induction of a T-cell immune response by antigen-presenting cells (APCs) occurs in three distinct stages. Initially, a nonspecific adhesion occurs between an APC and a T cell, followed by antigen-major histocompatability complex (MHC) of the APC crosslinkage with the T-cell receptor (TcR). The final step occurs when a second or costimulatory signal is delivered by the APC to the T cell, enhancing response. Presently, the best characterized second signal occurs when the B7.1 or B7.2 ligand of the APC binds to the CD28 receptor on the T cell, resulting in enhanced cellular activation *(12)*. The goal of genetic immunotherapy is to promote this T-cell response against cancer cells.

2. APPROACHES TO GENE THERAPY FOR CANCER

The approaches to gene therapy are as follows: (1) corrective gene therapy, (2) cytotoxic therapy, (3) immunotherapy, and (4) combination adjuvant therapy (Table 1).

2.1. Corrective Gene Therapy

Gene therapy can be used to correct any molecular aberrations in the control mechanism of cell proliferation. For example, replacement of a mutated tumor suppressor gene with a copy of the wild-type gene results in appropriate cell death. Alternatively, an oncogene can be inhibited either by transfecting the antisense cDNA so it binds to the mRNA of the oncogene or by adding a gene that regulates and inhibits the transcription of an oncogene.

2.2. Cytotoxic Therapy

Gene therapy can be used to augment cytotoxic therapy by either a drug sensitization or a resistance approach. In the drug sensitization approach, a gene is transfected to convert a prodrug into its active metabolite. This allows for drug conversion and a high level of active drug only in the tumor bed. One example is the herpes simplex virus thymidine kinase (TK) gene, which converts ganciclovir into its cytotoxic triphosphate. Another way to augment cytotoxic effects of chemotherapy is to use a drug resistance approach. A drug-resistant gene, such as multiple drug resistance (MDR1) gene, is added into cells that are sensitive to chemotherapy, such as hematopoietic stem cells, so they can resist the toxicity of chemotherapy. Therefore, higher doses of chemotherapy can be used since the most sensitive cells are now resistant to these levels of chemotherapy.

2.3. Immunotherapy

Immunotherapy can help decrease the immune suppression described above by "revving up" the immune system's tumor killing capabilities. Cytokine gene transfer is a method used to stimulate the immune system. Cytokine gene transfer is performed in vivo whereby tumor cells or immune cells, such as TILs and CTLs, are transfected in the body, upregulating the immune and anti-tumor response. Ex vivo cytokine gene transfer is performed after fibroblasts, immune cells (such as TILs, CTLs, or APCs) or irradiated cancer cells are removed from the body, and then these cells are placed back into the body to obtain high levels of a cytokine with a resulting immunological effect. Irradiated tumor cells are used not only to produce high levels of cytokine but also to provide tumor antigens for immune cells.

Table 1
Classification of Gene Therapy
Approaches

I. Corrective gene therapy
  A. Replace tumor suppressor gene
  B. Inhibit an oncogene
    1. Antisense cDNA
    2. Gene that regulate oncogene
II. Cytotoxic therapy
  A. Drug sensitization
  B. Drug resistance
III. Immunotherapy
  A. Cytokine gene transfer
    1. In vivo
    2. Ex vivo
  B. Vaccination
    1. Tumor-specific antigen
    2. Alloantigen
    3. Foreign antigen
  C. Costimulatory gene
IV. Combination/adjuvant therapy
  A. Adjuvant with chemotherapy
  B. Adjuvant with radiation therapy
  C. Adjuvant with surgery

Immune therapy can enhance the immune system's response to cancer cells by use of tumor-specific vaccines. After a tumor-specific antigen gene is injected into a cancer cell, the gene product helps the body recognize the tumor cell and reject it. The problem with HNSCC is that there are no reliably known tumor-specific antigens. Another vaccination approach is to add a gene that can produce an alloantigen. A third approach is simply adding a gene that produces a foreign antigen. Alloantigens and foreign antigens can also act as costimulatory molecules in the tumor cell so that the immune system recognizes tumor-specific antigens.

2.4. Genes Used in Combination Therapy

Ideally, gene therapy aims to introduce a gene into a cell's genome with a therapeutic benefit. The gene, which is under control of a promoter, is placed into a vector DNA, such as plasmids or viruses, which allow incorporation into the cell's genetic reproductive machinery. The gene then undergoes transcription and subsequent translation into a functional protein. There are many genes that can be used for gene therapy; only the genes that are currently being tested in HNSCC will be explored in detail here. Interleukin (IL)-2, IL-12, interferon (IFN)-α, and granulocyte-macrophage colony-stimulating factor (GM-CSF) are cytokines that enhance the immune response against tumors. The HLA-B7 gene is an alloantigen injected into tumors that helps the immune system recognize antigens on the tumor cells, expediting their destruction. The herpes simplex virus-TK gene converts the antiviral agent gancyclovir into its toxic triphosphate metabolite. After TK is transfected into tumor cells and gancyclovir is given to a patient, the activated drug not only kills the tumor cells but also allows for a killing of surrounding tumor cells (bystander effect), because of high levels of the activated drug that are produced locally. Two genes, p53 and E1A, have been used in corrective therapy in

HNSCC. The p53 gene has been transfected into tumor cells and has been shown to suppress growth. The E1A adenovirus gene functions to inhibit tumor growth by several pathways, including downregulation of an oncogene (HER-2/neu), reversion to an epithelial phenotype, loss of anchorage-independent growth, and decreased tumorgenicity in nude mice.

3. VECTORS

Crucial to gene therapy is the ability to target the culprit cell, enter the host nucleus, and exploit the host's ability to transcribe and translate genes into the desired protein. A *vector* is used so that a gene can be transfected into a cell and the gene can produce its protein product. The ideal vector would have a high efficiency (100% of cells are transfected), a high specificity (only tumor cells receive the gene), and a low toxicity. No known vector meets all these criteria. Vectors are classified as viral and nonviral (Table 2).

3.1. Viral Vectors

Of all *viral vectors* currently being studied, adenoviruses and retroviruses are most commonly used. These viruses are attenuated to transfect genes, but they cannot replicate or cause an infection. Eliminating their ability to replicate through genetic manipulation of the wild-type virus eliminates the pathogenicity of virus. Most viruses are replication deficient and need a packaging cell line to produce the virus. Adenovirus-associated virus (AAV), vaccinia virus, lentivirus, herpes simplex virus, and many others are currently being extensively studied in the preclinical setting.

3.1.1. ADENOVIRUS

The adenovirus (Ad) is the most commonly used virus in gene therapy. Ad is a double-stranded DNA virus that causes upper respiratory tract infections. Subgroup C, usually C2 or C5, is the most common adenoviruses used. A replication-deficient Ad after genetic modification, such as E1 deletion, is used to prevent pathological infection in the host. Replication-deficient Ad is grown in 293 human embryonic kidney cells, which have the missing Ad genes needed to replicate. Although adenoviruses infect almost all cell types including quiescent or actively dividing cells, adenoviruses have tropism for keratinocytes of the upper aerodigestive tract. After release of viral DNA, a nonreplicating extrachromasomal entity (episome) transcribes into RNA. The introduced gene persists for 7–42 d *(13)*. A potential risk is contamination with a replication-competent virus. Adenoviruses can be produced in large quantities and high titers. Adenoviruses have a high level of transduction and can transfect nondividing cells. The disadvantages of adenoviruses are the immune response against it and the fact that transfections are transient. The immune response to infected cells results in a loss of therapeutic gene expression *(14,15)*. The size of the gene is limited to 7–8 kb.

3.1.2. RETROVIRUSES

A retrovirus is a single-stranded RNA virus that replicates through DNA intermediates (reverse transcription). Retroviral vectors can permanently integrate in a random fashion into the host genome. All retroviruses, except HIV, integrate only in dividing cells. Retroviruses have high transduction efficiency. However, high titers are not achievable, which makes large-scale production difficult. The cell host range is limited because cells must be dividing in order to be transfected. Since retroviruses are integrated into the genome, a potential for genetic transformation exists by insertional mutagenesis. The size of the gene is limited to 6–10 kb.

Table 2
Vectors Used in Gene Therapy

Viral Vectors
    Adenovirus
    Retroviruses
    Adenovirus-associated virus (AAV)
    Lentivirus
    Vaccinia virus
    Herpes simplex virus
Nonviral Vectors
    Lipid complex
        Liposomes
    Peptide/protein
    Polymers
    Mechanical
        Electroporation
        Gene gun

3.2. Nonviral Vectors

Nonviral vectors use plasmid DNA to express a transgene. They are relatively easy to manufacture and use (Table 2). They have the added benefit of safety, as they avoid use of infectious agents. However, nonviral vectors have no cell specificity and usually lower transfection efficiency. DNA is a negatively charged molecule that is condensed by positively charged molecules (histones and polyamines). Free DNA is too large and has the wrong chemical characteristics to cross the cell membrane. Therefore, other molecules must be used to transfer DNA into the cell.

3.2.1. LIPID COMPLEX

Liposomes function by enabling a hydrophilic particle (DNA) to cross the lipophilic cellular membrane *(16)*. They are microscopic vesicles of lipid surrounding an aqueous compartment containing the genetic material. Cationic (positive charge) liposomes, as opposed to anionic (negative charge), are more frequently used since they can bind negatively charged DNA. The mechanism of DNA transduction by liposomes is thought to occur by fluid phase endocytosis but is not fully understood. The effectiveness of liposome-DNA complex to transfer DNA is based on proportions of each. Colipids, such as DOPE or cholesterol, are also added to facilitate liposome mediated transfection. Liposomes have no pathogenic or infectious potential and low immunogenicity; they are also inexpensive and easy to produce. Liposomes do not have the cell specificity and transfer efficiency of viruses, but they have less toxicity. Macrophages ingest and inactivate liposomes and transport them to the reticuloendothelial system. Liposomes are the most common nonviral vectors used in gene therapy.

3.2.2. PEPTIDE/PROTEIN AND POLYMERS

DNA-protein complexes use receptor-mediated pathways to transfer genes *(16)*. An example is polylysine conjugation to DNA-protein. The advantages include cell targeting, large gene size capacity, transfection of nonreplicating cells, and repeated administration. Polymers are more efficient in condensing DNA than liposomes. Polymer-based gene therapy is either a noncondensing or cationic-based system. Noncondensing polymers, such as polyvinyl pyrrolidone (PVP), bind to DNA and protect DNA from degradation, enhance tissue dispersion, and facilitate cellular uptake. Cationic polymer gene delivery can effectively condense DNA in order to transfect cells. PVP is currently under investigation with IL-12, IL-2, and IFN-α gene therapy trials.

Two mechanical gene-transducing techniques, electroporation and particle mediation, are also being studied. Electroporation uses short electrical pulses to induce a physical and transient permeabilization of cell membranes. Electroporation therapy in combination with chemotherapy (bleomycin) has been tested in patients with recurrent HNSCC *(17)* and has demonstrated tumor responses. Gene transfer using electroporation (electrogene therapy) is highly efficient, simple, and cost effective *(18)*. Using electrogene therapy, stable gene transfer and expression occurs only between the electrodes in many tissues, including tumor cells *(18)*. Electrogene therapy is currently being studied in eight trials. Particle-mediated gene transfection accelerates and bombards DNA-coated heavy metal (gold) particles to a sufficient velocity to penetrate target cells. Particle-mediated gene transfer has been used to transduce transgenes in animal models and has been shown to reduce tumor growth in mice when cytokine genes, such as interleukins and interferons *(19–24)*, are used.

4. GENE TRANSFER DELIVERY SITES

Genes can be delivered to the tumor, muscle, or nodes, intravascularly or systemically (Table 3). Most studies have used local intratumoral injections. Since head and neck cancer is a locoregional problem and access to most lesions is a relatively simple procedure using intratumoral injections, the head and neck area is a common site studied using gene therapy. Intravascular delivery, such as hepatic artery injections, systemic intravenous delivery, and immunogenic nodal site injections is also being studied.

Most clinical gene delivery approaches are based on direct intratumoral injections or ex vivo injection of lymphocytes, fibroblasts, or tumor cells. Some genes have been delivered into intracavitary spaces (peritoneal or thoracic cavity). Two mechanical delivery methods, electroporation and gene gun, are currently under investigation in preclinical models. These locally based delivery approaches are limited since distant disease failure is not addressed. Cytokine gene transfer into regional lymph nodes by direct injection has been used to overcome immune suppression. The regional draining lymph nodes can undergo ex vivo gene transfer after nodal lymphocytes are removed from the patient, transfected with the cytokine, and reintroduced into the patient. Intramuscular gene transfer of tumor antigens by direct injection or mechanical techniques has been used in tumor vaccination approaches, since APCs can uptake and process the antigen gene, present the antigen to T cells, and initiate an immune response against cancer cells. Intravascular administration of genetic agents allows for delivery into tissue supplied by an artery. Intrahepatic artery infusion of Ad-p53 has been examined in preclincal experiments and has been approved for phase I and II trials in patients with hepatic metastasis from colon cancer. Local delivery fails to treat distant disease and lesions that are not amenable to direct injection. Systemic delivery approaches (intravenous) allow for treatment beyond local disease. However, systemic delivery has to overcome toxicity and rapid degradation of the vector and has to target tumor cells. Three trials have been approved using intravenous delivery: (1) a pharmacokinetic, safety, and tolerability study of intravenous advexin; (2) intravenous injection of CV787, a PSA cytolytic adenovirus; and (3) intravenously administered liposome/IL-2.

Table 3
Delivery Approaches for Gene
Therapy

Local
Injection
Intratumoral
Mechanical
Electroporation
Gene gun
Regional
Intramuscular
Injection or mechanical
Nodal injection
Nodal ex vivo immunotherapy
Intraarterial
Systemic
Intravenous

5. GENE THERAPY TRIALS IN HNSCC

As of November 2003, 392 of the 601 approved gene therapy trials were for cancer in the United States. A review of all gene therapy trials can be found at the Office of Biological Activities of the NIH (http://www.nih.gov/od/oba/). Twenty-two trials using 12 different genes are being tested in recurrent HNSCC using intratumoral injections (Table 4). Many potential genes and gene therapy strategies that have been tested in vitro and in vivo have demonstrated tumor suppression or killing; however, only approaches that are currently being tested in human trials with HNSCC will be discussed in detail.

5.1. Gene Therapy Using the p53 Gene

The p53 gene regulates DNA repair, cell cycle progression, apoptosis, senescence, and genomic stability, along with many other cellular functions and is mutated in half of human cancers (2,25). In HNSCC, p53 mutations from tumor cells have been identified in histologically normal margins and have been correlated with a higher recurrence rate (26). Overexpression of p53 in head and neck cancer cells has demonstrated tumor growth suppression using in vitro and in vivo models (27,28). Using either mutated or wild-type p53 human HNSCC cell lines, exogenous wild-type p53 is dominant over its mutant gene and will select against proliferation. Twenty-three p53 gene therapy trials have been approved or have approval pending. Most of the experience is in patients with HNSCC and lung cancer. Two adenoviral-p53 agents are currently being tested. Advexin (Introgen) is the only agent that is tested in HNSCC. Advexin is a constructed adenoviral vector that contains the wild-type p53 gene driven by a cytomegalovirus (CMV) promoter.

5.1.1. Phase I Intratumoral HNSCC Trial (Ad-p53, or Advexin)

In a phase I trial, patients with recurrent HNSCC received multiple intratumoral injections of Ad-p53 and were monitored for adverse events, p53 expression, Ad-p53 in body fluids, antiadenoviral antibodies, and clinical responses (29). Thirty-three patients were injected (d 1, 3, 5, 8, 10, and 12 every 4 wk) with Ad-p53 using doses ranging between 1×10^6 and $1 \times$

Table 4
Clinical Gene Therapy Trials in Head and Neck Cancer

Gene	Vector	Institution (sponsor)	Trials	Results
p53	Adenovirus	M.D. Anderson (Introgen)	Phase I 1. Unresectable 2. Resectable	Safe Safe, no added surgical complications, 28% survival
p53	Adenovirus	Multicenter (Introgen)	Phase II (Three trials)	Response rate: 6% Antitumor activity: 26%
p53	Adenovirus	Multicenter (SWOG)	Phase II (Surgical adjuvant)	Ongoing
p53	Adenovirus	Multicenter (Introgen)	Phase III 5-FU/CDDP vs 5-FU/CDDP/ Ad-p53	Ongoing
p53	Adenovirus	Multicenter (Introgen)	Phase III MTX vs Ad-p53	Ongoing
BL7	Liposome	Univ. of Cincinnati Multicenter	Phase I Phase II	Safe Safe, two complete responses
BL7 + IL-2	Liposome	Multicenter	Phase II	Ongoing
E1A	Liposome	WSU and Rush Univ.	Phase I	Safe
E1A	Liposome	Multicenter	Phase II	Response rate: 5%
E1A	Liposome	Multicenter	Phase II	Ongoing
IL-2	Liposome	Johns Hopkins (Valentis)	Phase I	Safe
IL-2	Liposome	Multicenter (Valentis)	Phase II	Ongoing
TK	Liposome	Johns Hopkins	Phase I	Approved/not initiated
TK	Adenovirus	Johns Hopkins	Phase I	Approved/not initiated
EGFR	Liposome	Univ. of Pittsburgh	Phase I	Ongoing
IL-12	PVP	Multicenter (Valentis)	Phase I	Ongoing
IL-12 + IFN-γ	PVP	Multicenter (Valentis)	Phase II	Ongoing
IFN-α	PVP	Univ. of Pennsylvania (Valentis)	Phasc I	Ongoing
GM-CSF adenovirus		Univ. of Kansas	Phase I	Ongoing

Abbreviations: CDDP, cis-diaminedichloroplatinum; EGFR, epidermal growth factor receptor; 5-FU, 5-fluorouracil; GM-CSF, granulocyte/macrophage colony-stimulating factor; IFN, interferon; IL, interleukin; MTX, methotrexate; PVP, polyvinyl pyrrolidine; SWOG, Southwest Oncology Group; TK, thymidine kinase.

10^{11} plaque-forming units (PFU). No dose-limiting toxicity or related serious adverse events were noted.

5.1.2. PHASE II INTRATUMORAL HNSCC TRIALS

Two phase II monotherapy intratumoral injection multicenter trials *(30)* using two dosing schedules (low dose [d 1, 2, and 3 every 4 wk] or high dose [d 1, 3, 5, 8, 10, and 12 every 4 wk]) enrolled heavily pretreated, recurrent, and unresectable patients with HNSCC, respectively. Three and four lesions achieved a complete and partial response, respectively. The related adverse events were fever/chills, injection site pain, asthenia, nausea, and injection site bleeding. No treatment-related deaths were reported. The ongoing Advexin trials are: (1) refractory HNSCC (phase III, methotrexate vs advexin); (2) recurrent HNSCC (phase III, 5-fluorouracil/cis-diaminechloroplatinum [5-FU/CDDP] vs 5-FU/CDDP + Advexin); and (3) surgical adjuvant Advexin trial in advanced HNSCC (phase II).

5.1.3. SURGICAL ADJUVANT P53 GENE THERAPY

Using a model that simulated residual microscopic disease after gross tumor resection of squamous cell cancer, the feasibility of gene therapy as an adjuvant to surgical resection was demonstrated *(28)*. Nude mice were implanted subcutaneously with tumor cells and treated with Ad-p53 before gross tumor development. Ad-p53 therapy prevented tumor development since 2 of 30 (6.7%) mice grew tumors that were treated with Ad-p53, as opposed to 27 of 30 (90%) in the control group *(28)*. The primary mechanism of growth suppression was found to be apoptosis. Additional mechanisms of actions for Ad-p53 have been demonstrated, including Fas-mediated apoptosis and antiangiogenesis effects. In the single-center phase I trial, a cohort of 15 patients who had recurrent/refractory (failed multimodalities of therapy) cancer and were eligible for palliative surgical resection were enrolled *(29)*. These patients were resectable but thought to be incurable. Preoperatively, a patient's tumor was injected six times in a 2-wk period. Patients underwent a surgical resection and were given an intraoperative injection of Ad-p53 in the resected tumor bed and in the neck dissection site. Three days later, their drainage catheters were injected (retrograde) with Ad-p53. All patients had extensive surgery and required flaps for closure. The surgical complications (one vascular anastomotic failure and one delayed wound healing) were expected and unlikely to have been caused by Ad-p53 therapy. Therefore, this perioperative approach was found to be safe and well tolerated, with no significant added wound complications. Fever (six), injection pain (five), and flu-like (four) symptoms were the only complications observed in these patients. Otherwise, it was felt to be safe and well tolerated. In a follow-up report *(31)*, four (27%) patients were alive and free of disease at 18 mo and one other patient was alive with disease. Two died from other causes.

5.2. Allovectin (HLA-B7/β2-Microglobulin and DMRIE/DOPE) Gene Therapy

Class I MHC expression is a method of tumor-specific immunological gene therapy. Cancer cells are genetically altered to express a class I MHC. If the class I MHC that is used is a human antigen but is foreign to the individual, it would be an alloantigen. This alloantigen is capable of provoking an intense immune response. Then the class I MHC expression can also initiate immune responses throughout the tumor as a reaction to tumor-associated antigens. This theory was originally tested in a mouse tumor model. The tumors were treated with a foreign mouse class I MHC gene. MHC expression induced a CTL response to the MHC, as well as to other antigens present on the surrounding tumor cells that were not modified. Allovectin-7 encodes for the class I MHC HLA-B7 α-chain and β2-microglobulin. The β2-microglobulin allows for the synthesis and expression of the complete MHC on the cell surface. The plasmid DNA is complexed with a liposomal vector. A cationic lipid mixture DMRIE/DOPE (1,2-dimyristyloxypropyl-3-dimethyl-hydroxyethyl ammonium bromide/dioleoyl phosphytidal ethanolamine) was used. These results led to the development of the drug Allovectin-7 (Vical, San Diego, CA) for clinical investigations.

In a phase I trial *(32)*, nine patients with recurrent HNSCC who did not express HLA-B7 were treated with Allovectin-7 by direct intratumoral injection (10 mg) on d 0, 14, 42, and 56. Allovectin-7 contains a plasmid complementary DNA complexed with a cationic lipid, which results in expression of HLA-B7. No toxic effects of Allovectin-7 gene therapy were encountered. A partial response was found in four of nine patients. One patient has remained alive with no clinical evidence of disease but with persistent histological evidence of cancer. Analysis of tumor specimens from two of the patients who responded to therapy demonstrated HLA-B7 expression and apoptosis.

In a phase II trial *(33)*, 20 patients received 58 treatments with Allovectin-7 (10 mg) on d 0, 14, 42, and 56. All 20 patients received the first cycle of two injections. No drug-related adverse events were reported. Tumor progression resulted in one case of airway obstruction (tracheostomy tube placement) and another case of severe dysphagia (gastrostomy tube placement). At the 3-wk evaluation point, 11 patients had disease progression and all but 1 eventually died of their cancer, 4 patients had a partial response, and 5 patients had stable disease. At 16 wk, six patients had either a partial response or stable disease; five of these later progressed. One patient underwent surgery and remains alive and cancer free. Although two complete responses were noted, biopsies revealed persistent disease in these patients. In two tumor samples, expression of HLA-B7 and induction of apoptosis was shown.

5.3. Gene Therapy Using the E1A Gene

The adenovirus E1A gene is the first gene expressed in virus-infected cells and is a transcription factor. The E1A gene exhibits antitumor activity by downregulating oncogenes, such as HER2/neu, inducing apoptosis, inhibiting metastasis, and enhancing immune response against tumors *(34,35)*. E1A gene products have been shown to inhibit HER2 expression in cancer cells through inhibition of the HER2 promoter, resulting in suppression of tumor development and abolition of tumorigenicity and metastatic potential of HER2-transformed fibroblasts *(36–38)*. In vitro and in vivo experiments have demonstrated tumor growth suppression and increased survival using E1A gene therapy *(34)*.

Nine patients with HNSCC and nine with breast cancer were enrolled in a phase I trial *(39)*. One tumor nodule was injected with E1A/liposome on d 1, 2, and 3 and then weekly for 7 more weeks (10 injections total). No dose-limiting toxicity was observed in the four dose groups (15, 30, 60, and 120 μg DNA/cm tumor). Therefore, the maximum tolerated dose was not reached in this study. All patients tolerated the injections, although several experienced pain and bleeding at the injection site. E1A gene transfer was demonstrated in 11 of 11 tumor samples tested, and downregulation of HER2/neu was demonstrated in one of the six patients who overexpressed HER2/neu at baseline. HER2 could not be assessed post treatment in five of six specimens owing to severe necrosis. In one breast cancer patient, no pathologic evidence of tumor was found on biopsy of the treated tumor at wk 12. In 16 patients evaluated for response, 9 had stable disease, 5 had progressive disease, and 2 had minor responses. Since intratumoral E1A gene therapy was performed safely and patients tolerated the procedure well, a phase II trial was initiated.

In multicenter phase II trial of EIA-liposome therapy *(40)*, 24 patients with recurrent HNSCC were treated with E1A/liposome (30 μg/cm^3 tumor) on d 1, 2, and 3 and then weekly for 7 more weeks. Ten of 24 patients completed therapy, and 14 did not complete the protocol secondary to progression of tumor (11), voluntary withdrawal (1), and death (2). One of 21 (4.3%) patients had a complete response, while no partial responses, and two (8.3%) minor, and seven (29.2%) stable disease incidences were reported by bidimensional computed tomographic measurement. The common adverse events were asthenia (42%) and pain (33%), and no serious related adverse events were noted. E1A expression was detected in patients using reverse transcription-polymerase chain reaction and immunohistochemistry.

5.4. IL-12 Gene Therapy

IL-12 is an immunostimulatory cytokine with antitumor effects. IL-12 stimulates NK cells and augments CTL maturation along with induction of IFN-γ production. In a syngeneic mouse squamous cell carcinoma model, IL-12 gene therapy using irradiated tumor cells suppressed tumor growth *(41)*. A phase II trial of intravenous recombinant IL-12 was stopped early since significant toxicity was found *(42)*. Two phase I trials of IL-12 gene therapy using autologous fibroblasts by direct injection were approved and performed in HNSCC, breast cancer, and melanoma. In a phase I trial *(42)*, patients with solid cancers were injected with genetically engineered autologous fibroblasts that were transfected with the IL-12 gene. Fibroblasts from the patients were transduced using the retroviral vector carrying the human IL-12 gene. Two patients with HNSCC along with individuals with breast cancer (*n* = 6) and melanoma (*n* = 5) were treated. Fibroblast cultures were successfully established from the patients' dermis in 27 of 29 attempts (93%). In 21 of 21 attempts, IL-12 was transferred into fibroblasts, and expression of IL-12 protein was observed. No "untoward effects" were observed, and "reduction of the tumor size" was noted in one patient with HNSCC and in three patients with melanoma. Two IL-12 gene therapy trials using IL-12/PVP and IL-12/IFN-γ/PVP have been approved for HNSCC.

5.5. IL-2 Gene Therapy

IL-2 is a T- and NK-cell activation and growth factor that stimulates the antitumor immunological response *(43)*. Systemic administration has lead to tumor regression in some patients with significant toxicity in melanoma *(43)* and HNSCC *(44)*. High-dose localized IL-2 therapy is an attractive approach to overcome local immunosuppression and stimulate immunological tumor rejection along with the avoidance of systemic toxicity. Injection of IL-2 and a cationic liposome (DOTMA:cholesterol) in head and neck tumors of immunocompetent mice after subtotal surgical resection in mice resulted in tumor growth suppression, and no significant toxicity was noted *(45)*. Treated mice had increased IL-2 production as well as induction of murine IFN-γ and IL-12 compared with controls. Similar results were found using an adenoviral-IL-2 agent *(46)*. Although the completed phase I trial using IL-2/liposome has not yet been published, the phase II trial using IL-2/PVP is ongoing.

5.6. Herpes Simplex Virus–Thymidine Kinase

The herpes simplex virus–TK gene expresses an enzyme that phosphorylates a prodrug, ganciclovir, into a toxic compound. Furthermore, a "bystander effect" through the transfer of toxic metabolites via gap junctions intercellular communications has been described in which surrounding nontransduced cells are killed. Most studies are in glioblastoma; however, HNSCC has been studied using a combination of cytotoxic (TK) and immunological (IL-2) approaches in an in vivo model *(47–49)*. Mice receiving TK and IL-2 demonstrated a greater regression of tumors compared with controls and the group treated with TK only. The results of an approved TK-ganciclovir phase I trial in recurrent HNSCC are pending.

5.7. Antisense EGFR/Liposome

HNSCC cells overexpress epidermal growth factor receptor (EGFR), which is a tyrosine kinase cell surface receptor. Ligands, such as epidermal growth factor (EGF) and transforming growth factor (TGF)-α, which bind to EGFR stimulate mitogenesis and increases tumor growth and metastasis, with overexpression a predictor of poor outcomes in HNSCC *(50)*. Since EGFR protein is required to sustain the proliferation of HNSCC cells in vitro, downregulation of EGFR is a potential target in HNSCC. Intratumoral cationic liposome-mediated gene transfer of antisense EGFR gene into human head and neck tumor xenografts in nude mice resulted in inhibition of tumor growth, suppression of EGFR protein expression, and an increased rate of apoptosis *(50)*. Based on these preclinical data, a phase I trial using liposome-mediated antisense EGFR gene therapy was approved.

5.8. Interferon-α Gene Transfer Using PVP

IFN is an immunomodulator cytokine that has antitumor activity. IFN-α is the most widely used IFN. IFN-α2b is approved for use in high-risk melanoma and many other cancers. Response rates for patients with advanced head and neck cancer treated with IFN-α alone or with chemotherapy or IL-2 range between 18 and 54% *(44,51–54)*. However, significant toxicity has led some authors to suggest further investigations of less aggressive regimens. Preclinical data have demonstrated antitumor activity for interferon gene therapy *(55)*. A phase I trial is approved and is ongoing at the University of Pennsylvania using intratumoral IFN-α gene therapy.

5.9. GM-CSF-Based Gene Therapy

GM-CSF stimulates the proliferation of myeloid precursors and has a vital role in hematopoiesis of other cell lineages. Furthermore, GM-CSF has many other biologic effects on hematopoiesis and the immune system. The myeloproliferative effects of GM-CSF have led to its use in myelosuppressed patients. The additional biological effects have led to use of GM-CSF in many other diseases, such as immunotherapy for malignancies. Direct injections of the GM-CSF gene or ex vivo transduction of GM-CSF into irradiated tumor cells have been tested. An ex vivo transduction phase I trial in renal and prostate cancer *(56)* has shown immunological activity and limited toxicity. One patient with renal cancer responded. In HNSCC, breast and colon cancer, and sarcomas, a phase I trial using ex vivo transduced, irradiated cancer cells is ongoing.

6. FUTURE OF GENE THERAPY FOR CANCER

With the completion of the human genome project, many more genes will be available for transfer. However, genes that are currently used can produce all desired antitumor effects. The limitations of gene therapy can be overcome by combining genes with standard therapy, developing new vectors, and targeting vectors.

6.1. Combination With Standard Therapy

Gene therapy is also being used as an adjuvant to conventional therapies, such as chemotherapy, radiotherapy, and surgery. Gene transfer is currently being combined with chemotherapy (Ad-p53 and E1A), radiotherapy (Ad-p53, TK- and PSA-based vaccine), and surgery (Ad-p53). The best described adjuvant effect of gene transfer is p53. Chemotherapy and radiotherapy induce DNA damage, which leads to increases in p53 expression in normal cells and cell cycle arrest. If cells cannot repair the DNA damage, apoptosis will result through p53 pathways. In cancer cells that have an altered p53, cell cycle arrest and apoptosis can be avoided after exposure to chemotherapy and radiotherapy. Preclinical experiments have demonstrated synergy between chemotherapy and p53 *(57)* and E1A *(58)* overexpression. This synergy has led to the development of current ongoing trials using p53 gene transfer therapy and chemotherapy in HNSCC. The basis for surgical adjuvant gene therapy lies in the observation that tumor cells are present in the margin of resection even with histologically normal tissue. Since squamous cell-derived tumor cells have a higher level of adenoviral receptors than fibroblasts, adenovirus-based therapy can more easily transfect tumor cells in the tumor microenvironment. The favorable results of the phase I p53 gene therapy surgical adjuvant trial has led to the phase II trial in newly diagnosed HNSCC in which Ad-p53 gene therapy is given perioperatively.

6.2. New Vector Strategies

Although numerous vectors are in use for gene therapy and many more are under investigation, no existing vector meets the criteria of an ideal vector, which are a high efficiency (100% of cells are transfected), high specificity (only tumor cells receive the gene), and low toxicity. New vector strategies are based on novel vectors, replication-competent viruses, or modifications of existing vectors. Modified replication-competent adenoviruses (RCAs) are the most commonly used for cancer. RCAs consist of wild-type adenoviruses or modified viruses with or without an added gene or specific promoter of normal viral genes. One newer vector is AAV, a DNA virus that requires a helper virus in order to replicate. AAV can infect nondividing cells without causing pathological infection.

6.3. Targeting Vectors

Vectors can be targeted by (1) altering vector-target cell interaction or (2) targeting promoter gene transcription. Viruses infect cells through cell surface receptors on the target cells by binding to the cell and being endocytosed. Two adenovirus receptors, integrin and coxsackie-adenovirus receptor (CAR), are on target cells *(59)*. The methods of targeting cells are by altering vector coat proteins or by using a bifunctional crosslinker. The fiber protein on the adenovirus can be genetically altered to bind to specific tissue. Alternatively, a bifunctional crosslinker (protein or antibody) molecule can be introduced to bind to the adenovirus fiber, specifically to receptors on target cells. Tumor-specific targeting of transgene expression can be obtained by designing promoters of transcription. Promoters can be tissue specific (PSA), tumor selective (AFP), tumor endothelium directed (vascular endothelial growth factor receptor), cell cycle regulated (E2F), or treatment responsive (egr1-*early growth response*). Tissue-specific promoters, such as PSA, would express transgene only in certain tumor or normal cells.

REFERENCES

1. Fearon ER, Vogelstein B. A genetic model for colorectal tumorigenesis. [Review]. Cell 1990; 61:759–767.
2. Boyle JO, Hakim J, Koch W, et al. The incidence of p53 mutations increases with progression of head and neck cancer. Cancer Res 1993; 53:4477–4480.
3. Koch WM, Brennan JA, Zahurak M, et al. p53 mutation and locoregional treatment failure in head and neck squamous cell carcinoma. J Natl Cancer Inst 1996; 88:1580–1586.
4. Chomchai JS, Du W, Sarkar FH, et al. Prognostic significance of p53 gene mutations in laryngeal cancer. Laryngoscope 1999; 109:455–459.
5. Harris CC. Structure and function of the p53 tumor suppressor gene: clues for rational cancer therapeutic strategies. J Natl Cancer Inst 1996; 88:1442–1455.
6. Beckhardt RN, Kiyokawa N, Xi L, et al. HER-2/neu oncogene characterization in head and neck squamous cell carcinoma. Arch Otolaryngol Head Neck Surg 1995; 121:1265–1270.
7. Ibrahim SO, Vasstrand EN, Liavaag PG, Johannessen AC, Lillehaug JR. Expression of c-erbB proto-oncogene family members in squamous cell carcinoma of the head and neck. Anticancer Res 1997; 17:4539–4546.
8. Capaccio P, Pruneri G, Carboni N, et al. Cyclin D1 expression is predictive of occult metastases in head and neck cancer patients with clinically negative cervical lymph nodes. Head Neck 2000; 22:234–240.
9. Mineta H, Miura K, Takebayashi S, et al. Cyclin D1 overexpression correlates with poor prognosis in patients with tongue squamous cell carcinoma. Oral Oncol 2000; 36:194–198.
10. Bova RJ, Quinn DI, Nankervis JS, et al. Cyclin D1 and p16INK4A expression predict reduced survival in carcinoma of the anterior tongue. Clin.Cancer Res 1999; 5:2810–2819.
11. Myers JN, Whiteside T. Immunotherapy of squamous cell carcinoma of the head and neck. In: Myers EN, Suen J, eds. Cancer of the Head and Neck. Philadelphia: WB Saunders, 1995:805–817.
12. Guinan EC, Gribben JG, Boussiotis VA, Freeman GJ, Nadler LM. Pivotal role of the B7:CD28 pathway in transplantation tolerance and tumor immunity. Blood 1994; 84:3261–3282.
13. Mulligan RC. The basic science of gene therapy. Science 1993; 260:926–932.
14. Yang Y, Su Q, Wilson JM. Role of viral antigens in destructive cellular immune responses to adenovirus vector-transduced cells in mouse lungs. J Virol 1996; 70:7209–7212.
15. Yang Y, Wilson JM. Clearance of adenovirus-infected hepatocytes by MHC class I-restricted CD4+ CTLs in vivo. J Immunol 1995; 155:2564–2570.
16. Mahato RI, Smith LC, Rolland A. Pharmaceutical perspectives of nonviral gene therapy. Adv Genet 1999; 41:95–156.
17. Panje WR, Hier MP, Garman GR, Harrell E, Goldman A, Bloch I. Electroporation therapy of head and neck cancer. Ann Otol Rhinol Laryngol 1998; 107:779–785.
18. Hofmann GA, Dev SB, Nanda GS, Rabussay D. Electroporation therapy of solid tumors. Crit Rev Ther Drug Carrier Syst 1999; 16:523–569.
19. Rakhmilevich AL, Timmins JG, Janssen K, Pohlmann EL, Sheehy MJ, Yang NS. Gene gun-mediated IL-12 gene therapy induces antitumor effects in the absence of toxicity: a direct comparison with systemic IL-12 protein therapy. J Immunother 1999; 22:135–144.
20. Mahvi DM, Sheehy MJ, Yang NS. DNA cancer vaccines: a gene gun approach. Immunol Cell Biol 1997; 75:456–460.
21. Rakhmilevich AL, Turner J, Ford MJ, et al. Gene gun-mediated skin transfection with interleukin 12 gene results in regression of established primary and metastatic murine tumors. Proc Natl Acad Sci USA 1996; 93:6291–6296.
22. Sun WH, Burkholder JK, Sun J, et al. In vivo cytokine gene transfer by gene gun reduces tumor growth in mice. Proc Natl Acad Sci USA 1995; 92:2889–2893.
23. Mahvi DM, Sondel PM, Yang NS, et al. Phase I/IB study of immunization with autologous tumor cells transfected with the GM-CSF gene by particle-mediated transfer in patients with melanoma or sarcoma. Hum Gene Ther 1997; 8:875–891.
24. Mahvi DM, Burkholder JK, Turner J, et al. Particle-mediated gene transfer of granulocyte-macrophage colony-stimulating factor cDNA to tumor cells: implications for a clinically relevant tumor vaccine. Hum Gene Ther 1996; 7:1535–1543.
25. Hollstein M, Sidransky D, Vogelstein B, Harris CC. p53 mutations in human cancers. [Review]. Science 1991; 253:49–53.
26. Brennan JA, Mao L, Hruban RH, et al. Molecular assessment of histopathological staging in squamous-cell carcinoma of the head and neck [see comments]. N Engl J Med 1995; 332:429–435.
27. Liu TJ, Zhang WW, Taylor DL, Roth JA, Goepfert H, Clayman GL. Growth suppression of human head and neck cancer cells by the introduction of a wild-type p53 gene via a recombinant adenovirus. Cancer Res 1994; 54:3662–3667.

28. Clayman GL, el-Naggar AK, Roth JA, et al. In vivo molecular therapy with p53 adenovirus for microscopic residual head and neck squamous carcinoma. Cancer Res 1995; 55:1–6.
29. Clayman GL, el-Naggar AK, Lippman SM, et al. Adenovirus-mediated p53 gene transfer in patients with advanced recurrent head and neck squamous cell carcinoma. J Clin Oncol 1998; 16:2221–2232.
30. Bier-Laning CM, VanEcho D, Yver A, Dreiling L. A phase II multi-center study of AdCMV-p53 administered intratumorally to patients with recurrent head and neck cancer (#1712). Annual Meeting: Proceedings of the American Society of Clinical Oncology. 1999; 18:431a.
31. Clayman GL, Frank DK, Bruso PA, Goepfert H. Adenovirus-mediated wild-type p53 gene transfer as a surgical adjuvant in advanced head and neck cancers. Clin Cancer Res 1999; 5:1715–1722.
32. Gleich LL, Gluckman JL, Armstrong S, et al. Alloantigen gene therapy for squamous cell carcinoma of the head and neck: results of a phase-1 trial. Arch Otolaryngol Head Neck Surg 1998; 124:1097–1104.
33. Gleich LL. Gene therapy for head and neck cancer. Laryngoscope 2000; 110:708–726.
34. Yu D, Matin A, Xia W, Sorgi F, Huang L, Hung MC. Liposome-mediated in vivo E1A gene transfer suppressed dissemination of ovarian cancer cells that overexpress HER-2/neu. Oncogene 1995; 11:1383–1388.
35. Yu D, Hamada J, Zhang H, Nicolson GL, Hung MC. Mechanisms of c-erbB2/neu oncogene-induced metastasis and repression of metastatic properties by adenovirus 5 E1A gene products. Oncogene 1992; 7:2263–2270.
36. Zhang Y, Yu D, Xia W, Hung MC. HER-2/neu-targeting cancer therapy via adenovirus-mediated E1A delivery in an animal model. Oncogene 1995; 10:1947–1954.
37. Frisch SM. Antioncogenic effect of adenovirus E1A in human tumor cells. Proc Natl Acad Sci USA 1991; 88:9077–9081.
38. Frisch SM. E1a induces the expression of epithelial characteristics. J Cell Biol 1994; 127:1085–1096.
39. Yoo GH, Hung MC, Lopez-Berestein G, et al. Phase i trial of intratumoral liposome e1a gene therapy in patients with recurrent breast and head and neck cancer. Clin Cancer Res 2001; 7:1237–1245.
40. Villaret D, Glisson B, Kenady D, et al. A multicenter phase II study of tgDCC-E1A for the intratumoral treatment of patients with recurrent head and neck squamous cell carcinoma. Head Neck 2002; 24:661–669.
41. Myers JN, Mank-Seymour A, Zitvogel L, et al. Interleukin-12 gene therapy prevents establishment of SCC VII squamous cell carcinomas, inhibits tumor growth, and elicits long-term antitumor immunity in syngeneic C3H mice. Laryngoscope 1998; 108:261–268.
42. Lotze MT, Zitvogel L, Campbell R, et al. Cytokine gene therapy of cancer using interleukin-12: murine and clinical trials. Ann NY Acad Sci 1996; 795:440–454.
43. Atkins MB, Lotze MT, Dutcher JP, et al. High-dose recombinant interleukin 2 therapy for patients with metastatic melanoma: analysis of 270 patients treated between 1985 and 1993. J Clin Oncol 1999; 17:2105–2116.
44. Urba SG, Forastiere AA, Wolf GT, Amrein PC. Intensive recombinant interleukin-2 and alpha-interferon therapy in patients with advanced head and neck squamous carcinoma. Cancer 1993; 71:2326–2331.
45. Li D, Jiang W, Bishop JS, Ralston R, O'Malley BWJ. Combination surgery and nonviral interleukin 2 gene therapy for head and neck cancer. Clin Cancer Res 1999; 5:1551–1556.
46. O'Malley BWJ, Li D, Buckner A, Duan L, Woo SL, Pardoll DM. Limitations of adenovirus-mediated interleukin-2 gene therapy for oral cancer. Laryngoscope 1999; 109:389–395.
47. O'Malley BW, Cope KA, Chen SH, Li D, Schwarta MR, Woo SL. Combination gene therapy for oral cancer in a murine model. Cancer Res 1996; 56:1737–1741.
48. Sewell DA, Li D, Duan L, Schwartz MR, O'Malley BWJ. Optimizing suicide gene therapy for head and neck cancer. Laryngoscope 1997; 107:t–5.
49. O'Malley BWJ, Sewell DA, Li D, et al. The role of interleukin-2 in combination adenovirus gene therapy for head and neck cancer. Mol Endocrinol 1997; 11:667–673.
50. He Y, Zeng Q, Drenning SD, et al. Inhibition of human squamous cell carcinoma growth in vivo by epidermal growth factor receptor antisense RNA transcribed from the U6 promoter. J Natl Cancer Inst 1998; 90:1080–1087.
51. Benasso M, Merlano M, Blengio F, Cavallari M, Rosso R, Toma S. Concomitant alpha-interferon and chemotherapy in advanced squamous cell carcinoma of the head and neck. Am J Clin Oncol 1993; 16:465–468.
52. Trudeau M, Zukiwski A, Langleben A, Boos G, Batist G. A phase I study of recombinant human interferon alpha-2b combined with 5-fluorouracil and cisplatin in patients with advanced cancer. Cancer Chemother Pharmacol 1995; 35:496–500.
53. Hamasaki VK, Vokes EE. Interferons and other cytokines in head and neck cancer. Med Oncol 1995; 12:23–33.
54. Vlock DR, Andersen J, Kalish LA, et al. Phase II trial of interferon-alpha in locally recurrent or metastatic squamous cell carcinoma of the head and neck: immunological and clinical correlates. J Immunother Emphasis Tumor Immunol 1996; 19:433–442.
55. Ferrantini M, Belardelli F. Gene therapy of cancer with interferon: lessons from tumor models and perspectives for clinical applications [In Process Citation]. Semin Cancer Biol 2000; 10:145–157.
56. Nelson WG, Simons JW, Mikhak B, et al. Cancer cells engineered to secrete granulocyte-macrophage colony-stimulating factor using ex vivo gene transfer as vaccines for the treatment of genitourinary malignancies. Cancer Chemother Pharmacol 2000; 46(Suppl):S67–S72.

57. Inoue A, Narumi K, Matsubara N, et al. Administration of wild-type p53 adenoviral vector synergistically enhances the cytotoxicity of anti-cancer drugs in human lung cancer cells irrespective of the status of p53 gene. Cancer Lett 2000; 157:105–112.

58. Ueno NT, Yu D, Hung MC. Chemosensitization of HER-2/neu-overexpressing human breast cancer cells to paclitaxel (Taxol) by adenovirus type 5 E1A. Oncogene 1997; 15:953–960.

59. Nemerow GR. Cell receptors involved in adenovirus entry. Virology 2000; 274:1–4.

19

Chemoprevention
in Head and Neck Cancer

Nabil F. Saba, MD *and Fadlo R. Khuri,* MD

1. INTRODUCTION

Head and neck squamous cell carcinoma (HNSCC) is an aggressive epithelial malignancy that is the sixth most common neoplasm worldwide, with close to 5000 new cases diagnosed yearly in the United States (estimated to be 56,520 cases in 2004 *[1]*) and 600,000 worldwide according to the latest numbers from the International Agency for Research on Cancer, World Health Organization. HNSCC accounts for 2% of all cancer deaths in the United States *(2)* and is the most common epithelial neoplasm of the upper aerodigestive tract. It constitutes a major health care problem and is clearly associated with well-known risk factors such as tobacco smoking and alcohol use. The management of HNSCC is complex and the morbidity of treatment is life-long. Despite the numerous advances in its treatment, the long-term survival still does not exceed 45% and has only marginally improved over the last decades *(3)*.

The poor outcome of HNSCC is a result of multiple factors, including delayed detection and the development of multiple primary tumors. The observation that upper aerodigestive tract cancers undergo transformation in certain patients and not others is a reflection of probable alterations in the regional mucosa that are likely linked to certain genetic predisposition *(4)*. Prevention of new primary tumors seems to be a rational goal for improving patient outcome.

HNSCC is a heterogeneous disease with distinct patterns of behavior and represents a paradigm for cancer chemoprevention. The concept of field cancerization is the most accepted hypothesis for the cellular damage responsible for neoplastic transformation, making prevention of second primary tumors (SPTs) in initially cured patients one of the greatest challenges in therapy for oral squamous cell carcinomas. Given the extent of injury found as a result of environmental factors and the high incidence of SPT after curative treatment of early-stage carcinoma, the concept of chemoprevention is particularly attractive in the area of aerodigestive tract cancers (Table 1). Advances in the molecular biology of HNSCC, as well as the development of novel targeted therapies, have opened the door to an increased interest in the study of chemoprevention in these malignancies. The ability to identify etiologic factors has helped in improved identification and risk stratification. Therefore, novel cancer prevention strategies including lifestyle alteration and identification of biologic markers will play a key role in prevention of HNSCC. Randomized clinical trials over the last decade have produced significant results in reversing oral premalignant lesions and the occurrence of SPTs after definitive therapy for lung cancer and HNSCC *(5)*. Cancer incidence is still the main end

From: *Current Clinical Oncology: Squamous Cell Head and Neck Cancer*
Edited by: D. J. Adelstein © Humana Press Inc., Totowa, NJ

Table 1
Promising New Agents
for Chemoprevention

Newer retinoids (heteroatinoids)
COX-2 inhibitors
Farnesyl transferase inhibitors
Proteasome inhibitors (PS 341)
Bowman-Birk inhibitor concentrate (BBIC)
Nutritional supplements (green tea)

point of these phase III trials, yet it is conceivable that intermediate biologic markers may one day replace incidence as a major end point sparing the need for large and costly studies.

The application of selected biologic markers as intermediate end points that test the effectiveness of chemopreventive agents within a limited time frame will help in better defining the steps involved in carcinogenesis and evaluating the effects of different agents on tumor progression. It will also help in monitoring patient compliance. Markers of cell proliferation in normal and dysplastic epithelia of the oral cavity are serving as surrogate end point biomarkers for the different chemoprevention trials. When taken together, these strategies could bring chemoprevention of HNSCC to new frontiers.

Furthermore, the oral premalignant lesion model has been an important driving factor for the study of chemoprevention of tumors owing to the several research advantages it offers including ease of monitoring and sampling of lesions. The carcinogenesis process in HNSCC results from dysregulation in cellular proliferation and programmed cell death as a result of field exposure to carcinogens. The study of the genetic and molecular changes that accompany these cellular changes, and their translation into clinical and chemical interventions, forms the basis for chemoprevention studies.

2. THE MULTISTEP PROCESS OF CARCINOGENESIS

The evidence that HNSCC is a multistep process comes from findings of genetic alterations observed in the histologically defined premalignant lesions such as oral leukoplakia as well as the adjacent nonmalignant epithelium (6). The concept of field cancerization described earlier, where a carcinogen such as tobacco causes a diffuse insult to the epithelium of the aerodigestive tract (7), leading to multiple tumors or SPTs in the lung as well as the oral cavity (8), forms one important basis for chemoprevention in these tumors. These observations were the first to suggest that lung cancer and HNSCC are a result of a series of genetic defects accumulating in the normal bronchial epithelium as a result of tobacco exposure.

This multistep accumulation of successive genetic alterations that affects the whole exposed field, if better understood, will help provide us with the necessary knowledge for designing novel strategies that would halt or reverse the process of carcinogenesis. Furthermore, the activity of chemopreventive agents that target specific abnormalities can be accurately assessed using their specific effects on the biomarkers in question.

3. ORAL LEUKOPLAKIA

The association of white plaques or patches with carcinoma of the oral mucosa has been recognized for a long time. These whitish plaques may precede the appearance of cancer by months or years, or they may be found simultaneously with the diagnosis of carcinoma. The hyperkeratosis that characterizes epithelium in the vicinity of tumors produces the clinical appearance of white plaques. It is important to note, however, that carcinoma may not be preceded by plaques.

Lesions that precede the development of carcinoma may show cellular changes. The general changes seen in the epithelium are referred to as dysplasia. Severe grades of dysplasia may merge into carcinoma *in situ*, in which the whole thickness of the epithelium is involved.

The term *leukoplakia* is used to describe an oral mucosal white plaque that cannot be removed by scraping and cannot be classified as a disease entity by clinical or pathologic means. It is considered to be a potentially malignant lesion with a rate of transformation to malignancy ranging from 0.6 to 18%. Clinically it is in the same disease category as erythroplakia, which has a much higher transformation rate and is more likely on biopsy to be squamous cell carcinoma.

The term erythroplakia is used analogously to leukoplakia and designates lesions of the oral mucosa that are bright red velvety plaques that cannot be characterized clinically or pathologically as being caused by any other condition. High risk of malignant transformation of oral leukoplakia include the clinical presence of erythroplakia (erythroleukoplakia), found to be associated with a transformation rate four- to sevenfold the rate associated with homogeneous leukoplakia *(9,10)* and a verrucous-papillary hyperkeratotic pattern. These risk factors for transformation may warrant a more aggressive approach *(11)*. There is also evidence that the rate of transformation increases with increasing the follow-up period *(12)*, supporting the need for continued observation of these lesions even though clinical progression seems to be lacking.

The presence of dysplasia also seems to confer an increased risk of transformation, reported to be 13 to 45% *(11,13,14)*. Even though age confers an increased risk of malignancy, there does not seem to be a relation between age and malignant transformation of leukoplakia. Pain appears to be the initial complain of close to 25% of patients presenting with oral leukoplakia and seems to be prevalent in 50% of patients at the time of malignant transformation. Interestingly, smoking does not seem to confer an increased risk of transformation from leukoplakia to malignancy *(10,15,16)*, yet nonsmoking patients with leukoplakia have been noted to have five to eight times the risk of developing carcinoma *(10,16)*, an observation that is not explainable. Smoking cessation, on the other hand, is beneficial in terms of decreasing the rate of malignant transformation. There have also been suggestions that infection or colonization with *Candida albicans* may confer some risk for malignant transformation; however, the evidence is nonconclusive *(17)*.

Oral leukoplakia is associated with tobacco exposure; however, verrucous leukoplakia, which has a high rate of transformation to cancer, occurs predominantly in nonsmokers. On pathological examination, most leukoplakia show some degree of dysplasia, features of which remain somewhat subjectively recognizable, raising the need for a more reliable and reproducible molecular marker that would be predictive of transformation. Possible markers for transformation include DNA aneuploidy, as discussed in this chapter, as well as loss of heterozygosity based on microsatellite markers, p53 mutations, and other markers discussed in other parts of this chapter.

It has been shown that the nuclear DNA content of the lesion can predict the progression to oral carcinoma from leukoplakia *(18)*. In a study looking at DNA ploidy in 150 patients with epithelial dysplasia of the oral cavity, carcinoma developed in 3/105 patients (3%) with diploid lesions, 21/25 patients (84%) with aneuploid lesions, and 12/20 patients (60%) with tetraploid lesions. The cumulative disease-free survival rate for patients with diploid lesions was 97% compared with 16% of the aneuploid group ($p < 0.001$) *(18)*. These results support the acceptable practice of watchful waiting for patients with oral leukoplakia with normal DNA content, whereas they do not support such an approach for patients with aneuploid lesions. Whether intensive therapy of aneuploid lesions will improve survival and reduce the incidence and mortality from HNSCC in this patient group remains to be proved. Current chemopreventive strategies for HNSCC may improve the outcome of patients if the intervention comes at an early enough stage of the carcinogenesis process. In a follow up study by the same group, however, complete resections of aneuploid leukoplakia did not seem to reduce the risk of development of carcinoma and death from oral cancer in this patient population *(19)*. During the study period, patients with aneuploid leukoplakia had a 96% rate of primary cancer, a rate of new or subsequent cancer of 81%, and a death rate from cancer of 78%. The resection margin status did not seem to affect the risk of cancer development in this patient population. Subsequent cancers were more frequently multiple and at different sites in patients with aneuploid lesions than those with tetraploid lesions, and the stage of cancer was more advanced in the aneuploid group.

These findings suggest that all leukoplakia may not be premalignant after all and that aneuploidy may have the clinical significance of carcinoma. These patients need more aggressive interventions and more effective preventive approaches. Intriguingly, removal of lesions with clear margins did not improve the outcome for this population of patients. Aneuploidy seems therefore to be a sign reflecting an early and turning event in the process of carcinogenesis. Resection appears to be little more than a cosmetic approach for management of these lesions and, as was the case with retinoid use in dysplastic lesions, did not appear to improve the clinical outcome. Chemopreventive agents that may interfere with molecular events leading to the phenomenon of aneuploidy may be of help here. It is unclear whether smoking cessation will reverse the carcinogenesis process in aneuploid leukoplakia lesions. One possible future approach could be the use of cyclooxygenase inhibitors, as there seems to be an overexpression of cyclooxygenase-2 enzyme in aneuploid dysplasia compared with diploid or tetraploid variety *(20)*.

4. EPIDEMIOLOGY AND RELATION TO CARCINOGEN EXPOSURE

HNSCC risk increases linearly with tobacco smoking and is higher in heavy smokers compared with nonsmokers *(21)*. Even though tobacco and alcohol are major risk factors for HNSCC, inherited susceptibility is probably responsible for carcinogenesis as well and is most likely related to genomic stability, deregulated tumor suppressor and oncogenes, and impaired DNA repair mechanisms *(22)*. The latter has been demonstrated by finding that mutagen sensitivity confers a risk for HNSCC. The measurement of DNA repair capacity of the upper aerodigestive tract malignancies appears to have an important clinical relevance *(23)*. Individuals with identifiable risks may be the subjects of successful targeting by chemoprevention strategies.

Sensitivity to environmental carcinogens can be assessed through mutagen sensitivity assays, which quantitates chromosomal breaks with exposure to bleomycinin-cultured peripheral blood lymphocytes (PBLs). There is evidence that mutagen sensitivity (>0.8 chromosomal breaks per cell after in vitro exposure to bleomycin of cultured PBLs) carries an independent prognostic significance as a risk for development of HNSCC *(24,25)*. Mutagen hypersensitivity was also noted in 44% of patients with HNSCC in a retrospective evaluation of 278 patients. Mutagen hypersensitivity was associated with a relative risk of 2.67 of developing SPT4. The mean number of chromatid breaks per cell in patients who developed SPTs was significantly higher compared with those who did not develop SPTs (1.17 vs 0.98, $p < 0.04$). Other studies have confirmed these findings and also suggested mutagen sensitivity as a potential biomarker for SPT occurrence more than 3 yr after the primary tumor, as these patients had a higher mean breaks-per cell value (0.97) compared with patients with early SPTs (0.69; $p = 0.005$) (26). Increased sensitivity to benzo(a)pyrene diol epoxide in lymphoblastoid cells has also been associated with increased risk of HNSCC (27).

In the early 1990s, an Intergroup placebo-controlled, double-blind study examining the efficacy of 13-*cis*-retinoic acid (13-cRA) in prevention of SPTs assessed smoking status at enrollment and during the study. SPT development related to smoking status was marginally significant (5.7 vs 3.5%; $p = 0.035$). There was a significant difference in smoking-related SPT development in current, former and never smokers, indicating a significantly higher SPT rate in active vs never smokers and significantly higher smoking-related SPT rates in active vs never smokers (28).

Despite these findings, the role of continued smoking in the development of SPT is still under debate. The data are difficult to collect, and there is lack of biologic or biochemical confirmation.

5. GENOTYPIC AND PHENOTYPIC ALTERATIONS

Chromosome *in situ* hybridization, which measures the frequency of chromosome polysomy (cells with three or more chromosomes), has provided evidence that genetic instability occurs and increases along the path of progression from normal tissue to dysplasia and ultimately frank malignancy. Carcinogenesis in HNSCC seems to proceed through the acquisition of a series of genetic events in a multistep process that eventually leads to cancer. Several oncogene products are activated while tumor suppressor genes are inactivated, leading to uncontrolled cell growth (29).

Histologic progression from premalignant lesions to frank malignancy has been associated with degree of chromosomal polysomy, which is a simple measurement of gross genetic alterations identified by *in situ* hybridization (30). *In situ* hybridization has yielded evidence suggesting that polysomy results in genetic instability, which increases as cells progress histologically from normal to dysplastic epithelium and invasive carcinoma, suggesting that polysomy could be a useful marker for disease progression and genomic instability of premalignant lesions (30,31).

Allelic losses in specific regions have also been identified at 3p, 5q, 9p, 11q, 13q, 18q, and 17p (32) and appear to be important early events in head and neck tumorigenesis. Chromosomal losses and gains have also been identified consistently at different loci including 3q21, 5p, 7p, 8q, 11q13-23, 3p13-q24, 5q12-q23, 8p22-p23, 9p21-p24, and 18q22-23 (33). Deletions of chromosomes 3p, 5q, 9p, 11q, 13q, and 17p have been described in head and neck carcinogenesis. These loci are believed to carry tumor suppressor genes. Fragile histidine triad (FHIT), the tumor suppressor gene at 3p, is altered in 80% of HNSCC cell lines (34).

Loss of heterozygosity (LOH) has been observed in premalignant as well as malignant oral lesions and have been associated with an increased risk of malignant transformation (35). LOH at chromosome 3p or 9p occurs in approx 50% of oral premalignant lesions and is believed to play a role in regional clonal expansion of premalignant cells and the overall process of carcinogenesis (36). LOH at 9p21 and 3p14 has been linked to tumor suppressor genes p16$_{INK4A}$ as well as FHIT (34). FHIT is altered in 80% of HNSCC cell lines (34,37). Thirty-seven percent of patients with LOH at both loci developed HNSCC compared with only 6% of patients without LOH. Moreover, detection of LOH has genetically confirmed the concept of field cancerization through demonstration of transformation in cells in large areas of noncancerous mucosa *(38)*. LOH therefore hasthe potential for use in early detection of premalignant lesions with a high potential of transformation *(39)*. These studies and others looking at the expression of p16 in oral premalignant lesions suggest a major role of p16 in carcinogenesis *(40)*.

A high incidence of LOH was reported near the adenomatous polyposis coli gene at the 5q area, and was found in 80% of dysplastic epithelia, 67% of carcinoma *in situ*, and 50% of invasive carcinoma *(41,42)*. LOH on 13q occurs in approximately half of the tumors studied and is probably related to a tumor suppressor gene besides the retinoblastoma gene, as the latter has been rarely confirmed in these tumors *(43)*. Loss of chromosome 18, where several potential candidate genes exist such as the deleted in colon cancer gene (DCC) and deleted in pancreatic cancer DPG4 (all implicated in transforming growth factor-β), seems to be a later event in the process of carcinogenesis and has been documented in close to 60% of HNSCCs *(44,45)*.

Control of tumor suppressor genes leading to genomic instability has been reported in HNSCC. p53 is a tumor suppressor gene that is believed to function both in cell cycle check-point control and in one of the apoptotic pathways. Like other tumor suppressor genes, it is inactivated by deletion of an allele and mutation of the other. Alterations of p53, located at 17p13, are commonly found in HNSCC and occur in approx 50% of these tumors. Immuno-histochemical positivity has also been detected in 45% of dysplastic lesions, 29% of hyper-plastic lesions, and 21% of adjacent normal tissues *(46)*. p53 functions in cell regulation and survival and is activated in response to cellular stress. An association has been established between p53 mutation and cigarette smoking in HNSCC *(47)*. In premalignant lesions, p53 mutation appears to occur more frequently with histologic progression in head and neck tumors *(48)*. SPTs are more likely to occur if p53 is overexpressed in the initial HNSCC tumor *(49)*. Patients with HNSCCs whose tumors carry a p53 mutation are at higher risk for both SPT and recurrence and therefore shorter survival *(49)*. A higher level of polysomy found in premalignant lesions seems to be associated with p53 positivity, suggesting that an abnormal p53 function may interfere with the process of apoptosis, which in turn will allow accumula-tion of genetic insults to the cells manifested as chromosomal polysomy *(49)*.

Cell cycle control genes such as cyclin D1 plays an important role in the cell cycle transition from G1 to S, by contributing to phosphorylation and inactivation of the Rb gene product, thereby releasing E2F, which drives transcription of other downstream events *(50)*. The cyclin D1 protooncogene mapped to chromosome 11q13 encodes cyclin D1 protein, which promotes cell cycle progression through G1 and is overexpressed in 30 to 50% of head and neck tumors *(51)*. Gene amplification and protein overexpression have been described in premalignancies and associated with poor prognostic characteristics *(52,53)*. The p16 gene (discussed above), an inhibitor of the cyclin D/cyclin-dependent kinase complex is frequently inactivated in HNSCC and is the likely tumor suppressor gene at the 9p21-p24 locus as noted above *(54,55)*. Its loss is the most common genetic change found early in the progression of HNSCC, occur-ring at a frequency of about 80% *(56)*.

In addition to cyclin D1overexpression, epidermal growth factor receptor (EGF) is another amplified gene product of crucial importance. Upregulation of EGF occurs frequently in HNSCC and is an early event in the carcinogenesis process. It is considered a poor prognostic factor *(57)*. EGFR is the binding site for many growth factors that stimulate the proliferation of normal and neoplastic cells. A larger availability of these receptors appears to correlate with tumor progression. EGFR overexpression has been demonstrated in close to 85% of aerodigestive tumors. An increase in EGFR expression has also been noted in the process of progression from normal epithelium to frank malignancy, indicating its importance in HNSCC carcinogenesis. EGFR blockade in HNSCC cell lines and preclinical animal models shows inhibition of cell proliferation and tumor growth (58).

Hypermethylation has also been noted as a frequent genetic event in HNSCC. There is evidence that DNA methylation at CpG islands in the promoter region can silence certain critical genes contributing to tumorigenesis. Promoter hypermethylation of four genes including p16 was documented in 50% of HNSCC patients and was predictive for distant metastases as well as lymph node involvement (59). Aberrant p16 promoter methylation was seen in precursor lesions of squamous cell carcinomas of the lung, and its frequency increases with progression from hyperplasia to frank malignancy (60), a finding also confirmed in head and neck premalignant lesions (61). Further understanding of the loci in which methylation occurs can provide a potential marker for early cancer detection in the serum DNA of HNSCC patients (59).

6. THE CONCEPT OF CHEMOPREVENTION

Chemoprevention is defined as the use of pharmacologic or natural agents that prevent carcinogenesis by blocking genetic steps necessary for that process, or by reversing the progression to malignant phenotypes of already damaged cells (62). It inhibits the development of invasive cancer possibly by blocking DNA damage that initiates carcinogenesis or by reversing the progression of premalignant cells to malignant phenotypes. The development of HNSCC is a result of carcinogenesis, a multistep accumulation of genetic damage the end result of which is the occurrence of cancer. Identification of healthy individuals at risk for cancer and treatment of premalignant lesions prior to the occurrence of invasive cancer, as well as prevention of SPTs after initial treatment, all constitute important goals for chemoprevention strategies and can all be achieved through means that could arrest the process of carcinogenesis. Unlike other tumors, objective malignant and premalignant lesions are readily available for study and follow-up in HNSCC and may be sampled at different stages of carcinogenesis. Biopsied lesions could provide important information on the effectiveness of chemoprevention strategies.

6.1. The Biology of Carcinogenesis

Epithelial cancers result from a multistep process, as illustrated first in 1976 by the two-hit carcinogenesis process described in childhood malignancies using the retinoblastoma gene (63). Proof of this process in HNSCC comes from studies showing chromosomal abnormalities in premalignant lesions defined histologically, such as leukoplakia, as well as tumor cells. This multistep phenomenon was demonstrated by showing the same genetic abnormalities in cancer cells as well as in normal cells throughout the respiratory tract (6).

Field carcinogenesis, a concept described much earlier (7,8), describes the extensive development of a multifocal process of premalignant and malignant lesions scattered throughout the epithelial region exposed to a carcinogen.

As noted earlier, LOH provides a strong evidence for the multistep phenomenon. For example, the LOHs rate found in squamous dysplasia and carcinoma *in situ* were similar to those found in invasive carcinoma (35). Other observations associated the presence of LOH in premalignant oral leukoplakia lesions with a higher rate of progression to invasive carcinoma compared with non-LOH lesions *(64)*, stressing the importance of these early genetic alterations in premalignant lesions in the subsequent development of malignancy. Blocking or reversing cells and tissues from reaching the end stage of cancer is one primary focus of chemoprevention.

Smoking appears to be a major predictor for carcinogenesis and has been strongly linked in several chemoprevention trials to the occurrence of SPT *(65)*. However, a subpopulation of patients with HNSCC are never smokers in whom tobacco appeared to have little if any role in the carcinogenesis process. The cancer occurrence in this nonsmoking population may be linked to viruses such as human papillomavirus 16 and 18 *(66,67)*. As the incidence of SPT in this patient population is low, it suggests an alternate pathway for carcinogenesis in non-smokers.

6.2. Biomolecular Markers as Intermediate End Points

Attention has been devoted to the development of reliable genetic or molecular elements believed to be involved in the carcinogenesis process of HNSCC, in the hope that these would be reliable intermediate biomarkers that might objectively demonstrate the modulation effects of chemoprevention and be correlates to clinical responses. Surrogate end point biomarkers (SEBs) are detectable molecular, cellular, and tissue changes that take place during tumorigenesis and can be modulated by a chemopreventive agent. These would ultimately help in selecting effective chemoprevention strategies and also in completing clinical trials in a timely fashion. Those markers would also give us a further understanding of the process of carcinogenesis.

Each early phenomena in the process of carcinogenesis could be conceived of as markers for disease progression and could be used as selection criteria and possibly as intermediate biomarkers in chemoprevention trials. Some of these biomarkers are discussed in different sections of this chapter and include specific genotypic alterations detected through cytogenetics, tumor suppressor genes such as FHIT, and cell cycle control genes such as p16, p53 alterations, and DNA methylation. Another potential biomarker involves the testing of mutagen sensitivity.

In a prospective evaluation of the mean number of chromatid breaks per cell in cultured lymphocytes exposed to bleomycin as a possible predictor for SPT development in patients treated for HNSCC, significantly higher mean breaks per cell were noted in patients whose SPT occurred more than 3 yr after the first tumor, suggesting that mutagen sensitivity was a valid marker for the occurrence of late second malignancies *(68)*.

Some of the important findings in the area of intermediate biomarkers (in premalignancy trials) correlated retinoid acid receptor (RAR)-β with progression from premalignancy to malignant phenotypes in the carcinogenesis process. Upregulation of RAR-β seems to be correlated with the likelihood of improvement in premalignant lesions *(69)* and seems to be gradually lost during the carcinogenesis process *(70)*. RAR-β seems to be upregulated in patients treated with 13-cRA for oral leukoplakia and whose leukoplakia seems to be responding, whereas it was less likely to be upregulated in patients with no response *(69)*.

p53 has also been studied in relation to the carcinogenesis process and was found to be increased during the process of carcinogenesis and the progression from premalignant oral lesions to invasive cancer. Also, lesions with high p53 expression tended to be more resistant to 13-cRA and lacked RAR-β expression *(71,72)*. Patients with advanced premalignant lesions who respond to biochemoprevention seem to have persistent genetic abnormalities seen in the premalignant phenotype, suggesting that underlying mechanisms for carcinogenesis persists even in apparently normal tissues *(73)*.

Markers of cell proliferation in normal or dysplastic epithelia were also examined as a possible SEB in chemoprevention trials. Punch biopsies from different sites of the oral mucosa were analyzed for expression of proliferation markers including Mib-1, cyclin D1, and centromere-associated protein-F CENP-F *(74)*. No significant differences were detected between smokers and nonsmokers. There was a significant increment in the different markers, with an increase noted in high-grade dysplasia.

Based on this evidence, it seems that development of a molecular model for HNSCC that would ultimately help in guiding therapy and chemoprevention is possible. However, none of the biomarkers has been validated for use in chemoprevention trials. It is also possible that an effective chemopreventive agent may affect pathways downstream from the specific biomarker. Thus biomarkers as we know them presently run the risk of being the wrong marker for a specific chemopreventive agent occurring at an earlier or later stage than the one a particular agent is affecting. It seems that incorporating multiple biomarkers in models that systematically analyse them in correlation with clinical responses is needed to elucidate better their validity or lack of validity in chemopreventive studies.

6.3. Retinoids and Prevention of Oral Premalignant Lesions

Oral premalignant lesions offer a good model to test the principle of chemoprevention, as they have a clear association with known carcinogens and are easily monitored with readily available biopsies.

In vitro studies of retimoids have proved their ability to inhibit malignant transformation, an activity that seems to be related to their ability to modify cell growth, differentiation, and apoptosis of normal as well as premalignant and malignant cells in vitro and in vivo *(75,76)*. These effects are mostly mediated through the retinoid nuclear receptor, yet other mechanisms may be at play *(75)*.

Retinoids have an established effectiveness in reversing oral premalignant lesions *(77,78)*. Vitamin A deficiency was also linked to carcinogenesis in animals *(79)*.

Retinoids have played a major role in lung cancer chemoprevention and have been the focus of the largest chemoprevention trials in this disease (Table 2). They are potent regulators of gene expression and play an important role in regulating cell growth, apoptosis, and differentiation. They prevent the progression of premalignant cells to frank malignancies *(80)*. Retinoids are critical for epithelial differentiation and work through an elaborate family of cytoplasmic retinoic acid binding proteins *(81)*. It is thought that the anticarcinogenic effect of retinoids is a result of changes in specific genes. Retinoids exert their effect on gene expression by activating a signal transduction pathway in which the nuclear RARs play an essential role *(82)*. Once a retinoid reaches the cytoplasm, it is transported to the nucleus where it binds to the hormone binding domain of either RAR or retinoid x receptor (RXR), which are the two main subtypes of nuclear receptors. Subsequently, the ligand receptor complexes bind to DNA as homodimers or heterodimers and result in inhibition of protein kinase C.

Because each subtype (RAR and RXR) exhibits specific patterns of expression during embryogenesis, each is thought to regulate the expression of distinct genes *(82)*. The loss or abnormality of RAR-β,for example, seems to be frequently seen in lung cancer cell lines. There is also some evidence that the RAR-β has a tumor-suppressive function, as its loss has been documented in the bronchial epithelium of smokers *(83,84)*. Premalignant lesions that

Table 2
Randomized Premalignancy Clinical Trials Using Retinoids

Study	Patients	No. of patients	Drug	Results
Hong et al., 1986 (90)	Oral leukoplakia	44	13-cRA vs placebo	Regression of leukoplakia in 67% of patients vs 10% in placebo
Stich et al., 1988 (89)	Oral leukoplakia Betel nut chewers	65	Vitamin A	CR in 56% and lower rate of oral leukoplakia
Lippman et al., 1993 (91)	Oral leukoplakia to maintain remission after 13-cRA	70	HD 13-cRA for 3 mo LD 13-cRA or β-carotene for 9 mo	13-cRA better in maintenance than β-carotene
Costa et al., 1994 (145) (Italy)	Oral leukoplakia treated with laser in adjuvant setting	153	4 HPR for 1 yr or placebo	Lower rate of leukoplakia in 4-HPR group

Abbreviations: 13-cRA, 13-*cis*-retinoic acid; CR, complete response; HD, high dose; 4-HPR, *N*-4-hydroxycarbophenyl retinamide; LD, low dose.

respond to 13-cRA seem to have an increased RAR-β level (69,85), whereas restoration of RAR-β expression and reduction of metaplasia was noted in former smokers receiving 9-*cis*-retinoic acid (9-cRA), raising interest in investigating 9-cRA as a chemopreventive agent in prior smokers (86). Dysplastic lesions were, however, less likely to regress in current smokers taking retinols. The mechanism behind this observation is not known but it could be that tobacco has a contributing effect on the cellular metabolism of retinol (87). In addition, tobacco carcinogen can suppress RAR-β expression in cultured premalignant and malignant esophageal epithelial cells (88), confirming the persisting harmful effect of smoking.

Early interventional chemoprevention trials in oral premalignant lesions including leukoplakia and erythroplakia have been performed with a reported spontaneous regression of 30 to 40% of small hyperplastic leukoplakia lesions and a less than 5% risk of malignant transformation (9). Erythroplakia and dysplastic leukoplakia seem, on the other hand, to have a less than 5% rate of spontaneous regression and a 30 to 50% rate of progression to oral cancer (9). Oral micronuclei are fragments of extranuclear DNA believed to reflect genetic damage in a population of cells at high risk for transformation to malignancy. Epidemiologic and interventional studies in the 1970s have found a reduction in the frequency of oral micronuclei in patients taking β-carotene and retinol (89), in tobacco and betel nut chewers.

In a trial targeting nut chewers in India with well-differentiated oral leukoplakia comparing vitamin A at 200,000 IU/wk orally for 6 mo with placebo in 54 subjects, complete remission was observed in 12/21 patients (57.1%) on vitamin A, whereas only one complete remission was observed on the placebo arm, and 7/33 progressed. This finding prompted several investigational trials to examine the effect on oral leukoplakia of β-carotene alone, or in combination with other agents. It is of note, however, that the trials were not randomized and lacked a dose-response relationship. A spontaneous regression rate of 30 to 40% was noted (89).

Multiple randomized clinical trials with retinoids or β-carotene have been performed in upper aerodigestive tract tumors, and retinoids remain the most studied and active chemopreventive agents in the area of HNSCC. They have clearly been proved effective in reversal of early premalignant lesions. The first randomized clinical trial demonstrated a 67% response rate (16/24 patients) for 13-cRA compared with 10% for placebo, both administered for 3 mo. There was a greater reduction of dysplasia in the retinoid arm (54%) compared with the placebo arm (10%) *(90)*. Of interest was the considerable relapse rate of 50%, with evidence of recurrence within 2–3 mo after completion of therapy, suggesting the need for maintenance therapy. Mucocutaneous toxicity was significant.

To address the issues of relapse and toxicity, another follow-up trial was designed to evaluate the long-term effects of maintenance with retinoids and was concluded in 1993. Patients received 13-cRA at a dose of 1.5 mg/kg/d for 9 mo followed by a lower dose at 0.5 mg/kg/d for another 9 mo vs 9 mo of β-carotene at 30 mg/d. The reported initial response rate was comparable to that of the previous study at 55%; however a continued response was noted with the 13-cRA arm at 92 vs 45% for the β-carotene arm ($p = 0.001$). The lower dose of retinoic acid was also tolerated very well *(91)*. This trial indicated that maintenance retinoids at a low doses were more effective than β-carotene in maintaining the initial response to induction 13-cRA. A subsequent analysis however showed no significant difference in the development of HNSCC between the two arms *(91,92)*.

Another randomized trial used a synthetic retinoid (*N*-4-hydroxycarbophenyl retinamide [4-HPR])at 40 mg/d orally or topically vs placebo for 4 mo in 61 patients. Twenty-seven of 31 patients had major responses (87.1%), including several complete remissions, whereas a response rate of only 16.7% was noted on the placebo arm ($p = 0.01$). Toxicity consisted of some elevation in liver enzymes in two patients *(93)*.

In a randomized maintenance trial, 170 patients received systemic *N*-4-retinamide fenretidine (200 mg/d) or no intervention (control) as maintenance therapy for 1 yr following laser resection of oral leukoplakia. The local relapse rate or the occurrence of new lesions was 29% in the placebo arm vs 18% in the treatment arm ($p = 0.01$) *(94)*.

Other chemopreventive agents with potential use in HNSCC include green tea, which contains polyphenols with demonstrated chemopreventive benefits in animal studies *(95)*.

6.4. Biochemoprevention

Advanced premalignant lesions of the upper aerodigestive tract are associated with a defined risk of progression from moderate to severe dysplasia to invasive cancer at a rate of 36 to 50%. As noted, those lesions appear to be resistant to single-agent retinoid chemoprevention. Retinoid resistance has been reported and seems to be associated with p53 expression, increased degree of genomic instability, and lack of RAR-β upregulation following treatment with 13-c RA *(71)*. Biochemoprevention studies were devised to address the issue of retinoid resistance in advanced premalignant lesions of the upper aerodigestive tract. As noted, these advanced lesions are associated with a well-defined risk of progression to invasive carcinoma in oral as well as laryngeal tumors. Combination therapies using 13-cRA, α-tocopherol, and interferon (IFN)-α were designed.

In a trial of 36 patients with advanced premalignant lesions of the larynx and oral cavity defined as moderate or severe dysplasia or carcinoma *in situ*, biochemoprevention with 13-cRA (50 mg/m²/d) orally in combination with IFN-α (3 million IU/m² three times per week sc) and α-tocopherol (1200 IU daily orally) resulted in a 50% complete response in evaluable laryngeal premalignant lesions, with several documented durable complete responses for several months. However, among patients with oral cavity premalignant lesions, only transient partial responses were reported, and none had a durable complete response *(96)*. Biomarker analysis confirmed the negative prognostic value of p53 overexpression and revealed persistence of 9p21 in most lesions *(97)*.

The same combination has been highly effective in patients previously treated for locally advanced head and neck cancer *(98)*. This phase II study showed a 2-yr disease-free survival of 84% after completion of the definitive therapy.

The previous results, reported by Papadimitrakopoulou et al. *(96)*, have led to further investigations of the same combination in advanced laryngeal premalignant lesions, in which patients with either severe dysplasia or carcinoma *in situ* were treated for 1 yr with this combination, following which they were randomized to 4-HPR vs placebo. The results are awaited and will help to define the role of this combination better in aggressive laryngeal premalignant lesions. Further evidence from biologic studies that this combination can induce a complete phenotypic reversion and the observation at the clinical level of a reasonably well-tolerated combination with very few grade IV toxicities (National Cancer Institute [NCI] common toxicity criteria) made this a promising chemopreventive regimen in terms of effectiveness and tolerability for patients with aggressive laryngeal premalignant lesions *(73,96)*.

Still aggressive chemoprevention strategies does not seem to be effective in reversing advanced premalignant lesions of the oral cavity and the oropharynx and seems to be associated with substantial toxicity, suggesting a need for newer approaches and the use of other agents. Cyclooxygenase-2 inhibitors are among these other agents and are discussed in Subheading 6.7.

6.5. Primary Prevention of Tobacco Related Cancers

In lung cancer, primary chemoprevention trials using retinoids were also completed and proved the importance of smoking status of patients when these agents are tested. Smokers receiving β-carotene supplementation, alone or with α-tocopherol, had a reported increase in lung cancer incidence by about 18%. The Alpha Tocopherol Beta Carotene (ATBC) trial included 29,133 Finish male smokers. Participants received either daily α-tocopherol as a single agent at a dose of 50 mg or single-agent β-carotene at 20 mg, both agents, or placebo. The age range was 50–69 yr, and follow-up was for 5 to 8 yr. Participants smoked 5 to 8 cigarettes per day. α-Tocopherol alone did not appear to have an effect on lung cancer incidence, yet as noted there was an increased incidence in smokers *(99)*. In men who smoked more than 20 cigarettes a day, the negative effect was more pronounced, with an 8% worse mortality rate in the β-carotene group compared with participants who did not take β-carotene. The results observed in the ATBC trial were later confirmed by the Beta Carotene and Retinol Efficacy Trial (CARET), which enrolled 18,314 smokers and revealed a 28% increased incidence of lung cancer and a 17% higher overall mortality among participants who received β-carotene *(100)*. This trial included men and women aged 50–69 yr; most of them had at least a 20 pack/yr history of smoking. The end point was the same as in the ATBC trial. The study was terminated after an interim analysis revealed a 28% higher incidence of lung cancer and a 17% higher overall death rate in the β-carotene arm. Given the results of these studies, high-dose β-carotene is not recommended for high-risk smokers.

The harmful effects of β-carotene have not been observed in a similar large-scale preventive trial involving close to 22,071 mainly nonsmoking physicians *(101)*. This was a randomized 2 × 2 factorial trial that accrued 22,071 male physicians in the United States aged 40–84 yr; 11% were smokers, and 51% had a history of smoking. The follow-up period was 12-yr.

There were no adverse or beneficial effects on cancer incidence or mortality. Further data supported the role of continued smoking as an important factor in SPT development *(102)*.

6.6. Prevention of Second Primary Tumors

In retrospective analyses of HNSCC, the annual rate of SPT occurrence appears to range between 1.2 and 4.7%, and this appears to be a relatively fixed rate over time. Patients with HNSCC appear to have a significantly elevated risk for developing SPT regardless of their initial treatment. SPTs are a major cause of morbidity and mortality for the early stages of HNSCC, which are often treated with radiation and chemotherapy *(103)*, and appear to be the leading cause of cancer-related mortality in this patient population *(103)*. The origin of SPTs in HNSCC is debated. One possibility is that SPTs result from an independent genetic event, and another suggests mucosal spread from the primary tumor with subsequent transformation of genetically identical cells to the primary tumor. There seems to be no clear answer despite the availability of molecular testing and microsatellite analysis of the SPT *(104–107)*.

Based on the evidence shown for primary prevention using retinoids in oral leukoplakia, studies were conducted in the adjuvant setting to prevent SPTs in patients treated curatively for HNSCC (Table 3).

One such study used high-dose 13-cRA given with a chemopreventive intent in a placebo controlled randomized design for a total of 1 yr in 103 patients curatively treated for HNSCC. The primary end points (in addition to survival) were recurrence of primary disease and development of SPTs, defined as a different histologic type, or at a site greater than 2 cm from the previous disease, or occurring more than 3 yr after the initial diagnosis *(108)*. SPTs developed in 4% of treated patients over a follow-up period of 32 mo, whereas 24% of placebo patients developed SPTs over the same period ($p = 0.005$). Of the 14 SPTs that occurred at the time of initial analysis, 13 occurred in the tobacco-exposed fields of the upper aerodigestive tract, esophagus, and lungs. On a subset analysis of patients with high-risk tobacco exposure, the benefit seemed to persist in this subgroup of patients. In a subsequent analysis over a follow-up period of 4.5 yr there was a persistent reduction in SPTs among patients treated with 13-cRA compared with placebo ($p = 0.042$) *(109)*. More strikingly, a subset analysis of SPTs within the high risk tobacco exposed fields showed a persistent benefit in SPT prevention in these areas. Smoking-related SPTs occurred in 3/49 treated vs 13/51 placebo patients ($p = 0.008$). There was, on the other hand, substantial toxicity in this high-dose 13-cRA trial, as one-third of the treated patients required dose reduction or discontinuation of treatment because of grade II cheilitis, conjunctivitis, or skin toxicities. Also, as with studies in premalignant lesions, the benefit seems to be lost after the study period is over, as the SPT rates in both arms were reported to be equivalent 3 yr after completion of the trial.

Confirming the high rate of SPTs in HNSCC observed in the earlier trials, another study used a synthetic retinoid (etretinate) in patients treated for squamous cell carcinoma of the oral cavity or pharynx and found a reduction in SPTs over a period of 41 mo. Patients on this double-blind randomized multicentric trial were randomized to etretinate 50 mg/d for 1 mo, followed by 25 mg/d for 24 mo vs placebo. The study arms were equivalent in both primary tumor relapse and SPT occurrence, with 57/316 patients having SPTs and 45 of these SPTs occurring in the upper aerodigestive tract, lungs, or esophagus *(110)*.

Another trial used high-dose vitamin A in the adjuvant setting for patients with stage I non-small cell lung cancer (NSCLC). Ertinol palmitate at a dose of 300,000 IU/d was administered for 12 mo. Eighteen patients in the treatment group developed SPTs vs 29 in the control arm. Smoking-related SPTs occurred in 13 patients on the treatment arm, and 25 patients on the

Table3
SPT Prevention Trials

Study	Purpose	No. of patients	Drug	Results
Bolla et al., 1994 (110) (France)	Prevention of second primary in treated HNSCC	316	Etretinate or placebo for 2 yr	SPT 30% treatment 24% placebo
Han et al., 1990 (93)	Prevention of SPT	61	4-HPR vs placebo	87% CR in 4-HPR group vs 17% in placebo ($p <$ 0.01)
Hong et al., 1990 (108)	Prevention of SPT	103	13-cRA vs placebo for 12 mo	At 3 yr, 14% SPT vs 24%
van Zandwijk et al., 2003 (113) (Euroscan)	HNSCC and NSCLC SPT prevention	2592	Retinyl palmitate for 2 yr, N-acetyl-cysteine for 2 yr, both or neither	No difference in survival or SPT rate
Khuri et al., 2001 (28)	NSCLC SPT prevention	1483	13-cRA 30 mg/d for 36 mo or placebo	No difference in SPT rate, EFS, or OS. Higher recurrence in patients who continue to smoke
RTOG (0226)	HNSCC SPT prevention	136 projected sample	Celecoxib 400 mg bid for 2 yr	Study to open

Abbreviations: CR, complete response; EFS, event free survival; 4-HPR, 4-hydroxycarbophenyl retinamide; HNSCC, head and neck squamous cell carcinoma; NSCLC, non-small cell lung cancer; OS, overall survival; RTOG, Radiation Therapy Oncology Group; SPT, second primary tumor.

control arm, with a statistically significant difference ($p = 0.045$) (111). This difference, however, appears to have been lost 8 yr after completion of the study. So, similarly to the Hong et al. study (108), this study suggested that retinoids could prevent SPTs when administered to HNSCC or NSCLC patients. This protection was temporary, however, and in both studies the difference was lost with longer follow-up periods. The toxicity of retinoids seen in earlier leukoplakia studies was again confirmed in these prevention trials using high doses of retinoids (108,109).

Based on the positive results of Hong et al. (108), and in an attempt to clarify the results of Bolla et al. (110), the largest lung cancer chemoprevention trial so far was initiated by the NCI (intergroup NCI C91-002), a randomized, double-blind study. Patients who were definitively treated with surgery or radiation therapy for stage I and II SCC of the larynx, oral cavity, or pharynx were randomized to low-dose 13-cRA at 30 mg/d for 3 yr vs placebo followed by 4 yr of observation. The trial accrued 1486 participants and closed in June of 1999. Patients had to had a complete resection of stage I NSCLC 6 wk to 3 yr prior to enrollment. The primary objectives were to look at the rate of SPTs after complete resection of stage I NSCLC, overall survival on 13-cRA vs placebo, and toxicity of low-dose 13-cRA. After a median follow-up of 3.5 yr, there was no difference between the placebo and the 13-cRA groups in terms of recurrence rate, time to SPT, or mortality. Subsequent analysis suggested a possible protective effect of 13-cRA in never smokers and a harmful effect in current smokers *(28)*. The SPT rate in active smokers was found to be 5.1% annually. The rate in former smokers was 4.1%, and never smokers had a rate of 3%. This trial demonstrated that smoking plays an important role in SPT occurrence and unlike the prior studies, enrolled patients with early-stage disease, for whom SPTs were more likely to be survival determinants.

In another NCI intergroup phase III trial, patients with stage I NSCLC were randomized to receive isotretinoin 30 mg/d for 3 yr or placebo in a double-blinded fashion. After a median follow-up of 3.5 yr, there was no significant difference between the two groups in the time of SPT occurrence, the primary end point. Multivariate and subset analysis suggested a harmful effect of isotretinoin in current smokers *(112)*.

In a phase III multiinstitutional European study conducted by the European Organization for Research and Treatment of Cancer (EORTC; the EUROSCAN trial), retinyl palmitate and *N*-acetylcysteine efficacy was compared for SPT prevention after definitive treatment of head and neck or lung cancer. The study had a 2×2 factorial design and enrolled a total of 2592 patients with HNSCC and NSCLC. The four assigned treatment arms were retinyl palmitate (300,000 IU daily for 1 yr followed by 150,000 IU for a second year, *N*-acetylcysteine (600 mg/d for 2 yr), both, or no intervention. There was no reported survival advantage or SPT reduction after a median follow-up of 49 mo for both compounds, and for patients with HNSCC and lung cancer alike *(113)*. The study demonstrated no benefit of chemopreventive agents in patients with head and neck or lung cancer in terms of survival, event-free survival, or SPT occurrence.

The impact of active smoking on SPT occurrence was also demonstrated prospectively in a separate study in which low-dose 13-cRA was administered to patients treated for stage I or II HNSCC for up to 3 yr before participation. Patients were randomized to receive 13-cRA at 30 mg/d or a placebo for a total of 3 yr and were followed for 4 yr after completion of the chemopreventive phase. In all, 1384 patients were registered, and 1189 were evaluable and eligible. The annual SPT occurrence rate was 5.1%, with a higher rate observed in stage II HNSCC, compared with stage I. In addition, active smokers had a significantly higher rate of recurrence compared with former smokers ($p = 0.018$), with a nonsignificant difference noted between former and never smokers ($p = 0.11$). Of note is the better tolerability with the lower dose of 13-cRA *(28)*.

A phase III intergroup trial of isotretinoin to prevent SPTs in stage I and II HNSCC has been completed, and the results are to be published soon. In this trial patients with stages I or II HNSCC treated definitively with surgery and/or radiation therapy no fewer than 16 wk or more than 36 mo prior to enrollment were randomized, to receive either isotretinoid or placebo for 3 yr and were followed up for 4 additional years. There were 1190 patients enrolled and randomized with 590 on the isotretinoin arm and 600 on the placebo arm. Patients were stratified by stage, smoking status, and primary tumor site. With an estimated baseline annual SPT rate of 3%, the trial was designed to show a 50% reduction in SPT risk, with secondary end points being reduction in tobacco-related cancers (lung, HNSCC, esophagus, and bladder). With a median follow-up of 6 yr there did not seem to be a significant difference in SPT occurrence or overall survival between the two arms. The overall annual SPT rate was 4.6%, and most SPTs were smoking related, with the most common site being the lung (30.7%) followed by the oral cavity tumors (16.9%). Smoking-related SPT rates for the isotretinoin vs placebo groups were 3.0 and 3.3%, respectively. There was a reported decrease in recurrence of HNSCC on the isotretinoin arm that did not reach statistical significance. Multivariate analysis did reveal a pharyngeal site and current smoking to be significant predictors of SPT. Current smokers also had a worse survival rate compared with previous smokers or nonsmokers ($p = 0.0005$ and $p = 0.0002$, respectively). These unpublished data are the first to confirm in a prospective controlled trial the harmful effects of smoking on early-stage HNSCC patients.

6.7. Cyclooxygenase-2 Inhibitors

Nonsteroidal antiinflammatory agents (NSAIDs) have been shown to have a chemopreventive potential in HNSCC. Indomethacin administration has been associated with clinical benefits in HNSCC, namely, tumor regression *(114)*. This observation has led to an increased interest in NSAID use in HNSCC.

A broad range of laboratory investigations, animal models, and epidemiological studies provide evidence that inhibition of cyclooxygenase (COX)-2 pathways may have significant implications in cancer treatment. Cyclooxygenase catalyzes the conversion of 20-carbon unsaturated fatty acids to prostaglandin (PG) G2 and H2, the key steps in the synthesis of PGs *(115)*. Specific PG synthases are responsible for the subsequent catalysis of PGG2 and PGH2 to several groups. Prostaglandins are essential in most human tissues. Regulation of reproduction, immunity and vascular integrity is mediated by the paracrine and autocrine actions of PGs *(116)*.

There are at least two forms of the COX isoenzyme. COX-1 is thought to be responsible for PG biosynthesis and is constitutively expressed in most human tissues. COX-2, by contrast, is not normally expressed in most tissues but is induced by a wide spectrum of growth factors and cytokines in pathophysiological states *(117)*. In preclinical tumor models, upregulation of COX-2 results in changes in cellular migration, reduction in apoptosis, alteration in cell cycle progression, and promotion of angiogenesis, which can all contribute to a malignant phenotype. Epidemiologic and experimental evidence suggests that NSAIDs probably reduce tumorigenesis through the inhibition of COX *(118,119)*. Additional evidence for the role of COX in human tumors comes from the observations that epithelial malignancies (including colorectal, NSCLC, head, and neck, and pancreatic) form more PG than the normal tissue counterpart.

These observations indicate that inhibition of COX-2 and the resulting decrease in PG synthesis may prove useful in the prevention and treatment of some common human malignancies. Both nonselective blockade of COX and specific COX-2 blockade have been reported to reduce the number and size of polyps in patients with familial adenomatous polyposis, with a reduction of up to 30% by celecoxib compared with the untreated control group *(120)*. A growing body of evidence indicates that COX-2 plays a key role in lung cancer and can serve as a potential marker of prognosis in this disease. Because COX-2 inhibition has been demonstrated to interfere with tumorigenesis, the COX-2 enzyme may be an attractive target for therapeutic and chemoprevention strategies in lung cancer patients. COX-2, but not COX-1, seems to be expressed in human NSCLC cell lines and neither seem to be expressed in small cell lung cancer *(121)*. Furthermore, a substantial body of evidence indicates that COX-2 and PGs play an important role in tumorigenesis, with possible angiogenic stimulation as well as inhibition of apoptosis. COX-2 expression also seems to be a marker of poor prognosis in surgically resected stage I NSCLC.

Immunohistochemical analysis has revealed that COX-2 is expressed in both HNSCC and adjacent normal epithelium, with a mean level of COX-2 messenger RNA (mRNA) increased by close to 150 times in HNSCC compared with normal epithelial mucosa *(122)*. A higher level of COX-2 mRNA (around 50 times) was also noted in normal mucosa of HNSCC patients compared with healthy volunteers. eIFeE (a biomarker positive in individuals at high risk for relapse after definitive treatment for HNSCC) was correlated with the expression of COX-2 as a possible surrogate marker to predict response to COX-2 and relapse. Western blot analysis on mucosa of subjects at different stages of carcinogenesis and of normal mucosa, showed expression of eIF4E and COX-2 in all cancers and not in normal mucosa. There was a significant correlation between the expression of both markers ($p < 0.001$), all suggestive of a possible role of COX-2 inhibition in chemoprevention of HNSCC *(123)*.

Animal studies have suggested a potential role for topical use of COX-2 inhibitors as a chemopreventive strategy. Seventeen nude mice intradermally inoculated with carcinoma cells were divided into treatment group that received topical application of polymer-derived Celecoxib and no treatment. Tumor growth measured in 15 d favored the treatment group ($p < 0.001$) *(124)*. Other animal studies have looked at the potential chemopreventive role of celecoxib and explored a possible antiangiogenic mechanism of action. Celecoxib significantly delayed cell growth and reduced tumor volume. There was also a statistically significant difference in the quantity of new vasculature in the tumor sites between the two groups *(125)*.

COX-2 is also upregulated in a number of upper aerodigestive tract premalignant and malignant tumors. Based on the evidence presented, a number of chemoprevention trials in HNSCC using COX-2 inhibitors are under way. The Radiation Therapy Oncology Group (RTOG) is planning a phase II trial using celecoxib to prevent SPT in patients with HNSCC (RTOG 0226; Fig. 1). In this trial patients with HNSCC (excluding nasopharyngeal carcinomas) who have been disease free for a minimum of 16 wk and a maximum of 3 yr following completion of primary treatment will have biopsies of the oral mucosa for biomarker studies and then will receive celecoxib at 400 mg po bid for 2 yr. The results will be compared with historical controls for efficacy in reducing SPT as well as recurrences of the original primaries at 3 yr after follow-up. Results of this and other trials will be eagerly awaited to confirm or refute the value of COX-2 inhibitors as chemopreventive agents in HNSCC.

6.8. Protease Inhibitors

Ubiquitin-mediated protein degradation is an integral component of normal cellular processes, including apoptosis, signal transduction, gene transcription, and cell cycle regulation *(126)*. PS-341 is a dipeptidyl boronic acid that inhibits the proteasome 26S, whose function is to degrade proteins conjugated to the polypeptide ubiquitin through an ATP-dependent process. In vitro and in vivo studies have established the antitumor activity of PS-341 in hematologic malignancies including multiple myeloma as well as solid tumors including lung, postate, breast, colon, and pancreatic cancers and melanoma *(127)*. The total inhibition of 26S is lethal to most cell types; however, malignant cells are more sensitive than normal cells to proteasome inhibition. By its mechanism of inhibiting protein degradation, PS-341 targets a wide range of pathways that are relevant to tumor progression and drug resistance. The exact antitumor mechanism of PS-341 has not been elucidated, however. Potential targets affected by PS-341 in lung cancer include p27 *(128)*, p53, Bax *(129)*, cyclin D, E, and A, BCL-2, and nuclear factor (NF)-κB *(130)*.

The Bowman-Birk inhibitors (BBIs) come from dicotyledonous or monocotyledonous seeds and beans, and their amino acid sequence and structure have been worked out *(131)*. BBI concentrate administration was well tolerated and appeared to be nontoxic in phase I studies *(132)*.

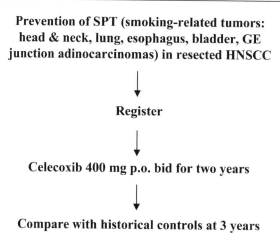

**Prevention of SPT (smoking-related tumors:
head & neck, lung, esophagus, bladder, GE
junction adinocarcinomas) in resected HNSCC**

↓

Register

↓

Celecoxib 400 mg p.o. bid for two years

↓

Compare with historical controls at 3 years

Fig. 1. Schema for secondary primary tumor (SPT) prevention trial using the cyclooxygenase (COX)-2 inhibitor celecoxib in resected head and neck squamous cell carcinoma (HNSCC) (RTOG 0226). GE, gastroesophageal.

The earliest known BBI was identified in soybeans by Bowman in the 1940s, and was purified by Birk in the early 1960s *(133)*. The BBI reported in the Armstrong study was BBI concentrate (BBIC), a mixture of the classic BBI and and four other soy PIs. There is some dietary and epidemiologic evidence supporting the notion that soybeans, cereals, and breads may be effective in reducing the risk of oral cancers *(134)*. A definite conclusion is, however, difficult to draw from such studies. More definite support for the protective effect of BBIs comes from preclinical evidence of their inhibition of transformation and carcinogenesis *(134)*.

In a phase IIa clinical trial of BBIC in patients with oral leukoplakia, BBIC was administered to 32 patients for 1 mo *(135)*. Toxicity and clinical and histologic response to the lesions were assessed. Oral mucosa protease activity (PA) and serum levels of micronutrients were assessed. Clinical response was determined by measurement of total lesion areas prior and following therapy. On the basis of these parameters, 31% of patients achieved a clinical response (two complete and eight partial) *(136)*. In a retrospective analysis of the pathologic specimens obtained from the phase IIa clinical trial, Armstrong et al. *(136)* looked at 32 sets of biopsy specimens before and after treatment with BBI and examined in a blinded fashion the expression of neu immunohistochemistry staining. The change in neu staining in control site biopsy was in an inverse relation to the change seen in the lesion area with BBI treatment. BBI appears therefore to modulate levels of neu and protease activity. BBIC was nontoxic, and the mean pretreatment total area of lesions decreased from 615 to 438 mm^2 after treatment (p < 0.004). A high pretreatment PA was associated with a greater PA decrease after treatment. Further studies are needed to elucidate better the mechanism of action of BBI as a chemopreventive agent and to understand better the role that neu, proteases, and their inhibitors may play in the process of oral premalignant lesion formation and progression. These results have opened the way for possible further investigation of BBI as an effective chemopreventive treatment on randomized clinical trials.

Despite these promising findings, the exact mechanism of action of BBI is yet to be defined and may include (in addition to targeting proteases) modulation of superoxide anion radical production, oncogene levels, DNA repair, immune effects, and arachidonic acid metabolism.

The clinical evidence of protease inhibition by BBIs remains unclear. Understanding the mechanism by which BBI exert their chemopreventive effect is key to launching additional studies and opens the door to a wide area of molecular and translational research.

6.9. Nutrition and Head and Neck Cancer

The topic of nutrition and HNSCC is underappreciated. There has been some interest in studying this area and using nutrition supplements as means to prevent HNSCC. Health care workers should also be aware of the widespread use of alternative nutritional supplements that may very well interfere with standard cytotoxic or targeted therapies.

In analyzing risk factors for oral cancer in young people, a recent case control study looked at 116 patients aged 45 or younger who had oral squamous cell carcinoma and 207 matched controls. The estimated risks associated with smoking or alcohol were low in this patient group, yet long-term consumption of fresh fruits and vegetables appeared to be protective for both sexes, suggesting that factors other than the known risks may be at play in this patient population with a relatively short exposure to known carcinogens *(137)*. Other similar studies have also found an inverse relation to risk of oral and pharyngeal cancer in young adults with high consumption of fresh vegetables, fruits, and β-carotene *(138)*. Other case control studies have linked glycemic index and load to risk of upper aerodigestive tract neoplasms *(139)*. Evidence also suggests that patients treated for early-stage oral squamous cell carcinoma have a significant deficiency in antioxidant nutrients compared with historical subjects *(140)*. Other studies have linked processed meat to risk of digestive tract as well as laryngeal neoplasms *(141)*. There seems to be evidence pointing to a protective role of vegetables including green and yellow vegetables and total and citrus fruit intake. All this information stems from epidemiologic studies, case control studies, and in vitro and animal studies *(142)*. Additional research at every level is clearly needed to define the role of these nutritional supplements better in preventing HNSCC and SPTs.

Among the nutritional substances with possible anticancer potentials is green tea. Green tea polyphenols were found to induce apoptosis in several tumors including oral cavity cancer cells *(143)*. Evidence suggests that green tea and its constituents induce apoptosis in oral carcinoma cells and are correlated with induction of some cell cycle regulators. Well-controlled clinical studies are yet to be initiated. Other preclinical studies have examined the potential anticancer effect of black raspberries and shown a potential inhibition of tumor formation in the oral cavity *(144)*.

7. CONCLUSIONS

Despite improvement in the diagnosis and management of HNSCC, the long-term survival of patients has changed minimally over the last three decades. There is a clear cost of long-term toxicity when chemoradiotherapy is used despite benefits in organ preservation as well as improvement in survival. Newer molecularly targeted therapies can be used in both the treatment and chemopreventive areas of HNSCC.

Continued biological investigations have helped us to understand the process of carcinogenesis, as well as the concept of field cancerization in HNSCC, with implications for accessibility to tissue sampling. These studies have pushed the area of chemoprevention in HNSCC forward.

Landmark trials with 13-cRA have demonstrated the possibility of chemoprevention in head and neck cancer. Retinoids alone and especially in combination with interferon in a biochemoprevention approach appear to have an effect on the development of SPTs in patients effectively treated for their initial cancers and in the prevention of cancer in patients with premalignant lesions. Newer agents targeting specific molecular abnormalities have been identified and may have a potential benefit. A better understanding of the alterations that affect premalignant lesions at the tissue and molecular levels is providing help in identifying cancer risk profiles and providing rational targets for chemopreventive measures. There are, however, obvious limitations, including the risks of assessing agents based on the wrong biomarkers, as it is always possible that agents may target other pathways parallel or downstream from a specific biomarker. More detailed and prospective studies perhaps relying on several biomarkers may be required to predict subsequent cancer development accurately.

REFERENCES

1. CFAF. Rates and Age—Adjusted to the 2000 US Standard Population. American Cancer Society, 2004.
2. Jemal A, Thomas A, Murray T, et al. Cancer statistics 2002. CA Cancer J Clin 2002; 52:23–47.
3. Vokes EE, Weicheelbaum RR, Lipman SM. Head and neck cancer. N Engl J Med 1993; 328:184–194.
4. Spitz MR. Epidemiology and risk factors for head and neck cancer. Semin Oncol 1994; 21:281–289.
5. Lippman SM, Benner SE, Hong WK. Cancer chemoprevention. J Clin Oncol 1994; 12:851–873.
6. Hung J, Kishimoto Y, Sujio K. Allele-specific chromosome 3p deletions occur at an early stage in the pathogenesis of lung carcinoma. JAMA 1995; 273:558–563.
7. Auerbach O, Gere JB, Forman JB. Changes in bronchial epithelium in relation to smoking and cancer of the lungs: a report of progress. N Engl J Med 1957; 256:97.
8. Slaughter DP, Southwick HW, Smejkal W. Field cancerization in oral stratifiedsquamous epithelium: clinical implications of multicentric origin. Cancer 1953; 273:558–563,
9. Silverman S, Gorsky M, Lozada F. Oral leukoplakia and malignant transformation: a follow-up study of 257 patients. Cancer 1984; 53:563–568.
10. Roed-Petersen B. Cancer development in oral leukoplakia: follow-up of 331 patients. J Dent Res 1971; 50:711 (abstract).
11. Silverman S Jr, Gorsky M, Lozada F. Oral leukoplakia and malignant transformation: a follow-up study of 257 patients. Cancer 1984; 53:563–584.
12. Banoczy J. Follow-up studies in oral leukoplakia. J Maxillofac Surg 1977; 5:772–776.
13. Mincer HH, Coleman SA, Hopkins KP. Observations and clinical characteristics of oral lesions showing histologic epithelial dysplasia. Oral Surg 1972; 33:389–392.
14. Banoczy J, Csiba A. Occurrence of epithelial dysplasia in leukoplakia. Oral Surg 1976; 42:766–774.
15. Silverman S J, Bhargava R, Mani NJ, et al. Malignant transformation and natural history of oral leukoplakia in 57,518 industrial workers in Gujarat, India. Cancer 1976; 38:1790–1795.
16. Einhorn J, Wersall J. Incidence of oral carcinoma in patients with leukoplakia of the oral mucosa. Cancer 1967; 20:2184–2193.
17. Renstrup G. Occurence of candida in oral leukoplakia. Pathol Microbiol Scand 1970; 78:421–424.
18. Sudbo J, Kidal W, Risberg B, et al. DNA content as a prognostic marker in patients with oral leukoplakia. N Engl J Med 2001; 344:1270–1278.
19. Sudbo J, Lippman SM, Lee JJ, et al. The influence of resection of aneuploidy on mortality in oral leukoplakia. N Engl J Med 2004; 350:1405–1413.
20. Sudbo J, Ristimaki A, Sondresen JE, et al. Cyclooxygenase-2 (COX-2) expression in high-risk premalignant oral lesions. Oral Oncol 2003; 39:497–505.
21. Rothman KJ, Cann CI, Flanders D, et al. Epidemiology of larynx cancer. Epidemiol Rev 1980; 2:195–209.
22. Shields PG, Harris CC. Molecular epidemiology and the genetics of environmental cancer. JAMA 1991; 266:681–687.
23. Spitz MR, Hogue A, Trizna Z. Mutagen sensitivity in upper aerodigestive tract cancer: a case-control analysis. Cancer Epidemiol Biomark Prev 1993; 2:329–333.
24. Spitz MR, Fueger JJ, Beddingfield NA. Chromosome sensitivity to bleomycin-induced mutagenesis, an independent risk factor for upper aerodigestive tract cancers. Cancer Res 1989; 49:4626–4628.
25. Spitz MR, Fueger JJ, Halabi S. Mutagen sensitivity in upper aerodigestive tract cancer: a case control analysis. Cancer Epidemiol Biomarkers Prev 2001; 2:329–333.
26. Cloos J, Braakhuis BJ, Steen I. Increased mutagen sensitivity in head and neck squamous cell carcinoma patients, particularly those with multiple primary tumors. Int J Cancer 1994; 56:816–819.

27. Wang LE, Sturgis EM, Eicher SA. Mutagen sensitivity to benzo(a)pyrene diol epoxide and the risk of squamous cell carcinoma of the head and neck. Clin Cancer Res 1998; 4:1773–1778.

28. Khuri FR, Kim ES, Lee JJ, et al. The impact of smoking status, disease stage, and index tumor site on second primary tumor incidence and tumor recurrence in head and neck retinoid chemoprevention trial. Cancer Epidemiol Biomark Prev 2001; 10:823–829.

29. Weinberg RA. Oncogenes, antioncogenes, and the molecular bases of multistep carcinogenesis. Cancer Res 1989; 49.

30. Voravud N, Shin DM, Ro JY, et al. Increased polysomies of chromosomes 7 and 17 during head and neck multistage tumorigenesis. Cancer Res 1993; 53:2784–2783.

31. Lee JS, Kim SY, Hong WK, et al. Detection of chromosomal polysomy in oral leukoplakia, a premalignant lesion. J Natl Cancer Inst 1993; 85:1951–1954.

32. Nawroz H, Van der Riet P, Hruban RH, et al. Allelotype of Head and Neck squamous cell carcinoma. Cancer Res 1994; 54:1152–1155.

33. Jin Y, Mertens F, Jin C, et al. Non-random chromosome abnormalities in short-term cultured primary squamous cell carcinomas of the head and neck. Cancer Res 1995; 55:3204–3210.

34. Mao L, Fan Y, Lotan R, et al. Frequent abnormalities of FHIT, a candidate tumor suppressor gene in head and neck cancer cell lines. Cancer Res 1996; 56:5128–5131.

35. van der Riet P, Nawroz H, Hruban RH. Frequent loss of cheromosome 9p21-22 early in head and neck cancer progression. Cancer Res 1994; 54:1156–1158.

36. Mao L, Lee JS, Fan YH. Frequent microsatellite alterations at chromosomes 9p21 and 3p14 in oral premalignant lesions and their value in cancer risk assessment. Nat Med 1996; 2:682–685.

37. Vigilio L, Shuser M, Gollin SM. FHIT gene alterations in head and neck squamous cell carcinoma. Proc Natl Acad Sci USA 1996; 93:9770–9775.

38. Califano J, van der Riet P, Westra W. Genetic progression model for head and neck cancer: implications for field cancerization. Cancer Res 1996; 56:2488–2492.

39. Guo Z, Yamaguchi K, Sanchez-Cespedes M. Allelic losses in oral test-directed biopsies of patients with prior upper aerodigestive tract malignancy. Clin Cancer Res 2001; 7:1963–1968.

40. Papadimitrakopoulou V, Izzo J, Lippman SM. Frequent inactivation of $p16_{INK4A}$ in OPL's. Oncogene 1997; 14:1799–1803.

41. Uzawa K, Yoshida H, Suzuki H. Abnormalities of the adenomatous polyposis coli gene in human oral squamous cell carcinoma. Int J Cancer 1994; 57:21–25.

42. Mao EJ, Oda D, Haigh WG, et al. Loss of adenomatous polyposis coli gene and human papilloma virus infection in oral carcinogenesis. Oral Oncol Eur J Cancer 1996; 32B:260–263.

43. Yoo GH, Xu HJ, Brennan JA. Infrequent inactivation of the retinoblastoma gene despite frequent loss of chromosome 13q in head and neck squamous cell carcinoma. Cancer Res 1994; 54:4603–4606.

44. Zhang Y, Feng X, We R, et al. Receptor associated Mad Homologues synergise as effectors of the TGF-beta response. Nature 1996; 383:168–172.

45. Kim SK, Fan Y, Papadimitrakopoulou V. DPC4, a candidate tumor suppressor gene, is altered infrequently in head and neck squamous cell carcinoma. Cancer Res 1996; 56.

46. Shin DM, Kim J, Ro JY. Activation of p53 gene expression in premalignant lesions during head and neck tumorigenesis. Cancer Res 1994; 54:321–326.

47. Brennan JA, Boyle JO, Koch WM. Association between cigarette smoking and mutation of p53 gene in squamous-cell carcinoma of the head and neck. N Engl J Med 1995; 332:712–717.

48. Boyle JO, Hakim J, Koch W, et al. The incidence of p53 gene mutations increases with progression of head and neck cancer. Cancer Res 1993; 53:4477–4480.

49. Shin DM, Lee JS, Lippman SM, et al. p53 expression: predicting recurrence and second primary tumors in head and neck squamous cell carcinoma. J Natl Cancer Inst 1996; 88:519–529.

50. Michalides R, van Veelen N, Hart A. Overexpression of cyclin D1 correlates with recurrence in agroup of fourty-seven operable squamous cell carcinomas of the head and neck. Cancer Res 1995; 55:975–978.

51. Williams ME, Gaffey MJ, Weiss LM. Chromosome 11q13 amplification in head and neck squamous cell carcinoma. Arch Otolaryngol Head Neck Surg 1993; 119:1238–1243.

52. Izzo JG, Papadimitrakopoulou VA, Hart A. Dysregulated cyclin D1 expression early in head and neck tumorigenesis: in vitro evidence of an association with subsequent gene amplification. Oncogene 1995; 17:2313–2322.

53. Motokura T, Bloom T, Kim HG. A novel cyclin encoded by BCL-1-linked candidate oncogene. Nature 1991; 350:512–515.

54. Serrano M, Hannon G, Beach D. A new regulatory motif in cell cycle control causing specific inhibition of cyclin D/CDK4. Nature 1993; 366:704–707.

55. Cairns P, Polascik TJ, Eby Y, et al. Frequency of homozygous deletion at p16/CDKN2 in primary human tumors. Nature 1995; 11:210–212.

56. Forastiere A, Koch W, Trotti A, et al. Head and neck cancer. N Engl J Med 2001; 345:1890–1900.

57. Grandis R, Tweardy DJ. Elevated levels of transforming growth factor alpha and epidermal growth factor receptor messenger RNA are early markers of carcinogenesis in head and neck cancer. Cancer Res 1993; 53:3579–3584.

58. Lomgo MN, Shin DM, Grandis JR. Targeting growth factor receptors: integration of novel therapeutics in the management of head and neck cancer. Curr Opin Oncol 2001; 13:1–8.

59. Sanchez-Cespedes M, Esteller M, Wu L. Gene promoter hypermethylation in tumors and serum of head and neck cancer patients. Cancer Res 2000; 60:892–895.

60. Belinsky SA, Nikula KJ, Palmisano WA, et al. Aberrant methylation of p16(INK4a) is an early event in lung cancer and a potential biomarker for early diagnosis. Proc Nat lAcad Sci USA 1998; 95:11,891–11,896.

61. Papadimitrakopoulou V, Mao L, Izzo J, et al. Multiple mechanisms of p16 inactivation in advanced premalignant lesions (APL) of the upper aerodigestive tract (UADT). Proc Am Assoc Cancer Res 2000; 41:224.

62. Sporn MB, Dunlop NM, Newton DL, et al. Prevention of chemical carcinogenesis by vitamin A and its synthetic analogs (retinoids). Fed Proc 1976; 35:1332–1338.

63. Knudson AG Jr, Hethcote HW, Brown BW. Mutation and childhood cancer: a probablistic model for the incidence of retinoblastoma. Proc Natl Acad Sci USA 1975; 72:5116–5120.

64. Mao L, Lee JS, Fan YH. Frequent microsatellite alterations at chromosome 9p21 and 3p14 in oral premalignant lesions and their value in cancer risk assessment. Nat Med 1996; 2.

65. Khuri F, Lee JJ, Lippman SM, et al. Isotretinoin effects on head and neck cancer recurrence and second primary tumors. Proc Am Soc Clin Oncol 2003; 22 (abstract 359).

66. Lopez-Amado M, Garcia-Caballero T, Lozano-Ramirez A, et al. Human papillomavirus and p53 oncoprotein in verrucous carcinoma of the larynx. J Laryngol Otol 1996; 10:742–747.

67. Gillison ML, Koch WM, Capone RB, et al. Evidence of a causal association between human papillomavirus and a subset of head and neck cancers. J Natl Cancer Inst (Bethesda) 2000; 92:709–720.

68. Cloos J, Leemans CR, van der Sterre ML, et al. Mutagen sensitivity as a biomarker for second primary tumors after head and neck squamous cell carcinoma. Cancer Epidemiol Biomarkers Prev 2000; 9:713–717.

69. Lotan R, Xu XC, Lippman SM. Suppression of retinoic acid receptor in premalignant oral lesions and its upregulation by isotretinoin. N Engl J Med 1995; 332:1405–1410.

70. Xu XC, Sozzi G, Lee JS, et al. Suppression of retinoic acid receptor beta in non-small cell lung cancer in-vivo: implications for lung cancer development. J Natl Cancer Inst 1997; 89:624–629.

71. Lippman SM, Shin DM, Lee JJ, et al. p53 and retinoid chemoprevention of oral carcinogenesis. Cancer Res 1995; 55:16–19.

72. Shin DM, Xu XC, Lippman SM, et al. Accumulation of p53 protein and retinoic acid receptor beta in retinoid chemoprevention. Cancer Res 1997; 3:875–860.

73. Mao L, El-Naggar AK, Papadimitrakopoulou VA. Molecular paradox of complete phenotypic response of advanced head and neck premalignancies to biochemoprevention. J Natl Cancer Inst 1998; 90:1545–1551.

74. Liu SC, Sauter ER, Clapper MI, et al. Markers of cell proliferation in normal epithelia and dysplastic leukoplakias of the oral cavity. Cancer Epidemiol Biomarkers Prev 1998; 7:597–603.

75. Lotan R. Retinoids in cancer chemoprevention. FASEB J 1996; 10:1031–1039.

76. Lotan R. Retinoids and apoptosis: implications for cancer chemoprevention and therapy. J Natl Cancer Inst 1995; 87:1655–1657.

77. Lee JS, Kim SY, Hong WK. Deletion of chromosomal polysomy in oral leukoplakia, a premalignant lesion. J Natl Cancer Inst 1993; 85:1951–1954.

78. Stich HF, Homby AP, Mathew B. Response of oral leukoplakias to the administration of vitamin A. Cancer Lett 1988; 40:93–101.

79. Wolbach SB, Howe PR. Tissue changes following deprivation of fat-soluble A vitamin. J Exp Med 1925; 62.

80. Wagner H, Ruckdeschel JC. Screening, early detection, and early intervention strategies for lung cancer. Cancer Control. J Moffitt Cancer Center 1995; 6:493–502.

81. Gudas L, Hu L. The reglation and gene expression by retinoids in normal and tumorigenic epithelial cells. Proc Annu Meet Am Assoc Cancer Res 1993; 34:588–589.

82. Sun SY, Lotan R. Retinoids and their receptors in cancer development and chemoprevention. Crit Rev Oncol Hematol 2002; 41:41–45.

83. Xu XC, Lee JS, Lee JJ. Nuclear retinoid receptor beta in bronchial epithelium of smokers before and during chemoprevention. J Natl Cancer Inst 1999; 91:1317–1321.

84. Khuri FR, Lee JS, Lippman SM. Modualtion of proliferating cell nuclear antigen in the bronchial epithelium of smokers. Cancer Epidemiol Biomarkers Prev 2001; 10:311–318.

85. Gebert JF, Moghal N, Frangioni JV. High-frequency of retinoic acid receptor beta abnormalities in human lung cancer. Oncogene 1991; 6:1859–1868.

86. Karp DD, Tsao AS, Kim ES. Non-small cell lung cancer: chemoprevention studies. Sem Thoracic Cardiovasc Surg 2003; 15:404–420.

87. Wang XD, Liu C, Bronson RT. Retinoid signaling and activator protein-1 expression in ferrets given beta-carotene supplements and exposed to tobacco smoke. J Natl Cancer Inst 1999; 91:760–761.

88. Song S, Xu XC. Effects of benzo[a]pyrene diol epoxide on expression of retinoic acid receptor-beta in immortalized esophageal epithelial cells and esophageal cancer cells. Biochem Biophys Res Commun 2001; 281:872–877.

89. Stich HR, Rosin MP, Hornby P, et al. Remission of oral leukoplakias and micronuclei in tobacco/betel quid chewers treated with beta-carotene and with beta-carotene plus vitamin A. Int J Cancer 1988; 42:195–199.

90. Hong WK, Endicott J, Itri LM. 13-cis-retinoic acid in the treatment of oral leukoplakia. N Engl J Med 1986; 315:1501–1505.

91. Lippman SM, Batsakis JG, Toth BB. Comparison of low-dose isotretinoin with beta carotene to prevent oral carcinogenesis. N Engl J Med 19993; 328:15–20.

92. Papadimitrakopoulou VA, Hong WK, Lee JS. Low-dose isotretinoin versus beta-carotene to prevent oral carcinogenesis: long term follow-up. J Natl Cancer Inst 1997; 89:257–258.

93. Han J, Jiao L, Lu Y. Evaluation of N-4-(hydroxycarbo-phenyl) retinamide as a cancer prevention agent and as a cancer chemotherapeutic agent. In Vivo 1990; 4:153–160.

94. Chiosa F, Tradatl N, Marazza M. Fenretinide (4-HPR) in chemoprevention of leukoplakia. J Cell Biochem Suppl 1999; 12F:255–2612.

95. Chiesa F, Tradaki N, Merazza M. Fenretidine (4-HPR) in chemoprevention of oral leukoplakia. J Cell Biochem 1993; 17F(Suppl):255–261.

96. Papadimitrakopoulou VA, Clayman GL, Shin DM, et al. Biochemoprevention for dysplastic lesions of the upper aerodigestive tract. Arch Otolaryngol Head Neck Surg 1999; 125:1083–1089.

97. Mao LM, El-Naggar A, Papadimitrakopoulou V, et al. Phenotype and genotype of advanced premalignant lesions after chemopreventive therapy. J Natl Cancer Inst 1998; 90:1545–1551.

98. Shin DM, Khuri FR, Murphy B. Combined interferone alpha, 13-cis-retinoic acid, and alpha tocopherol in locally advanced head and neck squamous cell carcinoma: novel bioadjuvant phase II trial. J Clin Oncol 2001; 19:3010–3017.

99. The alpha-Tocopherol BCCPsG. The effect of vitamin E and beta-carotene on the incidence of lung cancer and other cancers in male smokers. N Engl J Med 1994; 330:1029–1035.

100. Omenn GS, Goodman GE, Thornquist MD, et al. Effects of a combination of beta-carotene and vitamin A on lung cancer and cardiovascular disease. N Engl J Med 1996; 334:1150–1155.

101. Hennekens CH, Buring JE, Manson JE, et al. Lack of long-term supplementation with beta-carotene on the incidence of malignant neoplasms and cardiovascular disease. N Engl J Med 1996; 334:1145–1149.

102. Do KA, Johnson MM, Doherty DA, et al. Second primary tumors in patients with upper aerodigestive tract cancers: joint effects of smoking and alcohol. Cancer Causes Control 2003;14:131–138.

103. Vikram B. Changing patterns of failure in advanced head and neck cancer. Arch Otolaryngol 1984; 110:564–565.

104. Leong P, Resai B, Koch W, et al. Distinguishing second primary tumors from lung metastases in patients with head and neck squamous cell carcinoma. J Natl Cancer Inst (Bethesda) 1998; 90:972–977.

105. Bedi G, Westra W, Gabrielson E, et al. Multiple head and neck tumors: evidence for a common clonal origin. Cancer Res 1996; 56:2484–2487.

106. Califano J, Westra W, Meninger G, et al. Genetic progression and clonal relationship of recurrent premalignant head and neck lesions. Clin Cancer Res 2000; 6:347–352.

107. van Oijen MG, Leppers van der Straat FG, Tilanus MG, et al. The origins of multiple squamous cell carcinomas in the aerodigestive tract. Cancer (Phila) 2000; 88:884–893.

108. Hong WK, Lippman SM, Itri M. Prevention of second primary tumors with isotretinoin in squamous-cell carcinoma of the head and neck. N Engl J Med 1990; 323:795–801.

109. Benner SE, Pajak TF, Lippman SM. Prevention of second primary tumors with isotretinoin in patients with squamous cell carcinoma of the head and neck: long term follow-up. J Natl Cancer Inst 1994; 86:140–141.

110. Bolla M, Lefur R, Ton Van J, et al. Prevention of second primary tumors with etretinate in squamous cell carcinoma of the oral cavity and oropharynx. Results of a multicentric double-blind randomized study. Eur J Cancer 1994; 30A:767–772.

111. Pastorino U, Infante M, Maioli M. Adjuvant treatment for stage I lung cancer with high-dose vitamin A. J Clin Oncol 1993; 11:1216–1222.

112. Lippman SM, Lee JJ, Karp DD, et al. Randomized phase III intergroup trial of isotretinoin to prevent second primary tumors in stage I non-small cell lung cancer. J Natl Cancer Inst 2001; 18:605–618.

113. van Zandwijk N, Daleslo O, Pactorino U, et al. EUROSCAN, a randomized trial of vitamin A and N-acetylcysteine in patients with head and neck cancer or lung cancer. For the European Organization for Research and Treatment for Cancer, Head and Neck and Lung Cancer Cooperative Groups. J Nat Cancer Inst 2000; 92:977–986.

114. Panje WR. Regression of head and neck carcinoma with a prostaglandin-synthesis inhibitor. Arch Otoralyngol 1981; 107:658–663.

115. Dubois RN, Abramson SB, Crofford L. Cyclooxygenase in biology and disease. FASEB J 1998; 12:1063–1073.

116. Herschman HR, Xie W, Reddy S. Inflammation, reproduction, cancer and all that... The regulation and role of inducible prostaglandin synthase. Bioassays 1995; 17:1031–1037.

117. Eberhart CE, Coffey RJ, Rhadika A. Up-regulation of cyclo-oxygenase 2 gene expression in human colorectal adenomas and adenocarcinomas. Gastroenterology 1994; 107:1183–1188.

118. Waddell WR, Loughry RW. Sulindac for polyposis of the colon. J Surg Oncol 1983; 24:24.

119. Thun MJ, Namboodari MM, Heath CW Jr. Aspirin use and reduced risk of fatal colon cancer. N Engl J Med 1991; 325:1593–1596.

120. Staeinbach G, Lynch PM, Phillips RK. The effect of celecoxib, a cyclooxygenase-2 inhibitor, in familial adenomatous polyposis. N Engl J Med 2000; 342:1946–1952.

121. Tsoubouchi Y, Mukai S, Kawahito Y. Meloxicam inhibits the growth of non-small cell lung cancer. Anticancer Res 2000; 20:2867–2872.

122. Chan G, Boyle JO, Yang EK. Cyclo-oxygenase-2 expression is up-regulated in squamous cell carcinoma of the head and neck. Cancer Res 1999; 59:991–994.

123. Nathan CA, Leskov IL, Lin M, et al. COX-2 expression in dysplasia of the head and neck: correlation with eIF4E. Cancer 2001; 92:1888–1895.

124. Wang Z, Polavaram R, Shapshay SM. Topical inhibition of oral carcinoma cell with polymer delivered celecoxib. Cancer Lett 2003; 198:53–58.

125. Wang Z, Fuentes CF, Shashay SM. Antiangiogenic and chemopreventive activities of celecoxib in oral carcinoma cell. Laryngoscope 2002; 112:839–943.

126. Liu CW, Corboy MJ, De Martino GM, et al. Endoproteolytic activity of the proteasome. Science 2003; 299:408–411.

127. Adams J, Palombella VJ, Savsville EA, et al. Proteasome inhibitors: a novel class of potent and effective antitumor agents. Cancer Res 1999; 59:2615–2622.

128. Catzavellos C, Tsao MS, DeBoer G, et al. Reduced expression of the cell cycle inhibitor p27kip1 in non-small cell lung carcinoma: a prognostic factor independant of Ras. Cancer Res 1999; 59:684–688.

129. Li B, et al. Bax degradation by the Ubiquitin/proteasome-dependant pathway: involvement in tumor survival and progression. Proc Natl Acad Sci USA 2000; 97:3850–3855.

130. Sunwoo JB, Chen Z, et al. Novel proteasome inhibitor PS-341 inhibits activation of nuclear factor-kappa B, cell survival, tumor growth, and angiogenesis in squamous cell carcinoma. Clin Cancer Res 2001; 7:1419–1428.

131. Parakash B, Selvaraj S, MRN M, et al. Analysis of the amino-acid sequences of plant Bowman-Birk inhibitors. J Mol Evol 1996; 42:560–569.

132. Armstrong WB, Kennedy AR, Wan XS, et al. Single-dose administration of Bowman-Birk inhibitor concentrate in patients with oral leukoplakia. Cancer Epidemiol Biomarkers Prev 2000; 9:43–47.

133. Birk Y. The Bowman-Birk inhibitor. Trypsin and chymotrypsin inhibitor from soybeans. Int J Pept Protein Res 1985; 25:113–131.

134. Kennedy AR. Chemopreventive agents: protease inhibitors. Pharmacol Ther 1998; 78:167–209.

135. Armstrong WB, Kennedy AR, Wan XS, et al. Clinical modulation of oral leukoplakia and protease activity by Bowman-Birk inhibitor concentrate in a phase IIa chemoprevention trial. Clin Cancer Res 2000; 6:4684–4691.

136. Armstrong WB, Wan XS, Kennedy AR, et al, Development of the Bowman-Birk inhibitor of oral cancer chemoprevention and analysis of Neu immunohistochemical staining intensity with Bowman-Birk inhibitor concentrate treatment. Laryngoscope 2003; 113:1687–1702.

137. Llewelly CD, Linklater K, Bell J, et al. An analysis of risk factors for oral cancer in young people: a case-control study. Oral Oncol 2004; 40:304–313.

138. Rodriguez T, Altieri A, Chatenoud L, et al. Risk factors for oral and pharyngeal cancer in young adults. Oral Oncol 2004; 40:207–213.

139. Augustin LS, Gallus S, Franceschi S, et al. Glycemic index and load and risk of upper aero-digestive tract neoplasms (Italy). Cancer Causes Control 2003; 14:657–662.

140. Steward DL, Wiener F, Gleich LL, et al. Dietary antioxidant intake in patients at risk for second primary cancer. Laryngoscope 2003; 113:1487–1493.
141. Levi F, Pasche C, Lucchini F, et al. Processed meat and the risk of selected digestive tract and laryngeal neoplasms in Switzerland. Ann Oncol 2004; 15:346–349.
142. Chainani-Wu N. Diet and oral, pharyngeal, and esophageal cancer. Nutr Cancer 2002; 44:104–126.
143. Hsu SD, Singh BB, Lewis JB, et al. Chemoprevention of oral cancer by green tea. Gen Dent 2002; 2:140–146.
144. Casto BC, Kresty LA, Kraly CL, et al. Chemoprevention of oral cancer by black rasberries. Anticancer Res 2002; 22:4005–4015.
145. Costa A, Formelli F, Chiesa F, et al. Prospects of chemoprevention of human cancers with the synthetic retinoid fenretinide. Cancer Res 1994; 54(Suppl 7):2031s–2037s.

20

Quality of Life Outcomes in Head and Neck Cancer

Allen C. Sherman, PhD, Ehab Hanna, MD, FACS, and Stephanie Simonton, PhD

1. INTRODUCTION

Quality of life (QOL) has commanded growing attention within oncology in recent years. Adverse changes in functional and behavioral outcomes are a special concern in patients with head and neck squamous cell cancer (HNSCC), because these malignancies disrupt basic aspects of daily life such as eating, respiration, and communication. These difficulties are greatly amplified by demanding treatment toxicities. Thus, there is growing recognition that traditional clinical endpoints such as tumor response and disease-free survival need to be supplemented by indices of QOL. This development has been given further impetus lately by patient advocacy and by the introduction of improved QOL measures. In this chapter, we briefly discuss advances in QOL assessment, review research findings regarding acute and long-term QOL outcomes, and consider important determinants of risk and resilience.

2. ASSESSING QOL

Although definitions vary somewhat, health-related QOL is generally understood as a multidimensional construct that is rooted in the patient's perspective and that changes over time *(1–3)*. Some have defined it as the gap between one's current experience and one's wishes or expectations *(4,5)*. Performance status, a related concept, is an index of patients' functional capacities, e.g., their ability to eat solids, speak clearly, or ambulate independently *(5,6)*. In contrast, health-related QOL typically is construed as encompassing broader aspects of daily life. Important components include, among others, emotional and social well-being, as well as functional limitations and physical symptom burden. Sexual, vocational, and spiritual or existential domains are sometimes incorporated as well.

In recent years, a number of useful, psychometrically sound instruments have been developed to help assess these outcomes. For the most part, these measures are designed to capture the patient's perceptions rather than relying on the clinician's impressions, which is a notable consideration because it is the patient's experience that is of concern and because practitioners consistently underdiagnose salient difficulties *(7–11)*. Some measures are designed to have broad applicability for an array of different illnesses (e.g., the SF-36 *[12]*, Psychological Adjustment to Illness Scale *[13]*, Sickness Impact Profile *[14]*), whereas others target diffi-

From: *Current Clinical Oncology: Squamous Cell Head and Neck Cancer*
Edited by: D. J. Adelstein © Humana Press Inc., Totowa, NJ

culties associated more narrowly with a particular disease (e.g., Functional Living Index—Cancer [15]), a discrete disease site (e.g., Head and Neck Quality of Life Questionnaire [16]), or a specific treatment regimen (e.g., Head and Neck Radiotherapy Questionnaire [17]). In an effort to capitalize on the advantages of these divergent approaches, there has been a trend toward use of modular instruments (e.g., FACIT [18], EORTC QLQ [19–22]): a general or core measure captures multiple domains of functioning and allows comparisons across different diseases, while a site- or treatment-specific module ensures that unique concerns are addressed as well (23).

Table 1 offers a summary of some of the health-related QOL instruments that have been used with HNSCC patients, and notes a few of their respective advantages and disadvantages. No single instrument is ideal for all situations; investigators and clinicians should select those measures that best meet their specific needs (e.g., based on inclusion of particular toxicities, focus on brief vs more comprehensive assessment, and so on). Because different dimensions of QOL may deteriorate or improve at different rates, sole reliance on a single summary score can obscure important findings. Thus, instruments that provide scores in separate domains may offer richer information and greater sensitivity.

Although investigators have been understandably focused on adverse QOL outcomes, patients sometimes discover that their lives have shifted in more complex and unexpected ways in the aftermath of illness. Some individuals point to positive changes, such as altered priorities, closer relationships, stronger spirituality, or a heightened sense of meaning in life. Ideally, therefore, a comprehensive assessment of QOL might include the possibility of constructive as well as debilitating sequelae (29,30).

3. OVERVIEW OF QOL OUTCOMES IN HNSCC CANCER

The particular problems that patients encounter are of course shaped by the site and stage of disease, the treatment regimens they receive, and their phase in the trajectory of illness. Notwithstanding these distinctions, it is clear that individuals with HNSCC face dismaying burdens. A new diagnosis elicits concerns about survival, painful uncertainty about the future, and altered routines. Emotional distress and role disruption are common for both the patient (31,32) and the family (33–35). A number of studies demonstrate that physical and emotional spheres of functioning are significantly compromised relative to population norms, even prior to beginning taxing treatments (36,37). QOL is further eroded by demanding treatment toxicities, which may include radiotherapy-induced xerostomia, fatigue, and radionecrosis; surgery-related disfigurement, pain, and shoulder dysfunction; and chemotherapy-associated nausea, mucositis, and immunosuppression. For some, the challenges of treatment adherence or adjustment are exacerbated by a premorbid history of substance abuse, which is more prevalent among patients with HNSCC.

After completion of active treatment, patients may need to accommodate more enduring difficulties. These might include discouragement with ongoing fatigue; frustration with eating limitations; self-consciousness about disfigurement or tracheostomy care; or discomfort with speech difficulties, tracheoesophageal puncture (TEP) appliances, or electrolarynx devices. The end of active treatment sometimes elicits intensified distress or delayed grief (41), bringing new burdens just when patients expect to be feeling better and their support systems tend to recede. Long-term survivors may encounter additional challenges, such as fear of recurrence (38), sexual problems (39,40), or difficulties with nicotine or alcohol. For those with progressive disease, of course, symptom control and existential concerns take on greater

Table 1

Selected Measures Used to Assess Health-Related Quality of Life (QOL) Among Head and Neck Cancer Patients

Instrument	Description	Selected advantages/disadvantages
Generic QOL Measures		
SF-36 *(12)*	36-item patient-rated measure that yields scores for two summary scales, Physical Composite Summary and Mental Composite Summary, as well as eight scales: Physical functioning, Role functioning-physical, Bodily pain, General health, Vitality, Social functioning, Role functioning-emotional, Mental health Scored according to published algorithms from 0 (worst) to 100 (best) with 50 as mean for general US population An abbreviated version (SF-12) is available as well	Widely used, well-validated measure Norms available for general US population (age-related) and for various chronic illnesses, including cancer No coverage of HN-specific concerns
Psychological Adjustment to Illness Scale-Self Report (PAIS-SR) *(13)*	46-item patient-rated instrument that produces a Total score as well as scores in seven domains: Health attitudes, Vocational environment, Domestic environment, Sexual relations, Extended family, Social environment, Psychological distress	Covers diverse domains of functioning Norms available for cancer (mixed diagnoses) and other chronic illnesses No coverage of HN-specific concerns.
Sickness Impact Profile (SIP) *(14)*	136-item patient-rated measure that generates a Total score, two summary scales for Physical Impact and Psychological Distress, and 12 subscales: Ambulation, Mobility, Body care/movement, Eating, Work, Sleep/rest, Household management, Recreation/pastimes, Social interaction, Alertness behavior, Emotional behavior, Communication Scores range from 0 (best) to 100 (worst)	Broad assessment of diverse domains Lengthy measure No coverage of HN-specific concerns

(continued)

Table 1 (*continued*)

Instrument	Description	Selected advantages/disadvantages
Functional Living Index-Cancer (FLIC) (*15*)	22-item patient-rated scale that yields a Total score, encompassing three domains (physical well-being, psychological state, family interaction/sociability) Items are scored on a visual analog scale (VAS), with the total ranging from 22 (worst) to 154 (best)	Brief measure of cancer-related QOL Reliance on total score may obscure outcomes within specific domains (although some studies have used subscales) Does not assess HN-specific symptoms
Modular QOL instruments (generic and disease-specific)		
European Organization for Research and Treatment of Cancer Core Questionnaire and Head & Neck Module (EORTC-QLQ-C30, QLQ-H&N35) (*19–22*)	30-item patient-rated core instrument that assesses six functional scales (Physical, Role, Emotional, Social, Cognitive, Global QOL), three symptom scales (Fatigue, Pain, Nausea/Vomiting), and six single items 35-item HN-specific measure provides scores for 7 multiple-item scales (Pain, Swallowing, Senses, Speech, Social contact, Social eating, Sexuality) as well as 11 single items Scores are transformed from 1 to 100, with higher scores indicating better outcomes for the functional scales but poorer outcomes for the symptom and single-item scales	One of most widely validated QOL measures in oncology, with established cross-cultural utility across several European and North American countries Scandinavian population norms available Broad coverage of HN concerns Lengthy instrument; extensive reliance on single-item scores may be less reliable and sensitive relative to multiple-item scores
Functional Assessment of Chronic Illness Therapy General and Head & Neck Modules (FACIT-G, FACIT-HN) (*18*)	27-item patient-rated general module provides a Total score (FACIT-General) and four subscale scores (Physical well-being, Social well-being, Emotional well-being, and Functional well-being) The 11-item H&N module generates a Total score For all scales, higher scores indicate better functioning	Another commonly used, carefully constructed, well-validated measure Cancer norms available for both general and HN module Reliance on summary score for for the HN module may obscure outcomes within specific QOL domains

308

HN-specific QOL measures		
Head & Neck Quality of Life Questionnaire (HNQOL) (16)	20-item patient-rated instrument that generates a Total "overall bother" score as well as scores for four domains: Communication, Eating, Head and neck pain, and Emotional adjustment. It includes additional items regarding perceived response to treatment, and satisfaction with care Domains are scored from 0 (worst) to 100 (best)	Assesses important HN-related domains, using multiitem factor-derived scales Some concerns are not covered (e.g., shoulder dsfunction)
University of Washington Quality of Life Scale (UWQOL) (24,25)	Revised version includes 12 patient-rated items that generate a Total composite score (from 0 [worst] to 900 [best]) and scores for each item: Pain, Disfigurement, Activity, Recreation, Employment, Chewing, Swallowing, Speech, Shoulder disability, Appearance, Dry mouth, Saliva There is also a global QOL item, an item regarding incremental QOL changes over a specified time interval, and items inquiring about the perceived importance of each of the 12 domains	Revised scale includes broad coverage of salient HN-related domains; use of incremental change scores is a notable addition Reliance on single-item scores may be less sensitive and reliable than multiitem scales
Head & Neck Survey (H&NS) (26)	11-item patient rated-measure that provides a Total score and three domain scores: Eating/swallowing, Speech/Communication, and Appearance Scores range from 0 (worst) to 100 (best)	Brief measure that assesses important HN-related outcomes using multiitem scales Psychometric data very promising but limited thus far; some relevant concerns are not covered (e.g., pain)
HN-specific performance measures		
Performance Status Scale for Head and Neck Cancer (PSS-HN) (27)	Clinician-rated measure that yields three scores: Normalcy of diet, Understandability of speech, and Eating in public Scores range from 0 (worst) to 100 (best)	Widely employed, clinically useful performance scale Item content would appear to be somewhat more sensitive to surgical- than radiotherapy-related effects; possible that reliance on clinician ratings may be less sensitive than self-report (although observer ratings are a helpful complement to self-report)

(continued)

Table 1 (*continued*)

Instrument	Description	Selected advantages/disadvantages
Treatment-specific measures		
Head and Neck Radiotherapy Questionnaire (HNRQ) (*17*)	22-item measure that produces a Total (mean) score and six domain scores regarding radiotherapy-induced symptoms: Oral stomatitis, Throat irritation, Digestion, Skin toxicity, Energy, and Psychosocial changes Validated using clinician-rated items but subsequent studies have used patient-rated items	Covers acute toxicities associated with radiotherapy of HN region Initial data support validity but no data provided re: reliability By design, less sensitive to surgery-related sequelae
Xerostomia Questionnaire (XQ) (*28*)	8-item patient-rated measure of difficulties with dry mouth Yields a total score that is transformed to a scale ranging from 0 (best) to 100 (worst)	Brief, focused measure of xerostomia

310

immediacy. A growing research literature has characterized some of the difficulties that HNSCC patients experience at varying phases of illness.

4. RESEARCH FINDINGS REGARDING QOL

4.1. Short-Term Sequelae

Prospective studies point to a number of adverse changes over the course of active treatment and short-term recovery (i.e., through 1-yr post diagnosis). As one might anticipate, most investigations have documented marked deterioration in functional status and symptom burden from initial diagnosis through the acute treatment period *(36,37,39,42–50)*. Depending on the type of regimen, the nadir comes at 1–3 mo after starting treatment *(39,45–48)*, followed by a general improvement. Specific sequelae include, among others, difficulties with head and neck pain, swallowing, social eating, speech, sense of smell or taste, dry mouth, sticky saliva, appetite, nutritional concerns, weight loss, shoulder dysfunction, and fatigue, as well as broader disruptions in daily physical, role, and social functioning. By 1 yr, average scores for many symptoms have returned approximately to pretreatment baseline levels; commonly, however, there are many pockets of continued impairment, most notably including difficulties with xerostomia, sense of smell/taste, dysphagia, eating, speech, sticky saliva, fatigue, and physical functioning *(39,42,43,45,46,48,50–53)*.

Thus, a growing database indicates that physical spheres of functioning follow a pattern of acute deterioration and gradual recovery, with continued impairment in some domains. In contrast, psychosocial functioning evinces a different trajectory of recovery. Following the initial crisis of diagnosis, most prospective studies have found gradual improvements rather than declines in measures of emotional well-being *(36,39,42–44,46,50,51,54)* and distress *(42,52,53,55)*. Similarly, estimates of psychiatric morbidity tend to diminish somewhat by 1-yr follow-up *(42,45,51,56;* for an exception, *see* ref. *46)*. Nevertheless, levels of morbidity remain elevated relative to the general population, with 26 to 37% of patients exceeding cutoffs for psychiatric "caseness" on various screening instruments at 1 yr *(45,46,56)* and 19 to 25% exceeding cutoffs for clinical depression *(42–44,51)*.

4.2. Long-Term Sequelae

To what extent do adverse changes experienced in the posttreatment period carry over to long-term recovery? A number of prospective and cross-sectional investigations have examined QOL outcomes among HNSCC survivors 2–5 yr after treatment. In general, additional changes beyond the first year appear to be fairly modest. Patients tend to experience enduring difficulties with daily physical functioning and with specific head and neck symptoms, such as dry mouth, impaired taste/smell, sticky saliva, and dental problems *(51,55,57,58)*; the intensity of these difficulties generally is worse than their level at diagnosis. In contrast, emotional functioning *(51,57,58)*, life satisfaction *(55,59)*, and global QOL tend to improve *(51,57)* relative to the pretreatment period. For example, in a recent cross-sectional study *(22)*, 3-yr survivors fared significantly worse than age-matched population norms in day-to-day physical functioning and in an array of specific head and neck symptoms but had comparable scores in more general domains of functioning (e.g., self-perceived general health, social functioning, mental health, pain, vitality). The discrepancy between deterioration in some physical symptoms and improvement in emotional well-being has been noted by a number of investigators *(51,55;* *see* ref. *60* for conflicting results) and may, in part, reflect processes of psychosocial adaptation, improved coping, and response shift (i.e., the tendency of respondents to alter their judgments of QOL because of changes in internal standards or values *[61]*).

Nonetheless, despite a general trend toward improved mood over time, long-term survivors remain at heightened risk for emotional distress *(7,60,62)*, concerns that are rarely shared with the treating clinician *(7,10)*. Estimates of general psychiatric morbidity among long-term survivors range from 25 to 47% as assessed by various screening measures *(7,63–65)*; estimates of clinically meaningful depression range from 15 to 35% *(8,51,64–67)*. Moreover, other psychosocial domains may be disrupted as well, although they have received less scrutiny as yet. Some studies have documented long-term difficulties in sexual functioning (e.g., diminished interest, arousal, and activity) *(40,53)*, marital quality and communication *(53,68)*, family functioning *(60,69)*, health worries *(68)*, and substance abuse *(67)*. In sum, it appears that most patients adapt remarkably well to aggressive or disfiguring treatment, and many toxicities abate during the first year after diagnosis, but there may be multiple areas of continued concern over the long-term.

5. IMPACT ON THE FAMILY

Serious illness has a marked impact not only on the patient but also on the family system *(35)*. Growing interest has focused on the burdens experienced by the spouses or partners, who have long been neglected in both research and clinical care. The few studies conducted in the HNSCC setting suggest that levels of distress are even greater among the partners than among the patients themselves *(33,34)* and that the period of greatest perceived burden occurs during the first year of treatment, particularly among women *(70)*. One would anticipate that the difficulties families experience would also be influenced by their developmental phase in the life cycle (e.g., couple with young children vs elderly couple), by the social and economic context in which they live (e.g., access to health care, culturally informed health beliefs), and by the intensity of concurrent burdens they must accommodate (e.g., unemployment) *(35)*; as yet there have been few efforts to examine these variables among HNSCC families.

6. DETERMINANTS OF QOL OUTCOMES

6.1. Clinical Variables

As noted, QOL outcomes would be expected to vary with important clinical characteristics such as disease site, tumor stage, and type of treatment. Thus far there have been few randomized trials targeting QOL outcomes; in most observational studies type of treatment overlaps with disease site and stage, so it is not possible to disentangle their effects. Nonetheless, a number of descriptive studies suggest that different tumor sites are associated with differences in symptom burden. In general, patients with pharyngeal or oral cavity cancer tend to fare most poorly *(21,22,39,49,51,57,59,62,71)*. Problems with swallowing, nutrition, and pain are especially pronounced. Laryngeal cancer patients are more apt to struggle with speech, hoarseness, cough, and sticky saliva *(21,39,44,51,67,71)*. Among those with laryngeal cancer, patients with supraglottic tumors appear to experience more negative outcomes than their peers with glottic tumors, which are more common *(55,58)*. Among patients with oral cancer, there are preliminary indications that individuals with posterior sites demonstrated more adverse changes in social functioning than those with anterior sites *(37)*.

Patients with more advanced disease struggled with more extensive symptoms than those with earlier stage disease in a number of studies *(25,36,39,43,44,46,51,55,57,72–74)*, although not all *(22,48,53,56,62,75)*. In part, these findings may be due to differences in pain and dysphagia *(55)*. And of course, these results may also reflect group differences in treatments received.

As one would anticipate, individuals who undergo more extensive treatment typically experience greater QOL deficits than those who receive more limited therapies *(76)*. For example, in nonrandomized comparisons patients treated with combined modalities tended to fare more poorly than those who received surgery alone or radiotherapy alone *(43,44,51,55)*. Among laryngeal cancer patients, individuals treated with the most aggressive regimen—total laryngectomy with radical neck dissection—reported significantly worse outcomes in physical spheres of daily functioning than total laryngectomy patients who received less extensive neck dissection and than those who received other less aggressive modalities (i.e., conservation surgery alone or radiotherapy alone) *(77)*. Similarly, more extensive surgery was associated with more adverse QOL outcomes among patients with oral and pharyngeal cancers *(78)*, and more extensive neck dissection was linked with greater shoulder dysfunction among patients with mixed HN disease sites *(79)*.

In recent years growing interest has focused on organ conservation protocols, in particular those involving concurrent or sequential chemotherapy and radiation as an alternative to laryngectomy for individuals with advanced laryngeal cancer. If different regimens lead to comparable survival rates (e.g., refs. *80,81*), it is hoped that organ-sparing treatments will better preserve QOL. Unfortunately, thus far few comparison studies have directly examined this assumption regarding QOL outcomes. There is a pressing need for these comparisons, especially given advances in rehabilitation for laryngectomy patients and the fact that chemoradiation is associated with difficult toxicities of its own. In a long-term follow-up (mean 10.4 yr) of patients with advanced laryngeal cancer who had been randomized to *sequential* chemotherapy followed by radiation or to laryngectomy and radiation, those who had received surgery (as initial treatment or as salvage) reported significantly greater difficulties with mental health, emotional functioning, and pain *(82)*. The chemoradiation group was significantly older, and it is possible that this imbalance may have influenced the results (especially regarding emotional functioning). Somewhat surprisingly, the laryngectomy group did not fare worse in terms of speech difficulties at this long-term follow-up.

In our own work, we examined QOL differences among patients with advanced laryngeal or hypopharyngeal cancer who had been treated with *concurrent* chemoradiotherapy or with surgery and radiation *(83)*. We found relatively few group differences at long-term follow-up (mean 3 yr). The surgery group reported significantly greater difficulties with smell and taste, cough, and need for pain medication and marginally greater problems with social functioning. Those successfully treated with chemoradiotherapy were more apt to complain of dry mouth. Like Terrell and colleagues *(82)*, we did not find differences in speech difficulties, perhaps due in part to extensive use of TEP and voice rehabilitation and the long period since treatment. Additional comparison studies, using randomized, prospective designs and larger samples, would be helpful.

Other studies have compared outcomes among patients receiving *laryngectomy* and those treated with primary radiotherapy. These are nonrandomized investigations, and generally the radiotherapy patients had earlier stage disease. The most consistent findings in these studies involve greater speech deficits among the laryngectomy patients *(47,52,84,85)*. Fewer group differences emerged in other domains of functioning *(47,52,69,84–86)*. In a prospective study, for example, patients who received total laryngectomy (as initial treatment or as salvage) reported significantly greater difficulties with speech and marginally greater problems with cough and swallowing over the course of 2-yr follow-up, relative to radiotherapy patients, who generally had earlier stage disease *(52)*; pain was marginally greater for radiotherapy patients, and there were no significant differences in life satisfaction or distress. In a small cross-sectional study, patients who received salvage laryngectomy and tracheoesophageal prosthesis had significantly worse observer-ratings and self-ratings of voice quality and greater psychiatric morbidity than their radiation-treated counterparts, who were matched for disease stage, site, gender, and age *(84)*. The radiation group had greater hoarseness; other QOL outcomes were comparable. DeSanto and colleagues *(86)* reported poorer psychosocial outcomes among survivors who had undergone total or near-total laryngectomies relative to those who had received partial laryngectomies (i.e., no permanent tracheotomy); however, group differences in recruitment, gender, and time since treatment require caution in interpreting the findings.

Studies of long-term survivors of laryngectomy implied that individuals using different types of voice restoration (i.e., electrolaryngeal, esophageal, or tracheoesophageal speech) had roughly comparable levels of QOL and self-rated ability to communicate in everyday situations *(87,88)*; the very small samples *(87,88)* and use of unvalidated communication measures *(87)* contribute to the preliminary nature of the findings. For patients with early-stage laryngeal cancer, who are less likely to receive laryngectomy, there are preliminary indications that hyperfractioned radiation is tied to greater toxicities during the acute treatment period (e.g., problems with eating and taste) but better status by 1-yr follow-up, compared with conventional radiotherapy *(46)*.

Other investigations have begun to focus on QOL outcomes associated with different treatments for *oral cancers*. Among patients with oropharyngeal tumors, a nonrandomized study hinted at better outcomes for patients with advanced disease treated with accelerated radiotherapy (with or without chemotherapy) as opposed to primary surgery with postoperative radiotherapy *(89)*: there were fewer difficulties with speech, eating, diet, and pain and marginally better emotional and social functioning in the radiotherapy group. Conclusions are limited by notable group differences in gender and time since treatment. In an investigation of patients with oral or pharyngeal tumors, the addition of brachytherapy to treatment with external beam radiation (with or without surgery or chemotherapy) did not seem to generate greater QOL deficits relative to external beam radiotherapy alone *(45)*. A small comparison study among patients with base of tongue tumors suggested more favorable performance outcomes for those who received primary radiotherapy (i.e., external beam radiation plus brachytherapy) compared with those treated with primary surgery (and postoperative radiation) *(90)*. Finally, in a series of surgical studies, the worst QOL outcomes were demonstrated by patients with large bilateral defects (and therefore extensive, functionally important soft tissue loss) who received discontinuity resections of the mandible *(72,73)*.

6.2. Patient Variables

Responses to a particular treatment or disease site are characterized by considerable variability among patients. It is clear that QOL outcomes are strongly colored not only by clinical factors but also by the personal and social qualities that the patient brings to the illness. Findings regarding basic demographic variables have been mixed. Some studies reported greater difficulties among women in both psychosocial *(42,51,56,64,71,76,78)* and physical *(42,51,71,76)* spheres of functioning, including lower likelihood of acquiring esophageal speech following laryngectomy *(91)*. On the other hand, a Scandinavian study *(22)* noted poorer functioning in several domains among male rather than female survivors relative to population norms, and many investigations found few or no meaningful gender differences

(5,8,37,48,55,59,63,75,92). Older patients have often reported greater difficulties in general physical functioning *(37,44,51,57,71,76,77)*, sometimes in conjunction with disrupted speech *(44,76)* and sexuality *(39,57,71)*. Conversely, older individuals appear to be less vulnerable than their younger counterparts to psychosocial distress *(36,39,56,64,71,78)*. However, many investigations failed to find significant age effects *(8,48,59,63,67,72,75,85,92,93)*. Among the fewer studies that have examined the impact of education, one reported greater life satisfaction and perceived health for patients with more extensive education *(62)*, and two studies noted unexpectedly poorer outcomes among those with greater education *(76,77)*, but most investigations did not find significant associations with QOL outcomes *(5,8,44,48,63,85)*. Few investigations have focused on correlates of ethnic or socioeconomic differences.

Aside from basic demographic background, the patient's psychosocial resources and vulnerabilities may have a salient impact on adaptation to illness. Social support has long been recognized as a marker for improved physical and mental health *(94)*. Among long-term survivors, de Boer and colleagues *(76)* reported that more open communication within the family about illness was associated with more favorable outcomes on a broad range of psychosocial and physical measures (e.g., depression, anxiety, physical symptoms). Other investigators similarly found that increased perceived support was tied to improved medication adherence *(95)*, less distress *(91)*, increased life satisfaction *(55,59)*, and better daily functioning *(96)*. Interestingly, Mathieson et al. *(97)* reported that perceived support from the family physician (as opposed to oncologists, family, or friends) was associated with less depression and enhanced QOL. In contrast to findings regarding *perceived* social support (i.e., satisfaction with support), indices of *structural or network* support (i.e., marital status, number of social ties) have yielded mixed *(5,85)* or null *(8,56,63,66,91)* results with respect to QOL outcomes. That is, the quality of support may be more critical than the quantity. Notably, however, a recent Norwegian investigation of long-term survivors of laryngectomy found that patients who were more actively involved in the Norwegian Society of Laryngectomies, a widely used patient advocacy organization, had better QOL outcomes across multiple domains relative to their less engaged peers *(66)*.

Surprisingly few investigations have examined other personality or contextual factors that might influence adaptation to HNSCC. Studies have begun to explore optimism, health locus of control, sense of coherence, and coping. In a study of newly diagnosed Chinese patients undergoing radiotherapy for nasopharyngeal cancer, optimism mediated the impact of eating deficits on overall QOL *(54)*; that is, the extent to which treatment toxicities disrupted general QOL appeared to depend on the patient's level of optimism. In other studies, internal locus of control (i.e., perceptions that the course of illness is primarily influenced by oneself as opposed to external, chance, or religious factors) was tied to diminished anxiety, increased self-confidence regarding speech *(76)*, and greater self-reported treatment adherence *(95)*. Stronger sense of coherence (i.e., an appraisal that life is generally manageable, comprehensible, and meaningful) was linked with better psychosocial and physical outcomes at 12-mo follow-up in a small study of oral and pharyngeal cancer patients *(78)*.

Coping has been widely discussed but little studied in the HNSCC setting *(38,41,88,98,99)*. Blood et al. *(88)* found that patients with recent laryngectomies reported poorer adjustment and used different coping strategies than individuals further along in the recovery process. In particular, they relied more heavily on wishful thinking and self-blame and made less use of problem-focused coping. Unfortunately, the investigators did not report data concerning the associations between coping and adjustment. Patients using different types of alaryngeal speech (esophageal, tracheoesophageal, artificial larynx) did not differ in distress or coping.

In our own work *(41)*, we too found differences in distress and coping for patients at different phases of treatment. As expected, individuals receiving active treatment and those in the acute posttreatment period (i.e., within 6 mo of completing treatment) experienced significantly greater stress symptoms than patients who had not yet began treatment or who were long-term survivors. Moreover, the on-treatment and acute posttreatment groups reported significantly greater use of denial (e.g., "refusing to believe this has happened"), behavioral disengagement (e.g., "just giving up trying to deal with it"), and suppression of competing activities (e.g., "putting aside other activities to concentrate on this"). Denial and behavioral disengagement were associated with greater distress in most groups. Similarly, in an Indian study reliance on fatalistic or helpless coping responses was tied to greater distress *(38)*, whereas beliefs about "acting actively" were linked with favorable QOL outcomes in an Israeli study *(100)*. Research in other cancer or nonclinical settings also has generally supported the differential effectiveness of avoidant vs active coping in response to chronic stressors *(101,102)*. Patients who are actively engaged with their illness and treatment tend to manage more successfully.

7. METHODOLOGICAL ISSUES AND FUTURE DIRECTIONS

QOL research among HNSCC patients has grown appreciably in recent years, and studies are becoming more sophisticated. Salient improvements include the increased number of prospective studies, more consistent use of validated instruments, and greater focus on clinically homogenous populations (i.e., specific disease sites). These trends reflect an encouraging "sea-change" in the past decade.

Unfortunately, a number of methodological limitations still characterize a good deal of the research in this area. Most investigations are based on small samples; it is often difficult to obtain large samples in a single institution, particularly in prospective studies where attrition is a major challenge. Nonetheless, reliance on small samples results in statistically underpowered studies and ambiguous conclusions. Research has matured sufficiently to warrant greater movement toward collaborative group studies, as illustrated by a number of European investigations *(39,56,71,77)*. Some studies neglected to report basic demographic information (e.g., age, ethnicity, socioeconomic status), refusal or attrition rates, or differential refusal/ attrition rates across subgroups. Little work has targeted underserved ethnic minority or rural populations.

Despite intensified interest, there have been few published randomized clinical trials that have compared different treatment regimens on QOL endpoints (e.g., organ preservation vs primary surgery). Nor have there been many large, stratified, prospective observational studies designed to compare different subgroups descriptively (e.g., oral cavity vs laryngeal tumors, early stage vs advanced disease, etc.). In the absence of these, available observational studies offer preliminary hints about important subgroup differences. In many of these nonrandomized comparisons, however, it is not clear whether subgroups were equivalent on important confounding variables (e.g., tumor stage, gender, age), and when imbalances were identified, rarely were efforts made to address them through use of appropriate statistical controls.

Aside from moving toward more refined methodology, it would be helpful for future studies to extend the inquiry in new directions. Some QOL outcomes have received considerable attention in the HNSCC setting (e.g., difficulties with communication, dysphagia, eating). Other important domains, however, have received more limited scrutiny, such as problems with treatment adherence *(95)*, health behaviors *(67,82)*, fear of recurrence *(38)*, family functioning *(33)*, or the possibility of positive, adaptive life changes *(29,30)*. Moreover, there has been little focus on important factors that may influence risk of or resilience to QOL deficits, beyond the effects of basic demographic and medical variables. Factors that warrant increased attention include, among others, personal variables such as optimism *(103)* and substance abuse history; social factors such culturally determined meanings ascribed to illness and treatment; and coping resources such as religious/spiritual involvement *(104)*. Greater use of theoretical frameworks would also be helpful in guiding the inquiry *(28,103,105,106)*.

An additional challenge is to translate current research findings into improved clinical services. For example, difficulties with emotional distress, fatigue, pain, nutrition, and tobacco or alcohol dependence remain underdiagnosed and undertreated in oncology settings *(10,107,108)*. Suboptimal management of these symptoms may contribute not only to diminished QOL but also to disrupted treatment, prolonged hospitalization, and increased health care costs *(109,110)*. Practice guidelines, such as those issued by the National Comprehensive Cancer Network, call for routine screening and early intervention for a number of QOL deficits *(111–113)*. There is a pressing need to develop more effective screening and intervention programs for patients with HNSCC *(114)*.

8. CONCLUSIONS

In sum, individuals with HNSCC contend with considerable burdens. Most patients adapt well to these shifting challenges, but there are disruptions in multiple domains of physical and emotional functioning, some of which are marked and enduring. In the past decade notable advances have been made in assessing QOL changes among HNSCC patients. Investigators have made considerable progress in charting some of the difficulties commonly associated with different sites of HNSCC during active treatment and longer term recovery. It would be helpful for future studies to broaden the range of QOL outcomes that are examined, to extend the focus to underserved, culturally diverse patient groups, and to examine factors that may influence risk of psychosocial or physical morbidity. Increased efforts to develop systematic screening and early intervention programs might also enhance the quality of care for patients and families struggling with this demanding illness.

REFERENCES

1. Ganz PA. Quality of life and the patient with cancer: individual and policy implications. Cancer 1994; 74:1445–1452.
2. Gotay CC, Moore TD. Assessing quality of life in head and neck cancer. Qual Life Res 1992; 1:5–17.
3. De Boer MR, McCormick LK, Pruyn JFA, Ryckman RM. Physical and psychosocial correlates of head and neck cancer: a review of the literature. Orolaryngol Head Neck Surg 1999; 120:427–436.
4. Calman KC. Quality of life in cancer patients-an hypothesis. J Med Ethics 1984;10:124–127.
5. Long SA, D'Antonio L, Robinson EB, Zimmerman G, Petti G, Chonkich G. Factors related to quality of life and functional status in 50 patients with head and neck cancer. Laryngoscope 1996; 106:1084–1088.
6. Sherman AC, Simonton S, Adams DC, Vural E, Owens B, Hanna E. Assessing quality of life in patients with head and neck cancer: cross-validation of The European Organization for Research and Treatment of Cancer (EORTC) Quality of Life Head and Neck Module (QLQ-H&N35), Arch Otolaryngol Head Neck Surg 2000; 126:459–467.
7. Bjordal K, Freng A, Thorvik J, Kaasa S. Patient self-reported and clinician-rated quality of life in head and neck cancer patients: a cross-sectional study. Oral Oncol Eur J Cancer 1995; 31B:235–241.
8. D'Antonio LL, Long SA, Zimmerman GH, Peterman AH, Petti GH, Chonkich GD. Relationship between quality of life and depression in patients with head and neck cancer. Laryngoscope 1998; 108:806–811.

9. Mohide EA, Archibald DS, Tew M, Young,JE, Haines T. Postlaryngectomy quality-of-life dimensions identified by patients and health care professionals. Am J Surg 1992; 164:619–622.

10. Passik SD, Dugan W, McDonald MV, Rosenfeld B, Theobold DE, Edgerton S. Oncologists' recognition of depression in their patients with cancer. J Clin Oncol 1998; 16:1594–1600.

11. Slevin ML, Plant H, Lynch D, Drinkwater J, Gregory WM. Who should measure quality of life, the doctor or the patients? Br J Cancer 1988; 57:109–112.

12. Ware JE, Kosinski M, Dewey JE. How to Score Version Two of the SF-36 Health Survey. Lincoln, RI: QualityMetric, 2000.

13. Derogatis LR. The psychological adjustment to illness scale (PAIS). J Psychosom Res 1986; 30:77–91.

14. Bergner M, Bobitt RA. The sickness impact profile: development and final revision of a health status measure. Med Care 1981; 19:787–805.

15. Schipper H, Clinch J, McMurray A, Levitt M. Measuring the quality of life of cancer patients: the Functional Living Index—Cancer: development and validation. J Clin Oncol 1984; 2:472–483.

16. Terrell JE, Nanavati KA Esclamado RM, et al. Head and neck cancer-specific quality of life: instrument validation. Arch Otolaryngol Head Neck Surg 1997;123:1125–1132.

17. Browman GP, Levine MN, Hodson I, et al. The head and neck radiotherapy questionnaire: a morbidity/quality-of-life instrument for clinical trials of radiation therapy in locally advanced head and neck cancer. J Clin Oncol 1993 11:863–872.

18. Cella DF. Functional Assessment of Chronic Illness Therapy Manual, version 4. Evanston, Ill: Center on Outcomes, Research and Education (CORE), Evanston Northwestern Healthcare, 1997.

19. Aaronson NK, Ahmedzai S, Bergman B, et al. The European Organization for Research and Treatment of Cancer QLQ-C30: a quality of life instrument for use in international clinical trials in oncology. J Natl Cancer Inst 1993; 85:365–376.

20. Bjordal K, Hammerlid E, Ahlner-Elmqvist M, et al. Quality of life in head and neck cancer patients: validation of the European Organization for Research and Treatment of Cancer Quality of Life Questionnaire- H&N35. J Clin Oncol 1999;17:1008–1019.

21. Bjordal K, de Graeff A, Fayers PM, et al. A 12 country field study of the EORTC QOL-C30 (version 3.0) and the head and neck cancer specific module (EORTC QLQ-H&N35) in head and neck patients. Eur J Cancer 2000; 36:1796–1807.

22. Hammerlid E, Taft C. Health-related quality of life in long-term head and neck cancer survivors: a comparison with general population norms. Br J Cancer 2001; 84:149–156.

23. Hanna E, Sherman AC. Quality of life issues in head and neck cancer. Curr Oncol Rep 1999; 1:124–128.

24. Hassan SJ, Weymuller EA Jr. Assessment of quality of life in head and neck cancer patients. Head Neck 1993;15:485–496.

25. Weymuller EA Jr, Yueh B, Deleyiannis FWB, et al. Quality of life in patient with head and neck cancer: lessons learned from 549 prospectively evaluated patients. Arch Otolaryngol Head Neck Surg 2000; 126:329–335.

26. Gliklich RE, Goldsmith TA, Funk GF. Are head and neck specific quality of life measures necessary? Head Neck 1997; 19:474–480.

27. List MA, Ritter-Sterr C, Lansky SB. A performance status scale for head and neck cancer patients. Cancer 1990; 66:564–569.

28. Eisbruch A, Kim HM, Terrell JE, Marsh LH, Dawson LA, Ship JA. Xerostomia and its predictors following parotid-sparing irradiation of head and neck cancer. Int J Radiat Oncol Biol Phys 2001;50:695–704.

29. Tedeschi RG, Park CL, Calhoun LG, eds. Posttraumatic Growth: Positive Changes in the Aftermath of Crisis. Mahwah, NJ: Lawrence Erlbaum, 1998.

30. Antoni MH, Lehman JM, Kilbourn KM, et al. Cognitive-behavioral stress management intervention decreases the prevalence of depression and enhances benefit-finding among women under treatment for early-stage breast cancer. Health Psychol 2001; 20:20–32.

31. Baile WF, Gibertini M, Scott L, Endicott J. Depression and tumor stage in cancer of the head and neck. Psychooncol 1992;1:15–24.

32. Davies ADM, Davies C, Delpo MC. Depression and anxiety in patients undergoing diagnostic investigations for head and neck cancers. Br J Psychiatry 1986; 149:491–493.

33. Vickery LE, Latchford G, Hewison J, Beelew M, Feber T. The impact of head and neck cancer and facial disfigurement on the quality of life of patients and their partners. Head Neck 2003; 25:289–296.

34. Mathieson CM, Stam HJ. The impact of laryngectomy on the spouse: who is better off? Psychol Health 1991; 5:153–163.

35. Sherman AC, Simonton S. Family therapy for cancer patients: clinical issues and interventions. Family J 1999; 7:38–49.

36. Funk GF. Karnell LH, Dawson CJ, et al. Baseline and post-treatment assessment of the general health status of head and neck cancer patients compared with United States population norms. Head Neck 1997; 19:675–683.

37. Rogers SN, Humphris G, Lowe D, Brown JS, Vaughan ED. The impact of surgery for oral cancer on quality of life as measured by the Medical Outcomes Short Form 36. Oral Oncol 1998; 34:171–179.

38. Chaturvedi SK, Shenoy A, Prasad KMR, Senthilnathan SM, Premlatha BS. Concerns, coping, and quality of life in head and neck cancer patients. Support Care Cancer 1996; 4:186–190.

39. Bjordal K, Ahlner-Elmqvist M, Hammerlid E, et al. A prospective study of quality of life in head and neck cancer patients. part II: longitudinal data. Laryngoscope 2001; 111:1440–1452.

40. Siston AK, List MA, Schleser R, Vokes E. Sexual functioning and head and neck cancer. J Psychosoc Oncol 1997; 15:107–122.

41. Sherman AC, Simonton S, Adams DC, Vural E, Hanna E. Coping with head and neck cancer during different phases of treatment. Head Neck 2000; 22:787–793.

42. de Graeff A, de Leeuw JRJ, Ros WJG, et al. A prospective study on quality of life of laryngeal cancer patients treated with radiotherapy. Head Neck 1999; 21:291–296.

43. de Graeff A, de Leeuw JRJ, Ros WJG, Hordijk GJ, Blijham GH, Winnubst JAM. A prospective study on quality of life of patients with cancer of the oral cavity or oropharynx treated with surgery with or without radiotherapy. Oral Oncol 1999; 35:27–32.

44. de Graeff A, de Leeuw JRJ, Ros WJG, Hordijk G-J, Blijham GH, Winnubst JAM. Pretreatment factors predicting quality of life after treatment for head and neck cancer. Head Neck 2000; 22:398–407.

45. Hammerlid E, Mercke C, Sullivan M, Westin T. A prospective quality of life study of patients with oral or pharyngeal carcinoma treated with external beam irradiation with or without brachytherapy. Oral Oncol 1997; 33:189–196.

46. Hammerlid E, Mercke C, Sullivan M, Westin T. A prospective quality of life study of patients with laryngeal carcinoma by tumor stage and different radiation therapy schedules. Laryngoscope 1998; 108:747–759.

47. List MA, Ritter-Sterr CA, Baker TM, et al. Longitudinal assessment of quality of life in laryngeal cancer patients. Head Neck 1996; 18:1–10.

48. List MA, Siston A, Haraf D, et al. Quality of life and performance in advanced head and neck cancer patients on concomitant chemoradiotherapy: a prospective examination. J Clin Oncol 1999; 17:1020–1028.

49. Murry T, Madasu R, Martin A, Robbins KT. Acute and chronic changes in swallowing and quality of life following intraarterial chemoradiation for organ preservation in patients with advanced head and neck cancer. Head Neck 1998; 20:31–37.

50. Rogers SN, Lowe D, Brown JS, Vaughan ED. A comparison between the University of Washington Head and Neck Disease-Specific measure and the Medical Short Form 36, EORTC QOQ-C33 and EORTC Head and Neck 35. Oral Oncol 1998; 34:361–372.

51. de Graeff A, de Leeuw JRJ, Ros WJG, Hordijk G-J, Blijham GH, Winnubst JAM. Long-term quality of life of patients with head and neck cancer. Laryngoscope 2000; 110:98–106.

52. Morton RP. Laryngeal cancer: quality-of-life and cost-effectiveness. Head Neck 1997; 19:243–250.

53. Gritz ER, Carmack CL, de Moor C, et al. First year after head and neck cancer: quality of life. J Clin Oncol 1999; 17:352–360.

54. Yu CLM, Fielding R, Chan CLW. The mediating effect of optimism on post-radiation quality of life in nasopharyngeal carcinoma. Quality Life Res 2003; 12:41–51.

55. Morton RP. Studies in the quality of life of head and neck cancer patients: results of a two-year longitudinal study and a comparative cross-sectional cross-cultural survey. Laryngoscope 2003;113:1091–1103.

56. Hammerlid E, Ahlner-Elmqvist M, Bjordal K, et al. A prospective multicentre study in Sweden and Norway of mental distress and psychiatric morbidity in head and neck cancer patients. Br J Cancer 1999; 80:766–774.

57. Hammerlid E, Silander E, Hornestram L, Sullivan M. Health-related quality of life three years after diagnosis of head and neck cancer—a longitudinal study. Head Neck 2001; 23:113–125.

58. Nordgren M, Abendstein H, Jannert M, et al. Health-related quality of life five years after diagnosis of laryngeal carcinoma. Int J Radiation Oncol Biol Phys 2003; 56:1333–1343.

59. Morton RP. Life satisfaction in patients with head and neck cancer. Clin Ortolaryngol 1995; 20:499–503.

60. Rapoport Y, Kreitler S, Chaitchik S, Algor R, Weissler K. Psychosocial problems in head-and-neck cancer patients and their change with time since diagnosis. Ann Oncol 1993; 4:69–73.

61. Schwartz CE, Sprangers MAG, eds. Adaptation to Changing Health: Response Shift in Quality-of-Life Research. Washington, DC: American Psychological Association, 2000.

62. Bjordal K, Mastekaasa A, Kaasa S. Self-reported satisfaction with life and physical health in long-term cancer survivors and a matched control group. Oral Oncol Eur J Cancer 1995; 31B:340–345.

63. Bjordal K, Kaasa S. Psychological distress in head and neck cancer patients 7-11 years after curative treatment. Br J Cancer 1995; 71:595–597.

64. Espie CA, Freedlander E, Campsie LM, Soutar DS, Robertson AG. Psychological distress at follow-up after major surgery for intral-oral cancer. J Psychosom Res 1989; 33:441–448.

65. Tefler MR, Shepherd JP. Psychological distress in patients attending an oncology clinic after definitive treatment for maxillofacial malignant neoplasia. Int J Oral Maxillofacial Surg 1993; 22:347–349.

66. Birkhaug EJ, Aarstad HJ, Asrstad AKH, Olofsson J. Relation between mood, social support, and the quality of life in patients with laryngectomies. Eur Arch Otorhinolaryngol 2002; 259:197–204.

67. List MA, Mumby P, Haraf D, et al. Performance and quality of life outcome in patients completing concomitant chemotherapy protocols for head and neck cancer. Quality Life Res 1997; 6:274–284.

68. Kreitler S, Chaitchik S, Rapoport Y, Kreitler H, Algor R. Life satisfaction and health in cancer patients, orthopedic patients, and health individuals. Soc Sci Med 1993; 36:547–556.

69. Ramirez MJ, Ferriol EE, Domenech FG, Llatas MC, Suarez-Varela MM, Martinez RL. Psychosocial adjustment in patients surgically treated for laryngeal cancer. Otolaryngol Head Neck Surg 2003; 129:92–97.

70. Blood GW, Simpson KC, Dineen M, Kauffman SM, Raimondi SC. Spouses of individuals with laryngeal cancer: caregiver strain and burden. J Commun Disord 1994; 27:19–35.

71. Hammerlid E, Bjordal K, Ahlner-Elmqvist M, et al. A prospective study of quality of life in head and neck cancer patients. Part I: at diagnosis. Laryngoscope 2001; 111:669–680.

72. Schliephake H, Neukam FW, Schmelzeisen R, Varoga B, Schneller H. Long-term quality of life after ablative intraoral tumour surgery. J Cranio Maxillofac Surg 1995; 23:243–249.

73. Schliephake H, Ruffert K, Schneller T. Prospective study of the quality of life of cancer patients after intraoral tumor surgery. J Oral Maxillofac Surg 1996; 54:664–669.

74. Moore GJ, Parsons JT, Mendenhall WM. Quality of life outcomes after primary radiotherapy for squamous cell carcinoma of the base of tongue. Int J Radiation Oncol Biol Phys 1996; 36:351–354.

75. Bjordal K, Kaasa S, Mastekaasa A. Quality of life in patients treated for head and neck cancer: a follow-up study 7 to 11 years after radiotherapy. Int J Radiat Oncol Biol Phys 1994; 28:847–856.

76. de Boer MF, Pruyn JFA, van den Borne B, Knegt PP, Ryckman RM, Verwoerd CDA. Rehabilitation outcomes of long-term survivors treated for head and neck cancer. Head Neck 1995; 17:503–515.

77. Mosconi P, Cifani S, Crispino S, Fossati R, Apolone G. The performance of SF-36 health survey in patients with laryngeal cancer. Head Neck 2000; 22:175–182.

78. Langius A, Bjorvell H, Lind MG. Functional status and coping in patients with oral and pharyngeal cancer before and after surgery. Head Neck 1994; 16:559–568.

79. Kuntz AL, Weymuller EA Jr. Impact of neck dissection on quality of life. Laryngoscope 1999; 109:1334–1338.

80. Department of Veterans Affairs Laryngeal Cancer Study Group. Induction chemotherapy plus radiation compared with surgery plus radiation in patients with advanced laryngeal cancer. N Engl J Med 1991; 324:1685–1690.

81. Weber RS, Berkey BA, Forastiere A, et al. Outcome of salvage total laryngectomy following organ preservation therapy: the Radiation Therapy Oncology Group trial 91-11. Arch Otolaryngol Head Neck Surg 2003; 129:44–49.

82. Terrell JE, Fisher SG, Wolf GT. Long-term quality of life after treatment of laryngeal cancer. Arch Otolaryngol Head Neck Surg 1998; 124:964–971.

83. Hanna E, Sherman AC, Cash D, et al. Quality of life for patients following total laryngectomy versus chemoradiation for laryngeal preservation. Arch Otolaryngol Head Neck Surg 2004; 130:875–879.

84. Finizia C, Hammerlid E, Westin T, Lindstrom J. Quality of life and voice in patients with laryngeal carcinoma: a posttreatment comparison of laryngectomy (salvage surgery) versus radiotherapy. Laryngoscope 1998; 108:1566–1573.

85. Stewart MG, Chen AY, Stach CB. Outcomes analysis of voice and quality of life in patients with laryngeal cancer. Arch Otolaryngol Head Neck Surg 1998; 124:143–148.

86. DeSanto LW, Olsen KD, Perry WC, Rohe DE, Keith RL. Quality of life after surgical treatment of cancer of the larynx. Ann Otol Rhinol Laryngol 1995; 104:763–769.

87. Carr MM, Schmidbauer JA, Majaess L, Smith RL. Communication after laryngectomy: an assessment of quality of life. Otolaryngol Head Neck Surg 2000; 122:39–43.

88. Blood GW, Luther AR, Stemple JC. Coping and adjustment in alaryngeal speakers. Am J Clin Speech Lang Pathol 1992; 1:63–69.

89. Allal AS, Nicoucar K, Mach N, Dulguerov P. Quality of life in patients with oropharynx carcinomas: assessment after accelerated radiotherapy with or without chemotherapy versus radical surgery and postoperative radiotherapy. Head Neck 2003; 25:833–840.

90. Harrison LB, Zelefsky MJ, Armstrong JG, Carper E, Gaynor JJ, Sessions RB. Performance status after treatment for squamous cell cancer of the base of tongue—a comparison of primary radiation therapy versus primary surgery. Int J Radiat Oncol Biol Phys 1994; 30:953–957.

91. Stam HJ, Koopmans JP, Mathieson CM. The psychological impact of a laryngectomy: a comprehensive assessment. J Psychosoc Oncol 1991; 9:37–58.

92. Chaplin JM, Morton RP. A prospective, longitudinal study of pain in head and neck cancer patients. Head Neck 1999; 21:531–537.

93. Derks W, De Leeuw JRJ, Hordijk GJ, Winnubst JAM. Elderly patients with head and neck cancer: short-term effects of surgical treatment on quality of life. Clin Otolaryngol 2003; 28:399–405.

94. House JS, Landis KR, Umberson D. Social relationships and health. Science 1988; 241:540–545.

95. McDonough EM, Boyd JH, Varvares MA, Maves MD. Relationship between psychological status and compliance in a sample of patients treated for cancer of the head and neck. Head Neck 1996; 18:269–276.

96. Baker CA. Factors associated with rehabilitation in head and neck cancer. Cancer Nurs 1992; 15:395–400.

97. Mathieson CM, Logan-Smith LL, Phillips J, MacPhee M, Attia EL. Caring for head and neck oncology patients: does social support lead to better quality life? Can Fam Physician 1996; 42:1712–1720.

98. Dropkin MJ. Coping with disfigurement and dysfunction after head and neck cancer surgery: a conceptual framework. Semin Oncol Nurs 1989; 5:213–219.

99. Manuel GM, Roth S, Keefe FJ, Brantley BA. Coping with cancer. J Human Stress 1987; 13:149–158.

100. Kreitler S, Chaitchik S, Kreitler H, Rapoport Y, Algor R. Cogntive orientation and quality of life in cancer survivors. Int J Rehab Health 1996; 2:217–234.

101. Manne SL, Sabbioni C, Bovberg DH, Jacobsen PB, Taylor KL, Redd WH. Coping with chemotherapy for breast cancer. J Behav Med 1994; 17:41–55.

102. Suls J, Fletcher B. The relative efficacy of avoidant and nonavoidant coping strategies: a meta-analysis. Health Psychol 1985; 4:249–288.

103. Scheier MF, Carver CS. Optimism, coping, and health: assessment and implications of generalized outcome expectancies. Health Psychol 1985; 4:219–247.

104. Sherman AC, Simonton S. Religious involvement among cancer patients: associations with adjustment and quality of life. In: Plante TG, Sherman AC, eds. Faith and Health: Psychological Perspectives. New York: Guilford, 2001:167–194.

105. Folkman S, Greer S. Promoting psychological well-being in the face of serious illness: when theory, research and practice inform each other. Psycho-Oncology 2000; 9:11–19.

106. Nigg CR, Burbank PM, Padula C, et al. Stages of change across ten health risk behaviors for older adults. Gerontologist 1999; 39:473–482.

107. Zhukovsky DS, Gorowski E, Hausdorff J, et al. Unmet analgesic needs in cancer patients. J Pain Symptom Manage 1995; 10:113–119.

108. Irvine D, Vincent L, Graydon J, et al. The prevalence and correlates of fatigue in patients receiving chemotherapy and radiotherapy. Cancer Nurs 1994; 17:367–378.

109. Sherman AC, Simonton S, Latif U, Spohn R, Tricot G. Psychosocial adjustment and quality of life among multiple myeloma patients undergoing evaluation for autologous stem cell transplantation. Bone Marrow Transplant 2004; 33:955–962.

110. Katon W, Sullivan MD. Depression and chronic medical illness. J Clin Psychiatry 1994; 51:8–19.

111. Holland J. NCCN practice guidelines for the management of psychosocial distress. Oncology 1999; 13:113–147.

112. Atkinson A, Barsevick A, Cella D, et al. NCCN practice guidelines for cancer-related fatigue. Oncology 2000; 14:151–161.

113. Grossman SR, Benedetti C, Brooke C, et al. NCCN practice guidelines for cancer pain. Oncology 2000; 14:135–150.

114. Hammerlid E, Persson L-O, Sullivan M, Westin T. Quality of life effects of psychosocial intervention in patients with head and neck cancer. Otolaryngol Head Neck Surg 1999; 120:507–516.

21

Palliation of Head and Neck Cancer

Mellar P. Davis, MD, FACP

1. INTRODUCTION

Approximately 5% of all cancers arise from the head and neck region *(1,2)*. Patients with head and neck squamous cell cancers (HNSCC) have unique problems related both to the course of their disease and treatment. Pain from surgery and radiation is a particularly difficult problem and becomes a major problem with recurrence due to the high propensity for local erosive metastases in areas that are richly innervated *(3)*. Pain occurs in 31% of patients at presentation but becomes a progressive problem during therapy. Seventy-four percent will experience pain near the end of treatment, and at least one out of four will have significant chronic pain 2 yr after treatment *(4–6)*. Eating disturbances will peak near the end of treatment related to both the disease and the pain of mucositis. Most patients will lose at least 2 kg during treatment. The incidence of mucositis secondary to treatment is as high as 80%, and over half of those receiving intensive radiation combined with chemotherapy will have a grade 3–4 mucositis. Hospitalization owing to mucositis will occur in 16 to 33% of patients treated with radiation. Despite receiving analgesics and topical anesthetics, over one-third of treatment days will be spent in severe pain *(7,8)*.

Dysphasia occurs in nearly two-thirds of patients, and 90% of patients will have physical disfigurement owing to either disease and/or treatment, which becomes a barrier to socialization. Jaw dysfunction occurs in a significant minority, which limits eating and communication *(9)*.

Depression and anxiety play a significant role in quality of life of patients with HNSCC *(10)*. The most important psychosocial issues for these patients are worry, anxiety, mood disorders, fatigue, and depression *(11)*. Ongoing concerns include social interactions, recreational activities, and sexual function with disfigurement *(11)*.

Screening for HNSCC is ineffective if it is based on the seven warning signs of cancer published by the American Cancer Society. No symptom or symptom complex correlates with early-stage head and neck cancer with the exception of hoarseness associated with glottic primaries. Symptom duration is not an indicator of disease duration *(12)*. There are no well-developed screening criteria for patients "at risk" for head and neck cancer, and the at-risk population (males who abuses tobacco and alcohol) are not known to be highly compliant with screening.

The overall cure rate for HNSCC is 50%. Recurrences are associated with pain, progressive dysphasia, depression, anxiety, fatigue, anorexia, and cachexia *(13)*. There may be guilt with recurrences since most patients "author" their disease through alcohol and tobacco abuse.

From: *Current Clinical Oncology: Squamous Cell Head and Neck Cancer*
Edited by: D. J. Adelstein © Humana Press Inc., Totowa, NJ

The median survival of untreated HNSCC is 3–4 mo. Performance score and perhaps age are the most important prognostic factors *(14)*. The survival for recurrent cancer is months, and for distant metastases the average survival is 4 mo *(15)*.

Isolated lung metastases can be resected, with some patients enjoying long-term survival, although half of these may be lung primaries. Radiation therapy palliates the pain and dyspnea associated with bone and lung metastases, respectively. Chemotherapy unfortunately does not play a major role in influencing the course of metastatic cancer, or symptom control *(16)*.

2. PAIN

The three major signs of HNSCC at presentation are hoarseness, dysphasia, and pain. One-third to one-half of patients will have pain at diagnosis *(6,9)*. The high prevalence of pain is due to the rich innervation of the mouth, pharynx, and neck by cranial nerves V, IX, and X and cervical spinal nerves from C1 to 4 *(17)*. The highest frequency of pain occurs from cancers arising from the nasopharynx and oropharynx *(17)*. Pain is constant in 60% of patients, episodic or paroxysmal in 20%, and continuous with episodic flares in 20% *(9)*. Pain intensity increases with involvement of the skull and mandible *(9)*. Pain is predominantly mixed, that is, nociceptive and neuropathic *(3,17)*. However, one of four patients will have referred pain, which can mislead the physician and cause a delay in diagnosis or failure to find the primary *(17)*. The mean duration of pain prior to diagnosis is 4–6 mo but the duration does not correlate with tumor size *(9)*. The presence of pain at diagnosis is not prognostic. Neuropathic pain owing to tumor is most frequently caused by perineural involvement of the sensory afferents arising from cranial nerve V *(18)*. Fewer individuals (one of eight) will have cranial nerves IX and X involved. Atypical pain at presentation can be mistaken for dental pain, sinusitis, or temporomandibular joint dysfunction *(19)*.

Pain persists after treatment in 25 to 30% of patients who survive their cancer. Pain caused by treatment is largely neuropathic, although a minority will have myofacial pain or pain caused by temporomandibular joint dysfunction *(20)*. Treatment-related pain can also be pain in the shoulder or arm caused by neck dissection which interupts the spinal accessory nerve. Shoulder and arm pain from treatment correlates with the presence of pain at diagnosis. Patients who have a modified neck dissection rather than a radical neck dissection can also experience pain to the same degree in the neck and shoulder *(6)*. Sparing cranial nerves XI reduces long-term shoulder and neck pain and reduces the need for long-term analgesics *(10)*. Pain can increase during radiation therapy and can be complicated by mucositis. The pain may persist after radiation therapy and cause anxiety or fear about relapse *(5,20)*.

Seventy percent of patients with tumor recurrence experience pain prior to the discovery of their recurrence *(17)*. It is often associated with new nociceptive pain, although a minority will experience new neuropathic pain *(20)*. Pain usually occurs at the site of the primary cancer or near the surgical incision, although a minority will have referred pain with their initial recurrence. The median time from definitive treatment to relapse is 10 mo, but pain will precede recurrence by 2–4 mo *(17)*. Reasons for a delay in the diagnosis of recurrence are (1) the presence of persistent pain owing to treatment, which masks the pain of recurrence; and (2) the occult nature of recurrence, which defies detection by clinical examination, plain radiography, magnetic resonance imaging, and computed tomography *(21)*.

2.1. Pain Management

Patients with HNSCC have unique problems, which are barriers to pain management. Dysphagia may prevent the oral administration of analgesics. Large tablets of sustained-release opioids may be impossible to swallow. Many patients have a significant history of alcohol and tobacco use; hence this population is at a higher risk for substance abuse compared with the general cancer population (22). Finally there is a higher incidence of neuropathic pain, which is more refractory to opioids.

One of the advantages of opioids in the management of cancer pain is that opioids do not produce permanent organ damage. Toxicity is completely reversible with discontinuation of opioids. Opioids rarely cause respiratory depression in opioid-tolerant individuals. Opioid-induced respiratory depression is seen in patients with upper airway compromise or in opioid-naïve individuals who undergo a very rapid opioid titration. Addiction risks are present; however, in a medically supervised environment, psychological dependence can be managed with help from addiction specialists for those with a history of drug abuse. Methadone may be preferable owing to the risk of addiction and also methadone's presumed benefit in neuropathic pain. Opioids can induce analgesic tolerance and physical dependency, which is seen clinically as a withdrawal syndrome; hence incremental titration or stepwise dose reduction may be necessary depending on progression of disease or duration of therapy (23). Withdrawal symptoms are avoided by reducing doses by 50% every third day once pain has resolved. Finally, there are no ceiling doses to opioids (unlike nonopioid analgesics), and individual requirements, which are highly variable, can be accomodated without worrying about a particular "therapeutic" level. In general, opioids are more versatile than nonopioid analgesics because of the number of routes of administration.

Opioids are a family of agents that bind to three major receptors μ, δ, and σ (MOR, DOR, KOR) within the central and peripheral nervous system (24–28). The action of opioids leads to prevention of neurotransmitter release (substance P, calcitonin gene-related peptide, and glutamate), by preventing calcium influx in primary afferents and by blocking adenyl cyclase. Opioids cause hyperpolarization of postsynaptic second order afferent neurons by accelerating inward rectifying potassium channels (29). In the brainstem opioids facilitate inhibition of dorsal horn afferent processing through release of monoamines within the rostral ventromedial medulla and periaqueductal grey (30–36).

Opioids commonly used for cancer pain are morphine, methadone, fentanyl, oxycodone and hydromorphone (37) (Table 1). Meperidine and agonists/antagonists should be avoided. Step II "weak" opioids include hydrocodone (by virtue of being compounded to nonsteroid antiimflammatory agents [NSAIDs]) and tramadol. Codeine is metabolized to morphine and hence has little benefit over low doses of morphine. Oxycodone when compounded to NSAIDs has dose limitations owing to the NSAID and is considered a step II opioid by virtue of the dose limitations imposed by the NSAID (37–39).

Opioid choices are based on clinical experience, opioid versatility, side effects, patient history (previous response to opioids), history of substance abuse, organ dysfunction, comorbidity, comedications, and cost. Morphine is the drug of choice by virtue of its (1) versatility, and extensive clinical experience (2). There is simply no other opioid that has proved to be superior to morphine (38,39). The type of pain does not appear to influence the choice of opioids, although randomized trials have found methadone, levorphanol, and fentanyl to be effective for neuropathic pain (40–42). Although patients with HNSCC have complex pain syndromes and may require higher doses of opioids, on average, pain control is possible in most individuals with morphine (43).

Dosing intervals for immediate-release opioids are usually at 4 h (37,38) Sustained-release opioids are given at 12–24 h depending on the commercial product. Morphine, oxycodone, and (in some countries) hydromorphone are available as sustained-release products. Methadone is both an immediate- and a sustained-release substance by virtue of its prolonged half-life and hence fulfills both roles inexpensively (44).

Table 1
Opioid Equivalents

Opioid	Oral (mg)	Parenteral (mg)
Morphine	30	10
Oxycodone	20–30	
Fentanyl	—	200–250 µg
Methadone	6–7[a]	3[a]
Hydromorphone	6	3[b]

[a]Methadone has a dose-related potency ratio to morphine: for daily oral morphine doses <90 mg 1:4, 90–300 mg 1:8, and >300 mg but <1000 mg 1:12 and >1000 mg 1:20.

[b]Reported equivalents of parenteral hydromorphone to oral methadone have been reported to be 1:1 owing to a significant degree of analgesic non-cross tolerance.

Methadone has unique pharmacokinetics and as a result should be dosed differently than morphine. Several strategies have been reported *(44)*. Since methadone is generally used as a second-line opioid, total daily morphine equivalents are calculated, and one-tenth of the daily dose up to 30 mg as a single dose is given every 3 h as needed for pain control. Patients will build a dose by using a q 3 h "as needed" strategy over 4–5 d, at which time the total methadone dose can be calculated based on d 4 and 5, divided by 4, and given at 12-h intervals. Other dosing schemas are available and could be used depending on the clinical situation *(45)*.

Opioid side effects should be anticipated. Constipation should be treated proactively with laxatives and stool softeners. Nausea, which occurs in 10 to 40%, requires antiemetics, but not routinely, since nausea occurs in a minority. Treatment of nausea is with metoclopramide 10 mg prior to meals and at bedtime or haloperidol 1 mg q 4 h as needed. Nausea from opioids usually resolves over several days despite continued dosing. A few patients will have intractable nausea, for which opioid rotation is necessary *(37,46)*.

Sedation and mental clouding may occur for a few days and then clear. In general, patients on stable doses of opioids are able to drive. Visual hallucinations, myoclonus, and overt cognitive failure are dose limiting, and if the patient is in persistent pain, opioid route conversion, opioid rotation, or opioid sparing with the addition of an adjuvant analgesic are effective strategies that improve pain and resolve neurotoxicity *(37,47)*. Respiratory depression, as mentioned previously, is rare. Pain stimulus acts as an opioid antagonist within the brainstem *(22)*. Clinically significant respiratory depression is preceded by sensorium changes and accompanied by miosis. Respiratory rates of 8–10 per minute in an alert individual do not represent opioid toxicity, and opioids should not be reduced. Respiratory depression may be potentiated by cancer-related upper airway obstruction. In addition, sudden relief of pain, rapid titration in the opioid naïve, and the development of hepatic or renal failure in the face of stable opioid dosing may lead to respiratory depression *(37)*. Reversal of respiratory depression is best done by titrating naloxone 0.4 mg diluted in 10 mL of a normal saline given parenterally at 1 mL/min (40 µg) until return of sensorium and a respiratory rate of more than 10/min *(22)*. Patients on sustained-release opioids or methadone may require a continuous infusion of naloxone, as the half-life of naloxone is only 0.5 h. The hourly dose of naloxone is the same as the dose that reversed sensorium, infused hourly until the sustained-release opioid or methadone clears *(48,49)*.

Spinal opioids have been used with some success in individuals whose pain fails to respond to opioid titration or rotation *(50–52)*. Intraventricular therapy may be preferred owing to the location of pain in the head and neck region.

Adjuvant analgesics will be necessary for many patients with HNSCC. A prospective trial involving patients with recurrent cancer whose pain failed to respond to acetominophen plus codeine or oxycodone showed that patients responded to a combination of methadone, plus a tricyclic antidepressant and either a NSAID or acetaminophen *(53)*. The addition of NSAIDs to an opioid can improve pain relief and reduce the need for opioid titration *(54)*. It has been assumed that NSAIDs and corticosteroids are ineffective in the treatment of neuropathic pain. There are few data to substantiate this claim. It is known that NSAIDs do block production of nitric oxide and prostaglandins, which are secondary mediators of the N-methyl-D-aspartate (NMDA) receptor *(55)*. The NMDA receptors are important mediators of neuropathic pain and spinal-generated "wind-up" pain *(56)*.

As previously mentioned, neuropathic pain is common in HNSCC patients. Many agents have been reported to reduce neuropathic pain (Table 2) *(57)*. Among the tricyclic antidepressants, the preferred adjuvants are secondary amine tricyclic antidepressants (desipramine, nortriptyline), since there are fewer anticholinergic side effects with secondary amines and less xerostomia. Of the classical antiseizure medications, phenytoin and carbamazepine are associated with a significant number of drug interactions. Gabapentin and valproic acid are preferred *(58)*. Topical lidocaine in the form of a sustained-release patch in an area of mononeuropathy will relieve pain without being systematically absorbed. Intraspinal opioids alone are usually ineffective in opioid-refractory neuropathic pain. However, spinal opioids plus bupivicaine and/or clonidine will relieve pain unresponsive to opioids alone *(59)*.

3. DYSPHAGIA AND WEIGHT LOSS

Swallowing requires transfer of a food bolus through a series of channels or chambers separated by valves *(60)*. There is a shared pathway with respiration, which must be isolated before swallowing. Each chamber has an entrance and an exit valve whose function must be coordinated with muscular propulsion *(60)*. Swallowing dysfunction may arise from (1) failed or discoordinated propulsion, (2) a failure of the valve to open or close, or (3) a failure to coordinate valve function with propulsion.

The frequency of dysphagia at the time of diagnosis ranges from 34 to 66% *(60–63)*. More than 40% of patients are aspirating oral contents at diagnosis and poorly protect their airways. Clinical assessment alone inadequately predicts those who are aspirating *(64)*. Pneumonia may be the initial presentation of those who have a significant degree of dysphagia.

Swallowing dysfunction at presentation increases with stage of disease. Patients with oral and pharyngeal cancers have greater swallowing difficulties than those with laryngeal cancer *(62,63)*. Patients with oral cancers have dysphagia to the extent of oral tongue, base of tongue, and soft pallate involvement *(65)*. Patients with HNSCC and dysphagia will have (1) longer oral and pharyngeal transit times, (2) greater oral and pharyngeal food residue, (3) shorter cricopharyngeal opening duration, and (4) lower swallowing efficiency *(62,63)*. Swallowing difficulties are perceived by patients to be more problematic than loss of speech *(66)*.

Surgery leads to dysphagia, acutely, owing to pain and soft tissue swelling; dysphagia may continue long term because of scarring, denervation, and deconditioning *(60)*. The greatest difficulty with swallowing arises from extensive oral and pharyngeal resections with flap reconstruction followed by postoperative radiation therapy. Most patients undergoing such

Table 2
Neuropathic Pain Analgesia

Sodium channel blockers
    Carbomazepine
    Oxycarbamazepine
    Phenytoin
    Topiramate
    Lamotrigine
    Lidocaine
    Mexiletine
    Tricyclic antidepressants
Modulators of descending inhibition
    Antidepressants
    Opioids
    Tramadol
Modulators of central sensitization valproic acid
    Gabapentin
    Lamotrigine
    Oxycarbazepine
    Levetracetam
    Ketamine
    Memantine

therapy will experience dysphagia, and only 50% will be able to maintain their weight without supplemental enteral feeding. The amount of oral tongue and base of tongue resected inversely correlates with swallowing efficacy (65). Reconstruction of the soft palate and superior pharynx reduces dysphagia; however, postoperative radiation therapy after reconstruction can curtail or reduce the gains in swallowing made by reconstructive surgery (62,63,67).

During radiation or radiation therapy plus chemotherapy, most patients will experience mucositis and dysphagia. Nutritional failure will be such that 20 to 25% will require enteral nutrition to complete therapy, and a smaller percentage will require permanent feeding tubes in order to survive (60,68–74). Patients undergoing aggressive chemoradiotherapy to "preserve" head and neck function will experience dysphagia to a greater extent than patients receiving radiation therapy alone. Nearly 75% will require feeding tubes, and one-third will require permanent gastric tubes for nutritional support. By videofluoroscopy, 65 to 80% will have abnormal propulsion of a moderate to severe degree, which will persist in 20% for more than 6 mo posttreatment (75–78). Finally, postradiation xerostomia increases the patient's perceived difficulty with swallowing (79).

Weight loss in a patient with HNSCC is due to (1) reduced personal hygiene, (2) mechanical obstruction by tumor, (3) cancer cachexia, (4) temporary treatment sequelae, or (5) permanent loss of function owing to sensory and muscle loss from treatment (80). Prior to treatment most patients with HNSCC will have lost weight on average 6–7 kg, or approx 10% of total body weight (81).

Percutaneous fluoroscopic gastrostomy or esophagogastrostomy and early institution of nutritional support during combined therapy will prevent weight loss (71,82). Enteral nutritional therapy should be considered early, particularly for those patients who have (1) lost 5% or more of their baseline weight prior to treatment, (2) are undergoing chemoradiotherapy in order to "preserve" organ function, or (3) are to undergo large oropharyngeal resections including a significant portion of the tongue and soft palate with reconstruction followed by radiation. Patients with laryngeal cancers who are undergoing single-modality therapy are followed expectantly. Patients should be advised that the ability to swallow can be lost and require permanent gastrostomy for feeding. Both a dietician and a speech pathologist should be involved early in rehabilitation for these patients to maximize nutritional support and facilitate the recovery of swallowing function *(83)*.

An important differential to weight loss in HNSCC is cancer cachexia. Weight loss owing to caloric deprivation will respond to nutritional therapy, whereas the inflammatory-mediated weight loss of cancer cachexia is refractory to caloric replacement *(84)*. Caloric replacement in advanced cancer cachexia will not only fail to maintain or improve weight but will also fail to improve quality of life and survival *(85–88)*. Most patients will have several etiologies to account for weight loss, including mucositis, xerostomia, taste changes, dysphagia, nausea, vomiting, anorexia, pain, depression, delirium, and recurrent cancer *(86)*.

Evaluation of nutritional status includes three measurements: (1) dietary factors, including appetite, weight, activity, food habit, food aversions, taste changes, and symptoms related to digestion (dyspepsia, bloating, satiety); (2) clinical indicators of nutritional deficiencies (anthropometric changes); (3) biochemical indicators of visceral protein deficiency and elevated C-reactive protein; and (4) bioelectric impedance. There are gender differences to the degree of weight loss, and weight loss does not necessarily correlate with the degree of appetite loss. In the United States, the body mass index may be normal and yet a significant degree of nutritional deficiency may be present owing to the prevalence of premorbid obesity. Bioelectric impedance is an important advance in the assessment of nutrition, particularly if it includes capacitance and phase angle *(89–92)*.

Treatment of pain, depression, mucositis, nausea, vomiting, xerostomia, and delirium may improve caloric intake in individual patients. Recurrent pneumonia from aspiration may accelerate weight loss and to deconditioning *(86)*. Both are potentially reversible with antibiotics and exercise.

A clear diagnosis of cancer cachexia is made by presence of substantial weight loss in the face of advanced or recurrent cancer and with the exclusion of reversible causes. In these individuals there is a metabolic shift that results in decreased anabolism and increased catabolism, which is orchestrated by a series of cytokines, principally tumor necrosis factor (TNF)-α, interleukin (IL)-1 and -6. At best, this group of patients will only partially respond to nutritional therapy. Neither quality of life nor survival will be improved with nutritional therapies alone in advanced cancer *(88,93)*.

It may be difficult to impossible to determine whether weight loss is caused by caloric deprivation or cancer cachexia in individual patients. A trial in nutritional support would be reasonable for those individuals with a good performance score and who are good candidates for further antitumor therapy. Even in this situation, survival is not usually improed by nutritional support. If, during nutritional support, the patient sustains a complication owing to fluid overload, electrolyte abnormalities, hyperglycemia, or recurrent infections or fails to respond to nutritional therapy with improved performance status, quality of life or does not have treatment options such as chemotherapy, additional radiation, or surgery, then nutritional support should be curtailed. This requires both education of families and an open discussion with compassion. Gastrostomy could be maintained for hydration and drug delivery to facilitate terminal care.

Table 3
Treatment for Anorexia and Cachexia

Central appetite stimulants
    Progesterone
    Cannabinoids
    Corticosteroids
    Olanzapine
    Mirtazapine
Anabiolic steroids
Branched chain amino acids
ATP
Creatinine
Insulin
Exercise
Antiinflammatory agents
    NSAIDS
    O-3 fatty acids
    Macrotide antibiotic
    Statins
    Thalidomide
Propanolol
Angitension-converting enzyme inhibitors
Melatonin

Certain agents have been used (with some success) to reverse anorexia and cachexia (Table 3). The evidence is strongest with progesterone and is meager for other agents *(93,94)*. Additional studies are necessary to confirm the benefits of combination therapy, that includes agents which block cytokines and tumor cachexins and stimulate anabolism. Combination therapies are probably going to be necessary to significantly alter the multifaceted nature of cancer cachexia (Table 3).

4. ORAL COMPLICATIONS AND SIDE EFFECTS

Three oral complications are common to patients with HNSCC. Mucositis is an acute and painful side effect of treatment, which for the most part resolves. Both dysgeusia and xerostomia are chronic, usually treatment-related, side effects. Xerostomia in particular is a major determinant of quality of life *(95,96)*.

4.1. Mucositis

Mucositis is a major adverse effect of radiation that often leads to reduced or shortened treatment. The pain, dysphagia, and soreness of mucositis leads to accelerated nutritional failure *(74)*. The addition of chemotherapy to radiation increases the risk of mucositis and also severity *(7,97)*. The threshold for mucositis with radiation is approx 20 Gy of standard once-daily radiation therapy.

Mucositis is initiated by an inflammatory process generated from reactive oxygen species released within the submucosa, which initiates an inflammatory reaction. In addition, the normal cell cycle of the basal stem cells, which require a 4-d regeneration time to replace desquamated keratinocytes, is blocked by radiation. The mucosa epithelium is three to four cells thick, so the usual observable mucositis owing to radiation therapy will be seen around d 12 of standard radiation *(98)*. The dose fraction, field size, and radiation schedule determines the incidence and degree of mucositis *(98)*. Hyperfractionated radiation, smoking during radiation, and simultaneous chemotherapy increase the risk of mucositis and delay recovery *(99)*.

Chemotherapy-associated mucositis is most commonly associated with antimetabolites like methotrexate as well as, etoposide, melphalan, doxorubicin, vinblastine, and taxanes *(98)*. Mucositis varies in severity depending on dose and schedule. Patients receiving a combination of cisplatin and 5-fluorouracil are at highest risk for mucositis.

Certain patient populations are at greater risk for mucositis from antitumor therapy than others. Patients who are receiving stem cell transplants, those with collagen vascular diseases, and those with HIV are at high risk for mucositis *(100)*.

4.1.1. Pathogenesis

Mucositis occurs on a continuum from mild erythemia to white desquamation to pseudomembrane formation and ulceration *(98,100)*. Neutropenia during mucositis increases the risk of septicemia and fungemia and may secondarily worsen mucositis by adding infection to local inflammation. The stages of mucositis are (1) inflammation, (2) epithelial desquamation, (3) ulcer formation, and (4) healing. The inflammatory stage is both a submucosal and an intrathelial event in which submucosal proinflammatory cytokines play a major role *(98)*. The generation of reactive oxygen species, by either radiation or chemotherapy, leads to rapid expression of early response genes, such as C-JUN, C-FOS, and ERG-1, as well as activation of transcription factor nuclear factor (NF)-κB, proteasome 26S, the H-SNK gene, and vascular adhesion molecules. There is increased expression and release of proinflammatory cytokines from the endothelium and stromal cells owing to upregulation of the transcription factors NF-κB. IL-1 and TNF-α lead to cellular infiltration and apoptosis of mucosal cells *(98)*. The pathobiology of mucositis eventually rises to the epithelial surface, which thins, leading to erythemia and ulceration *(98)*. Reduced salivary flow owing to acinar cell damage increases the contact time of chemotherapy agents to epithelial surfaces if chemoradiotherapy is used and produces further damage. In addition, salivary immunoglobins such as IgG, IgA, and IgM are reduced, predisposing to bacterial colonization and leading to systemic infections. The oral flora changes such that α-hemolytic streptococcus, *Streptococcus oralis*, *Streptococcus milie*, and *Candida* species dominant *(98)*.

4.1.2. Prevention

There are no formal guidelines to prevent mucosal injury, no proven prophylactic therapies, and no universally accepted treatment guidelines for managing mucositis *(98–100)*. Basic strategies include (1) pain relief, (2) efforts to hasten healing, and (3) prevention of infectious complications.

1. Antiinflammatory therapy. Chamomile has been used with little benefit to prevent chemotherapy mucositis. Benzydamine, which is not available in the United States, attenuates TNF-α production, inhibits nitric oxide production and release, has antimicrobrobial activity, and stabilizes cellular membranes. Benzydamine has been effective in reducing radiation-induced erythemia and mucosal ulceration *(98,101)*.
2. Antimicrobials. Chlorohexidine is ineffective in preventing or managing chemotherapy-induced mucositis. Prophylactic partially absorbed antifungals may reduce oral *Candida* colonization and systemic infections *(98)*. Combinations of antimicrobials such as polymyxin, tobramycin, and amphotericin-B lozenges or bacitracin, gentamicin, and clotrimazole have

mixed results in chemotherapy- and radiation-induced mucositis *(98)*. The combination of sucralfate plus ciprofloxacin or ampicillin plus chlortrimazole troches has been reported to reduce radiation induced mucositis *(102)*. Metaanalysis suggests that narrow-rather than broad-spectrum antibacterial agents are more effective *(103,104)*.

3. Biologic modifiers. Promising but unproven benefits have been reported with certain biologic modifiers. These agents, such as IL-1, IL-11, transforming growth factor (TGF)-β, and keratinocyte growth factors, either reduce epithelial cell sensitivity to radiation or stimulate repair *(98)*. Colony-stimulating factors (CSFs) may reduce mucositis caused by chemotherapy. Local application of granulocyte/macrophage-CSF and granulocyte-CSF have marginally improved mucositis associated with bone marrow transplant *(98)*. Thalidomide, through reduction of TNF-α, may also decrease mucositis, although more studies are needed.

4. Cryoprotective agents. Prostaglandins, vitamin E, and the free radical scavenger amifostine have been used to reduce chemotherapy- and radiation-induced mucositis. Amifostine is more effective in preventing xerostomia than mucositis *(98,99)*.

5. Propantheline. Propantheline may reduce chemotherapy mucositis by reducing the duration of etoposide exposure to mucosal surfaces. Pilocarpine stimulates acinar cell saliva production and reduces chemotherapy contact to surface epithelium *(98,105,106)*.

6. Ice chips. Cryotherapy 30 min before 5-fluorouracil reduces mucositis, probably because of vasoconstriction and reduced mucosal exposure. This will only be effective with drugs that have a short half-life. Continuous 5-fluorouracil infusions commonly used in HNSCC chemotherapy will preclude the benefits of cryotherapy *(98,107)*.

To summarize, the only preventive approachs to mucositis that can be recommend are (1) ice chips for bolus 5-fluorouracil and (2) benzydamine for radiation-induced mucositis. The expert opinion of the Symptom Control Committee of the National Cancer Institute Canada, Clinical Trials Group, is that there is enough evidence to support the use of benzydamine HCl as the appropriate control arm when studying radiation mucositis *(99)*. It is unlikely that agents acting only on the surface epithelium or altering bacterial colonization will significantly influence the course of mucositis.

4.1.3. TREATMENT

Although single-agent trials demonstrate some benefit, evidence-based recommendations cannot be given owing to differences in methodology and outcome measures. The use of "magic mouthwash" consisting of diphenhydramine, Nystatin, and distilled water or magnesium or aluminum salts, although commonly employed, has not undergone formal evaluation *(99)*.

Chemotherapy-induced mucositis, unlike that caused by radiation, is generally limited to nonkeratinized surfaces *(98)*. Fungal and viral infections are commonly misdiagnosed in patients with chemotherapy-induced mucositis. Viral infections usually produce crops of punctuate vesicles involving the keratinized surfaces of the mucosa, including the hard palate, gingiva, and dorsal tongue *(98)*. In neutropenia patients, cultures of involved surfaces and exfoliate cytology may be necessary to rule out opportunistic infections.

Evaluation of mucositis in clinical trials depends in large part on the visual changes, observed on mucosal surfaces. Fortunately, there is good interobserver reliability and strong correlation between objective and subjective measures, including pain and swallowing function *(108,109)*. However, it is the patient centered outcome of pain and swallowing that is the important determinant to the quality of life and outcome of mucositis rather than observed mucosal damage *(110)*.

Scoring of chemotherapy-induced mucositis takes into account objective and subjective findings and functional disability *(108,109)*. The sum of the scores is probably more accurate in gauging the disability and severity of mucositis than relying simply on the appearance of the mucosa.

Once mucositis has been established, anesthetic agents, benzydamine, topical doxepin, coating agents, and systemic analgesics (in the form of either NSAIDS or opioids) may palliate pain until the epithelium recovers. The use of opioids by patient controlled analgesia is not superior to standard opioid dosing strategies *(110)*. The pain of mucositis will respond to tricyclic antidepressants, but to a lesser extent than to opioids. The antifungal agent fluconazole and antiviral agents such as acyclovir and valacyclovir may reduce secondary associated infectious complications *(98)*. Antifungals and antibacterial agents will reduce pain if there are secondary infections but will not significantly modify the course of mucositis. Patients with significant nutritional deficiency prior to treatment and in whom chemoradiotherapy is indicated should have gastrostomy placed before therapy rather than when symptoms are severe since it is anticipated that this group of patients will have significant mucositis and further nutritional failure during treatment.

4.2. Dysgeusia

The perversion of taste is common in advanced cancer but is particularly common in HNSCC patients because of its association with xerostomia *(98–100)*. Radiation and the resultant loss of taste buds accentuates the problem. Owing to age and comorbidity, patients with HNSCC are frequently on multiple medications which also cause dysgeusia (Table 4).

The treatment of dygeusia is not well developed since it is a "orphan" symptom and rarely studied. However, three options are available to physicians: (1) treat xerostomia, (2) alter the drug regimen by removing offending medications, and (3) try zinc (Table 4). Zinc deficiency has been associated with dygeusia, and many patients with HNSCC are nutritionally depleted, and zinc may be helpful. Evidence for the routine use of zinc to treat dygeusia is still lacking *(100)*.

4.3. Xerostomia

The role of saliva in oral health and disease relates to its fluid content and individual components, which in turn are determined by the relative input from the parotid, submandibular, submaxillary, and lingual glands. Water accounts for 99% of saliva *(96,112)*. The serous component contains vital substances such as bactericidal thiocyanate, statherins, histatins, and lactoferrin. It also contains antibodies such as secretory IgA as well as proteolytic enzymes including α-amylase, lysozyme, and peroxidase, which contain oral flora. The surface epithelium is maintained by epidermal growth factor. The electrolyte content is hypotonic owing to ductal epithelium electrolyte absorption from serous acinar cell secretion. Saliva is particularly rich in bicarbonate, which buffers acidic content *(96,112)*. Bicarbonate is necessary to maintain dental enamel. Normal saliva pH ranges between 6.5 and 7.4. Calcium and phosphate are necessary for dental mineralization *(96)*. Mucin is an important component, as it plays a role in lubricating and coating mucosal surfaces, which prevents epithelial dehydration, facilitates mastication, and swallowing, and enhances taste and speech *(112)*. Finally, the saliva washes away bacteria and food debris, minimizes bacterial overgrowth, and as a result reduces the risk of mucositis and dental caries that can be generated by release of bacterial enzymes and secondary inflammation *(112)*.

Ninety percent of saliva comes from the parotid, submandibular, and submaxillary glands and only 10% from small labial and buccal glands *(112)*. The parotid produces serous fluid, and the submandibular gland secretes both serous fluid and mucin. The viscosity of saliva will

Table 4
Medications Associated With Dysgeusia

Angitension-converting enzyme inhibitors
Antibiotics
Antidepressants
Benzodiazepines
Bronchodilators
Antihypertensives
H_2 blockers
Diuretics
Opioids
Proton pump inhibitors
NSAIDS
Steroids

From ref. *100*.

therefore depend on the contribution of each gland. Loss of parotid function increases saliva's viscosity *(112)*. In an unstimulated state two-thirds of saliva is derived from submandibular glands, but with oral stimulation the parotid accounts for nearly half the volume of saliva *(96)*. In health, about 1.5 L of saliva are produced daily, and basal secretion rates range between 0.3 and 0.5 mL/min. The rate of baseline saliva production depends mostly on the input of parasympathetics *(112)*.

The central nervous system salivary center is located within the pons and medulla. Saliva production is positively influenced by both sympathetic and parasympathetic activity, though parasympathetic activity is more important *(112)*. Sympathetic stimulation produces a thick mucin-containing saliva, whereas parasympathetics produce a watery saliva with high enzyme content *(112)*. The saliva center is influenced by higher brain centers and external factors such as sight, thought, and smell, which stimulate saliva flow *(112)*.

4.3.1. SYMPTOMS

The subjective feeling of a dry mouth does not necessarily correlate with the objective evidence of reduced salivary flow *(96,112,113)*. The content of saliva may play as much of a role in the sensation of xerostomia as the amount. However, normal individuals will complain of a dry mouth when baseline saliva is reduced by 50%. Qualitative changes of saliva related to mucin content are associated with xerostomia *(114)*. Xerostomia has been reported in 25% of women and 16% of men in the general population; it increases to more than 30% of palliative medicine and 77% of hospice patients *(112,114)*. Advanced cancer patients rate xerostomia as the third or fourth most common problem. In more than 80% it is moderate to severe in intensity *(114)*. The frequency of xerostomia in advanced cancer correlates with performance scores and the number of medications, but not age *(114)*. The at-risk population of cancer patients includes those on offending medications such as opioids, diuretics, and tricyclic antidepressants, with advanced disease. Xerostomia is clustered with oral discomfort, dysgeusia, dysphagia, and dysphonia as well as anorexia *(114)*. Xerostomia in cancer appears to correlate with reduced basal levels of saliva production but not decreased production with stimulation *(114)*. The risk for xerostomia is multiplied if there is large field radiation to the head and neck or if chemotherapy and radiation are used simultaneously *(112)*.

Radiation-induced xerostomia depends on the volume of gland radiated and the radiation dose *(96)*. A 50% reduction in basal saliva flow is observed with parotid doses of 20 Gy. Some recovery of function occurs up to doses of 52 Gy. Fully radiated parotid glands (above 60 Gy) will remain permanently hypofunctional *(96)*. Radiation fields that include 50% or more of the parotid gland will increase xerostomia *(96)*.

The serous acinar cells are more radiosensitive than ductal or endothelial cells. Mucin-secreting cells are more radioresistant than serous acinar cells even though both types of cells divide slowly and would be predicted to be relatively radioresistant *(96)*. The different radiosensitivities may be related to heavy metals located within the acinar cell secretory granules *(96)*.

There is a time-related bimodal loss of salivary function with radiation. Transient recovery occurs immediately after radiation followed by progressive loss *(96)*. The perception of recovery by patients may be related to both adaptation to reduced saliva and hypertrophy of surviving glandular tissue *(96)*.

Qualitative changes in saliva occur with time. Saliva becomes more viscous owing to the relative loss of serous content. Saliva color will change to yellow or brown. There is a temporary increase in secretory IgA, albumin, lactoferrin, lysozyme, and myeloperoxidase during radiation. This is followed by a loss of these proteins with time. Serum levels of α-amylase increase during radiation, reflecting glandular damage, whereas amylase diminishes in saliva. Epidermal growth factor diminishes during radiation, and bicarbonate and calcium content decrease as pH decreases *(96,112)*. Mucin content gradually declines with time.

As a result of the qualitative changes in salvia, recurrent dental infections and caries become a major problem (Table 5). Decreased pH is associated with overgrowth of *Streptococcus mutans*, lactobacilli, and *Candida* species. Reduction in immunoglobulin content, as well as reduced saliva, allows for increased colonization on mucosal surfaces *(96)*. Dental caries are increased owing to loss of mineralization from a decreased pH and calcium content and secondarily from an increase in cariogenic bacteria *(96,112)*. The loss of antimicrobial peptides and enzymes facilitates further bacterial colonization. Patients will avoid vegetables and dry and sticky foods, and become nutritionally depleted owing to mouth sensitivity. Dentures become incredibly uncomfortable *(96)*.

Chemotherapy alone will cause xerostomia. If neutropenia occurs, the risk of sepsis from oral organisms becomes a significant problem. Chemotherapy will thin mucosal surfaces and reduce IgA, compounding the risk for oral infections and sepsis *(112)*. Decreased saliva with each cycle of chemotherapy will prolong the chemotherapy contact time with oral mucosa and increase the risk of mucositis with subsequent cycles *(96)*. During chemotherapy, microorganisms will multiple and double in concentration as saliva flow diminishes. This increases the risk for periodontal infections *(96)*. Chemotherapy variably influences the protein content of saliva and fortunately does not have a permanent effect on saliva *(96)*. However, infections are a major cause of death in cancer patients undergoing aggressive chemotherapy and stem cell transplant, and in many the offending organism arises from oral colonization *(112)*.

4.3.2. Treatment

Treatment for xerostomia consists of dietary modifications, saliva stimulation, saliva substitutes, and dental prophylaxis. If there is any residual salivary function, then stimulation is better than saliva substitutes *(112)*.

4.3.2.1. Dietary Recommendations. Tepid, nonspicy foods are better tolerated since oral hypersensitivity is a common accompanying problem. Foods should have a soft texture.

Table 5
Complications of Xerostomia

Oral pain and hypersensitivity
Nutritional failure
Caronal and root caries
Anaerobic infections
Oral candidasis
Dysgeusia
Dysphonia
Dysphagia

From ref. *112.*

Patients should avoid citric acid and fruit juices with low pH since these not only can increase pain but also can accelerate loss of dental enamel. Chewing gum prior to meals stimulates saliva and may improve tolerance to meals; if this fails, a saliva substitute may do the same *(113)*. Prolonged mastication reduces or retards gland atrophy and stimulates saliva flow through baroreceptors *(112)*. Sweets also stimulate saliva through local baroreceptors but will promote enamel demineralization and cariogenesis *(112)*. Gustatory stimulation (taste) increases saliva flow independent of mastication. By combining both stimuli (mastication and taste), saliva production will occur in most individuals *(112)*.

4.3.2.2. Saliva Stimulation. Chewing gum (if there is residual gland function), improves saliva flow. Both V6 (Stimoral) and Fredent (Wrigley, Chicago, IL) contain a buffering system and are sugarless *(113)*. Chewing gum, which contains monocalcium phosphate monohydrate, will promote mineralization and improve oral pH *(112)*.

The problem with chewing gum is that it may further worsen tempromandibular joint dysfunction. The practice is inappropriate for edentulous individuals *(112)*.

4.3.2.3. Saliva Stimulation and Drug Therapy. Pilocarpine HCL, a parasympathomimetic drug, has been effective in xerostomia caused by various medications and radiation. Evidence for its benefit after radiation therapy, however, is relatively meager, although half of patients will state they have some benefit *(112)*. Subjective benefits may not be associated with objective evidence of saliva production. The best results occur with prolonged use (more than 8 wk), and the usual doses are 2.5–5 mg three times daily *(112)*.

The subjective benefits of pilocarpine will last only a few hours *(113)*. The composition of saliva with pilocarpine differs from normal owing to the imbalance of parasympathetic to sympathetic input from the drug. Side effects of pilocarpine are lacrimation, sweating, urinary frequency, cramps, colic, and rhinitis *(112)*. Topically applied pilocarpine in the form of pastilles may be better tolerated owing to reduced systemic absorption *(112)*.

Cerumeline is a cholinergic agent with selective affinity for M1 and M3 muscarinic receptors. Cerumeline reduces systemic effects compared with other muscarinic agents since it does not bind to M2 and M4 receptors found in the heart and lungs *(113)*. Other parasympathetic drugs include bethanechol chloride, methacholine, carbachol, and the anticholinesterases distigimine and pyridostigmine. It is not known whether these other parasympathetic agents work in patients who fail to respond to pilocarpine.

4.3.2.4. Saliva Substitutes. Normal saliva is both complex and difficult to replace. Substitutes range from simple aqueous formulations to carboxymethylcellulose polymers and mucin-containing solutions. Sips of water relieve xerostomia for short periods. The duration of benefit is only approx 12–18 min *(112)*. Milk has chemical and physical properties that mimic saliva. Milk acts as a buffer, improves dental mineralization (owing to its calcium and phosphate content), is nutritional, and is relatively inexpensive. Patients with lactase deficiency will not tolerate milk *(112)*. Biotene and Oral Balance (Laclede Professionals, Rochodominguez, CA) contain antimicrobial enzymes and enhance mouth wetting compared with saline or water alone *(113)*.

Polymers include Glanosone, Xerolube (Colgate/Scherer, Canton, MA), Orex, and Saliment (Ferring, Denmark) *(113)*. Polymers as well as mucin-containing substitutes usually have calcium phosphate and fluoride for enamel remineralization and sugar alcohols *(112)*. Neither substitute, however, provides antibacterial or immunological protection *(112)*. Salinum contains a water-soluble extract of linseed, which is an alternative to mucin-containing substitutes *(112)*.

Mucin-containing saliva substitutes (Saliva Orthana, Nycomed Pharma) contains natural porcine mucin *(113)*. Mucin substitutes are generally better tolerated than polymers except for those containing hydroxypropylmethylcellulose.112 For a mucin substitute to be effective, the entire mucosa needs to be sprayed, and a small pool of substitute should be left on the dorsal of the tongue. A dental appliance can act as a reservoir. Porcine-containing substitutes may not be acceptable to individuals of Jewish or Muslim faith *(112)*.

Glycerin and glycerol-containing oral solutions and commercial mouthwashes, which contain detergents, cause oral mucosal dehydration and are to be avoided *(112)*.

4.3.2.5. Antibacterial Agents. Chlorohexidine and hexidene have broad antimicrobial activity and may retard the development of dental plaque. Both may prevent gingivitis, but at the cost of tooth discoloration *(112)*. There is very little evidence that prophylactic antibiotics or antifungals are beneficial in the treatment of xerostomia, and they can lead to colonization of resistant organisms *(112)*.

5. SYSTEMIC SYMPTOMS OF CANCER

The systemic symptoms associated with recurrent HNSCC are protean. In a comprehensive, prospective study involving 1000 patients referred to the palliative medicine program at The Cleveland Clinic, the median number of symptoms per individual with cancer was 11 (range 1–27) *(114)*. The 10 most prevalent symptoms in all cancer patients are pain, fatigue, weakness, anorexia, lack of energy, dry mouth, constipation, early satiety, dyspnea, and significant weight loss. The prevalence of these symptoms ranges from 50 to 84%. In a second prospective study by the same group, sleep problems occurred in 50% of patients, nausea and vomiting in 40%, and depression in 32% when patients were queried with initial consultation *(112)*. There are subtle gender differences in symptom prevalence. Females with advanced cancer experience more early satiety, nausea, and vomiting, and males experience more dysphagia, hoarseness, and weight loss as well sleep disorders *(115)*. Symptom severity and prevalence is associated with reduced performance status *(115)*.

Prognosis is related to the symptom clusters. Patients experiencing gastrointestinal symptoms (dysphagia and early satiety) have reduced survival. The gastrointestinal cluster of symptoms and gender have nearly the same influence on survival as performance status *(116)*. Other prognostic or unfavorable indicators are anorexia, weight loss, dyspnea, cognitive failure, lymphopenia, and leukocytosis *(117)*. A Palliative Prognostic Score can be generated using symptom clusters, Karnofsky performance score, clinician-estimated survival, and white blood cell count, which is relatively accurate *(117)*.

5.1. Fatigue

Cancer-related fatigue is associated with anemia, endocrine disorders (hypothyroidism), depression, insomnia, uncontrolled pain, and poor nutrition *(118)*. Physicians should treat reversible causes of fatigue and uncontrolled pain before considering pharmacologic management. There is a high positive correlation between fatigue and depression in cancer patients, and symptoms overlap. Current qualitative instruments for fatigue may not be able to separate the two symptoms *(119)*. Nonpharmacological approaches to the management of fatigue include graded exercise programs to reduce deconditioning and stress reduction through meditation, yoga, massage, and visual imagery *(118)*. Methylphenidate can reduce cancer related fatigue. Doses are 5 mg in the morning and 5 mg at noon, titrated to 10–20 mg twice daily up to 1 mg per kilogram body weight. Methylphenidate will reduce opioid sedation, nausea, pain, and anxiety and will improve appetite and depression *(120,121)*. Interestingly, paroxetine, a selective serotonin reuptake inhibitor (SSRI) does not have a significant influence on cancer- or treatment-related fatigue *(122)*. Therefore, even though methylphenidate treats depression, its benefits may be independent of its antidepressant activity.

5.2. Depression

The prevalence of depression in the general population is 6–10%, but it is much higher in the cancer population, ranging between 20 and 30%. Depression is underrecognized and is a major contributor to suffering *(123)*. Somatic manifestations of depression, such as fatigue, loss of energy, weight loss, insomnia, or hypersomnia and anorexia overlap with cancer symptoms such that clinicians must depend on the psychological symptoms of mood, sense of worthlessness, helplessness or guilt, thoughts of self-harm, to make a diagnosis *(123)*. Screening questionnaires have a high specificity for depression but a low positive predictive value *(123)*. Risk factors for depression include gender (females), young age, past history of depression, lack of social support, reduced functional status, uncontrolled pain, brain metastases, hypercalcemia, corticosteroids, cytokine treatment, and existential distress over the meaning of life *(124)*.

Treatment of depression requires a combination of supportive psychotherapy and antidepressant medications *(124)*. Psychotherapy involves facilitating emotional expression, cognitive reconstruction, and acquisition of coping skills *(123)*. Psychotropic medications include tricyclic antidepressants, SSRIs, mirtazapine, and psychostimulants. The problem with tricyclic antidepressants is the anticholinergic side effects, risk for arrhythmias, and drug interactions. Secondary amine tricyclics, such as nortriptyline and despiramine, are to be preferred over teriary tricyclics since the secondary amines are less anticholinergic. Although SSRIs do not have anticholinergic side effects, they do have significant drug interactions and may initially worsen anorexia and nausea *(124)*. Mirtazapine has fewer side effects than tricyclic antidepressants and SSRIs and may improve sleep and appetite. There are few drug interactions with mirtazapine *(125)*. Initial doses are 15 mg at night, which can be increased to 45 mg depending on response. Methylphenidate has an advantage owing to its rapid onset of action, which can be seen be seen within days *(126–128)*. Initial doses are the same as for fatigue. Side effects include overstimulation, anxiety, insomnia, paranoia, and confusion *(124)*. Psychostimulants should not be used in delirious patients.

5.3. Delirium

Delirium is present on admission in 20% of advanced cancer patients, and nearly one-third will develop delirium during hospitalization *(129)*. The diagnosis of delirium significantly worsens life expectancy. The median survival for delirious patients is 21 d *(130)*. Delirium is independently associated with male gender, central nervous system metastases, poor performance score, poor predicted survival by clinicians, and progesterone treatment *(130)*. Effective screening tools include the Memorial Delirium Assessment Scale, the Confusion Assessment Method, and the Bedside Delirium Scale *(131–133)*. Hyperalert agitated patients will distress relatives, who in turn demand either sedation for their loved one or that all medications be discontinued *(132)*. Some physicians will adopt a nihilistic approach to the management of delirium and simply sedate the patient without bothering to look for reversible causes. Medications, (opioids, anticholinergics, and benzodiazepines), electrolyte abnormalities, infections, azotemia, dehydration, and hypoxemia are reversible causes of delirium. Opioid rotation and minimizing psychoactive agents may reverse delirium without the need for neuroleptics. Alcohol and nicotine withdrawal are other reversible but poorly recognized causes for delirium during hospitalization *(132–134)*. Except for delirium caused by alcohol and hypnotic withdrawal, neuroleptics are the treatment of choice. Haloperidol 0.5–10 mg orally or parenterally per day improves most delirium *(135)*. For hypoalert delirium, 1 mg twice daily and as needed may be adequate, whereas the agitated patient, particularly if paranoid, will require 5 mg parenteral,y as a single dose and 1 mg hourly until calm. Second-line agents are the atypical antipsychotics resperidone and olanzapine, particularly for patients who develop extrapyramidal reactions to haloperidol or who fail to respond to haloperidol in high doses *(134)*. Olanzapine has been reported to be beneficial in the treatment of delirium associated with advanced cancer *(134)*. Initial doses are 5 mg q 12 h with 2.5 mg once or twice daily for the elderly. Additional doses should be available as needed. A dissolvable disk formulation of olanzapine facilitates treatment for those with dysphagia *(125)*.

5.4. Early Satiety

Early satiety is a common and often neglected symptom. Early satiety reduces food intake and accelerates weight loss. Metoclopramide increases esophageal peristalsis, accelerates gastric emptying, and shortens small bowel transit time *(136)*. By improving gastric motility, metoclopramide will diminish satiety, bloating, nausea, and hiccups, which in turn may improve nutritional intake. Usual doses are 10 mg by mouth before meals and at bedtime or 40–60 mg iv or sc over 24 h *(136–138)*. Common side effects are akathesia, dystonia, and somnolence. Ondansetron should not be given with metoclopramide owing to the risk of cardiac arrythmias. Doses will need to be reduced by half with renal and hepatic failure *(136)*.

Low doses of erthyromycin (50–100 mg) before meals or the newly released $5HT_4$ agonists may improve gastric motility and reduce early satiety.

5.5. Nausea and Vomiting

Nausea and vomiting in advanced cancer is more dreaded than pain *(139)*. Nausea caused by medications, electrolyte disturbances, or metabolic abnormalities is usually constant, unrelieved by vomiting, and not associated with colic or abdominal pain *(139)*. Nausea and vomiting associated with gastric outlet obstruction or small bowel obstruction crescendos to the point of vomiting followed by a short period of relief. Colic and visceral pain frequently accompany nausea and vomiting associated with bowel obstruction *(139)*.

There are a paucity of studies available to guide antiemetic choices *(140)*. Physicians frequently use antiemetic guidelines for chemotherapy-induced nausea and vomiting which little rationale *(141)*. Initial treatment has most frequently been with either haloperidol or metoclopramide *(137–139)*. Doses of single agents should be optimized before other medications are added. Metoclopramide doses are similar to those used for satiety. Metoclopramide should be avoided in patients with bowel obstruction. Haloperidol doses are 5 mg parenterally over 24 h with a provision for a rescue dose of 1 mg q 4 h as needed. Corticosteroids, antihistaminics, antimuscarinics, and $5HT_3$ antagonists (with phenothiazines or butyrophenones) have been used in patients who fail to respond to single agents. Cannabinoids or broad-spectrum (atypical) neuroleptics such as olanzapine work when metoclopramide or haloperidol fail. Olanzapine has been reported to relieve refractory nausea and vomiting in advanced cancer *(142,143)*.

Treating the underlying causes of nausea and vomiting such as hypercalcemia, bowel obstruction, or brain metastases or switching offending medications should be done while one is treating the symptom *(139)*.

6. MANAGING THE ACTIVELY DYING PATIENT

Patients who are dying need (1) symptom relief, (2) the presence of family members and significant others, (3) reassurance by physical touch, and (4) truth telling *(144)*. Autonomy should be preserved and extended into the dying phase through advanced directives. The spiritual life with a sense of completeness can be fostered through liturgy and sacrament or by individualized or personalized ritual if the patient is not closely tied to a religious community *(144,145)*. The dying process should not be prolonged through technology. Pharmacology should be directed to symptom management only and extraneous medication deleted. Such extraneous medications include diuretics, antihypertensives, antidepressants, and lipid-lowering agents *(144,145)*.

We have used three drugs to manage symptoms at the end of life: (1) opioids for pain and dyspnea, (2) phenothiazines (chlorpromazine) for nausea and delirium, and (3) antimuscarinics (glycopyrrolate) for terminal secretions *(144)*. Opioids should not be tapered during the dying process. Patients are nonverbal but still experience pain that may cause terminal restlessness. Family education that includes signs and symptoms of dying and medical management, is an important part of care. Families may mistake the dying process for medication toxicity and demand discontinuation of all medications. Hygiene and physical care should be maintained at the highest degree. Patients should not be subject to invasive treatments or procedures and should be reassured that they are not a burden. Families and patients are encouraged to reminisce in order to provide a sense of completeness to life. Death should not be portrayed as a failure but as a final stage in the development and growth that occurs throughout life *(144)*.

7. SUMMARY

Patients with HNSCC face unique problems, which include treatment sequelae and a greater incidence of neuropathic pain, dysphagia, xerostomia, and mucositis than most cancer patients. In addition, such patients are predisposed to psychological drug dependence, which complicates their management. Many carry the guilt of authoring their disease.

HNSCC patients experience a significant risk for local recurrence compounded by systemic symptoms at relapse, which require polypharmacy to manage. A multidisciplinary approach to cancer care will facilitate optimal outcomes for these patients. The interchange among oncologists, radiologists, and palliative medicine specialists is critical to this process.

REFERENCES

1. Tarvainen L, Suuronen R, Lindqvist C, et al. Is the incidence of oral and pharyngeal cancer increasing in Finland? An epidemiological study of 17, 383 cases in 1953–1999. Oral Dis 2004; 10:167–172.
2. Sanderson RJ, Ironside JAD. Squamous cell carcinomas of the head and neck. BMJ 2002; 325:822–827.
3. Potter J, Higginson IJ, Scadding JW, et al. Identifying neuropathic pain in patients with head and neck cancer: use of the Leeds Assessment of Neuropathic symptoms and signs scale. J R Soc Med 2003; 96:379–383.
4. Whale Z, Lyne PA, Papanikolaou P. Pain experience following radical treatment for head and neck cancer. Eur J Oncol Nurs 2001; 5:112–120.
5. Epstein JB, Stewart KH. Radiation therapy and pain in patients with head and neck cancer. Eur J Can B Oral Oncol 1993; 29B:191–199.
6. Chaplin JM, Morton RP. A prospective, longitudinal study of pain in head and neck cancer patients. Head Neck 1999; 21:531–537.
7. Trotti A, Bellm LA, Epstein JB, et al. Mucositis incidence, severity and associated outcomes in patients with head and neck cancer receiving radiotherapy with our without chemotherapy: a systematic literature review. Radiol Oncol 2003; 66:253–262.
8. Weissman DE, Janjan N, Byhardt RW. Assessment of pain during head and neck irradiation. J Pain Symptom Manage 1989; 4:90–95.
9. Chua KS, Reddy SK, Lee MC, et al. Pain and loss of function in head and neck cancer survivors. J Pain Symptom Manage 1999; 18:193–202.
10. Terrell JE, Welsh DE, Bradford CR, et al. Pain, quality of life and spinal accessory nerve status after neck dissection. Laryngoscope 2000; 110:620–626.
11. De Boer MF, McCormick LK, Pruyn JF, et al. Physical and psychosocial correlates of head and neck cancer: a review of the literature. Otol Head Neck Surg 1999; 120:427–436.
12. Dolan RW, Vaughan CW, Fuleihan N. Symptoms in early head and neck cancer: an inadequate indicator. Otol Head Neck Surg 1998; 119:463–467.
13. Kidder TM. Symptom management for incurable head and neck cancer. Wis Med J 1997; 96:19–24.
14. Kowalski LP, Carvalho AL. Natural history of untreated head and neck cancer. Eur J Cancer 2000; 36:1032–1037.
15. Al-Othman MO, Morris CG, Hinerman RW, et al. Distant metastases after definitive radiotherapy for squamous cell carcinoma of the head and neck. Head Neck 2003; 25:629–633.
16. Buckley JG, Ferlito A, Shaha AR, et al. The treatment of distant metastases in head and neck cancer—present and future. Orl J Otor Relat Spec 2001; 63:259–264.
17. Smit M, Balm AJM, Hilgers FJM, et al. Pain as sign of recurrent disease in head and neck squamous cell carcinoma. Head Neck 2001; 23:372–375.
18. Boerman RH, Maassen EM, Joosten J, et al. Trigeminal neuropathy secondary to perineural invasion of head and neck carcinomas. Neurology 1999; 53:213–216.
19. Marshall JA, Mahanna GK. Cancer in the differential diagnosis of orofacial pain. 1997; 41:355.
20. Vecht CJ, Hoff AM, Kansen PJ, et al. Types and causes of pain in cancer of the head and neck. Cancer 1992; 70:178–184.
21. Wong JK, Wood RE, McLean M. Pain preceding recurrent head and neck cancer. J Orofac Pain 1998; 12:52–59.
22. Thompson AR. Opioids and their proper use as analgesics in the management of head and neck cancer patients. Am J Otol 2000; 21:244–254.
23. Cox BM, Crowder AT. Receptor domains regulating mu opioid receptor uncoupling and internalization: relevance to opioid tolerance. Mol Pharmacol 2004; 65:492–495.
24. Pasternak GW. The pharmacology of mu analgesics: from patients to genes. Neuroscientist 2001; 7:220–231.
25. Pasternak GW. Insights into mu opioid pharmacology the role of mu opioid receptor subtypes. Life Sci 2001; 68:2213–2219.
26. DeHaven-Hudkins DL, Dolle RE. Peripherally restricted opioid agonists as novel analgesic agents. Curr Pharm Des 2004; 10:743–457.
27. Pol O, Puig MM. Expression of opioid receptors during peripheral inflammation. Curr Top Med Chem 2004; 4:51–61.
28. Janson W, Stein C. Peripheral opioid analgesia. Curr Pharm Biotech 2003; 4:270–274.
29. Von Zastrow M. Opioid receptor regulation. Neuromol Med 2004; 5:5–58.
30. Millan MJ. The induction of pain: an integrative review. Prog Neurobiol 1999; 57:1–164.

31. Urban MO, Gebhart GF. Central mechanisms in pain. Med Clin North Am 1999; 83:585–596.
32. Christie MJ, Connor M, Vaughan CW, et al. Cellular actions of opioids and other analgesics: implications for synergism in pain relief. Clin Exp Pharacol Physiol 2000; 27:520–523.
33. Jensen TS. Opioids in the brain. Acta Anaesth Scand 1997; 41:123–132.
34. Urban MO, Gebhart, GF. Supraspinal contributions to hyperalgesia. Proc Natl Acad Sci USA 1999; 96:7687–7692.
35. Pasternak GW. Pharmacological mechanisms of opioid analgesics. Clin Neuropharmacol 1993; 16:1–18.
36. Dickenson AH. Plasticity: implications for opioid and other pharmacological interventions in specific pain states. Behav Brain Sci 1997; 20:392–403.
37. Walsh D. Pharmacological management of cancer pain. Semin Oncol 2000; 27:45–63.
38. Bruera E, Kim HN. Cancer pain. JAMA 2003; 290:2476–2479.
39. Bruera E, Fainsinger RL. Pharmacologic treatment of cancer pain. N Engl J Med 1997; 336:962–963.
40. Rowbotham MC, Twilling L, Davies PS, et al. Oral opioid therapy for chronic peripheral and central neuropathic pain. N Engl J Med 2003; 348:1223–1232.
41. Morley JS, Bridson J, Nash TP, et al. Low-dose methadone had an analgesic effect in neuropathic pain: a double-blind randomized controlled crossover trial. Pall Med 2003; 17:576–587.
42. Dellemijn PL, Van Duijn H, Vanneste JA. Prolonged treatment with transdermal fentanyl in neuropathic pain. J Pain Symptom Manage 1998; 16:220–229.
43. Mercadante S. Opioid responsiveness in patients with advanced head and neck cancer. SCC 1998; 6:482–485.
44. Davis MP, Walsh D. Methadone for relief of cancer pain: a review of pharmacokinetics, pharmcodynamics, drug interactions and protocols of administration. SCC 2001; 9:73–83.
45. Nicholson A. Methadone for cancer pain. Cochrane Database System Rev 2004; 2:CD003971.
46. McNicol E, Horowicz-Mehler N, Fisk RA, et al. Management of opioid side effects in cancer-related and chronic noncancer pain: a systematic review. J Pain Symptom Manage 2003; 4:231–256.
47. Mercadante S, Portenoy RK. Opioid poorly-responsive cancer pain. Part 3 Clinical strategies to improve opioid responsiveness. J Pain Symptom Manage 2001; 21:338–354.
48. Goldfrank L, Weisman RS, Errick JK, et al. A dosing nomogram for continuous infusion intravenous naloxone. Ann Emerg Med 1986; 15:566–570.
49. Berkowitz BA. The relationship of pharmacokinetics to pharmacological activity: morphine, methadone and naloxone. Clin Pharmacokinet 1976; 1:219–230.
50. Andersen PE, Cohen JI, Everts EC, et al. Intrathecal narcotics for relief of pain from head and neck cancer. Arch Otol Head Neck Surg 1991; 117:1277–1280.
51. Dennis GC, DeWitty RL. Long-term intraventricular infusion of morphine for intractable pain in cancer of the head and neck. Neurosurgery 1990, 26:404–407.
52. Cramond T, Stuart G. Intraventricular morphine for intractable pain of advanced cancer. J Pain Symptom Manage 1993; 8:465–473.
53. Carrol EN, Fine E, Ruff RL, et al. A four-drug pain regimen for head and neck cancers. Laryngoscope 1994; 104:694.
54. Curatolo M, Sveticic G. Drug combinations in pain treatment: a review of the published evidence and a method for finding the optimal combination. Best Pract Res Clin Anaesth 2002; 16:507–519.
55. Cashman JN. The mechanisms of action of NSAIDs in analgesia. Drugs 1996; 52(suppl 5):13–23.
56. Parsons CG. NMDA receptors as targets for drug action in neuropathic pain. Eur J Pharm 2001; 429:71–78.
57. Beydoun A, Backonja MM. Mechanistic stratification of antineuralgic agents. J Pain Symptom Manage 2003; 25(5 suppl):S18–30.
58. Backonja M, Glanzman RL. Gabapentin dosing for neuropathic pain: evidence from randomized, placebo-controlled clinical trials. Clin Ther 2003; 25:81–104.
59. Vielhaber A, Portenoy RK. Advances in cancer pain management. Hematol Oncol Clin North Am 2002; 16:527–541.
60. Simental AA, Carrau RL. Assessment of swallowing function in patients with head and neck cancer. Curr Oncol Rep 2004; 6:162–165.
61. Colangelo LA, Logemann JA, Rademaker AW. Tumor size and pretreatment speech and swallowing in patients with resectable tumors. Otol Head Neck Surg 2000; 122:653–651.
62. Pauloski BR, Logemann JA, Rademaker AW, et al. Speech and swallowing function after anterior tongue and floor of mouth resection with distal flap reconstruction. J Speech Hear Res 1993; 36:267–276.
63. Pauloski BR, Logemann JA, Rademaker AW, et al. Speech and swallowing function after oral and oropharyngeal resections: one-year follow-up. Head Neck 1994; 16:313–322.
64. Rosen A, Three TH, Kaufman R. Prediction of aspiration in patients with newly diagnosed untreated advanced head and neck cancer. Arch Otol Head Neck Surg 2001; 127:975–979.

65. McConnel F, Logemann JA, Rademaker AW, et al. Surgical variables affecting postoperative swallowing efficiency in oral cancer patients: a pilot study. Laryngoscope 1994; 104:87.

66. Mady K, Sader R, Hoole PH, et al. Speech evaluation and swallowing ability after intra-oral cancer. Clin Ling Phon 2003; 17:411–420.

67. Yamamoto Y, Sugihara T, Furuta Y, et al. Functional reconstruction of the tongue and deglutition muscles following extensive resection of tongue cancer. Plast Reconstr Surg 1998; 102:993–998.

68. Al-Othman MO, Amdur RJ, Morris CG, et al. Does feeding tube placement predict for long-term swallowing disability after radiotherapy for head and neck cancer? Head Neck 2003; 25:741–747.

69. Schweinfurth JM, Boger GN, Feusel PJ. Preoperative risk assessment for gastrostomy tube placement in head and neck cancer patients. Head Neck 2001; 23:376–382.

70. Magne N, Marcy PY, Foa C, et al. Comparison between nasogstric tube feeding and percutaneous fluoroscopic gastrostomy in advanced head and neck cancer patients. SpringerLink Internet Article.

71. Marcy PY, Magne N, Bensadoun RJ, et al. Systematic percutaneous fluoroscopic gastrostomy for concomitant radiochemotherapy of advanced head and neck cancer: optimization of therapy. Support Care Center 2000; 8:410–413.

72. Beaver ME, Matheny KE, Roberts DB, et al. Predictors of weight loss during radiation therapy. Otol Head Neck Surg 2001; 125:645–648.

73. Urban KG, Terris DJ. Percutaneous endoscopic gastrostomy by head and neck surgeons. Otol Head Neck Surg 1997; 116:489–492.

74. Snyderman CH. Nutrition and head and neck cancer. Curr Oncol Rep 2003; 5:158–163.

75. Eisbruch A, Lyden T, Bradford CR, et al. Objective assessment of swallowing dysfunction and aspiration after radiation concurrent with chemotherapy for head and neck cancer. Int J Radiat Oncol Biol Phys 2002; 53:23–28.

76. Lazarus CL, Logemann JA, Pauloski BR, et al. Swallowing disorders in head and neck cancer patients treated with radiotherapy and adjuvant chemotherapy. Laryngoscope 1996; 106:1157–1166.

77. Pauloski BR, Rademaker AW, Logemann JA, et al. Swallow function and perception of dysphagia in patients with head and neck cancer. Head Neck 2002; 24:555–565.

78. Eisenhuber E, Schima W, Schober E, et al. Videofluoroscopic assessment of patients with dysphagia: pharyngeal retention is a predictive factor for aspiration. AJR 2002; 178:393–398.

79. Logemann JA, Smith CH, Pauloski BR, et al. Effects of xerosteomia on perception and performance of swallow function. Head Neck 2001; 23:317–321.

80. Johns ME. The nutrition problem in head and neck cancer. Otol Head Neck Surg 1980; 88:691–694.

81. Lees J. Incidence of weight loss in head and neck cancer patients on commencing radiotherapy treatment at a regional oncology centre. Eur J Cancer Care 1999; 8:133–136.

82. Body JJ. The syndrome of anorexia-cachexia. SCC 1999; 11:255–260.

83. Baredes S, Blitzer A. Nutritional considerations in the management of head and neck cancer patients. Otol Clin North Am 1984; 17:725–733.

84. Davis MP, Dickerson D. Cachexia and anorexia: cancer's covert killer. SCC 2000; 8:180–187.

85. Body JJ. Metabolic sequelae of cancers (excluding bone marrow transplantation). Curr Opin Clin Nutr Met Care 1999; 2:339–344.

86. Strasser F, Bruera ED. Update on anorexia and cachexia. Hematol Oncol Clin North Am 2002; 16:589–617.

87. McCarthy DO. Rethinking nutritional support for persons with cancer cachexia. Bio Res Nurs 2003; 5:3–17.

88. MacDonald N, Easson AM, Mazurak VC, et al. Understanding and managing cancer cachexia. Pall Care 2003; 197:143–161.

89. Sarhill N, Walsh D, Nelson K, et al. Bioelectrical impedance, cancer nutritional assessment, and ascites. SCC 2000; 8:341–343.

90. Sarhill N, Mahmoud F, Walsh D, et al. Evaluation of nutritional status in advanced metastatic cancer. SCC 2003; 11:652–659.

91. Toso S, Piccoli A, Gusella M, et al. Altered tissue electric properties in lung cancer patients as detected by bioelectric impedance vector analysis. Nutrition 2000; 16:120–124.

92. Toso S, Piccoli A, Gusella M, et al. Bioimpedance vector pattern in cancer patients without disease versus locally advanced or disseminated disease. Nutrition 2003; 19:510–514.

93. Davis MP. New drugs for the anorexia-cachexia syndrome. Curr Oncol Rep 2002; 4:264–274.

94. Davis MP, Dreicer R, Walsh D, et al. Appetite and cancer-associated anorexia: a review. J Clin Oncol 2004; 22:1510–1517.

95. Hammerlid E, Taft C. Health-related quality of life in long-term head and neck cancer survivors: a comparison with general population norms. Br J Cancer 2001; 84:149–156.

96. Jensen SB, Pedersen AM, Reibel J, et al. Xerostomia and hypofunction of the salivary glands in cancer therapy. SCC 2003; 11:207–225.

97. Haddad R, Wirth L, Costello R, et al. Phase II randomized study of concomitant chemoradiation using weekly carboplatin/paclitaxel with or without daily subcutaneous amifostine in patients with newly diagnosed locally advanced squamous cell carcinoma of the head and neck. Semin Oncol 2003; 30:84–88.

98. Hoffman HT. Clinical review. Head Neck 2003; 25:1057–1070.

99. Wright JR, McKenzie M, DeAngelis C, et al. Radiation induced mucositis: co-ordinating a research agenda. Clin Oncol 2003; 15:473–477.

100. Jackson KC, Chambers MS. Oral mucosal problems in palliative care patients. J Pharm Care Pain Sx Cont 2000; 8:143–161.

101. Epstein JB, Schubert MM. Oropharyngeal mucositis in cancer therapy. Review of pathogenesis, diagnosis and management. Oncology 2003; 17:1767–1779.

102. Matthews RH, Ercal N. Prevention of mucositis in irradiated head and neck cancer patients. J Exp Ther Oncol 1996; 1:135–18.

103. Sutherland SE, Browman GP. Prophylaxis of oral mucositis in irradiated head and neck cancer patients: a proposed classification scheme of interventions and meta-analysis of randomized controlled trials. Int J Radiat Oncol Biol Phys 2001; 49:917–930.

104. Symonds RP. Treatment-induced mucositis: an old problem with new remedies. Br J Cancer 1998; 77:1689–1695.

105. Awidi A, Homsi U, Kakail RI, et al. Double-blind, placebo-controlled cross-over study of oral pilocarpine for the prevention of chemotherapy-induced oral mucositis in adult patients with cancer. Eur J Canver 2001; 37:2010–2014.

106. Ahmed T, Engelking C, Szalyga J, et al. Propantheline prevention of mucositis from etoposide. Bone Marrow Transplant 1993; 12:131–132.

107. Cascinu S, Fedeli A, Fedeli SL, et al. Oral cooling (cryotherapy), an effective treatment for the prevention of 5-fluorouracil-induced stomatitis. Eur J Cancer B Oral Oncol 1994; 30B:234–236.

108. Sonis ST, Eilers JP, Epstein JB, et al. Validation of a new scoring system for the assessment of clinical trial research of oral mucositis induced by radiation or chemotherapy. Cancer 1999; 85:2103–21013.

109. Sonis ST, Elting LS, Keefe D, et al. Perspectives on cancer therapy-induced mucosal injury. Cancer 2004; 100(9 Suppl):1995–2025.

110. Dodd MJ. Defining clinically meaningful outcomes in the evaluation of new treatments for oral mucositis: a commentary. Cancer Invest 2002; 20:851–852.

111. Worthington HV, Clarkson JE, Eden OB. Interventions for treating oral mucositis for patients with cancer receiving treatment. Cochrane Library 2003; 1.

112. Holmes S. Xerostomia: aetiology and management in cancer patients. SCC 1998; 6:348–355.

113. Nieuw Amerongen AV, Veerman ECI. Current therapies for xerostomia and salivary gland hypofunction associated with cancer therapies. SCC 2003; 11:226–231.

114. Davies AN, Broadley K, Beighton D. Xerostomia in patients with advanced cancer. J Pain Symptom Manage 2001; 22:820–825.

115. Walsh D, Donnelly S, Rybicki L. The symptoms of advanced cancer: relationship to age, gender, and performance status in 1,000 patients. SCC 2000; 8:175–179.

116. Walsh D, Rybicki L, Nelson KA, et al. Symptoms and prognosis in advanced cancer. SCC 2002; 10:385–388.

117. Maltoni M, Amadori D. Prognosis in advanced cancer. Hematol Oncol Clin North Am 2002; 16:715–729.

118. Escalante CP. Treatment of cancer-related fatigue: an update. SCC 2003; 11:79–83.

119. Jacobsen PB, Donovan KA, Weitzner MA. Distinguishing fatigue and depression in patients with cancer. Semin Clin Neuropsych 2003; 8:229–240.

120. Bruera E, Driver L, Barnes EA, et al. Patient-controlled methylphenidate for the management of fatigue in patients with advanced care: a preliminary report. J Clin Oncol 2003; 21:4439–4443.

121. Sarhill N, Walsh D, Nelson KA. Methylphenidate for fatigue in advanced cancer: a prospective open-label pilot study. Am J Hosp Pall Care 2001; 18:187–192.

122. Morrow GR, Hickok JT, Roscoe JA, et al. Differential effects of paroxetine on fatigue and depression: a randomized, double-blind trial from the University of Rochester Cancer Center Community Clinical Oncology Program. J Clin Oncol 2003; 21:4635–4641.

123. Lloyd-Williams M. Depression—the hidden symptom in advanced cancer. J R Soc Med 2003; 96:577–581.

124. Pessin H, Potash M, Breitbart W. Diagnosis, assessment and treatment of depression in palliative care. In: Lloyd-Williams M, ed. Psychosocial Issues in Palliative Care. Oxford: Oxford University Press, 2003.

125. Davis MP, Khawam E, Pozuelo L, et al. Management of symptoms associated with advanced cancer: olanzapine and mirtazapine. Exp Rev Anticancer Ther 2002; 2:365–376.

126. Homsi J, Walsh D, Nelson K. Psychostimulants in supportive care. SCC 2000; 8:385–397.

127. Homsi J, Walsh D, Nelson KA, et al. Methylphenidate for depression in hospice practice: a case series. Am J Hosp Pall Care 2000; 17:393–398.
128. Homsi J, Nelson KA, Sarhill N, et al. A phase II study of methylphenidate for depression in advanced cancer. Am J Hosp Pall Care 2001; 18:403–407.
129. Gagnon P, Allard P, Masse B, et al. Delirium in terminal cancer: a prospective study using daily screening, early diagnosis, and continuous monitoring. J Pain Symptom Manage 2000; 19:412–426.
130. Caraceni A, Nanni O, Maltoni M, et al. Impact of delirium on the short term prognosis of advanced cancer patients. Italian Multicenter Study Group on Palliative Care. Cancer 2000; 89:1145–1149.
131. Grassi L, Caraceni A, Beltrami E, et al. Assessing delirium in cancer patients: the Italian versions of the Delirium Rating Scale and the Memorial Delirium Assessment Scale. J Pain Symptom Manage 2001; 21:59–68.
132. Lawlor PG, Bruera ED. Delirium in patients with advanced cancer. Hematol Oncol Clin North Am 2002; 16:701–714.
133. Sarhill N, Walsh D, Nelson K, et al. Assessment of delirium in advanced cancer: the use of the bedside confusion scale. Am J Hosp Pall Care 2001; 18:335.
134. Burns A, Gallagley A, Byrne J. Delirium. J Neurol Psychiatry 2004; 75:362–367.
135. Bruera E, Neumann CM. The uses of psychotropics in symptom management in advanced cancer. Psych-Oncol 1998; 7:346–358.
136. Walsh D, Doona M, Molnar M, et al. Symptom control in advanced cancer: important drugs and routes of administration. Semin Oncol 2000; 27:69–83.
137. Bruera E, Belzile M, Neumann C, et al. A double-blind, crossover study of controlled-release metoclopramide and placebo for the chronic nausea and dyspepsia of advanced cancer. J Pain Symptom Manage 2000; 19:427–435.
138. Bruera E, Seifert L, Watanabe S, et al. Chronic nausea in advanced cancer patients: a retrospective assessment of a metoclopramide-based antiemetic regimen. J Pain Symptom Manage 1996; 11:147–153.
139. Davis MP, Walsh D. Treatment of nausea and vomiting in advanced cancer. SCC 2000; 8:444–452.
140. Glare P, Pereira G, Kristjanson LJ, et al. Systematic review of the efficacy of antiemetics in the treatment of nausea in patients with far-advanced cancer. SCC 2004 [Epub ahead of print].
141. Rousseau P. Antiemetic therapy in adults with terminal disease: a brief review. Am J Hosp Pall Care 1995; 12:13–18.
142. Jackson WC, Tavernier L. Olanzapine for intractable nausea in palliative care patients. J Pall Med 2003; 6:251–255.
143. Srivastava M, Brito-Dellan N, Davis MP, et al. Olanzapine as an antiemetic in refractory nausea and vomiting in advanced cancer. J Pain Symptom Manage 2003; 25:578–582.
144. Davis MP, Frandsen J, Dickerson D, et al. Prescribing for the dying patient: principles and practice. JTO 2002; 1:32.
145. Nelson KA, Walsh D, Behrens C. The dying cancer patient. Semin Oncol 2000; 27:84–89.

Index